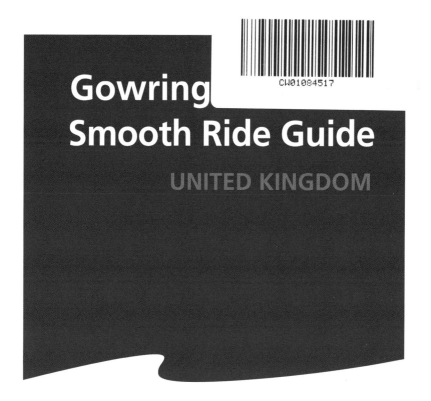

Gowring
Smooth Ride Guide

UNITED KINGDOM

*"Indispensable travel planning
handbooks for people with
mobility difficulties"*

gowrings
mobility

SMOOTH RIDE GUIDES
UNITED KINGDOM
By July Ramsey

Researchers: July Ramsey, Ian Wilcox and Liza Grant
Editor: Ann Innes
Publishers: Gowrings Mobility
Design & Production: Colleagues Direct Marketing
Printed in the EC

ISBN 0-9521982-9-0

The contents of this publication are believed correct at the time of going to press, but some details are likely to have changed. The publishers would greatly appreciate comments, criticism and suggestions for the next revision.

Please write to:
July Ramsey,
Smooth Ride Guides,
Duck Street Barns, Duck Street,
Furneux Pelham, Herts SG9 0LA.

PICTURE CREDITS
We would like to thank the following organisations for kindly allowing us to reproduce the photographs used in this publication.

AMBER VALLEY TOURISM
ASHMOLEAN MUSEUM, OXFORD
ASTLEY HALL MUSEUM
BADDESLEY CLINTON
BEARSTED WINE
BEDE'S WORLD
BEKONSCOT MODEL VILLAGE
BELFAST CONFERENCE AND VISITORS BUREAU
BIRDLAND PARK
BIRMINGHAM BOTANICAL GARDENS
BIRMINGHAM CONFERENCE & VISITOR BUREAU
BIRMINGHAM MARKETING DEPARTMENT
BLACKPOOL TOURISM DEPT.
BRISTOL TOURISM & CONFERENCE BUREAU
BURRELL COLLECTION
CAMELOT THEME PARK
CHATSWORTH HOUSE TRUST
CHESTER CITY COUNCIL TOURISM DEVELOPMENT UNIT
COMPTON ACRES
CORNWALL TOURIST BOARD
COTSWOLD WILDLIFE PARK
COVENTRY & WARWICKSHIRE PROMOTIONS
CUMBRIA TOURIST BOARD
DARTINGTON CRYSTAL
DERBY CITY COUNCIL
DOVER DISTRICT COUNCIL
EARTH CENTRE
EAST OF ENGLAND TOURIST BOARD
ENGLISH WINE CENTRE
ESSEX COUNTY COUNCIL TOURISM SECTION
FITZWILLIAM MUSEUM, UNIVERSITY OF CAMBRIDGE
GUERNSEY TOURISM
HATFIELD HOUSE
HATTON COUNTRY WORLD
HEDGEHOG HOSPITAL
HEREFORDSHIRE TOURISM
HIGHLANDS OF SCOTLAND TOURIST BOARD
HISTORIC SCOTLAND
ISLE OF MAN TOURISM
JERSEY TOURISM
KNOLL GARDENS
LEEDS CASTLE ENTERPRISES
LEEDS CITY COUNCIL
LEEDS DEPARTMENT OF LEISURE TOURISM
LONGTON BRICKCROFT

LONG SHOP STEAM MUSEUM
LOWESTOFT MARITME MUSEUM
MARBLES UK (River & Rowing Museum, Henley)
MARKETING MANCHESTER
MERSEY TOURISM
MUSEUM OF ST. ALBANS
THE NATIONAL TRUST
NATIONAL GALLERY OF SCOTLAND
NATURAL HISTORY MUSEUM
NATIONAL HORSE RACING MUSEUM
NORTHERN IRELAND TOURIST BOARD
NORTH LINCOLNSHIRE COUNCIL TOURISM TEAM
NORTHUMBRIA TOURIST BOARD
NOTTINGHAM CASTLE MUSEUM
PAIGNTON ZOO
ROMNEY, HYTHE & DYMCHURCH RAILWAY
ROYAL BOTANIC GARDENS KEW
ROYAL COLLECTION ENTERPRISES
copyright HM Queen Elizabeth ll
ROYAL HORTICULTURAL SOCIETY, ROSEMOOR
ROYAL HORTICULTURAL SOCIETY, WISLEY
ROYAL NATIONAL ROSE SOCIETY
SANDRINGHAM ESTATE,
by Gracious Permission of HM The Queen
SCOTTISH TOURIST BOARD
SEA LIFE AQUARIUM
SHETLANDS ISLAND TOURISM
SHROPSHIRE TOURISM
SOUTH EAST ENGLAND TOURIST BOARD
SOUTHERN TOURIST BOARD
SOUTH SOMERSET TOURISM & CULTURAL SERVICES
SOUTH WARWICKSHIRE TOURISM
SPOTLIGHT PUBLIC RELATIONS
STOKE-ON-TRENT TOURISM GROUP
SUFFOLK TOURISM
SURREY TOURISM
THRIGBY HALL WILDLIFE GARDEN
UNIVERSITY BOTANIC GARDEN, CAMBRIDGE
UNIVERSITY OF NEWCASTLE MUSEUM OF ANTIQUITIES
WALES TOURIST BOARD
WESTONBIRT ARBORETUM
WHIPSNADE WILD ANIMAL PARK
WIND IN THE WILLOWS ATTRACTION
WORCESTER CITY COUNCIL
YORK TOURISM BUREAU

CONTENTS

3

4

Foreword

by *Glenn J Shaw, FRGS*

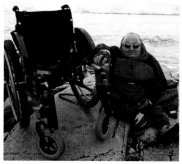

First landing in Antarctica, Portal Point

"As a keen traveller, explorer and adventurer who is also a wheelchair user, I was thrilled to be asked to write a few words about this book.

Having explored some of the world's most dangerous yet beautiful places our planet has to offer, there is nothing more frustrating than arriving at a venue only to find there are no accessible bathroom facilities, suitable car park or worse still, as a wheelchair user you can't even get into the building or attraction in the first place!

This said, there are many wonderful places to visit in the UK which do take the needs of wheelchair users into account. Planning a trip and searching out the places that cater for everyone avoids disappointment and wasted time.

This guide offers a 'hands on' practical addition to any disabled traveller's rucksack or car glove box and who knows, it could be the catalyst for some great adventures closer to home."

Glenn Shaw is an ordinary young man, with a compulsion to do extraordinary things despite being in a wheelchair since birth.

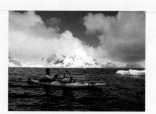

Kayaking in perfect conditions

He has trekked in the Himalayas, travelled in North America by ski and dogsled, and kayaked in the Middle East. Glenn suffers from a condition known as 'Brittle Bones'. He knows that the slightest knock can result in a broken limb but Glenn is an adventurer.

He first made headlines in 1997 when he set out to reach the Nepalese Base Camp of Mount Everest, the world's highest mountain. That attempt ended at an altitude of almost 4000 metres when Glenn suffered a dramatic fall breaking his legs in a total of eight places.

Glenn received a Fellowship to the Royal Geographical Society in 1999. In 2001, he was a recipient of a Winston Churchill Memorial Trust Fellowship that enabled him to undertake a voyage by sea kayak around part of the Antarctic coastline.

Glenn feels he has unfinished business and not one to give up, plans a second attempt on Everest in 2003. Follow Glenn's attempt on www.glennshaw.com

"With every part of the UK covered, there are ideas for days out for disabled people in every part of the country"

Glenn J Shaw FRGS, Adventurer

Gowrings Mobility – A Brief History

Gowrings Mobility is the UK's longest established company manufacturing and supplying vehicles adapted for wheelchair passengers. The company started in the 1960s by marketing small numbers of vehicles based on the Austin Mini Van. By the 1970s production volumes had grown to 50 and the Mini was replaced by the Austin Metro. During the early 1980s a more sophisticated conversion was introduced, with a cut, low floor, offering much easier wheelchair access.

Following a decision to relocate to their purpose designed 45,000 square feet factory and showroom, Gowrings Mobility experienced vigorous growth. The year ending March 2002 saw just under 1,000 vehicles delivered, reaffirming our position as UK market leader.

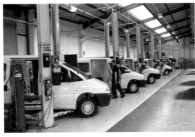

As a company we have had a huge influence on the progress of the disabled vehicle industry, working with government bodies on improving standards and driving down the end-user price throughout the industry due to the manufacturing changes we have implemented.

The new factory

> **❝Mobility is not a luxury – it is essential to the quality of life.❞**

Linda Ling - MD

What we do

For almost 40 years, we have built an unrivalled reputation for providing wheelchair passengers with the largest range of cost effective conversions in the UK.

Gowrings Mobility's extensive range of vehicles includes models from Renault, Citroen, Ford, Vauxhall, Chrysler and Mercedes.

We enjoy a close working relationship with all manufacturers and suppliers, in order to reduce costs and improve specifications and delivery lead times. From the initial design and production to marketing and after sales servicing, our partnerships ensure standards are consistently at a high level.

The way we work

A personal service

What makes us different from many companies is that we truly operate as a customer centric organisation. We are passionate about the difference our products and services make to our customers' lives.

Our research shows that 97% of our customers would recommend us. They particularly commend us as being customer friendly and for offering a comprehensive service. We feel this is testament of the exceptional service we provide.

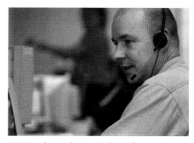

We're always happy to hear from you

not just specialists in the range of vehicles and conversion options but also in understanding how personal requirements and situations need tailor-made solutions. Our additional services encompass advice on finance options plus advising on any mobility related enquiry.

Expert advice

We believe we have an in-depth knowledge of our market and a high level of expertise. We are equipped to offer professional advice, which addresses individual needs. Our Sales Consultants are

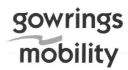

❝You were like a family to us all the way...❞

Derrick Bonfield

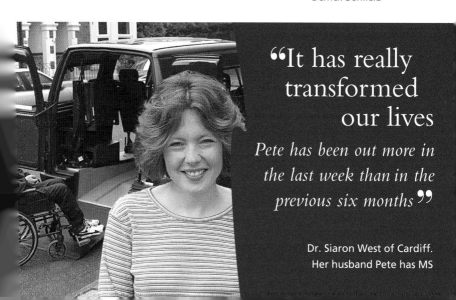

❝It has really transformed our lives

Pete has been out more in the last week than in the previous six months ❞

Dr. Siaron West of Cardiff. Her husband Pete has MS

We are happy to come to you

Our team of demonstrators will visit you in your own home, spending time with you to ensure that the vehicle is suitable for the whole family. This service is highly popular with many people who find it difficult to travel. It enables you, wherever you are in the country, to really try out the car – with your extra medical equipment or luggage if necessary – to ensure that you make the right choice.

Uniquely, our demonstrators are not members of our sales team; they are semi-retired gentlemen who will let you take your time. You will never feel pressurised into making a decision.

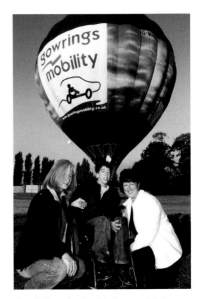

Our Balloon is wheelchair accessible too

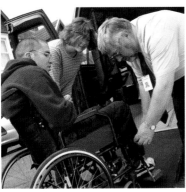

With you all the way

We like to keep our customers informed and talk to them through all stages of the purchasing process. You will be introduced to a member of our Customer Care team, who will work with your chosen local dealer to provide immediate support for any issues, large or small, and at any time in the future.

Peace of mind

Once you have placed your order, we will keep you informed about its progress and agree a convenient delivery date. We pay great attention to the delivery, which is direct to your home. A member of staff will make sure you are familiar with all the features and controls of your new vehicle, and stay with you until you feel confident to set off driving.

"It was wonderful to be independent again, we recommend your company to anyone who needs a wheelchair accessible vehicle"

Mr & Mrs Collins, Bristol

Gowrings Mobility in the Community

Research shows that many wheelchair users without their own vehicles face difficulties using public transport, making trips to the shops, meeting friends or attending hospital appointments. The various organisations they rely on have to select the right vehicles to ensure they offer first class services.

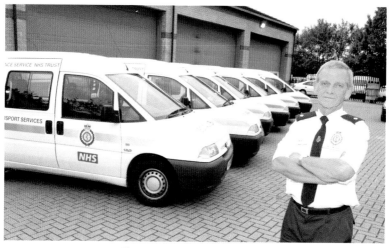

Citroen Dispatches supplied to West Midlands Ambulance Service

"We are extremely pleased with the new vehicles. They are practical, reliable and look great"

Greater Manchester Ambulance Service
Chief Executive, John Burnside

Whether we are liaising with care homes, charities, community transport providers, ambulance services, taxi operators or special needs schools, our focus remains on providing superior vehicles with a service to match.

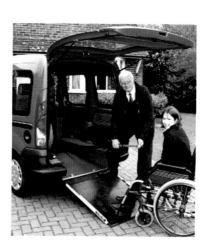

"The fuel consumption..., is almost halved. These vehicles not only raise standards in transportation but they improve conditions for users, too"

Councillor Dick Walsh,
Argyll and Bute Council

Introducing the new line of Gowrings Mobility products

3 Great Swivel Seats, new from Gowrings Mobility

If you find it difficult transferring into a front car seat, a Gowrings Mobility Swivel Seat is the ideal solution. We have introduced a range of swivel seats that make getting in and out of a car much easier.
Our seats are designed to be fitted to a wide range of cars. They can be removed and fitted to subsequent cars.

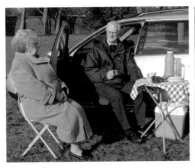 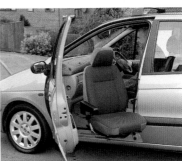

> "The seat has made travel possible again, widening horizons and boosting confidence"
>
> Mrs F, Yorkshire

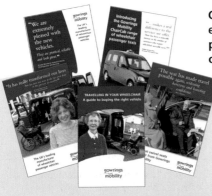

Gowrings Mobility is continuously extending its range of mobility products to benefit a wider range of customers.

Further Information

We have a selection of brochures and leaflets that we can send to you

For more information regarding the Gowrings Mobility range of products contact

Lo-Call 0845 608 8020
www.gowringsmobility.co.uk

gowring mobilit

In support of '2003 European Year of People with Disabilities,' Gowrings Mobility is donating £1 from the sale of each book to charity. This will be divided equally between The Princess Royal Trust for Carers, The Stroke Association and the MS Society

Multiple Sclerosis literally means 'Many Scars, and the scarring results from the bodies own immune system attacking the central nervous system. The damage that this causes means that the nerves are unable to carry messages to other parts of the body.

This makes MS a very unpredictable illness with every person's experience different, for some it is characterised by periods of acute illness and then complete recovery whilst for others it is chronically disabling.

We don't yet have a cure for MS, and we don't yet know what causes it.

The MS Society

The MS Society is a UK-wide charity dedicated to providing support to people who have MS, their families, friends, colleagues and carers. We are a society run by people with MS, from local welfare officers through to trustees, and we do everything we can to ensure that we work in partnership, and where necessary on behalf of, everyone affected by MS to ensure that they reach their full potential.

We are a research, care and campaigning organisation, and some of our work includes running a national MS Helpline, providing MS Specialist Nurses, providing information and publications, providing welfare grants, awareness advertising, parliamentary lobbying, funding research and providing respite care.

The Princess Royal Trust for Carers

The Princess Royal Trust for Carers exists to make it easier for carers to cope by providing information, support and practical help via national network of over 100 independently-managed Carers Centres across the UK. A Carer is someone who cares, unpaid, for people who cannot manage without help because of disability, illness or frailty. For further information please contact us on **020 7480 7788** or **www.carers.org/mobility**

The Stroke Association

Stroke is the major cause of severe disability in adults in England and Wales; the most common cause epilepsy in older people; the second most common cause of dementia; and a frequent cause of depression. This adds up to 300,000 people who are currently disabled by stroke.

The Stroke Association is the major charity working exclusively for people who have had strokes and their families in England and Wales. We aim to reduce the effects of stroke on patients, their families, carers and the community by:

Developing and providing services

Supporting research

Spreading knowledge in relation to prevention

Improving standards of care through training and education

Constantly urging government and other authorities to do more in the field of Stroke.

To find out more about how you can support us and those affected call **0207 566 0300.**

NATIONAL ACCESSIBILITY CRITERIA FOR ACCOMMODATION AND ATTRACTIONS

CATEGORY 1 [♿] Accessible to a wheelchair-user travelling independently.

CATEGORY 2 [♿] Accessible to a wheelchair-user travelling with assistance.

CATEGORY 3 [🚶] Accessible to a wheelchair-user or someone with limited mobility,
able to walk a few paces and up a maximum of three steps.

The minimum requirements for each of the three categories of accessibility are as follows.

ACCOMMODATION – CATEGORY REQUIREMENTS

PUBLIC ENTRANCE

CATEGORY 3 [🚶]	CATEGORY 2 [♿]	CATEGORY 1 [♿]
1. A public entrance must be accessible to wheelchair users from a setting down point or a car park.		
2. If an establishment has a car park, a reservable parking space should be available for a disabled guest on request.		1. If there is a car park, there must be a level reservable space with a minimum width of 3.6m for each bedroom meeting the Category 1 requirements.
3. The route from the parking point or space to the entrance must be sound and free from obstacles. Deep gravel, cobbles or pot-holed surfaces are unlikely to be acceptable.		2. The route from parking point or space to the entrance must be level or ramped.
4. Entrance door must have a clear opening of not less than 70cm.		
5. Where there is no ramp, there must be no more than three steps at any one point to the entrance.	1. Where there is no ramp there must be no more than single steps to the entrance.	3. The threshold at the entrance must be no higher than 2cm.
6. Within the reception area there must be an unobstructed space of not less than 110x70cm.		

INTERIOR GENERAL

CATEGORY 3 🏃 | ## CATEGORY 2 ♿ | ## CATEGORY 1 ♿

CATEGORY 3	CATEGORY 2	CATEGORY 1
1. Public passageways that lead to a restaurant, dining room, lounge, TV lounge (unless TV is provided in the bedroom), bar, disabled guest's bedroom and bath-room (if other than en suite), should be not less than 75cm wide. The immediate approach to the entrance must include no more than three steps.	1. Public passageways that lead to a restaurant or dining room, lounge, TV lounge (unless TV is provided in the bedroom), bar, disabled guest's bedroom and bathroom (if other than en suite), should not be less than 80cm wide and not less than 120cm opposite the doors to the rooms a disabled guest will be required to use.	
2. Doors to the rooms referred to above should have a clear opening of not less than 70cm.	2. Doors to the rooms referred to above should have a clear opening of not less than 75cm.	
3. There must be no more than three steps at any one point in the corridors a disabled guest will be required to use or at the entrance of the rooms referred to above.	3. There must be no more than single steps at any one point in the corridors or to the rooms a disabled guest will be required to use.	1. All routes to be used by a disabled guest must be level or ramped.
		2. Access to a restaurant or dining room, lounge, bar, bedroom, bath-room and WC (where not en suite) must be level or ramped with thresholds that are no higher than 2cm.
	4. In the restaurant or dining room there must be at least one accessible table with a clear underspace of at least 65cm. Blocks to lift the table when required, are acceptable. Where three or more bedrooms meet the requirements for Category 2 or 1, at least two such accessible tables should be provided.	
4. If a disabled guest is required to use a lift, the door should have a clear opening of not less than 70cm and the interior of the lift should be not less than 110cm deep by 70cm wide.	5. If a disabled guest is required to use a lift, the door should have a clear opening of not less than 75cm and the interior of the lift should be not less than 120cm deep by 80cm wide.	
5. Have no more than three steps at any point along the route or more than three steps in each 50m.		3. Where a disabled guest is required to use a lift it must have automatic doors with controls 140cm or less above the floor.

13

BEDROOM (Only one bedroom should meet these requirements.)

CATEGORY 3	CATEGORY 2	CATEGORY 1
	1. There must be unobstructed space of not less than 110cm x70cm.	
	2. On at least one side of the bed there must be space of not less than 80cm to allow for lateral transfer.	
		1. The surface of the bed must be between 45-54cm above the floor.
		2. Door handles, light switches, TV controls, curtain pulls, wardrobe rails, etc. should be accessible and not more than 140cm above the floor.
		3. Light switch and telephone (where provided) should be no more than 50cm from the bed.

14

WC

CATEGORY 3	CATEGORY 2	CATEGORY 1
1. The WC must be en suite or on the same floor as a disabled guest's bedroom.		
2. Toilet paper must be within reach of the seat.		
	1. There must be a lateral transfer space to the WC of not less than 80cm.	
	2. The rim of the WC seat must be between 45-50cm above the floor.	
	3. There must be a horizontal or angled support rail opposite the transfer space, between 20-30cm above the seat.	
3. Where the WC is separate from the bathroom there must be a washbasin in the same room.	4. If separate from the bedroom, there must be an unobstructed interior space of not less than 100x70cm and a washbasin with clear underspace.	1. The horizontal or angled support rail opposite the transfer space must be no more than 50cm from the centre of the seat.

BATHROOM. Categories 1 and 2. (Only one bathroom, separate or en suite with the bedroom(s) above, should meet these requirements.)

CATEGORY 3	CATEGORY 2	CATEGORY 1
1. The bathroom must be en suite or on the same floor as a disabled guest's bedroom.		1. The door handle and light switch must be 140cm or less above floor level.
	1. There must be an unobstructed interior space, clear of the door swing, of not less than 100x70cm.	2. The horizontal or angled support rail at the far side of the bath must be no more than 30cm above the rim.
2. Where a bath is provided it should have a horizontal or angled support rail on the far side (recommended height is 25cm above the rim).		
	2. Where a bath is provided there must be space alongside of not less than 80cm to allow for lateral transfer.	3. The rim of the bath must be 45-50cm above floor level.
3. Where only a shower is provided, it must have a seat (recommended height 45-50cm above the floor) and a support rail on the far wall (recommended height 25cm above the top of the seat and a maximum of 50cm from the centre of seat).		
	3. Where only a shower is provided, it must have a level entry, i.e. no rim, a lateral transfer space of not less than 80cm, and a seat.	4. Where only a shower is available, the controls must be 140cm or less above floor level.
4. Where there is a step into the shower, it should have a rise of no more than 19cm.		
5. There must be a washbasin within the bathroom or bedroom.	4. The washbasin, either within the bathroom or bedroom, must have sufficient clear underspace and/or lever taps to enable it to be used by someone in a wheelchair.	

KITCHENS (Self-catering-units only.)

CATEGORY 3 🧍	CATEGORY 2 ♿	CATEGORY 1 ♿
		1. There must be a minimum clear floor space of 120cm in front of units and work surfaces.
		2. At least one work surface or table should have a clear underspace between 65-80cm.
		3. The hob should be not more than 80cm high, have a clear underspace below or alongside, and accessible controls.
		4. The oven should have front controls and base between 65cm and 80cm above floor level.
		5. The sink should have level taps and a clear underspace.
		6. The base of wall cupboards and shelves should not be more than 120cm above floor level.
		7. Light switches and door handles should not be more than 140cm above floor level.
		8. Power socket should be unobstructed and not more than 140cm above floor level (extension sockets acceptable).
		9. A fire extinguisher or fire blanket, not more than 140cm above floor level, should be sited between hob and doorway and be accessible.

ATTRACTIONS – CATEGORY REQUIREMENTS

APPROACH

CATEGORY 3	CATEGORY 2	CATEGORY 1
1. A public entrance must be accessible to wheelchair users from either a setting down point or a car park. Any such setting down point must have a firm level surface regardless of whether or not there is a car park.		
2. If an attraction has a car park but no setting down point, two dedicated car parking spaces plus one for every 50 spaces up to a maximum of 20 dedicated spaces should be provided. Dedicated spaces should be as close as possible to the entrance but no farther than 100m.		1. If there is no general car park, there must be at least two dedicated parking spaces, each with a minimum width of 360cm, capable of being reserved in advance.
3. All such dedicated spaces must be clearly signposted and marked using the international wheelchair symbol.		2. If there is a car park, each dedicated space must have a minimum width of 360cm (that may include wheelchair transfer space with an adjoining dedicated space).
4. The car park surface of dedicated spaces and the route to the nearest public entrance must be firm, sound and free from obstacles. Rough grass, deep gravel, cobbles and pot-holed surfaces are not acceptable.		
5. The route to the nearest entrance from dedicated parking spaces must have no more than three steps at any one point and no more than three per 50m. Steps should have risers no greater than 19cm, treads no less than 25cm deep and 75cm wide. Where there are two or more steps a handrail must be provided.	1. The route to the entrance from dedicated parking spaces must be no more than 100m and must have no more than single steps at any one point and no more than three such steps per 50m. Steps may have risers no greater than 19cm, treads no less than 120cm deep and 75cm wide. There must be a clear space not less than 360cm between each step.	3. The route to the entrance must not include steps and must not be steeper than 1:15. Long slopes must have level resting places 150cm long at no more than 10m intervals.

continued overleaf

17

6. Where provided, paths must be not less than 75cm wide and passing places not less than 150cm x 150cm must be provided at intervals of not less than 25m.	2. Where provided, paths must be not less than 90cm wide and passing places not less than 150cm x 150cm must be provided at intervals of not less than 25m.	
7. Slopes on the route must be not steeper than 1:12 at any point and level resting places 150cm long must be provided at 10m intervals on paths or slopes that exceed 15m in length.		
NB: Requirements 4, 5, 6, & 7 may be waived where a regular shuttle transport plies between the car park and the entrance, provided the transport has no more than three steps and is capable of carrying a folded wheelchair.	NB: Category Three waiver applies, provided the vehicle has a wheelchair lift.	NB: Category Two waiver applies

ENTRANCE

CATEGORY 3	CATEGORY 2	CATEGORY 1
1. The immediate approach to the entrance must not have more than three steps.	1. The immediate approach to the entrance must not have more than three single steps with a minimum space of 120cm between each step.	1. The immediate approach to the entrance must be level or ramped with a gradient not exceeding 1:15, with a level landing 120cm deep clear of any door swing, and with level resting places 150cm long at no more than 10m intervals.
2. Thresholds must not exceed 5cm and must be adequately tapered if they exceed 2cm.	2. Ramps must be no steeper than 1:12. The steeper gradient of 1:10 for internal ramps less than 1.5m long is not acceptable.	2. Thresholds must not exceed 2cm.
3. Ramps should be no steeper than 1:12 with level resting places 150cm long at no more than 10m intervals. NB: For internal ramps 1:12 is the preferred gradient except for ramps of less than 1.5m where 1:10 is acceptable. Ramps must be of solid construction, well maintained with a slip-resistant surface.		

continued overleaf

4. The entrance door or gate must have a clear opening of not less than 67cm. If the normal entrance is via a turnstile or kissing gate, an alternative nearby entrance with a clear opening of no less than 67cm must be available.

FACILITIES including WCs, retail units, bars. (If an attraction includes one or more of these facilities, at least one or more of each facility must be accessible.)

The route to each accessible facility must

CATEGORY 3	CATEGORY 2	CATEGORY 1
1. Have a firm, sound surface, free from obstacles.	1. The route to each accessible facility must have no more than single steps at any point with a minimum space of 120cm between each step and no more than three steps in each 50m.	
2. Contain no incline or ramp steeper than 1:12 except for internal ramps less than 1.5m long where 1:10 is acceptable. Level resting places 150cm long must be provided at no more than 10m intervals on paths or slopes that exceed 15m in length	2. The route to each accessible facility must contain no incline or ramp steeper than 1:12. The steeper gradient of 1:10 for internal ramps less than 1.5m long is not acceptable.	1. The route to each accessible facility must be level or ramped with gradients not exceeding 1:15.
3. Have no more than three steps at any point along the route or more than three steps in each 50m.	3. The route to each accessible facility must have corridors or paths (where present) not less than 90cm wide.	
4. Have corridors or paths (where present) not less than 75cm wide.		
5. Have no doors along the route with clear opening widths of less than 67cm or clear approaches less than 110cm deep.		
6. Have no more than three steps at the entrance. Where there are two or more steps a handrail must be provided.		

19

continued overleaf

7. Where the route requires the use of a lift or lifts, their doors should have clear openings of not less than 67cm and internal dimensions of not less than 110cm deep by 70cm wide.

4. Where the route requires the use of a lift or lifts, their doors must have clear opening widths of not less than 75cm and internal dimensions not less than 140cm deep by 110cm wide. Controls for the lift must not be more than 140cm above the floor or landing.

4. If an attraction has only one WC, it must be an accessible unisex facility.

2. If an attraction contains more than one WC facility, all those located on Category 1 accessible routes must contain an accessible unisex facility.

5. If an attraction has more than one WC facility, at least 50% of those on Category 2 access routes must be accessible unisex WC facilities.

6. Within an accessible WC:
a) There must be no more than a single step at the entrance.
b) The entrance must not be locked and must have a clear opening width of not less than 75cm and a clear approach not less than 120cm deep.
c) There must be unobstructed interior space of not less than 110cm x 70cm.
d) There must be a lateral transfer space to the WC of not less than 80cm.
e) The rim of the WC seat must be between 45cm and 50cm above the floor.
f) A toilet paper dispenser must be within easy reach of the WC.
g) There must be a horizontal support rail 65 to 75cm above the floor on the wall opposite the transfer space and positioned between 40 and 50cm from the centre of the seat.
h) A hinged support rail must be located on the transfer side.
i) There must be a washbasin within the WC with clear underspace to allow access to a wheelchair user.
j) A soap dispenser must be located within reach of a wheelchair user at the washbasin.
k) A hand dryer and/or paper towel dispenser must be within reach of a

3. All such accessible WC facilities must be unisex and conform to Part T Building Regulations (Scotland only). Door widths must provide a clear opening width of 80cm.

continued overleaf

	wheelchair user at the washbasin. l) A light switch must not be more than 140cm above the floor.	
	7. Within an accessible catering outlet and/or bar; a) There must be no more than a single step at the entrance. b) The entrance must have a clear opening width not less than 75cm and a clear approach not less than 120cm deep. c) There must be at least two, plus one in 10, accessible tables with a clear underspace at least 70cm high, 60cm wide and 45cm deep.	
	8. Within an accessible shop; a) There must be no more than a single step at the entrance. b) The entrance must have a clear opening width not less than 75cm and a clear approach not less than 120cm deep. c) Where there are aisles they must be at least 90cm wide.	

FEATURES (Displays, exhibits, rides etc. within an attraction.)

The route to the feature must:

CATEGORY 3	CATEGORY 2	CATEGORY 1
1. Have a firm, sound surface, free from obstacles.		
2. Contain no incline or ramp steeper than 1:12 except for internal ramps less than 1.5m long where 1:10 is acceptable. Level resting places 150cm long must be provided at no more than 10m intervals on paths or slopes that exceed 15m in length.	2. The route to each accessible feature must contain no incline or ramp steeper than 1:12. The steeper gradient of 1:10 for internal ramps less than 1.5m in length is not acceptable.	
3. Have no more than three steps at any point along the route or more than three steps in each 50m.	1. There should be no more than single steps at any one point with a minimum space of 120cm between each step.	1. The route to each accessible feature must be level or ramped with gradients not exceeding 1:15. continued overleaf

4. Have corridors or paths, where present, not less than 75cm wide.	3. There should be no corridors or paths, where present, less than 90cm wide.	
5. Have no doors along the route or at the entrance with clear opening widths of less than 67cm or clear approaches less than 110cm deep.		
6. Have no more than three steps at the entrance. Where there are two or more steps, a handrail must be provided.		3. Entrances and interiors of accessible features must be level or ramped with gradients not exceeding 1:15 and thresholds must be no higher than 2cm.
7. Where the route requires the use of a lift or lifts, their doors should have clear openings of not less than 67cm and internal dimensions of not less than 110cm deep by 70cm wide.		2. Where the route requires the use of a lift or lifts, their doors must have clear opening widths of not less than 75cm and internal dimensions not less than 140cm deep by 110cm wide. Controls for the lift must not be more than 140cm above the floor or landing.

The symbols shown in grey are categories that Smooth Ride Guides has devised and have been awarded where appropriate by Smooth Ride Guides inspectors.

CODE EXPLANATIONS – ATTRACTIONS

SD = set down	CP = carpark	E = entrance
RF = route to facilities	L = lift	C = catering
S = shop	WC = toilet	RFE = route to features
G = garden		

CODE EXPLANATIONS – THEATRES, CONCERT HALLS, SPORTS VENUES

RE = route to entrance	ED = entrance door	INT = interior
AUD = auditorium	SS = stadium seating	B/R = bar or restaurant

FINDING YOUR WAY

AIRPORTS
How to travel by air with a wheelchair.

AIR CARRIER ACCESS RULES
www.faa.gov/acr/dat.htm
Usually you can use your own wheelchair so far as the boarding point of the aircraft, where you transfer to a special aisle chair. If you are able to walk a short distance, you should request a seat near the entrance doors. Your own wheelchair will be stored for immediate availability on arrival. You have a choice about preboarding although the airline probably will want to preboard you, so arrive at the airport early.

TYPES OF WHEELCHAIR
1. Normal hand-propelled chairs.
2. Electric wheelchairs, including scooters with wet acid batteries.
3. Electric wheelchairs, including scooters with dry cell or seal gel batteries. Check with the airline if you have type 2 because the battery could be removed and placed in the hold. If so you should be at the airport at least three hours before departure. Most power-operated wheelchairs have safety batteries, but the leads must be disconnected from the terminal and capped to avoid shorting. Pre-boarding may be necessary and there could be a delay on arrival. The airline is responsible for ensuring your battery is reconnected and the chair is working on arrival at your destination. Electric scooter battery requirements are the same as for wheelchairs.
Notes: Wide aisles = more than 90cm wide.
High tables = more than 65cm underspace.
Trained staff = trained in disability awareness.

ABERDEEN AIRPORT
Dyce AB21 7DU
Tel: (01224) 722331   Fax: (01224) 725751
Setting down point near entrance:
15 non-reservable disabled badge spaces, pre-arranged assistance or by telephone in car park from car park to check in. Route to entrance has no lifts: accessible revolving entrance with special controls for wheelchair users and alternative non-automatic side door with level route to check-in. 3 unisex adapted WCs (1 main concourse, 1 main departures, 1 international departures). 2 Restaurants, 4 bars. Ramp down to departure lounge. Shop with ramp, ramp from check-in to departures: First aid at information desk. Wheelchairs available.

ALDERNEY AIRPORT (Channel Islands)
The Blaye, Alderney
Tel: (01481) 822624   Fax: (01481) 623005
Very small airport, setting down point near entrance. No disabled badge parking. Level route to entrance, no lifts. Accessible non-automatic door. Route to check-in level, no lifts. 2 separate WCs (150 x 150cm with rail next to WC, not hinged, outward opening door). Cafeteria on same level as check-in. No shop or bar. Accessible route from check-in to departure. Accessible public phones. No printed information. Medical and first aid available but no trained staff. Wheelchairs available. Can stay in own wheelchair until boarding.

BARRA AIRPORT Western Isles
Eoligarry, Isle of Barra HS9 5UA
Tel: (01871) 890212   Fax: (01871) 890220
Setting down point near entrance. No Disabled badge parking. Informal assistance given. Level route to accessible entrance and check-in, no lifts. 1 unisex adapted WC (300 x 300cm, support rail next to WC, hinged rail, outward opening door). Restaurant with high tables. 1 accessible shop, no aisles. Accessible route from check-in to departures. No wheelchairs possible on board. Accessible public phones. No printed information. Medical and first aid available but no trained staff. No wheelchairs available. Can stay in own wheelchair until boarding.

BELFAST CITY AIRPORT
Sydenham By-Pass, Belfast BT3 9JH
Tel: (02890) 457745 Fax: (02890) 738455

Setting down point near entrance. 8 non-reservable disabled badge spaces. Assistance by prior arrangement. Accessible non-automatic entrance route to check-in level. Level route from check-in to departure. Level entrance to arrivals. Ramped entrance to departures (less than 1:12, slip resistant, 200cm wide), no steps. 4 unisex adapted WCs (1 departure area, 1 boarding lounge, 1 arrival hall, 1 arrivals waiting, 200 x 180cm, support rail next to WC, hinged support rail, 2 with outward opening doors). 3 Restaurants, 3 bars all with level access and low tables, but not low counters. Accessible shops with wide aisles. Ambulift available, but generally carried. Public phones not accessible. No printed information. First aid trained staff. Wheelchairs available. Can stay in own wheelchair until boarding.

BELFAST INTERNATIONAL AIRPORT
Belfast BT29 4AB
Tel: (02894) 484848/484313
Fax: (02894) 423883

Setting down point near entrance. 16 non-reservable disabled badge spaces. 24hr. porterage. Level route to entrance, no steps. Accessible entrance with automatic door, level route to check-in. 8 accessible lifts. 11 separate WCs all over airport (5ft2), support rails, hinged support rails, outward opening doors. 2 restaurants, 6 bars, all accessible, 1 with ramp, high tables. Accessible shops with wide aisles. Accessible route from check-in to departures via lift. Alternative, 6 gates with bridge, Ambulift and chairlift. Accessible public phones. Printed information available. Medical and first aid available, trained staff. Wheelchairs available. Can stay in own wheelchair until boarding. Information supplied by member of Transport Advisory Committee of Disability Action for Northern Ireland.

BIRMINGHAM INTERNATIONAL AIRPORT
Birmingham B26 3QJ

Tel: (0121) 7678275 Fax: (0121) 7677357

Setting down point near entrance. Unreservable disabled badge spaces. Bus from long-stay car park. Level route to entrance. Accessible, automatic door. Level route to check-in. 22 lifts conform to specs. 23 adapted unisex WCs (measurements unavailable, both supports, outward opening doors). 5 bars, 9 restaurants (table height unavailable). Shops with level access. Accessible route to check-in, sometimes via lift. Accessible public phones. Printed information available. Medical and first aid available. Staff trained in disability awareness, some special staff employed. Wheelchairs available. Can stay in own wheelchair until boarding.

BOURNEMOUTH INTERNATIONAL AIRPORT
Christchurch, Dorset BH23 6SE
Tel: (01202) 364000/364170
Fax: (01202) 364179

Setting down point near entrance. 5 non-reservable disabled badge spaces. Assistance provided, minibus available. Level route to entrance. Automatic accessible main entrance door. Level route to check-in, no lifts. 3 unisex adapted WCs (smallest 165 x 235cm, support rail, hinged support rail, outward opening doors. 2 bars, 1 restaurant with high tables. Shops with wide aisles. Accessible route from check-in to departure. Lifts for boarding. Accessible public phones, will lower other phones. Printed information available. Medical and first aid available, trained staff. Wheelchairs available. Can stay in own wheelchair until boarding.

BRISTOL INTERNATIONAL AIRPORT
Bristol BS49 3DY
Tel: (0870) 1212747 Fax: (0870) 1244747
www.bristolairport.co.uk

New terminal completed March 2000. Setting down point near entrance. 76 non-reservable disabled badge space. Full assistance from car park to entrance by prior notice. Level route to entrance. Automatic accessible main entrance door. Level route to check-in. 1 accessible lift. 4 unisex adapted WCs (smallest 162 x

172cm support rail next to WC, no hinged support rail, inward opening door). 1 restaurant, 3 bars, main restaurant has high tables. Shops with wide aisles. Accessible route from check-in to departures. Boarding via lifts. Accessible public phones. Printed information available. Medical and first aid available. Staff disabled-aware. Wheelchairs available. can stay in own wheelchair until boarding. Bristol International Flyer; dedicated bus from Bristol Temple Meads railway station and bus station.

CARDIFF INTERNATIONAL AIRPORT
Vale of Glamorgan CF62 3BD
Tel: (01446) 711111   Fax: (01446) 711675
www.cardiffairportonline.com
Setting down point near entrance. Some disabled badge spaces. Assistance provided on request through travel agent. Level route to entrance. 2 lifts. Accessible automatic entrance door. Level route to check-in. 4 lifts (104 x 134cm, controls 130-150cm above floor and **not accessible** but to be addressed). 4 adapted unisex and separate WCs (standard sizes, both support rails, outward opening doors). 2 restaurants, 2 bars, all with high tables. Shops with wide aisles. Accessible route from check-in to departure. Boarding via airbridges or lifts. Accessible public phones. Printed information. Medical and first aid available. Most staff are trained. Wheel-chairs available. Special staff employed. Can stay in own wheelchair until boarding. Ambulift for boarding aircraft. Minicom facility at Information Desk.

CARLISLE AIRPORT
Carlisle CA6 4NW
Tel: (01228) 573641   Fax: (01228) 573310
Setting down point near entrance. No disabled badge spaces. Assistance provided. Level route to entrance. No lifts. Automatic accessible entrance door. Level route to check-in. No lifts. No adapted WCs. 1 bar/ restaurant with high tables. No shops. Accessible route from check-in to departure. No airbridges or lifts. 8 accessible public phones. No printed information. Medical and first aid

available. Staff trained in disability awareness. No special staff. Wheelchair available. Can stay in own wheelchair until boarding.

DUNDEE AIRPORT
Riverside Drive, Dundee DD2 1UH
Tel: (01382) 643242   Fax: (01382) 641263
Setting down point near entrance. 2 non-reservable disabled badge spaces, tel: 01382 641263 with arrival time for assistance. Level route to entrance. Automatic accessible main entrance door. Level route to check-in. No lifts. 3 unisex-adapted WCs to part M (1 landside, 1 airside departures, 1 baggage reclaim, with support rail next to WC, hinged support rail, outward opening doors). No bars, restaurants or shops. Accessible route from check-in to departures. Accessible public phones. No printed information. Trained staff. Wheelchairs available. Can stay in own wheelchair until boarding.

EAST MIDLANDS AIRPORT
Castle Donnington, Derbyshire DE74 2SA
Tel: (01332) 852852/852885
Fax: (01332) 852899
Setting down point near entrance and 2 disabled pick up points: 30 reservable disabled badge spaces. Phone information desk for assistance from car park to check-in. Level route to entrance, no steps. Automatic accessible main entrance door. Level route to check-in. 2 accessible lifts. 9 adapted unisex WCs, varying sizes, none less than 140cm, all with both support rails, most with outward opening doors. 4 bars, 2 restaurants. Shops accessible, but not all with wide aisles. Accessible route from check-in to departures. Pre-boarded by ambulift. 20 accessible public phones. Printed material available. Medical and first aid available, trained staff. Wheelchairs available. Can stay in own wheelchair until boarding. On site taxi firm can provide wheelchair-accessible transport.

EDINBURGH AIRPORT
Edinburgh EH12 9DN
Tel: (0131) 3331000   Fax: (0131) 3333181

Setting down point near entrance. 10 non-reservable disabled badge spaces. No assistance from car park to check-in. Route level to entrance (low, wide, slip-resistant ramp over road). Automatic accessible entry door. 4 accessible lifts. 3 unisex adapted WCs conforming to BAA specs, support rail, hinged support rail, outward opening doors. 2 bars, 3 restaurants with high tables. Accessible shops with wide aisles. 4 accessible phones. Check-in to departure via lift. Boarding by airbridges where necessary. No printed information. First aid available. Wheelchairs available. No trained staff. Can stay in own wheelchair until boarding.

EXETER AND DEVON AIRPORT
Exeter, Devon EX5 2BD
Tel: (01392) 367433 Fax: (01392) 445539
Assistance provided from set-down point into terminal with slip-resistant ramp. 7 reservable disabled badge parking spaces. Level automatic entrance door. Level route to check-in. 3 adapted unisex WCs (1 check-in, 1 arrivals, 1 departures), 140 x 240cm with support rail, hinged support rail, outward opening doors. 1 restaurant, 1 bar with high tables. Level shops with wide aisles. Accessible route from check-in to departure. Specially designed lift-on. Accessible phones. First aid available. No trained staff. Wheelchairs available. Can remain in own wheelchair until boarding.

GLASGOW PAISLEY AIRPORT
Paisley PA3 2ST
Tel: (0141) 8484 778 Fax: (0141) 848 4354
E-mail:customercomments_glal@baa.com
The new multi-storey car park has over 100 blue badge spaces located over five floors. Level 2 is fast-track with direct link bridge access to the first floor of the terminal building, at an additional cost. Help phones are located on each floor adjacent to the blue badge spaces, as well as in Car Park 1 and on the forecourt outside Door 2. Passengers with reduced mobility can request assistance into the terminal building from these phones. Level route to entrance. For long stay

(more than four days) contact NCP on (0870) 000 1000 to arrange long term rates in Car Park 2 (blue badge holders only).
Setting down point near entrance. 34 non-reservable disabled badge spaces. Fax in advance for assistance (0141) 8484354. Level route to entrance.
11 accessible unisex toilets with support rails, hinged support tail and outward opening doors throughout airport. 4 babychange rooms throughout airport, with babychange units in most accessible toilets.
4 restaurants, 3 bars, with low level tables. Shops with wide aisles. Accessible route from check-in to departures via lift and/or ramp. Boarding by airbridge or ambulift. Accessible public phones and e-mail phones. e-mail public telephones throughout building. Text phone manned 24hours - (0141)848 4848. Printed information available. First Aid available. Wheelchairs available. Can stay in own wheelchair until boarding.

GLASGOW PRESTWICK INTERNATIONAL AIRPORT
Aviation House, Prestwick KA9 2PL
Tel: (01292) 479822/511234
Fax: (01292) 511010
Setting down point near entrance. 30 non- reservable disabled badge spaces. Prior notice for assistance recommended. Ramped entrance (1:50, slip-resistant, 250cm wide), no steps or lifts. Automatic accessible entrance door. Level route to check-in. Lift if arriving by train, 2 lifts at rail station (car interiors 97 x 133cm, controls 130cm high). 1 WC in concourse confirming to spec, 6 unisex and separate WCs to part M, 200 x 200cm, support rail next to WC, hinged support rail, outward opening or sliding doors. 2 bars, 2 restaurants with high tables. Shops with wide aisles. Accessible route from check-in to departures. Boarding via specially adapted vehicle if necessary. Public phones not accessible. No printed information. Medical and first aid available. Wheelchairs available Staff not trained, but aware. Can stay in own wheelchair until boarding. This airport is

used every year by those making pilgrimages to Lourdes, it handles large numbers of passengers with mobility difficulties, and is recognised for its sensitive, friendly handling.

STATES OF GUERNSEY AIRPORT
Channel Islands
La Villiaze, Forest, Guernsey
Tel: (01481) 37766/37267
Fax: (01481) 39595

Setting down point near entrance: 3 non-reservable disabled badge spaces. Staff available for assistance. Level route to entrance. Automatic accessible door. Level route to check-in. No lifts. 1 unisex-adapted WC, 280 x 170cm, support rail next to WC, hinged support rail, inward opening door. 1 bar, 1 restaurant with high tables. Shops with wide aisles. Accessible route from check-in to departures. Manually lifted on board. Public phones not accessible. No printed information. Medical and first aid available. Staff not trained. Wheelchairs available. Can stay in own wheelchair until boarding. New terminal with upgraded facilities will be completed and operational early in 2004.

HUMBERSIDE INTERNATIONAL AIRPORT
Kirmington, Lincolnshire DN39 6YH
Tel: (01652) 688456   Fax: (01652) 680524

Setting down point near entrance. 6 non-reservable disabled badge spaces. Assistance preferably pre-arranged. Level route to entrance. No steps or lifts. Automatic accessible entrance door. 4 unisex-adapted WCs, smallest 170 x 133cm, all with support rails next to WC, hinged support rails and outward opening doors. 1 bar, 1 restaurant with some high tables. Shops with wide aisles. Accessible route from check-in to departures. Boarding by Ambulift. Accessible public phones. Printed information available. Medical and first aid available. Trained staff. Wheelchairs available. Can stay in own wheelchair until boarding.

INVERNESS AIRPORT
Inverness, Scotland IV1 2JB

Tel: (01667) 464000   Fax: (01667) 462041

Setting down point near entrance. 2 non-reservable disabled badge spaces. Contact airline for assistance. Level route to entrance. Automatic accessible main entrance door. No lifts. 1 unisex-adapted WC, 300 x 200cm, both support rails, outward opening doors, on ground floor. 1 bar, 1 restaurant with high tables. Shops with wide aisles. Level route from check-in to departure. Boarding via Ambulift. Accessible public phones. No printed information. First aid available. Wheelchairs available. Trained staff. Can stay in own wheelchair until boarding.

ISLE OF MAN AIRPORT
Ballasalla, Isle of Man IM0 2AS
Tel: (01624) 821603   Fax: (01624) 821611
www.iom-airport.com

Setting down point near entrance. 10 non-reservable disabled badge spaces. No assistance from car park to entrance. Ramped route to entrance (less than 1:12, slip resistant, 200cm wide, no steps, no lifts). Accessible entry door. 4 lifts, all conform to specs. 4 adapted WCs, 150 x 205cm, both support rails, outward opening door. 2 bars, 2 restaurants with high tables. Shops with wide aisles. Check-in to departure via lift. Boarding by lift, Ambulift, airline staff assist PRM. Accessible public phones. Printed information available. First aid. Some staff trained. Wheelchairs available. Staff prefer passenger to transfer to airport chairs. Major refurbishment in 1999.

ISLES OF SCILLY AIRPORT
St. Mary's, Isles of Scilly, Cornwall
TR21 0NG
Tel: (01720) 422677   Fax: (01720) 423302

Setting down point near entrance. No disabled badge spaces. Duty crew available for assistance. Ramp to entrance (1:10, not slip resistant, 112cm wide, no steps, no lifts). Automatic accessible main entrance door. No lifts in terminal. 1 unisex-adapted WC, 240 x 150cm, both support rails, inward opening door. 1 bar/restaurant with high tables. Short ramp between lounge and buffet area.

No shops. Accessible route from check-in to departure. Accessible public phones. No printed information. First aid available. No trained staff. Wheelchairs available. Can stay in own wheelchair until boarding.

JERSEY STATES AIRPORT Channel Islands
St. Peter, Jersey JE1 2BY
Tel: (01534) 492266/490999
Fax: (01534) 498084

Setting down point near entrance. 6 non-reservable disabled badge spaces. Assistance through customer service agents. Level route to entrance. Automatic accessible main entrance door. 2 lifts conforming to specs. 5 adapted unisex WCs, 162 x 140cm, both support rails, outward opening doors. 2 bars, 2 restaurants with high tables. Shops with wide aisles. Level route from check-in to departures. No airbridges or Ambulifts. Accessible public phones. No printed information. Limited first aid available Sat/Sun. Staff not trained, but special staff employed.

KIRKWALL AIRPORT
Orkney, Scotland KW15 1TH
Tel: (01856) 872421   Fax: (01856) 871252

Small split-level airport. New terminal under consideration but no decision taken when inspected in May 1999. Set-down point near entrance. 1 non-reservable disabled badge space. No assistance. Level route to entrance. Accessible automatic entrance door. No lifts in terminal. 1 unisex-adapted WC, 330 x 140cm, support rail next to WC, no hinged support rail, inward opening door. 1 restaurant with high tables. No shops. Route from check-in to departures not accessible inside, requires exit and re-entry to building. Boarding via Ambulift. Accessible public phones. No printed information. Limited first aid. No trained staff. Wheelchairs available. Can stay in own wheelchair until boarding.

LANDS END AERODROME
St. Just, Penzance, Cornwall TR19 2BL
Tel: (01736) 788771

Very small airport with limited facilities.

Setting down point near entrance. No designated parking. Level entrance. Non-automatic door. Level route to check-in. No lifts. No adapted WC. 1 unisex WC 75 x 130cm without handrails in Skybus lounge. 1 restaurant, level access, low tables. No shops. Level route from check-in to departure. Accessible public phones. Limited first aid available. Some staff are trained. Wheelchairs available.

LEEDS BRADFORD INTERNATIONAL AIRPORT
Leeds, West Yorks LS19 7TU
Tel: (0113) 2509696   Fax: (0113) 2505426

Setting down point near entrance. 30 non-reservable disabled badge spaces. Assistance available. Level route to entrance. Automatic accessible entry door. Level route to check-in. 3 lifts conforming to specs. 5 unisex adapted WCs, 245 x 2175cm, both support rails, outward opening doors. 2 restaurants, 3 bars with high tables. Shops with wide aisles. Accessible route from check-in to departures. Boarding via airbridge and lifts. Accessible public phones. No printed information. First aid available. Trained staff. Wheelchairs available. Special company Airway to assist special needs passengers. Can stay in own wheelchair until boarding.

LERWICK SUMBURGH AIRPORT
Uirkig, Shetland, Scotland
Tel: (01950) 460204   Fax: (01950) 460218

Set-down point near entrance. 5 reservable disabled badge spaces. Assistance provided. Level route to entrance. Accessible automatic entrance door. No lifts in terminal. 1 adapted unisex WC to part M, outward opening door. 1 bar, 1 restaurant. Shops with wide aisles. Level route from check-in to departure. Boarding via Ambulift. No accessible public phones. No printed information. First Aid. No trained staff. Wheelchairs available. Can stay in own wheelchair until boarding.

LERWICK TINGWALL AIRPORT
Toll Clock, Lerwick, Shetland ZE1 0PE
Tel: (01595) 744872   Fax: (01595) 744869

Set-down point near entrance. No disabled badge spaces. Assistance by airline staff. Level route to entrance. Non-automatic accessible entrance door. No lifts. 1 unisex adapted WC, 148 x 242cm, both support rails, outward opening door. No bars or restaurants. No shops. No public phones. No printed information. No trained staff. No wheelchairs available. Tingwall is the base for an inter-island service via Loganair using a seven-seater B/N Islander aircraft that also is used as an air ambulance.

LIVERPOOL AIRPORT
Liverpool, Merseyside L24 1YD
Tel: (0151) 2884000   Fax: (0151) 2884120
Setting down point near entrance. 3 non-reservable disabled badge spaces near entrance, 6 in NCP 100m. away, under review, request assistance when booking flight. Ramped entrance, gradient unknown, no steps, no lifts. Automatic accessible main entrance door. Level route to check-in. 1 lift conforming to specs. 3 unisex-adapted WCs, both support rails, outward opening door. 2 restaurants, 2 bars with high tables. Shops with wide aisles. Accessible route from check-in to departures. Boarding by Ambulift. Some accessible public phones. First aid available. Fire service have trained staff. Wheelchairs available. Can stay in own wheelchair until boarding. In 1998 this airport was nominated for an Ease award for services to disabled passengers judged on public response.

LONDON CITY AIRPORT
Royal Docks, London E1
Tel: (020) 7 6460092/6460088
Fax: (020) 7 4745747
Setting down point near entrance. 6 non-reservable disabled badge spaces. No assistance provided from car park to check-in. Level route to entrance. Accessible automatic entrance door. Level route to check-in. No lifts. 5 unisex adapted WCs (146 x 200cm, both support rails, outward opening doors). 2 bars, 2 restaurants with high tables. Shops with wide aisles. Accessible route from check-in to departures via lift. Board by lift.

Accessible public phones. No special information. Some special staff. First aid available. Wheelchairs available. Can stay in own wheelchair until boarding.

LONDON GATWICK AIRPORT
Crawley, West Sussex RH6 0NP
Tel: (01293) 503124   Fax: (01293) 504177
Setting down point near entrance. More than 100 non-reservable disabled badge spaces. Help points to request assistance. Route to main entrance with automatic door is level. Slip-resistant ramps elsewhere. Lifts to some entrances. Route to check-in varies by terminal entrance. More than 70 lifts all confirming to specs. Many unisex-adapted WCs of varying sizes, most with both support rails and outward opening doors. Many bars and restaurants, all with accessible tables. Shops with wide aisles. Routes from check-in to departures are accessible. Lift for route to UK departures in South Terminal. Boarding via Ambulifts and airbridges. Printed information available.

29

Stansted offers the finest of facilities for disabled people.

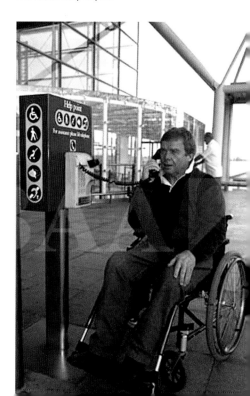

First aid available. Key operational staff trained. Wheelchairs available. Can stay in own wheelchair until boarding. Annual accessibility audits.

LONDON HEATHROW AIRPORT
Heathrow Travel-Care, Room 1308, Queens Building, Heathrow Airport, Hounslow, Middlesex TW6 1BZ
Tel: (020) 8 7457495
Fax: (020) 8 7454161
Minicom: (020) 8 7457565
This organisation provides social work and counselling at LHR and produces Travellers' Information Guide – Special Needs Edition, a comprehensive guide to all aspects of LHR. It covers getting to and from the airport, parking, arrival, terminal layouts, checking-in, security check, connections, in the air, useful phone numbers and contacts. We strongly recommend a copy be obtained from: Passenger Relations, Public Affairs, Heathrow Airport Ltd. Heathrow Point, 234 Bath Road, Harlington, Middlesex UB3 5AP, Tel: (0208) 745 7127 . SRG is always happy to answer specific queries, call us on (01279) 777966.

LONDON STANSTED AIRPORT
Stansted, Essex CM24 1QW
Tel: (01279) 662041/662039
Fax: (01279) 662066
Minicom: (01279) 663725
Setting down point near entrance. 24-hour short stay and 104 long stay unreservable disabled badge spaces. Assistance provided on request from help point. Level and ramped route to entrance. Lifts to entrance level. Automatic accessible door. Level and ramped route to check-in desks. Several lifts all conforming to specs. 14 adapted unisex WCs conform to Part M (both supporting rails, outward opening doors). 5 bars, 8 restaurants, all with accessible tables. Accessible shops. Route from check-in to departures accessible, sometimes via lift. Boarding via airbridge and lifts. Accessible public phones. Printed information available. Some tactile/Braille signage. Medical and

first aid available. Some staff trained. Wheelchairs available. Some special staff employed. Buses from long-stay car parks are low floor.

MANCHESTER AIRPORT
Manchester M90 1QX
Tel: (0161) 4893000
Fax: (0161) 4893813/3647
Setting down point near entrance. Non-reservable disabled badge spaces. Phone for assistance. Level route to entrance. Also lifts to entrance level. Automatic accessible main entrance door. Level route to check-in. 6 lifts conform to specs. Unisex-adapted WCs, number unknown. More than 20 restaurants and bars with high tables. Shops with wide aisles. Accessible route from check-in to departures, one route via lift. Boarding via airbridges and lifts. Accessible public phones. No printed information. Medical and first aid available. No trained staff. Wheelchairs available. Can stay in own wheelchair until boarding, special staff.

NEWCASTLE AIRPORT
Newcastle upon Tyne NE13 8BZ
Tel: (0191) 2144444/2143451
Fax: (0191) 2143351
Setting down point near entrance 50 non-reservable disabled badge spaces. Phone from car park for assistance. Level route to entrance. Automatic accessible entrance door. 4 lifts conform to specs. 9 separate WCs, 220 x 140cm, both support rails, outward opening doors. 2 restaurants, 2 bars with high tables. Shops with wide aisles Accessible route from check-in to departures. Boarding by airbridge or lift. Accessible public phones. Printed information available. First Aid available. Trained staff. Wheelchairs available. Can stay in own wheelchair until boarding.

NEWQUAY CORNWALL AIRPORT
c/o Plymouth City Airport Ltd, Roborough House, Crownhill, Plymouth, Devon PL6 8BW
Tel: (01752) 209571/772752
Fax: (01752) 774885
Set-down point near entrance.

Designated non-reservable disabled badge spaces. No assistance provided. Level route to entrance. Automatic accessible main entrance. No lifts. 2 adapted unisex WCs to part M, 174 x 146cm, both support rails, outward opening doors. 1 bar/restaurant with high tables. No shops. Accessible route from check-in to departure. Boarding by lift. Accessible public phones. No printed information. First aid available. No trained staff. Wheelchairs available. Can stay in own wheelchair until boarding.

NORWICH AIRPORT
Amsterdam Way, Norwich NR6 6JA
Tel: (01603) 420650/411923
Fax: (01603) 487523

Set-down point near entrance. 30 non-reservable disabled badge spaces, assistance available if previously arranged with duty airport manager. Level route to entrance. Accessible entrance door. Level route to check-in, no lifts. 2 unisex-adapted WCs, both support rails, outward opening doors. 2 bars, 2 restaurants with high tables. Shops with wide aisles. Accessible route from check-in to departures. Boarding by lifts. No printed information. First aid available. Trained staff. Wheelchairs available. Passengers must transfer to airport wheelchair at check-in. Terminal on one level and very user-friendly.

PLYMOUTH CITY AIRPORT
Roborough House, Crownhill,
Plymouth PL6 8BW
Tel: (01752) 772752
Fax: (01752) 774885

Setting down point near entrance. 4 non-reservable disabled badge spaces. Assistance from car park to check-in available on request. Level route to entrance, then one step to accessible automatic entrance door. Level route to check-in, no lifts. 1 adapted unisex WC at check in, conforming to part M, 280 x 167cm with both support rails and outward opening doors. 1 bar, 1 restaurant with high tables. No shops. Accessible route from check-in to departure. Accessible public phones. First

aid available. Wheelchairs available. Can stay in own wheelchair until boarding.

SOUTHAMPTON INTERNATIONAL AIRPORT
Southampton, Hants SO18 2NL
Tel: (02380) 620021/627099
Fax: (02380) 629300

Setting down point near entrance. 30 reservable disabled badge spaces: Assistance provided on request. Level route to entrance. No lifts. Accessible automatic entrance door. Level route to check-in. 1 lift conforms to all specs. 4 adapted unisex WCs conforming to Part M (both support rails, outward opening doors). 2 bars/2 restaurants with high tables. Accessible shops. Accessible route from check-in to departure. Boarding by lift. Accessible public phones. Text phones available. Hearing loops throughout. Printed information available. First aid available. Special staff employed. Staff training in disability awareness. Wheelchairs available. Can stay in own wheelchair until boarding.

SOUTHEND AIRPORT
Southend on Sea, Essex SS2 6YF
Tel: (01702) 608100   Fax: (01702) 608110

Setting down point near entrance. 6 non-reservable disabled badge spaces. Assistance by prior request. Level route to entrance. Manual accessible entrance door, no lifts. 1 adapted unisex WC, support rail next to WC, no hinged support rail, outward opening door. 1 bar, 1 restaurant with high tables. No shops. Accessible route from check-in to departures. Boarding by carry-on. Accessible public phones. First aid available. Wheelchairs available. Can stay in own wheelchair until boarding.

STORNOWAY AIRPORT
Stornoway, Isle of Lewis, Western Isles,
Scotland HS2 0BN
Tel: (01851) 707400   Fax: (01851) 707408
www.hial.co.uk

New terminal now open. Setting down point near entrance. 6 disabled badge spaces. Assistance available. Main entrance accessible without ramps. Level route to check-in. No lifts in terminal. Two purpose built disabled facility toilets

- one in main concourse, one in departures. 1 bar, 1 restaurant with high tables. Shops with wide aisles. Accessible route from check-in to departures. Boarding by lift. Phone access if required. Trained First aid staff available. Quiet room available. Wheelchairs available. Can stay in own chair until boarding. Induction loop for hard of hearing. Electronic access doors.

TEESSIDE INTERNATIONAL AIRPORT
Darlington, North Yorks DL2 1LU
Tel: (01325) 332811 Fax: (01325) 332810
Setting down point near entrance. 12 non-reservable disabled badge spaces. Prior notice for assistance. Level route to entrance with ramped kerbs. Accessible main entrance door. Level route to check-in. No lifts in terminal. 3 unisex, 2 separate WCs, 146 x 196cm, both support rails, outward opening doors. 1 bar, 1 restaurant with high tables. Shops with wide aisles. Accessible route from check-in to departures. Boarding by lift. Accessible public phones. First aid available. No trained staff. Wheelchairs available. Can stay in own wheelchair until boarding.

TRESCO HELIPORT Isles of Scilly
Tresco, Isle of Scilly, Cornwall TR24 0QQ
Tel: (01720) 422970   Fax: (01720) 422807
Tresco is a small island without buses, lorries, cars etc. Heliport is small but can accommodate electric wheelchairs, as can the helicopter. Most of terminal building is level but where stepped, staff will come to a passenger, e.g. at check-in. No lifts, public phones, WCs, restaurants or bars. Wheelchairs are taken from the terminal on tractors or by road.

WICK AIRPORT
Wick, Caithness, Scotland KW1 4QP
Tel: (01955) 602215   Fax: (01955) 605946
Very small airport. Setting down point near entrance. 2 non-reservable disabled badge spaces. Assistance available. Level route to entrance. Automatic accessible entrance door. No lifts. 1 unisex adapted WC to part M, 165 x 165cm, both support rails, outward opening doors: 1

café with high tables. No shops. Accessible route from check-in to departures. No accessible public telephones: 1 wheelchair available. No trained staff. Can stay in own wheelchair until boarding.

AIRLINES
AER LINGUS
Tel: (0353) 1 7052222
Fax: (0353) 1 7053832
Minicom: (0353) 1 8863666
e-mail: aerweb@aerlingus.ie
www.aerlingus.ie

UK Routes
City of Derry – Birmingham, Blackpool, Bristol, Channel Islands, Exeter, Glasgow, Isle of Man, London Gatwick, Manchester.
Subscribes to Carefree Journeys & Holidays guide for disabled people, with several pages detailing trip tips for passengers with special needs.
Also information sheet for Passengers Requiring Special Assistance available in Aer Lingus offices and travel agencies. Medical Form required. Advise reservations staff when booking of nature/degree of disability. Check-in 1 hour prior to departure. Wet-cell batteries cannot be carried.
Special seat allocation:
A330-rows 12-16 and 27-29 AC-HK
A321-row 3 DEF & Economy aft row 20
B737-400/500-row 3 DEF and last row
Fokker 50-row 2 and 10AC
BAE146-row 2ABC and 19AC
These seats have moveable armrests and seat belt extensions only.
With prior notice, special medical apparatus can be offered if compatible with safety regulations. Details to be given through reservations staff to medical centre at airport. A330 aircraft has specially designed WC. Meals for special dietary and medical requirements are available.

AURIGNY AIRLINES
Tel: (01481) 822886
Fax: (01481) 823344

Routes: Alderney/Jersey/Guernsey hops, plus Stansted-Guernsey, Manchester - guernsey, East Midlands - Guernsey (seasonal).No literature for disabled travellers. Medical Form not required. Advise reservations staff when booking of nature/degree of disability because type of aircraft may preclude travel. Check-in minimum 30 minutes prior to departure on inter-island routes, 60 minutes on regional services. Wheelchairs available, request on booking, for transfer to/from aircraft. Transportation of personal electric chairs not possible. Special seat allocation. No moveable armrests, leg rests or harnesses. Seat belt extensions are available. No clinical air pumps/Stoma masks. No specially designed WC. No aisle wheelchairs. No special telephone number for disabled travellers.

BRITISH AIRWAYS
Head Office: Waterside, PO Box 365 Harmondsworth, Middlesex UB7 0GB
Tel: Admin/Reservations: (0345) 222111
www.british-airways.com
Minicom: (0345) 007706
UK routes: London Heathrow-Aberdeen, Belfast, Edinburgh, Glasgow, Islay, Jersey, Kirkwall, Manchester, Newcastle, Shetland (Sumburgh), Stornoway Wick.
London Gatwick-Aberdeen, Bristol, Edinburgh, Glasgow, Guernsey, Inverness, Jersey, Manchester, Newcastle, Newquay, Plymouth, Stornoway.
London City-Sheffield
Aberdeen-Belfast Int'l, Birmingham, Bristol, Cardiff, Glasgow, Leeds Bradford, Manchester, Newcastle, Newquay, Plymouth, Shetland (Sumburgh), Southampton, Stornoway.
Belfast City-Edinburgh, Glasgow, Guernsey, Jersey, Liverpool, Manchester, Sheffield, Southampton.
Belfast Int'l-Birmingham, Cardiff, Edinburgh, Glasgow, Manchester, Newcastle, Southampton.
Birmingham-Edinburgh, Glasgow, Inverness, Kirkwall, Newcastle, Shetland (Sumburgh), Stornoway, Wick.
Bristol-Edinburgh, Glasgow, Guernsey, Jersey, Manchester, Newcastle, Plymouth
Cardiff-Edinburgh, Glasgow.

Edinburgh-Glasgow, Guernsey, Inverness, Kirkwall, Manchester, Newquay, Plymouth, Southampton, Stornoway, Wick.
Glasgow-Inverness, Islay, Kirkwall, Manchester, Newquay, Plymouth, Southampton, Stornoway.
Guernsey-Manchester.
Inverness-Kirkwall, Shetland (Sumburgh), Stornoway.
Jersey-Manchester.
Kirkwall-Shetland (Sumburgh), Stornoway.
Leeds Bradford-Southampton.
Londonderry-Glasgow, Manchester.
Manchester-Newquay, Plymouth, Southampton.
Newcastle-Newquay, Plymouth, Southampton.
Shetland (Sumburgh)-Shetland (Lerwick/Tingwall), Wick.
For all routes call reservations on the number above for full clarification. Specific literature for both disabled passengers and staff. No medical form required if stable disability. Airline offers Special Services Desks and Meet & Greet service, advise at least two days prior to flight. Also includes special procedures on check-in, lounge facilities, assistance through the airport and boarding the aircraft. Allow additional 30 minutes above normal check-in time for special services application. Wheelchairs are available on request, both from check-in to aircraft, and in-flight. Electric wheelchair restrictions; passengers must transfer to a ground wheelchair operated by the airline at check-in. Taken through terminal in this chair. Own wheelchair taken at check-in and battery removed. Chair and battery loaded into hold of aircraft and stored separately for duration of flight. On arrival chair is re-assembled and delivered to baggage hall. Special seats are allocated at time of booking, although on day of flight, alterations to seating plan can be made. These seats have moveable armrests and seat belt extensions also are available. No clinical air pumps or Stoma masks available. No adapted WCs on domestic services although most have emergency cord and grab bars. Long-haul flight aircraft have specially designed WC. No aisle

33

wheelchairs, except on long- haul. Special meals provided, advance notice required. The only special phone number for disabled passengers is the minicom: (0345) 007706.

BRITISH MIDLAND
Donington Hall, Castle Donington, Derby DE74 2SB
Tel: (01332) 854000   Fax: (01332) 854632
www.britishmidland.com
UK Routes: East Midlands-Aberdeen, Belfast, Edinburgh, Glasgow, Jersey. Aberdeen-Manchester. Belfast-Heathrow (T1). Edinburgh-Heathrow (T1), Manchester. Glasgow-Leeds Bradford, Manchester. Teesside-Heathrow (T1). No literature for disabled passengers. Medical form usually not required. Disabled passengers normally pre-boarded and disembarked last. Normal check-in time as per timetable, but if assistance required do allow additional time for this. Wheelchairs available for transfer from check-in to aircraft. Non-spillable batteries can be carried provided the battery is disconnected and securely attached to the wheelchair and terminals insulated to prevent short circuit. Spillable batteries can be carried provided the wheelchair can be handled and secured in an upright position and meets conditions for non-spillable batteries. Dedicated rows on each aircraft. Seats in these rows have moveable armrests. No clinical air pumps or Stoma masks. Assist handle provided in each WC. No aisle wheelchairs available in cabin. Special meals include diabetic, gluten-free, low sodium/salt, low cholesterol and low calorie that can be provided if pre-ordered before 1600hrs on day prior to departure. No special telephone/fax number for disabled passengers. General customer enquiries are able to assist.

JERSEY EUROPEAN AIRWAYS
Hangar 3, Exeter Airport, Exeter, Devon EX5 2BD
Tel: (Reservations) (0990) 676676
Fax: (01392) 366151
www.jersey-european.co.uk
UK Routes: Guernsey-Belfast City,

Birmingham, Exeter, Jersey, Glasgow, London Gatwick, London Luton, Southampton, London City-Leeds/Bradford, Jersey, Aberdeen. No literature for disabled travellers. Medical form not required. No special procedures. Normal check-in. Dry cell battery electric chairs acceptable with advance notice. Special seat no: 00 allocated close to exit. Seat has moveable armrests, leg rests, seat belt extension, quadriplegic harness. No clinical air pumps or Stoma masks. No specially designed WC. No aisle wheelchairs. Special meals available for dietary and medical requirements. No special telephone/fax numbers.

KLM
ETS Ltd, Amsterdam Way, Norwich, Norfolk NR6 6HA
Tel: (Reservations) (08705) 074074
Fax: (01603) 778111
www.klmuk.com
UK routes: No literature for disabled travellers. Medical form usually not required, although FREMEC form sometimes is needed when extreme circumstances apply. Normal check-in. Seats have moveable armrests, leg rests and seatbelt extensions, but no quadriplegic harnesses. Stoma masks not available, passengers should carry their own. No specially designed WC. No wheelchairs in cabin. Only dietary meals available. All agents trained to deal with special needs through usual booking numbers as above.

MANX AIRLINES
Isle of Man (Ronaldsway) Airport, Ballasalla, Isle of Man IM29 2JE
Tel: (Reservations) (01624) 824313 or (0345) 256256   Fax: (01624) 826031
UK routes: Isle of Man-Aberdeen, Birmingham, Cardiff, Edinburgh, Glasgow, Guernsey, Jersey, Leeds Bradford, Liverpool, London Heathrow, London Luton, London Stansted, Manchester, Southampton. Cardiff-Jersey No specific literature for disabled passengers, except safety Braille cards on aircraft. No medical form required unless

passenger had to get medical clearance for travel. All disabled passengers are pre-boarded. Check-in no later than 45 minutes prior to departure. Wheelchairs have to be within size and with totally disconnected battery, dry cell only. Specific seating in rows 1/2 or nearest to exit, but not at emergency exits. Seats have seat belt extensions and on some aircraft moveable arm rests. No clinical air masks or Stoma pumps. No adapted WCs on aircraft. No aisle wheelchairs on board for use in cabin. Special meals are available, that should be pre-booked when reserving seat: Tel: (01624) 826006 Fax: (01624) 826004.

RYANAIR
Dublin Airport, Co. Dublin, Eire
Tel: Reservations (0353) 1 6097800
Fax: (0353) 1 6097801
UK routes: London Stansted-Glasgow Prestwick.
No specific literature for disabled passengers. No medical form required. Full assistance to wheelchair-bound passengers travelling in their own wheelchairs. Advise when booking of any special needs. Check-in at least one hour prior to departure. No wheelchair transfer provided from check-in to aircraft. No restrictions regarding transport of personal electric chairs. Rows 2 and 3 on aircraft are prioritised for disabled passengers. Moveable arms rests and seat belt extensions available in these rows. No clinical air pumps or Stoma masks. No specially adapted WCs. No aisle wheelchairs for use in cabin. Airline does not offer meals. No special phone number for disabled passengers.

RAILWAYS
For all bookings, seat reservations, information about all stations, tel: (018457) 413775.

www.railtrack.co.uk/travel/
Timetables on-line.
Crossing London: London Transport operates a Stationlink bus service between Paddington, Marylebone, Euston, St. Pancras, Kings Cross, Liverpool Street,

Fenchurch Street, London Bridge, Waterloo and Victoria. The buses have adapted low floors and ramps. There are also Airbus services from Kings Cross, Victoria, Euston and Paddington stations to Heathrow Airport, serving all terminals, that are accessible.
For information contact:

TRAVELINE
Public Transport Information
Tel: (0870) 608 2608
www:traveline.org.uk

LONDON TRANSPORT UNIT FOR DISABLED PASSENGERS
172 Buckingham Palace Road,
London SW1 9TN
Tel: (020) 7 918 3312

TRAIN OPERATORS

ANGLIA RAILWAYS
Assistance: Tel: (01473) 693333

CENTRAL TRAINS
Assistance: Tel: (08457) 056027
www.centraltrains.co.uk

CHILTERN RAILWAYS
Mobility Impaired: Tel: (01296) 332113/4
www.chilternRailways.co.uk

CONNEX SOUTH CENTRAL/
CONNEX SOUTH EASTERN
Customer Services: Tel: (08706) 030405
Fax: (08706) 030505
Minicom: (01233) 617621

FIRST GREAT EASTERN RAILWAY
Special Needs: Tel: (08459) 505000

FIRST GREAT WESTERN TRAINS CO.
Special Needs: Tel: (0845) 7413775

GREAT NORTH EASTERN RAILWAY
Special Needs: Tel: (08457) 225444

FIRST NORTH WESTERN TRAINS
Special Needs: Tel: (0845) 6040231

HEATHROW EXPRESS
Disabled Assistance: Tel: (0845) 6001515

35

C2C Rail
Special Needs: Tel/Minicom: (01702) 357640

MERSEYRAIL
Special Needs: Tel: (08457) 125678

MIDLAND MAINLINE
Special Needs: Tel: (08457) 125678

ARRIVA TRAINS NORTHERN
Special Needs: (0845) 6008008

SILVERLINK
Special Needs:
County Customers: Tel: (0845) 601 4868
Metro Customers: Tel: (0845) 601 4867
Minicom: (08457) 125 988

SOUTHWEST TRAINS
Special Needs: Tel: (0845) 6050440

THAMES TRAINS
Special Needs: Tel: (0118) 9083607
www.thamestrains.co.uk

THAMESLINK
Special Needs: Tel: (020) 7 620 6333
Minicom: (020) 7 620 5561

VALLEY LINES
Special Needs: (02920) 449944

VIRGIN TRAINS
Special Needs: (0845) 7443366

WALES & BORDERS
Special Needs: Tel: (0845) 3003005
Minicom: (0845) 7585469

WEST ANGLIA GREAT NORTHERN (WAGN)
Special Needs: (0345) 226688
Minicom: (0345) 125988

ROAD
NATIONAL EXPRESS COACH
Tel: (08705) 80 80 80
www.gobycoach.com
Network of long-distance buses and coaches. Site includes timetable, fares and booking on-line. NE cannot carry battery-operated wheelchairs, only folding types in the boot. Normally require seven days' notice. Coaches have some features to help disabled passengers; kneeling facility, reserved seats closest to entrance, guide and hearing dogs carried free. Details of journey are logged with driver to ensure awareness of special needs. Staff at manned stations on hand to help.

FERRIES
All companies stress the importance of stating one's needs when booking, sea travel is less uniform than air travel. Tides etc, particularly on smaller vessels, can make a difference as to which deck boarding for passengers with mobility difficulties is assigned. Therefore certain facilities may not be available during all voyages. All companies seem to be disabled-aware and all stress that their crew will be more than happy to help. **Many companies also offer discounts for disabled passengers.**

CALEDONIAN MACBRAYNE
The Ferry Terminal, Gourock, Renfrewshire PA19 1QP
Tel: (Reservations) (0990) 650000
Fax: (01475) 635235
e-mail: reservations@calmac.co.uk
www.calmac.co.uk
UK routes: Firth of Clyde islands and peninsulas. Islay, Colonsay and Gigha. Mull and Inner Hebrides. Isles of Skye, Raasay and Small Isles. Outer Hebrides. No specific literature. No medical form required. Let car marshall know details of travel in advance. Lift from vehicle deck to passenger area that is on one level. Older ships have no accessible WC or restaurant. Each new ship is more accessible. Access from shore to vessel is via car deck.
The nature of the routes requires this service to be more than just a car ferry, cargo, coffins, etc also are carried.

CONDOR FERRIES LIMITED
Condor House, New Harbour Road South, Hamworthy, Poole, Dorset BH15 4AJ
Tel: (Reservations) (0845) 3452000

Fax: (01305) 760776
UK routes: Weymouth and Poole-Guernsey and Jersey.
No specific literature, but brochure gives detailed information on vessels. No medical form required. Advance notice required. Lift from vehicle deck to main passenger area. Accessible WC with alarm. Restaurants on some vessels are accessible but if not, there is at-seat service. Discounts available through the DDA.

ISLE OF MAN STEAM PACKET CO. Owned by Sea Containers
Tel: (Reservations) (01624) 661661
Fax: (01624) 645697
e-mail: res@steam-packet.com
www.steam-packet.com
UK routes: Liverpool-Isle of Man, Heysham-Isle of Man, Heysham-Belfast. No specific literature. No medical form required. Advance notice required. Lift from vehicle deck to main deck that is on one level. 1 adapted WC, 2 adapted cabins. Accessible restaurant. Movement from ship to shore and vice versa is accessible.

ISLES OF SCILLY STEAMSHIP CO.
Quay Street, Penzance, Cornwall TR18 4BD
Tel: (01736) 362009
UK route: Penzance-St. Mary's.
No specific literature. No medical form needed. No special procedures for boarding. No lift. Main passenger area on one level except buffet, but staff are helpful. 1 adapted WC, smaller than regulation size but accessible by some wheelchairs. No special access from shore to vessel or vice versa.

NORSE IRISH FERRIES
Victoria Terminal 2, West Bank Road, Belfast BT3 9JN
Tel: Reservations: (02890) 779090
Fax: (012890) 775520
www.Norse-Irish-Ferries.co.uk
Liverpool Office: North Brocklebank Dock, Bootle, Merseyside L20 1BY
Tel: (Reservations) (0151) 944 1010
Fax: (0151) 922 0344
UK route: Liverpool-Belfast.

No specific literature. No medical form required. Notice recommended. Lift from vehicle deck to main passenger area that is on one level. 1 accessible WC and restaurant. Disabled friendly access from shore to vessel.

ORKNEY FERRIES LTD
Shore Street, Kirkwall, Orkney, Scotland KW15 1LG
Tel: (Reservations) (01856) 872044
Fax: (01856) 872921
UK routes: Mainland (Kirkwall)-all 10 islands. No specific literature. No medical form required. Notify in advance. No special boarding procedures. Lifts on some vessels. Some vehicles decks have some facilities on that level. No special access to shore from vessel and vice versa.

P & O IRISH SEA LTD
Cairnryan, Nr. Stranraer, Wigtownshire, Scotland DG9 8RF
Tel: (Reservations)
(0870) 2424777/(028)2887 2195
Fax: (01581) 200282
UK route: Cairnryan-Larne (N. Ireland). No specific literature. No medical form required. May be boarded anytime during embarkation. Lifts from vehicle deck to main passenger area that is on one level. Accessible WCs and restaurant. Minibus available ship to shore.

P & O SCOTTISH FERRIES LTD
PO Box 5, Jamiesons Quay, Aberdeen AB11 5NP
Tel: (Reservations) (01224) 572615
Fax: (01224) 574411
UK routes: Aberdeen-Lerwick, Stromness and Scrabster-Stromness. No specific literature. No medical form required. Boarding depends on availability of lifts. Lifts connect vehicle deck and main passenger area that are on different levels. Accessible WC and restaurant. No minibus but short distance from quayside to vessel.

RED FUNNEL FERRIES
12 Bugle Street, Southampton SO14 2JY

Tel: (Reservations) (0870) 444 8898
Tel: (Special Needs) (0870) 444 8890
Fax: (0870) 444 8897
e-mail: sales@redfunnel.co.uk
www.redfunnel.co.uk
UK route: Southampton-Isle of Wight.
Specific literature available. No medical
form required. No special boarding
procedures, but inform terminal staff of
requirements. Lift sometimes available
from vehicle deck to main passenger area
that is on one level and accessible, except
for upper deck area. Accessible WCs and
restaurants/buffet. No special access from
shore to vessel and vice versa.

SEA CAT Owned by Sea Containers, see Isle
of Man Steam Packet Co.
General Booking Tel: (08705) 523523
UK Route: Isle of Man-Belfast.

SEA CAT SCOTLAND Owned by Sea
Containers, see Isle of Man Steam Packet Co.
General Booking Tel: (08705) 523523
UK routes: Stranraer and Troom-Belfast.

STENA LINE
Charter House, Park Street, Ashford,
Kent TN24 8EX
Tel: (Reservations) (08705) 707070
Fax: (01233) 202231
Minicom: (01233) 615678
www.stenaline.co.uk
UK routes: Stranraer-Belfast (HSS).
No specific literature. No medical form
required. Boarding depends on disability.
Lifts from vehicle deck to main passenger
area that is one level on new high-speed
vessels. Accessible WCs and restaurants.
Ramps from shore to vessel.

WIGHTLINK LTD
Wightlink House, 70 Broad Street,
Portsmouth, Hants PO1 2LB
Tel: (0870) 582 7744
Tel: (023) 9281 2011
Call in advance for assistance
Fax: (023) 9285 5257
www.wightlink.co.uk
UK routes: Portsmouth-Fishbourne.
Portsmouth Harbour-Ryde Pier Head.
Lymington-Yarmouth.
Information in general timetable. No

medical form necessary. No special
boarding procedures. Some vessels have
lifts from vehicle deck to main passenger
areas, some of which are on one level.
Accessible WC on board and in terminals.
Accessible restaurant. No special access
from shore to vessel or vice versa.
Passengers should contact road staff for
assistance on arrival. Disabled persons
travel card available with discounts for
travel, and is well worth applying for.

MAJOR UNITED KINGDOM ORGANISATIONS CONCERNED WITH DISABILITY

ARTHRITIS CARE
18 Stephenson Way, London NW1 2HD
Tel: (020) 7 3806500 Fax: (020) 7 916 1505
Free Helpline: (0808) 8004050 12-4pm
www.arthritiscare.org.uk
Advice and practical help for people with
arthritis.

ARTSLINE
54 Chalton Street, London NW1 1HS
Tel/Mincom: (020) 7 388 2227
Fax: (020) 7 3832653
e-mail: access@artsline.co.uk
London's major information and advice
centre for disabled people on arts and
entertainment. Produces excellent
comprehensive series of guidebooks on
theatres, cinemas, arts venues, museums
etc. Also produces guide to access at
Edinburgh cinemas. For access
information to all of these contact
Artsline.

ASSOCIATION FOR SPINA BIFIDA AND
HYDROCEPHALUS (ASBAH)
Asbah House, 42 Park Road,
Peterborough PE1 2UQ
Tel: (01733) 555988   Fax: (01733) 555985
e-mail: info@asbah.org
www.asbah.org

BRITISH COUNCIL OF DISABLED PEOPLE
(BCODP)
Litchurch Plaza, Litchurch Lane,
Derby DE24 8AA
Tel: (01332) 295551

Fax: (01332) 295580
Minicom: (01332) 295581
e-mail: general@bcodp.org.uk
www.bcodp.org.uk
National umbrella organisations for groups controlled by disabled people.

BRITISH POLIO FELLOWSHIP
Eagle Office Centre, The Runway, South Ruislip, Middlesex HA4 6SE
Tel: (020) 8 8421898
Fax: (020) 8 8420555
e-mail: british.polio@dial.pipex.com
Charity supporting people with polio, runs own holiday accommodation.

BRITISH RED CROSS SOCIETY
9 Grosvenor Crescent, London SW1X 7EJ
Tel: (020) 7 235 5454
Fax: (020) 7 235 3501
www.redcross.org.uk

CYSTIC FIBROSIS TRUST
11 London Road, Bromley, Kent BR1 1BY
Tel: (020) 8 464 7211
Fax: (020) 8 313 0472
www.cftrust.org.uk

DEPARTMENT OF TRANSPORT MOBILITY UNIT
1/11 Gt. Minster House, 76 Marsham Street, London SW1P 4DR Tel: (020) 7 893 3000
Deals with implementation of transport provisions of the DDA plus access to pedestrian environment.

DIAL UK
St. Catherine's Hospital, Tickhill Road, Balby, Doncaster, South Yorks DN4 8QN
Tel/Minicom: (01302) 310123
Fax: (01302) 310404
e-mail: dialuk@aol.com
www.dial.org.uk
Supports many local disability information and advises services.

DISABILITY RIGHTS COMMISSION HELPLINE
Tel: (08457) 622633
Minicom: (08457) 622644
e-mail: drc-gb.org
www.drc-gb.org

DISABILITY INFORMATION TRUST
Mary Marlborough Lodge, Nuffield Orthopaedic Centre, Headington, Oxford OX3 7LD
Tel: (01865) 227600
Assessment and testing of disability equipment and publishing of in-depth information.

DISABLED DRIVERS ASSOCIATION
Ashwellthorpe, Norwich, Norfolk NR16 1EX
Tel: (01508) 489449   Fax: (01508) 488173
e-mail: DDAHQ@aol.com
www.dda.org.uk
Fights to improve mobility and access for disabled people. Publishes excellent Magic Carpet magazine.

DISABLED DRIVERS MOTOR CLUB
Cottingham Way, Thrapston, Northants NN14 4PL
Tel: (01832) 734724   Fax: (01832) 733816
e-mail: ddmc@ukonline.co.uk
Helps and encourages disabled people to gain mobility.

DISABLED LIVING FOUNDATION
380-384 Harrow Road, London W9 2HU
Tel: (020) 7 289 6111   Fax: (020) 7 266 2922
Minicom: (020) 7 432 8009
e-mail: dlf@dlf.org.uk
www.dlf.org.uk
Aims to make everyday life easier for people with disabilities.

DISS
Harrowlands, Harrowlands Park, Dorking, Surrey RH4 2RA
Tel: (01306) 875156   Fax: (01306) 741740
Minicom: (01306) 742128
e-mail: diss@diss.org.uk
Disability information service that has developaed the data base, DissBASE, an invaluable source of information.

ENGLISH HERITAGE
Customer Services, PO Box 570, Swindon, Wilts SN2 2UR
Tel: (0870) 3331181   Fax: (01793) 414926
www.english-heritage.org.uk
Produces a comprehensive *Guide for Visitors with Disabilities* to all its properties.

HOLIDAY CARE
2nd Floor, Imperial Buildings, Victoria Road,
Horley, Surrey RH6 7PZ
Tel: (01293) 774535   Fax: (01293) 784647
Minicom: (01293) 776943
Reservations: (01293) 773716
e-mail: holiday.care@virgin.net
www.holidaycare.org.uk
Central source of holiday and travel
information for disabled people and
carers. Offers details on accessible
accommodation, attractions and transport
and help with reservations.

HOTELIERS FORUM
(Part of Disability Partnership Initiative)
Nutmeg House, 60 Gainsford Street,
London SE1 2NY
Tel: (020) 7 403 9433
Fax: (020) 7 403 3957
e-mail: hoteliers@disabilitypartnership.co.uk
www.disabilitypartnership.co.uk
Aims to make the hospitality sector a
leader in disability equality in the fields of
service provision and employment.

LONDON TRANSPORT UNIT FOR DISABLED PASSENGERS
172 Buckingham Palace Road,
London SW1W 9TN
Tel/Minicom: (020) 7 918 3312
Fax: (020) 7 918 3876
e-mail: lt.udp@ltbuses.co.uk
www.londontransport.co.uk
Dedicated to securing better access to
London's public transport system and
providing information to mobility
impaired passengers.

MOTABILITY
Goodman House, Station Approach, Harlow,
Essex CM20 2ET
Tel: (01279) 635666   Fax: (01279) 632035
www.motability.co.uk

NATIONAL MULTIPLE SCLEROSIS SOCIETY
372 Edgeware Road, Staples Corner,
London NW2 6ND
Tel: (020) 8438 0700
e-mail: info@mssociety.org.uk
www.mssociety.org.uk
Provides information and support for
people affected by MS.

MULTIPLE SCLEROSIS SOCIETY IN SCOTLAND
The Rural Centre, West Mains, Ingleston,
Newbridge, Edinburgh EH28 8NZ
Tel: (0131) 472 4106   Fax: (0131) 472 4099
45 branches throughout Scotland aiming
to provide and promote welfare of people
with MS and their families.

MUSCULAR DYSTROPHY GROUP
7-11 Prescott Place, London SW4 6BS
Tel: (020) 7 720 8055   Fax: (020) 7 498 0670
e-mail: info@muscular-dystrophy.org
www.muscular-dystrophy.org

NATIONAL CENTRE FOR INDEPENDENT LIVING
250 Kennington Lane, London SE11 5RD
Tel: (020) 7 587 1663
Fax: (020) 7 582 2469
Minicom: (020) 7 587 1177
e-mail: ncil@ncil.org.uk
www.ncil.org.uk

NATIONAL INFORMATION FORUM
PP 10/101 BT Burne House, Bell Street,
London NW1 5BZ
Tel: (020) 7 402 6681
Fax: (020) 7 402 1259
e-mail: niforum@talk21.com
www.nif.org.uk
Works for improved provision of disability
information.

NATIONAL TRUST DISABILITY UNIT
36 Queen Anne's Gate, London SW1H 9AS
Tel: (020) 7 222 9251
Fax: (020) 7 222 5097
e-mail: accessforall@nttrust.org.uk
www.nationaltrust.org.uk
Welcomes and provides for disabled
visitors at a majority of its properties.
Produces an excellent access guide.

QUEEN ELIZABETH'S FOUNDATION FOR DISABLED PEOPLE
Leatherhead Court, Woodlands Road,
Leatherhead, Surrey KT22 0BN
Tel: (01372) 841100   Fax: (01372) 844657
e-mail: webmaster@gedf.org
www.qefd.org
National charity serving over 100,000
disabled people annually.

PHAB
Summit House, Wandle Road, Croydon,
Surrey CR0 1DF
Tel: (020) 8 667 9443   Fax: (020) 8 681 1399
e-mail: info@phabengland.co.uk
www.phabengland.org.uk
Works for the integration of people with
and without physical disabilities within the
community through social clubs and
activities and through holidays and courses.

ROYAL ASSOCIATION FOR DISABILITY AND
REHABILITATION (RADAR)
12 City Forum, 250 City Road,
London EC1V 8AF
Tel: (020) 7 250 3222
Fax: (020) 7 250 0212
Minicom: (020) 7 250 4119
e-mail: radar@radar.org.uk
www.radar.org.uk
National charity working for disabled
people. Produces many publications
relating to civil rights, mobility,
employment and travel, with excellent UK
and worldwide holiday guides and holiday
fact packs.

SCOPE
6 Market Road, London N7 9PW
Tel: (020) 7619 7296   Fax: (020) 7619 7380
www.scope.org.uk
For people with cerebal palsy, scope
offers a wide range of projects and
professional help.

SPINAL INJURIES ASSOCIATION
76 St. James Lane, London N10 3DF
Tel: (020) 8 444 2121
Fax: (020) 8 444 3761
Freephone Helpline: (0800) 980 0501
e-mail: sia@spinali.co.uk
www.spinal.co.uk
This National Charity exists because life
does not stop when you become
paralysed. Offers advice on all aspects of
disability. Comprehensive web site with
items such as lists of disabled living
centres.

TRIPSCOPE
The Vassall Centre, Gill Avenue
Bristol BS16 2QQ
Tel: as London

e-mail: tripscopesw@cableinet.co.uk
Provides a nationwide travel and
transport information service for disabled
and elderly people.

TOURISM FOR ALL
3 Broomfield Hall, Enmore,
Somerset, TA5 2DZ
Tel: (01278) 671863
e-mail: jenny@tourismforall.org.uk
www.tourismforall.org.uk
Works to create and support mainstream
tourism, hospitality and leisure industries
that are accessible to all customers and
staff, irrespective of disability, age or
income. It is a UK-wide umbrella
organisation which provides a national
focus and co-ordinating role.
It is a consortium of members who
include commercial operators, voluntary
organisations, local and central
government bodies, tourism industry and
individual members,

SPECIALIST TOUR/HOLIDAY ORGANISATIONS

ACCESS TRAVEL (LANCS) LTD
6 The Hillock, Astley, Lancs M29 7GW
Tel: (01942) 888844   Fax: (01942) 891811
e-mail: des@access-travel.co.uk
www.access-travel.co
Arranges an extensive variety of holidays
to many destinations for disabled people.

A.T.S. Travel Ltd
1 Tank Lane, Purfleet, Essex RM19 1TA
Tel: (01708) 863198
Fax: (01708) 860514
e-mail: aatstravel@aol.com
www.assistedholidays.com
Specialist agency arranging tailor-made
holidays throughout UK, Europe and
worldwide.

Bendriff Trust, Bendrigg Lodge, Old Hutton,
Kendal, Cumbria, LA8 0NR
Tel: (01539) 723766
Fax: (01539) 722446
e-mail:bendriff@msn.com
Two countryside properties in the Lake
District and Yorkshire Dales. Activities
include archery, camping, orienteering,

adventure course, zip-wire and tube slide, caving, canoeing, sailing.

CAMPING FOR THE DISABLED
c/o National Mobility Centre,
Unit 2, Atcham Estate, Shrewsbury,
Shropshire SY4 4YG
Tel: (01743) 463072
e-mail: mis@nmcuk.freeserve.co.uk
Publish a list of adapted campsites.

CAN BE DONE LIMITED
11 Woodcock Hill, Harrow, Middlesex,
HA3 OXP
Tel: (0208) 907 2400   Fax: (0208) 9091854
e-mail: holidays@canbedone.co.uk
www.canbedone.co.uk
Individually tailored holidays and tours designed to be accessible for wheelchair users and for touring at a leisurely pace.

CHALFONT LINE HOLIDAYS
4 Providence Road, West Drayton,
Middlesex UB7 8HJ
Tel: (01895) 459540   Fax: (01895) 459549
e-mail: holidays@chalfont-line.co.uk
www.chalfont-line.co.uk
Escorted holidays for disabled people in UK and abroad. Specially adapted coach with side lift, clamped wheelchair spaces.

Churchtown Outdoor Adventure Centre
Lanlivery, Bodmin, Cornwall,PL30 5BT
Tel: (01208) 872148   Fax: (01208) 873377
e-mail: churchtown@saqnet.co.uk
Converted farmstead with accessible accommodation for groups, families and individuals of all abilities. Respite care, specialist equipment and care support is available.

LEONARD CHESHIRE FOUNDATION
30 Millbank, London SW1P 4QD
Tel: (020) 7 802 8200
Fax: (020) 7 802 8250
e-mail: info@london-cheshire.org.uk
www.leonard-cheshire.org
Runs holiday properties for disabled persons.
There are 10 regional offices.

DISABLED LIVING
Redbank House, 4 St. Chad's Street,

Cheetham, Manchester M8 8QA
Tel: (0161) 214 5959 Fax: (0161) 835 3591
e-mail: information@disabledliving.co.uk
Group holiday provision for disabled people of all ages in both UK and abroad.

GROOMS HOLIDAYS
For Self-Catering and Boating Holidays
PO Box 36, Cowbridge,
Vale of Glamorgan CF71 7GB
Tel: (01446) 771311   Fax: (01446) 775060
e-mail: gmo@cwcom.net
www.johngrooms.org.uk/holidays

DISABLED HOLIDAY DIRECTORY
6 Seaview Crescent, Goodwick,
Pembrokeshire, SA64 OAZ
Tel: (01348) 875 592
e-mail: sian@disabledholidaydirectory.co.uk
www.disabledholidaydirectory.co.uk
Independently run small company which produces a directory specialising in all types of accommodation with disabled access. Worldwide listings.

CAR HIRE – LYNX HAND CONTROLS
Mansion House, St. Helens Road, Ormskirk,
Lancs. L39 4QJ
Tel: (01695) 573816   Fax: (01695) 581500
e-mail: info@lynxcontrols.com
www.lynxcontrols.com
Produces hand control equipment that can be fitted to a hire car. Suitable only for someone with a lower limb disability. Also supplies push-pull systems if the need arises. Lynx works with most of the major car hire companies as well as many smaller firms covering all the UK.

SPECIAL FAMILIES HOME SWAP REGISTER
Erme House, Station Road, Plympton,
Devon PL7 2AU
Tel: (01752) 347577   Fax: (01752) 344611
e-mail: med_serv@globalnet.co.uk
www.mywebpage.net/special-families/index
Subscription based allowing swapping of specially adapted homes UK wide. Short breaks, full length holidays and visits.

SPEYSIDE TRUST
Badaguish Centre, Aviemore, PH22 1QU
Tel: (01479) 861285   Fax: (01479) 861258
e-mail: badaguish@cali.co.uk
Respite care activity holiday and courses for unaccompanied individuals or small

groups with learning/physical or multiple disabilities. 24 hour care/assistance provided. Forest setting with extensive camping, games and adventure play facilities. Bunkhouse or campsite accommodation.

THE STACKPOLE CENTRE
Home Farm, Pembroke, SA71 5DQ
Tel: (01646) 661425
Fax: (01646) 661456
Facilities include indoor pool and activities include canoeing, abseiling, horse riding, fishing. Self-catering cottage or group house accommodation and b&b full board.

WHEELCHAIR TRAVEL LTD
1 Johnston Green, Guildford, Surrey GU2 6XS
Tel: (01483) 233 640   Fax: (01483) 237 772
e-mail: info@wheelchair-travel.co.uk
www.wheelchair-travel.co.uk
Comprehensive private transport service for wheelchair users including self-drive rental accessible minibuses, Fiat Fiorino cars and hand-controlled cars, accessible luxury taxis, tour/airport transfers.

WINGED FELLOWSHIP TRUST
Angel House, 20-32 Pentonville Road
London N1 9XD
Tel: (020) 7 833 2594   Fax: (020) 7 278 0370
e-mail: admin@wft.org.uk
www.wft.org.uk
Operates five fully accessible holiday centres at Netley (Hants), Chigwell (Essex), Nottingham and Southport (Merseyside). See under separate counties.

SPECIALIST SPORTS/ OUTDOOR ASSOCIATIONS

BRITISH DISABLED FLYING CLUB
Pantiles, The Street, Tendering,
Essex CO16 0BL
Tel/Fax: (01255) 830198
e-mail: deltaftrot@aol.com
http://fly.to/bdfc

BRITISH DISABLED WATER SKI ASSOCIATION
The Tony Edge National Centre,
Heron Lake, Hythend, Wraysbury,
Middlesex TW19 6HW
Tel: (01784) 483664   Fax: (01784) 482747
e-mail: info@bdwsa.org.uk
www.bdwsa.org.uk
Centres throughout the UK, open between April and October. The aim is to introduce newcomers to the sport who, because of their disabilities, would not have considered this challenge possible. Accessible changing facilities and WCs, wetsuits and lifejackets included.

BRITISH MOTORSPORTS ASSOCIATION FOR THE DISABLED
Bullsland Farm, Bullsland Lane,
Chorleywood, Hertfordshire, WD3 5BG
Tel: (01923) 285554
Fax:(01923) 285553
e-mail: david@justwebs.co.uk
www.justmobility.co.uk/bmsad

BRITISH SKI CLUB FOR THE DISABLED
Springmount, Berwick St. John, Shaftesbury, Dorset SP7 0HO
Tel: (01747) 828515

BRITISH WHEELCHAIR ATHLETICS ASSOCIATION
Tel: (01937) 572668
2a Westoff Lane, South Hiendley, Barnsley, Yorkshire, S72 9DE
The Association is committed to develop new athletes who have to use a wheelchair for mobility reasons, with a physical ability.

BRITISH WHEELCHAIR SPORTS FOUNDATION
Guttman Road, Stoke Mandeville, Bucks HP21 9PP
Tel: (01296) 3995995
Fax: (01296) 424171
email: enquiries@britishwheelchairsports.org
www.britishwheelchairsports.org
National organisation for wheelchair sport in the UK. Based at the national wheelchair sports centre at Stoke Mandeville, the Foundation exists to provide, promote and develop opportunities for men, women and children with disabilities to participate in recreational competitive wheelchair sport.

DISABILITY SPORTS ENGLAND
Solecast House,
13-27 Brunswick Place, London N1 6DX
Tel: (020) 7 490 4919
Fax: (020) 7 490 49146532

GREAT BRITAIN WHEELCHAIR RUGBY
ASSOCIATION
Contact: Ross Morrison, 1 Sunbury Court,
Fareham, Hants, PO15 6HB
Tel: (01329) 513506
www.gbwra.org.uk

HANDICAPPED ANGLERS TRUST
Angling Link, 9 Yew Tree Road, Delves,
Walsall, West Midlands, WS5 4NQ
Tel/Fax: (01922) 860912
e-mail: terry@anglinglink.co.uk

HANDICAPPED SCUBA ASSOCIATION
United Kingdom, Ireland & Switzerland,
Lwyn Onn, Pentrefoelas,
Betws-Y-Coed,Conwy, Wales LL24 OTW
Tel: (0800) 026 5071
info@hsa-international.co.uk

JUBILEE SAILING TRUST
Jubilee Yard, Hazel Road, Woolstone,
Southampton, Hants S019 7GB
Tel: (01703) 449108   Fax: (01703) 449145
e-mail: info@jst.org.uk
www.jst.org.uk
This is a UK based organisation which
aims to promote the integration of able-
bodied and physically disabled people
through adventure tall ship sailing
holidays.

NATIONAL ASSOCIATION OF SWIMMING
CLUBS FOR THE HANDICAPPED
The Willows, Mayles Lane, Wickham,
Hants PO17 5ND
Tel: (01329) 833689

NATIONAL HANDICAPPED SKIERS
ASSOCIATION
e-mail: rhona@lineone.net
www.complete-skier.com/skier/bssf.html

NATIONAL WHEELCHAIR TENNIS
ASSOCIATION
c/o Secretary, BWTTA, 3 Brentford,
Wellingborough, Northants NN8 3TE

www.britishwheelchairsports.org/associate/
tatennis.htm

RIDING FOR THE DISABLED ASSOCIATION
Avenue R, National Agricultural Centre,
Kenilworth, Warwicks CV8 2LY
Tel: (0247) 669 6510
Fax: (0247) 669 6532
e-mail: rdahq@riding-for-disabled.org.uk
www.riding-for-disabled.org.uk
Aims to provide riding and driving
opportunities to disabled people.

RYA SAILABILITY
The Stables, Blind Burn Hall, Wark, Hexham,
Northumberland NE48 3HE
Tel: (01434) 230464 or
Romsey Road, Eastleigh, Hants SO50 9YA
Tel: (01703) 627400   Fax: (01703) 620545
www.rya.org.uk/sailability
In Hexham, RYA owns Sea Legs, a
catamaran adapted for disabled people.
Available for charter with qualified
skippers available on request. Sailability
also offers other water-based holidays.

UPHILL SKI CLUB
Head Office: 6a Emerson Close, Saffrom
Walden, Essex CB10 1HL
Tel: (01799) 525 406
e-mail:info@uphillskiclub.co.uk
Registered charity, committed to
providing winter sports activities for
disabled people.

44

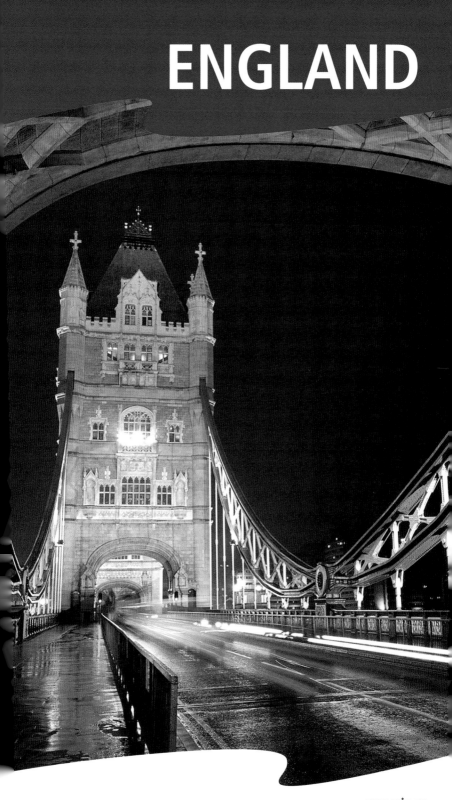

ENGLAND

*Tower Bridge. Still one of the most
impressive buildings on the London skyline.*

gowrings
mobility

MAJOR TOURIST BOARDS

BRITISH TOURIST AUTHORITY AND ENGLISH TOURISM COUNCIL
Thames Tower, Black's Road, London W6 9EL
Tel (020) 8563 3000
Fax: (020) 8563 0302
www: www.visitbritain.com
www: britannia.com/
www.englishtourism.org.uk

BTA/ETB also run immediate response query line called SCOOT. Tel: (0800) 192 192.

CUMBRIA TOURIST BOARD
(County of Cumbria, including Lake District)
Ashleigh, Holly Road, Windermere,
Cumbria LA23 2AQ
Tel: (01539) 444444
Fax: (01539) 444 041
e-mail: mail@cumbria tourist board.co.uk
www.golakes.co.uk

EAST OF ENGLAND TOURIST BOARD
(Counties of Beds., Cambs., Essex, Herts.,
Norfolk and Suffolk)
Toppesfield Hall, Hadleigh, Suffolk IP7 5DN
Tel: (01473) 822922
Fax: (01473) 823063
e-mail:
englandtouristboard@compuserve.com
www.visitbritain.com/east-of-england

EAST MIDLANDS TOURIST BOARD
(Counties of Derby, Leics., Lincs.,
Northants and Notts.)
Exchequergate, Lincoln LN2 1PZ
Tel: (01522) 531 521   Fax: (01522) 532 501

HEART OF ENGLAND TOURIST BOARD
(Counties of Cherwell, Glos., Hereford and
Worcs./Salop, Staffs., War., West Midlands
and West Oxon.)
Woodside, Larkhill Road, Worcester WR5 2EF
Tel: (01905) 763436   Fax: (01905) 763450
www.visitbritain.com

LONDON TOURIST BOARD
(Greater London area)
26 Grosvenor Gardens, London SW1W 0DU
Tel: (020) 7932 2000
Fax: (020) 7932 0222
www.londontown.com

NORTH WEST TOURIST BOARD
(Counties of Cheshire, Gtr. Manchester,
Lancs., Merseyside and High Peak District of
Derbys.)
Swan House, Swan Meadow Road, Wigan
Pier, Wigan, Lancs. WN3 5BB
Tel: (01942) 821222
Fax: (01942) 820002
e-mail: info@nwtb.u-net.com
www.visitbritain.com/north-west-england

NORTHUMBRIA TOURIST BOARD
(Counties of Cleveland, Durham,
Northumberland and Tyne & Wear)
Aykley Heads, Durham DH1 5UX
Tel: (0191) 821222
Fax: (0191) 3860899
www.ntb.org.uk

SOUTH EAST ENGLAND TOURIST BOARD
(Counties of east Sussex, Kent,
Surrey and west Sussex).
The Old Brew House, Warwick Park,
Tunbridge Wells, Kent TN2 5TU
Tel: (01892) 540766
Fax: (01892) 511008
e-mail: enquiries@seetb.org.uk
www.seetb.org.uk

SOUTHERN TOURIST BOARD
(Counties of Berks., Bucks., east and north
Dorset, Hants.. Oxon. and Isle of Wight)
40 Chamberlayne Road, Eastleigh,
Hants SO50 5JH
Tel: (01703) 620006
Fax: (01703) 620010
www.visitbritain.com

WEST COUNTRY TOURIST BOARD
(Counties of Cornwall, Devon, west Dorset,
Somerset, Wilts. and Isles of Scilly)
60 St. Davids Hill, Exeter, Devon EX4 4SY
Tel:(0870) 442 0880   Fax: (0870) 0881
www.westwestcountynow.com
e-mail:info@westcountyholidays.com

YORKSHIRE TOURIST BOARD
(Counties of north, south and west Yorks.,
and Humberside)
312 Tadcaster Road, York YO2 2HF
Tel: (01904) 707961   Fax: (01904) 701404
e-mail:info@YTB.org.uk
www.ytb.org.uk

BEDFORDSHIRE

BEDFORD

County town with modern shopping centre and open market twice a week. Entertainment in Corn Exchange, whilst more leisurely pursuits include viewing the embankment gardens and the many historical buildings.

TOURIST INFORMATION CENTRE

10 St. Paul's Square, Bedford MK40 1SL
Tel: (01234) 215226

DISABILITY INFORMATION SERVICE (ABOVE SHOPMOBILITY)

First Floor, 1 The Howard Centre, Horne Lane, Bedford MK40 1HU
Tel/Fax: (01234) 349988
Mincom: (01582) 470968
e-mail: disbeds@cwcom.net
Provides wide range of information for disabled people and those who support them.

Bedford CC publish booklet Community Transport Handbook with much relevant information, available from TIC or BCC (Transport) Tel: (01234) 228399/228337

TRAVELLINE

Tel: (0870) 6082608

Arriva – The Shires, Marchwood House, 934-974 St. Albans Road, Garston, Watford, Herts WD2 6NN
Tel: (01923) 673121

BEDFORD SHOPMOBILITY

1 The Howard Centre, Horne Lane, Bedford MK40 1UH
Tel: (01234) 348000

TRAINS

Midland Main Line:
Special Needs: Tel: (0114) 2537654
Minicom: (0845) 7078051

Silverlink,
Customer Relations
Station Road, Cambridge, CB1 2JW
Special Needs:
County Customers: (0845) 601 4868
Metro Customers: (0845) 601 4867
Minicom: (08457) 125 988
www.silverlink-trains.com
Thameslink:
Special Needs: Tel: (0207) 6206333
Minicom: (0207) 6205561
Stationlink bus: Tel: (0207) 9183312

TAXIS:

Ampthill Taxis: Tel: (01525) 841841
A - K Cars: Tel: (01234) 215030
AGS Taxis: Tel: (012134) 771960

BRITISH RED CROSS

Bedfordshire Branch,
Emerald Court Pilgrim Centre
Brickhill Drive, Bedford MK41 7P
Tel: (01234) 349166

ATTRACTIONS

BEDFORD MUSEUM
Castle Lane, Bedford MK40 3XD
Tel: (01234) 353323
Fax: (01234) 273401
www.bedfordmuseum.org
Housed in former brewery, the museum is within the grounds of Bedford Castle, beside the Great Ouse river embankment. Wide range of exhibits and collections tell human and natural history of north Bedfordshire, together with delightful rural room sets and Old School Museum. Located close to 2 town centre car parks.

SD ♿ CP n/a E ♿ RF ♿
L ♿ S ♿ WC 🚹

JOHN BUNYAN MUSEUM and LIBRARY
Mill Street, Bedford MK40 3EU
Tel/Fax: (01234) 213722
Contains most of known possessions of John Bunyan and many editions of his 60 recognised works including "The Pilgrim's Progress" in 168 foreign languages.

SD ♿ CP ♿ E ♿ RF ♿ L ♿
C ♿ S 🚹 RFE 🚹 WC n/a

BROMHAM MILL
Bridge Road, Bromham,
Bedford MK43 8LP
Tel: (01234) 824330
By the river Great Ouse, this C17th restored water mill offers flour milling demonstrations, and has an art gallery with exhibition programmes and craft displays. Upstairs gallery not accessible.

SD ♿ CP ♿ E ♿ via fire door.
RF ♿ C ♿ S ♿ WC 🚹

RIVERSIDE WALK
2 miles easy going, all hard paths suitable for wheelchairs. Starting from the north west bank at Town Bridge, the walk follows a route to the edge of town marked by County Bridge and returns along the Embankment Gardens. Follow the path from the Bridge (Charter Walk) past red brick Shire Hall designed by eminent Victorian architect Alfred Waterhouse, alongside being the market place. This path (Queen's Walk) takes you past the Star Club and walking towards County Bridge you pass the moorings at Queens Reach, before the path takes you up to the bridge past the river-front development of Sovereign Quay.

BIGGLESWADE
Known as a busy market-gardening area with many historical pubs from its days as a flourishing coach stop.

ATTRACTION
SWISS GARDEN
Biggleswade Road, Old Warden, Biggleswade
Tel: (01761) 627666
Go back to early C19th when interests in ornamental gardening and picturesque architecture were first combined. Within 10 acres wander among splendid shrubs and rare trees at the centre of which is the tiny romantic Swiss Cottage, although there are other exotic structures. There is also a fernery and grotto. A wheelchair route around the garden is available, together with loan of wheelchairs.

SD ♿ CP 🚹 E ♿
C 🚹 WC ♿ RFE ♿

DUNSTABLE
The town was built at the junction of Watling Street and the prehistoric Icknield Way with the wonderful, Windy Downs offering amazing views.

ATTRACTION
WHIPSNADE WILD ANIMAL PARK
Dunstable LU6 2LF
Tel: (01582) 872171
Fax: (01582) 872649
www.whipsnade.co.uk
One of Europe's largest conservation centres with over 2,500 animals set in 600 acres of beautiful parkland. Many of the animals are endangered species. See the park by car and explore wherever you wish to stop, or on foot. Wheelchairs available.

SD ♿ CP ♿ E ♿ RF ♿
C 🚹 S 🚹 WC ♿ RFE ♿

LEIGHTON BUZZARD
Large, pleasant market town with many buildings of interest.

ATTRACTIONS
LEIGHTON BUZZARD RAILWAY
Page's Park Station, Billington Road, Leighton Buzzard LU7 8TN
Tel: (01525) 373888
Fax: (01525) 377814
info@buzzrail.co.uk
www.buzzrail.co.uk
5.5-mile train ride through mix of housing, industry and open countryside, following original authentic route created in 1919. Trip lasts for one hour.
One carriage capable of carrying up to four wheelchairs, operating on 11.15, 12.45, 14.15 and 15.45 departure trains.

SD ♿ CP 🚹 E 🚹 RF 🚹
C ♿ S ♿ WC 🚹 RFE ♿

MEAD OPEN FARM
Stanbridge Road, Billington, Nr. Leighton Buzzard LU7 9HL
Tel: (01525) 852954
info@meadopenfarm.co.uk
www.meadopenfarm.co.uk
Working family farm with wide range of traditional animals and rare breeds. Pet's corner with lots of hands-on activities. Falconry displays, tractor trailer rides and children's play area. Surface in yard area is flat concrete with slight slope. Paddocks are flat with grass surface – accessible in dry weather – no steps at any point.

SD 🦽　CP 🦽　E 🦽　RF 🦽　WC 🦽
C 🦽　S 🦽

LUTON
Largest town in the county with delightful parks.

HOTEL
THISTLE LUTON　
Arndale Centre, Luton LU1 2TR
Tel: (0870) 333 9138
Fax: (0870) 49238
e-mail: luton@thistle.co.uk
www.thistlehotels.com/luton
No. of Accessible Rooms: 1
Accessible Facilities: Lounge, Restaurant (1st floor, via accessible lift). Large, modern property located in central Luton, next door to the Arndale Shopping Centre.

LUTON MUSEUM and ART GALLERY
Wardown Park, Luton LU2 7MA
Tel: (01582) 546722　Fax: (01582) 546763
e-mail: burgessl@luton.gov.uk
Victorian mansion in Wardown park with exhibits on natural and cultural history of the area, including development of hat industry in C19th and C20th. NB: Entrance via door to left of front entrance. Wheelchairs available.

SD 🦽　CP 🦽　E 🦽　RF 🦽
C 🦽　S 🦽　WC 🚹

STOCKWOOD CRAFT MUSEUM and GARDENS
Stockwood Country Park, Farley Hill, Luton LU1 4BH
Tel: (01582) 738714

Exterior exhibits include sculpture, period and winter gardens, plus interior exhibition galleries. Wheelchairs available.

P 🦽　E 🚹　C 🦽　S 🚹
WC 🦽　RFE 🦽　WC 🚹　craft museum

WOODSIDE WILDFOWL PARK
Mancroft Road, Slip End Village, Luton LU1 4DG
Tel: (01582) 841044
A vast farm shop, poultry centre, children's farm and leisure complex with daily handling, feeding and learning about poultry. Wheelchairs available.

SD 🦽　CP 🚹　E 🦽　RF 🦽
C 🚹　S 🦽　WC 🚹

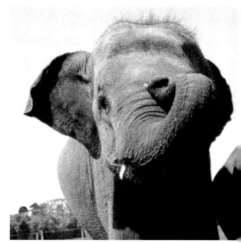

Full access for all at Whipsnade Wild Animal Park.

SANDY
Small, but growing town in pleasant countryside. Home of the Royal Society for the Preservation of Birds.

ATTRACTION
RSPB, THE LODGE NATURE RESERVE and VISITOR CENTRE.
The Lodge, Sandy SG19 2DL
Tel: (01767) 680551　Fax: (01767) 683508
e-mail: thelodge@rspb.org.uk
UK headquarters of the RSPB with heathland, woodland and meadow, lakes and formal gardens. Several exotic trees

including the Atlas Cedar. Useful map of areas of access available. Main car park is next to shop and reception centre and is surfaced with rolled stone. Secondary parking for special needs visitors is 45 m from the lake hide. The reception centre and shop are accessed from main car park by concrete path and 8m 1:16 ramp. The reception centre and shop are on ground level. As they are housed in a listed building the internal layout is cramped in places but staff are available to help with purchases. There is one adapted toilet accessed via a ramp.

There are a number of paths of varying lengths and surfaces throughout the reserve; terrain is steeply undulating in places. Lake hide is 500 m from main car park, special needs visitors may drive to parking bays 12 m from hide; eight adapted places giving views over the lake and birdfeeders. One wheelchair is available for free loan.

SD ♿ CP ♿ RF ♿ S ♿
WC ♿ RFE ♿

WOBURN
Old village situated in picturesque wooded countryside.

HOTEL
THE INN AT WOBURN
George Street, Woburn MK17 9PX
Tel: (01525) 290441   Fax: (01525) 290432
No. of Accessible Rooms: 7 new cottages on ground floor. 18 ground floor rooms two of which have rooms especially for disabled guests, one with roll-in shower. Whole hotel is wheelchair friendly. Accessible Facilities: Lounge, Dining room. Originally an inn, now completely modernised, located in town centre.

ATTRACTION
WOBURN SAFARI PARK
Woburn Park, Woburn MK17 9QN
Tel: (01525) 290407   Fax: (01525) 290489
350 acres of Safari Park with varied animal species collection and extensive leisure park. Parking is provided for disabled

badge holders in the main Leisure Area car park. A map of wheelchair routes is available when you purchase your ticket. A limited number of wheelchairs are available from the 'Junglies' gift shop. Alternatively you can pre-book by phoning the shop direct on (01525) 290826. Contact number at top to find out about special rates for disabled groups.

SD ♿   CP ♿   RF ♿
C ♿   S ♿   WC ♿

BERKSHIRE

WEST BERKSHIRE TOURISM
The Wharf, Newbury, Berkshire, RG14 5AS
Tel: (01635) 30267
Fax: (01635) 519562
e-mail: tourism@westberks.gov.uk.co
www.westberks.gov.uk

ASCOT
Famous for its racecourse, started by Queen Anne in 1711. The Ascot Gold Cup was first presented in 1807. Few of the original buildings remain.

SPORTING VENUE
ASCOT RACECOURSE
Ascot, Berks. SL5 7JN
Admin: (01344) 878505
Booking-Box Office: (01344) 876876
Fax: (0870) 4601238
e-mail: enquiries@ascot.co.uk
www.ascot.co.uk
NB. June meeting pre-booked, ticket only. No pre-booking for other meetings.
CP ♿   RTE ♿   ED ♿
INT ♿ (assistance available)   L ♿
WC ♿ (except no hinged support rail). Located in Royal Enclosure, Grandstand and Silver Ring.
SS ♿ open – platform designated.
Route to Grandstand is tarmac, slight gradient to grandstand, out onto lawned area
and platform.   B/R ♿

BRACKNELL
Berkshire's only new town.

TOURIST INFORMATION CENTRE
The Look Out Discovery Park, Nine Mile Ride,
Bracknell RG12 7QW
Tel: (01344) 869896   Fax: (01344) 869343
The Look Out Discovery Park is set in 2,600
acres of Crown Estate woodland. It is
situated opposite the Coral Reef Complex.

HOTEL
COPPID BEECH HOTEL
John Nike Way, Binfield,
Nr. Bracknell RG12 8TF
Tel: (01344) 303333 Fax: (01344) 301200
No. of Accessible Rooms: 16. Shower
Accessible Facilities: Lounge, Restaurant,
Leisure Club with Pool, Sauna, Spa Alpine-
style hotel with extensive leisure facilities.

LEISURE FACILITY
CORAL REEF, BRACKNELL'S WATER WORLD
Nine Mile Ride, Bracknell RG12 7JQ
Tel: (01344) 862525 Fax: (01344) 869146
e-mail: coral.reef@bracknell-forest.gov.uk
Various pools for adults and children.

SD ♿ CP ♿ E ♿ RF ♿ L ♿
C ♿ S ♿ WC ♿

ATTRACTION
THE LOOK OUT DISCOVERY CENTRE
Nine Mile Ride, Bracknell RG12 7JQ
Tel: (01344) 354400 Fax: (01344) 354422
e-mail: lookout@bracknell-forest.gov.uk
www.bracknell-forest.gov.uk/lookout
Over 70 interactive exhibits, much hands-
on, to entertain both children and adults.

CP ♿ E ♿ RF ♿ L ♿
C ♿ S ♿ WC ♿

MAIDENHEAD
Pleasant residential town popular for
boating on the Thames. Walks along
the towpath are rewarding.

TOURIST INFORMATION CENTRE
The Library, St. Ives Road,
Maidenhead SL6 1QU
Tel: (01628) 796502 Fax: (01628) 796408

ATTRACTION
COURAGE SHIRE HORSE CENTRE
Cherry Garden Lane, Maidenhead Thicket,
Maidenhead SL6 3QD
Tel: (01628) 824848
Free guided tours of prize-winning shire
horses, dray rides, farriers shop, harness
maker displays, small animal and bird area.
Situated on the A4 two miles west of
Maidenhed - Junction 8/9 M4, Junction 4
M40, A4130 (Remenham Hill) out of
Henley.

SD ♿ CP 🚹 E ♿ C n/a
S ♿ WC 🚹 RFE 🚹

NEWBURY

TOURIST INFORMATION CENTRE
The Wharf, Newbury RG14 5AS
Tel: (01635) 30267 Fax: (01635) 51962
www.westberks.gov.uk/tourism

SPORTING VENUE
NEWBURY RACECOURSE
The Racecourse, Newbury RG14 7NZ
Admin and Booking-Box Office:
(01635) 40015
Fax: (01635) 528358
E-mail: info@newbury-racecourse.co.uk
www.newbury-racecourse.co.uk

CP ♿ RE ♿ ED ♿ INT ♿
L ♿ WC ♿ SS ♿ B/R 🚹

READING
County town with fine Georgian
buildings.

TOURIST INFORMATION CENTRE
Church House, Chain Street, Reading
RG1 2HX
Tel: (0118) 9566226 Fax: (0118) 9399885

READING BOROUGH COUNCIL
Town Hall, Blagrave Street,
Reading RG1 1QH
Tel: (0118) 9399873

ACCESS OFFICER
Civic Centre, Reading RG1 7TD
Tel: (0118) 955 3621 Fax: (0118) 955 3738

DIAL-A-RIDE Berkshire
Readibus: Tel: (0118) 9310000

DISABILITY INFORMATION NETWORK
Freepost (RG2750), Brakenhale School,
Rectory Lane, Bracknell RG12 7BA
Tel: (01344) 301572
Minicom: (01344) 427757
e-mail: ask@brin.freeserve.co.uk
www.bdin.freeserve.co.uk
Maintains a comprehensive disability-
related library with wide range of
information, including holidays.

TRAVELINE
Tel: (0870) 606268

BUSES
Reading Buses, The Travel Shop, 9 Duke
Street, Reading
Tel: (0118) 9594000
Fax: (0118) 9575379
Minicom: (0118) 9027630
e-mail: info@reading-buses.co.uk
Some vehicles are fitted with kneeling
facility and some routes operated by Super
Low Floor vehicles.

TAXIS
Hackney Carriages: Tel: (0118) 9670670
30 FX4s.

Checkers Cars: Tel: (0118) 9595959
1 FX4 with ramp, clamps and straps.

TRAINS
First Great Western – Special Needs:
Tel: (0845) 7413775
Thames Trains – Special Needs:
Tel: (0118) 9083607
www.thamestrains.co.uk
Virgin Trains – Special Needs:
Tel: (0845) 7443366
Minicom: (0845) 7443367
Wales & West – Special Needs:
Tel: (0845) 3003005
Minicom: (0845) 7585469

CAR PARKS
6-hour free disabled badge parking in
Broad Street Mall.
Tel: (0118) 9390900
Minicom: (0118) 9390700

SHOPMOBILITY
Readibus, 2nd Floor, Broad Street Mall,
Reading RH2 0JX
Tel: (0118) 9310000
Minicom: (0118) 9310000

HOTEL
COURTYARD BY MARRIOTT
Bath Road, Padworth, Reading RG7 5HT
Tel: (0118) 971 4411
Fax: (0118) 971 4442
No. of Accessible Rooms: 2. Bath
Accessible Facilities: Lounge, Restaurant.

READING HOLIDAY INN
Caversham Bridge, Richfield Avenue,
Reading RG1 8BD
Tel: (0118) 9259988   Fax: (0118) 9391665
No. of Accessible Rooms: 1.
Accessible Facilities: Ramped access to
Lounge and Restaurant. Purpose-built
hotel located next to Caversham Bridge,
overlooking River Thames.

RENAISSANCE READING HOTEL
Oxford Road, Reading RG1 7RH
Tel: (0118) 9586222   Fax: (0118) 9597842
www.renaissancehotels.com
No. of Accessible Rooms: 1. Bath.
Accessible Facilities: Lounge, Restaurant
Deluxe hotel in town centre close to
pedestrianised shopping and
entertainment.

WINDSOR
Famous for its castle, home of British
monarchs for almost 900 years.
Recently restored after 1992 fire.
Largest inhabited castle in the world.
Known also for Eton, England's
famous public school. An attractive
town with Georgian and Victorian
buildings, many interesting walks.

TOURIST INFORMATION CENTRE
24 High Street, Windsor SL4 1LH
Tel: (01753) 743900   Fax: (01753) 743904
HOTEL
OAKLEY COURT HOTEL
Windsor Road, Water Oakley,
Windsor SL4 5UR

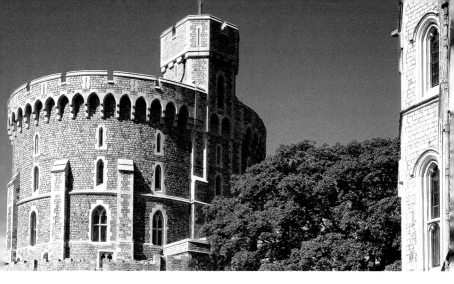

Windsor Castle – originally built by the Normans and restored in the 1990's after the fire.

Tel: (01753) 609988   Fax: (01628) 637011
e-mail:oakleyct@atlas.co.uk
No. of Accessible Rooms: 2
Accessible Facilities: Lounge, Restaurant
(both via ramps). Victorian Gothic
mansion set in 35 acres overlooking River
Thames. Used in the 60s as location for
Hammer Horror films.

ATTRACTIONS
LEGOLAND WINDSOR
Winkfield Road, Windsor SL4 4AY
Tel: (0990) 040404   Fax: (01753) 626300
www.legoland.co.uk
Set in 1,500 acres of Windsor Great Park
with many hands-on activities, rides,
themes, playscapes and millions of Lego
bricks. Also peaceful areas with restaurants
and facilities. Legoland's award winning
facilities enable guests with disabilities the
best possible enjoyment and accessibility.
The park is based on a hill, but is serviced
by a hill train, which transports guests
from the top to the bottom of the park
and vice versa. An advisory leaflet will help
visitors maximise LEGOLAND's special
needs facilities and is available in advance
from the Reservations Centre (08705 04
04 04). This leaflet is also available from
Guest Services at The Beginning.
Wheelchair hire is also available but it is
advisable to call first.

WINDSOR CASTLE
Windsor SL4 1NJ
Tel: (0207) 3212233   Fax: (0207) 9309625
e-mail:information@royalcollection.org.uk
www.royal.gov.uk
Originally built for William the Conqueror
900 years ago to guard western approach
to London. The castle is one of three
official residences of the Queen. It is the
largest inhabited castle in the world and
the oldest in continious occupation. State
apartments contain fine works of art,
armour, pictures and interiors. NOTE: NO
PARKING FACILITIES.
All areas within precincts of Castle
accessible, except Queen Mary's Dolls
House and some semi state rooms within
State Apartments open only in winter.
Principal restored areas that form year-
round visitor route are accessible. Lift
available to State Apartments.

ST GEORGE'S CHAPEL
Situated inside Windsor Castle this is one
of the most beautiful church buildings in
England. The building work started in
1475 and took 50 years to construct. Ten
monarchs are buried here including
Edward IV, Henry VIII with his favourite
wife, Jane Seymour.

SD n/a   CP n/a   E   RF
L &   WC &

BRISTOL

Thriving ancient city-port developed originally for wool export and C18th slave trading, with resultant fine terraces and grand buildings built on the ensuing riches. Clifton, once a village on the steep cliffs above the port, is the most attractive part, and location of the university. Brunel's famous suspension bridge is located here.

TOURIST INFORMATION CENTRE
St. Nicholas Church, St. Nicholas Church Street, Bristol BS1 1UE
Tel: (0117) 9260767   Fax: (0117) 9297703
e-mail: bristol@tourism. gov.uk
www.tourism.bristol.gov.uk

TRAVELINE
Tel: (0820) 6082608

BUSES
Easyrider: Tel: (0117) 9778759
General Bus/Park & Ride Information:
Tel: (0870) 6082608

TAXIS
Bristol Hackney Cabs: Tel: (0117) 9538638
15 adapted vehicles.
Peter's Taxis: Tel: (0117) 9714141
2 adapted vehicles.
Streamline Taxis: Tel: (0117) 9264001

TRAINS
First Great Western – Special Needs:
Tel: (0845) 7413775
Virgin Trains – Special Needs: (0845) 7443366
Minicom: (0845) 7443367
Wales & West: (0845) 3003005
Minicom: (0845) 7585469

CAR PARKS
Some free unlimited Disabled badge parking.
Tel: (0117) 9223006

SHOPMOBILITY
Unit 26, Castle Gallery,

The Galleries, Broadmead, Bristol BS1 3XE
Tel: (0117) 9226342

HOTELS
BRISTOL MARRIOTT ROYAL HOTEL 🚶
College Green, Bristol BS1 5TA
Tel: (0117) 9255100   Fax: (0117) 9251515
No. of Accessible Rooms: 2
Accessible Facilities: All public areas, except pool. Quality city centre hotel next to the cathedral restored to former Victorian glory with contemporary luxury.

CROWNE PLAZA BRISTOL 🚶
Victoria Street, Bristol BS1 6HY
Tel: (0117) 9769988   Fax: (0117) 9255040
No. of Accessible Rooms: 2
Accessible Facilities: Lounge, Restaurant
Modern hotel in city centre close to Temple Meads Railway station.

THISTLE BRISTOL 🚶
Broad Street, Bristol BS1 2EL
Tel: (0117) 9291645   Fax: (0117) 9227619
No. of Accessible Rooms: 6. Bath
Accessible Facilities: Restaurant.
Quality hotel in the centre of the city.

ATTRACTIONS
@BRISTOL
Anchor Road, Harbourside, Bristol BS1 5DB
Tel: (0845) 345 1235   Fax: (0117) 915 7200
e-mail: information@at-bristol.org.uk
www.at-bristol.org.uk
Millenium project now alive, with three attractions: Wildwalk that recreates the extraordinary diversity of the natural world, Explore that entices visitors to delve into science stories that seek to explain how the world works and an IMAX theatre which has a screen four storeys high and digital surround sound. Also Open Spaces-at-Bristol, with public art, including light features and sculptures, tree-lined seating areas, plus shops, cafes and restaurants.
Designated Car Parking available in large underground car park close to lift access to main square. Smooth path links all facilities with clear route throughout exhibitions. Pedestrian area and pedestrian routes continue throughout the site across 66 acres.

SPECIAL ARRANGEMENTS: If your vehicle is above 2 metres high please call security in advance of your visit on 0117 9157254 to arrange parking. Wheelchair hire can be arranged but please book in advance.

CP ⑂ E ⑂ RF ⑂ C ⑂
S ⑂ WC ⑂ L ⑂

BRISTOL INDUSTRIAL MUSEUM
Princes Wharf, City Docks, Bristol BS1 4RN
Tel: (0117) 9251470 Fax: (0117) 9297318
Displays of motor and horse-drawn vehicles, plus locally built aircraft. Railway exhibits include an industrial locomotive. Local port displays also.

SD ⑂ CP 大 E 大 RF 大
C n/a S ⑂ WC 大

BRISTOL ZOO GARDENS
Clifton, Bristol BS8 3HA
Tel: (0117) 9738951 Fax: (0117) 9736814
e-mail: information@bristolzoo.org.uk
www.bristolzoo.org.uk
Over 300 species of wildlife in delightful gardens, notable for gorilla exhibit, walk-through aviary. Also aquarium reptile house, bug and twilight worlds.

SD ⑂ CP 大 E ⑂ RF ⑂
C 大 S 大 WC 大 RFE 大

SS GREAT BRITAIN
Great Western Dock, Gas Ferry Road,
Bristol BS1 6TY
Tel: (0117) 9260680 Fax: (0117) 9255788
The first ocean-going, propeller-driven, iron ship in history, designed by Brunel and built and launched in Bristol in 1843. Now being restored to original appearance.

SD ⑂ CP 大 E ⑂ RF ⑂ C ⑂
S ⑂ WC 大 RFE ⑂

THEATRE
BRISTOL OLD VIC
King Street, Bristol BS1 4ED
Admin: (0117) 9493993
Booking-Box Office: (0117) 9877877
Minicom: (0117) 9264388
Fax: (0117) 9493996
e-mail:admin@bristol-old-vic.co.uk
www.bristol-old-vic.co.uk
Complies Part M, Building Regulations.

SD ⑂ CP 大 Nearest Public CP – Queen

Charlotte Street, Disabled badge spaces.　No Taxi
Rank RE ⑂　ED ⑂　INT ⑂
L ⑂ (wheelchair lift)　WC ⑂ (Adapted,
unisex, on ground floor)　AUD ⑂　B/R ⑂
Additional Notes: Concessionary prices for you and companion. Level entrance to steps (lift), level to wheelchair spaces.

BUCKINGHAMSHIRE

CHILTERN MULTIPLE SCLEROSIS CENTRE
Scarlett Avenue, Halton, Aylesbury HP22 5PG
Tel: (01296) 696133

BEACONSFIELD
Old town with historical buildings separated from the new town by over 0.25 miles of wooded country.

ATTRACTION
BEKONSCOT MODEL VILLAGE
Warwick Road, Beaconsfield HP9 2PL
Tel: (01494) 672919
Fax: (01494) 675284
e-mail: info@bekonscot.co.uk
www.bekonscot.org.uk
Oldest model village in the world founded in 1929. It portrays rural England in the 1930s with six villages each with their miniature population going about their daily routines. Many moving models including a gauge-1 model railway that runs throughout the 1.5-acre site. Width of some of the paths is a little narrow.
Just off Junction 2 of the M40.

SD ⑂　CP 大　E ⑂　C ⑂
S n/a　WC 大　RFE 大

BURNHAM
Fairly large residential village known for its forest of Burnham Beeches, one of the country's finest beauty spots.

HOTEL
THE GROVEFIELD HOTEL　　大
Taplow Common Road, Burnham SL1 8LP

Tel: (01628) 603131   Fax: (01628) 668078
www.macdonaldhotels.co.uk/grovefield-hotel
No. of Accessible Rooms: 2. Bath
Accessible Facilities: Lounge, Restaurant,
Bar. Elegant property set in seven acres
of lawns surrounded by woodland.
Originally the country retreat of John
Fuller, of brewing fame and still retains
many original architectural features.

HIGH WYCOMBE
Large town of importance since
Roman times. Now a modern town
surrounded by many areas of natural
beauty.

ATTRACTION
HUGHENDEN MANOR ESTATE (NT)
High Wycombe HP14 4LA
Tel: (01494) 755573
Home of Benjamin Disraeli, Victorian
Prime Minister from 1848 until his death
in 1881. House contains many personal
items: lovely walks in surrounding park
and colourful gardens.

SD n/a   CP 🚶   E 🚶   FR 🚶
C 🚶   S 🚶   WC 🚶   RFE 🚶

MILTON KEYNES
New town built in 1960s, arranged
on grid/roundabout system,
surrounded by pleasant countryside.

TOURIST INFORMATION CENTRE
The Food Centre, 411 Secklow Gate East,
Central Milton Keynes MK9 3NE
Tel: Fax: (01908) 235050

BRITISH RED CROSS
Westfield Road, Bletchley,
Milton Keynes MK2 2RA
Tel: (01908) 370996
They also operate a range medical
equipment (including wheelchairs) short-
term loan service.

BUSES
No easy access/low-floor buses at present,
but planned. Information on services:

Community Information Centre, Central
Library, 555 Silbury Boulevard,
Milton Keynes MK9 3HL
Tel: (01908) 254055   Fax: (01908) 254086

TAXIS
Hackney Carriages: Tel: (07802) 847503
mark@wheelchairtaxi.co.uk
www.wheelchairtaxi.co.uk
2 London-style cabs - wheelchair taxi
service, no private hire cars available.

TRAINS
Connex: Customer Services:
Tel: (0870) 6030405
Fax: (0870) 6030505
Minicom: (01233) 617621
Silverlink – Special Needs:
Tel: (01923) 207818
Fax: (01923) 207023
Minicom: (01923) 256430
Virgin Trains – Special Needs:
Tel: (0845) 7443366
Minicom: (0845) 7443367

CAR PARKS
Free unlimited disabled badge parking.

SHOPMOBILITY
Shopping information Centre, CMK
Shopping Building, Midsummer Arcade,
Milton Keynes.   Tel: (01908) 670231

HOTEL
HILTON NATIONAL   🚶
Timbold Drive, Kents Hill Park,
Milton Keynes MK7 6HL
Tel: (01908) 694433 Fax: (01908) 695533
No. of Accessible Rooms: 2. Bath
Accessible Facilities: Lounge, Restaurant
Bright, modern hotel close to the M1.

MILTON KEYNES CENTRE FOR
INTEGRATED LIVING
330 Saxongate West, Central Milton
Keynes, MK9 2ES
Tel: (01908) 231344
E-mail:mkcil@aol.com
Help people with disabilities to lead an
integrated life in the community. Display
area for disabled equipment. Extensive
kitchen and bathroom showing gadgets
for disabled people.

CAMBRIDGESHIRE

CAMBRIDGESHIRE TOURISM
The Old Library, Wheeler Street
Cambridge CB2 3QB
Tel: (01223) 322640
Fax: (01223) 457588
Comprehensive Guide to Cambridge for
Disabled People covering most of what
one needs to know.

BRITISH RED CROSS
2 Shaftesbury Road, Cambridge CB2 2BW
Tel: (01223) 354434

CAMBRIDGE PASSENGER TRANSPORT INFORMATION LINE
Tel: (01223) 717740

DIRECTIONS PLUS
Affiliated to DIAL. Disabled persons
information project with factsheet with
much information covering whole country.
Tel: (01223) 569600
Textphone: (01223) 569601
Fax: (01223) 506470
e-mail: info@directions.plus@dial.pipex.com
www.direction-plus.org.uk

BUSES
Stagecoach Cambus:. Tel: (01223) 423578
Whippet Coaches: Tel: (01480) 463792
Community Transport: Tel: (01223) 717755
Park & Ride: (01223) 718167

HICOM
Histon and Impington Community Minibus
may be available for hire:
Neil Davis
Tel: (01223) 232514/233349
All these companies operate some low
floor buses on some routes.

TAXIS
Camtax: Tel: (01223) 313131
2 FX4s with ramps, 1 minibus with ramps,
clamps and straps. N.B. Pre-book.
Regency: Tel: (01223) 311311
1 Nissan Cargo.

TRAINS
Anglia Railways: Assistance:
Tel: (01473) 693333
Minicom: (01603) 630748 or
(0845) 6050600
Central Trains: Assistance:
Tel: (0845) 7056027
www.centraltrains.co.uk
West Anglia Great Northern: Special Needs
– Tel: (08457) 818919
Minicom: (08457) 125988
www.wagn.co.uk

SHOPMOBILITY
5th Floor, Lion Yard Car Park
Tel: (01223) 457452
Grafton Centre East
Tel: (01223) 461858
Textphone: (01223) 457050

CAMBRIDGE MOBILITY
Wheelchair Hire
Tel: (01223) 844666

CAMBRIDGE
Ancient university town with row of
colleges lining the River Cam and
overlooking the Banks on the other
side of the river. This area of lawns
and trees is delightful. Modern
shopping in historical surroundings
adds to the unique atmosphere
created by the university, river and
gardens.

HOTELS
CROWN PLAZA HOTEL
Downing Street, Cambridge CB2 3DT
Tel: (01223) 464466
Fax: (01223) 464440
No. of Accessible Rooms: 2. Bath
Accessible Facilities: Lounge, Restaurant,
gym. Modern city centre hotel with
reserved car park

SORRENTO HOTEL
196 Cherry Hinton Road, Cambridge
CB1 7AN
Tel: (01223) 243533
Fax: (01223) 213463
www.sorrentohotel.com

No. of Accessible Rooms: 1. Bath
Accessible Facilities: Lounge, Restaurant
(ramped at 1:11), conservatory. Medium-
sized private and family-run hotel 1.5 miles
from city centre. Progressive staff.

ATTRACTIONS
ANGLESEY ABBEY GARDENS and LODE MILL
(NT), Lode CB5 9EJ
Tel/Fax: (01223) 811200

Gardens and ground floor of Mill
accessible, Abbey not so. Founded in 1135
as a religious house, becoming a secular
property by C16th. Purchased by the first
Lord Fairhaven in 1926. He created a
superb landscaped garden with great
statuary and trees for all seasons and a
working water mill.

SD 🚷 CP 🚶 RF 🚶   C 🚶
S 🚶   WC 🚶 RFE 🚷

CAMBRIDGE UNIVERSITY BOTANIC GARDEN
Cory Lodge, Bateman Street,
Cambridge CB2 1JF
Tel: (01223) 336265
Fax: (01223) 336278
e-mail: enquiries@botanic.cam.ac.uk
www.botanic.cam.ac.uk

Founded in 1762, in its present site since
1846, there are 40 acres including nine
national collections. Also a Winter Garden,
Chronological Bed, Scented Garden and a
collection of native British plants.
Glasshouses contain sub-tropical and
tropical plants.

SD 🚷 CP 🚶 E 🚷   RF 🚷 L n/a
C 🚶   S 🚶   WC 🚶

The imposing frontage of
The Fitzwilliam Museum.

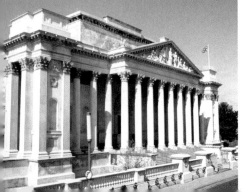

CHILFORD HALL VINEYARD
Linton, Cambridge CB1 6LE
Tel: (01223) 892641
Fax: (01223) 894056
www.chilfordhall.co.uk

Award winning vineyard in East Anglia
and home to one of the region's most
respected producers. The first vines were
planted in 1972 and covers 18-acres.
Wine-tasting and buying, plus winery tour
to learn how English wine is produced.

SD 🚷 CP 🚶 E 🚷   RF 🚶 C 🚶
S 🚶   WC 🚶

THE FITZWILLIAM MUSEUM
Trumpington Street, Cambridge CB2 1RB
Tel: (01223) 332900
Fax: (01223) 332923

Small, personal museum which is
currently undergoing major refurbishment
expected to be completed in 2004. At
time of writing limited displays of
antiquities on ground floor available.
Upper floor houses five galleries of
paintings from all periods. Admittance at
rear of building where set down is
available. From Trumpington Street,
approach by lane opposite Brown's
Restaurant. N.B. Lift dependant on
available staff to operate.

SD 🚷 CP n/a E 🚷 RF 🚷 L 🚷
C 🚷   S 🚶   WC 🚶

IMPERIAL WAR MUSEUM
Duxford Airfield, Duxford,
Nr. Cambridge CB2 4QR
Tel: (01223) 835000
Fax: (01223) 837267
www.iwm.org.uk

Former Battle of Britain fighter station and
home to Europe's largest collection of
historic aircraft. Experience the American
Air Museum and Land Warfare
exhibitions.

SD 🚷 CP 🚷 E 🚷   RF 🚷 L n/a
C 🚷   S 🚷   WC 🚷 RFE 🚷

ELY
Famous for its great cathedral,
there are also pleasant walks and
beautiful views.

TOURIST INFORMATION CENTRE
Oliver Cromwell's House,
29 St. Mary's Street, Ely CB7 4HF
Tel: (01353) 662062

HOTEL
TRAVELODGE 🚶
Witchford Road, Ely CB6 3NN
Tel/Fax: (01353) 668499
No. of Accessible Rooms: 2. Bath
Accessible Facilities: Restaurant.
Spacious accommodation in modern
building located at roundabout of A10
and A142.

ATTRACTION
ELY CATHEDRAL
Chapter House, The College, Ely CB7 4DL
Tel: (01353) 667735
Fax: (01353) 665658
Magnificent Norman cathedral set amidst
medieval monastic buildings.
SD ♿ CP 🚶 E ♿ (South door)
RF ♿ (except Refectory door that is ramped at 1:6)
C ♿ S ♿ WC 🚶 RFE ♿

HUNTINGDON
Attractive county town with narrow
main street, stretches of Georgian
buildings,

TOURIST INFORMATION CENTRE
Princes Street, Huntingdon PE18 6PH
Tel: (01480) 388588
Fax: (01480) 388591

SPORTING VENUE
HUNTINGDON STEEPLECHASES LTD
The Racecourse, Brampton,
Huntingdon PE18 8NN
www.huntingdon-racecourse.co.uk
Booking-Box Office: (01480) 453373
Fax: (01480) 455275
CP ♿ RE ♿ ED ♿
WC 🚶 (Members Enclosure)
SS 🚶 Wheelchair platform designated. Route via
Paddock Enclosure Grandstand near main entrance.
B/R ♿

PETERBOROUGH
Known as a market town with a fine
cathedral, historic buildings and good
shops.

HOTELS
PETERBOROUGH MARRIOTT ♿
Lynch Wood, Peterborough Business Park,
Peterborough PE2 6GB
Tel: (01733) 371111
Fax: (01733) 236725
No. of Accessible Rooms: 2
Accessible Facilities: Lounge, Restaurant.
Modern hotel located opposite East of
England Showground.

PETERBOROUGH MOAT HOUSE 🚶
Thorpe Wood, Peterborough PE3 6SG
Tel: (01733) 289988
Fax: (01733) 262737
No. of Accessible Rooms: 1
Accessible Facilities: Lounge, Restaurant
Modern hotel on outskirts of town,
overlooking 500-acre country park.

ATTRACTION
NENE VALLEY RAILWAY
Wansford Station, Stibbington,
Peterborough PE8 6LR
Tel: (01780) 784444
Fax: (01780) 784440
The golden age of steam – 7.5 mile track
following River Nene meandering from HQ
at Wansford Station to Peterborough
passing through the 500-acre ferry
Meadows Country Park.
SD ♿ CP ♿ E ♿ RF ♿ L n/a
C ♿ S ♿ WC ♿ RFE ♿

PEAKIRK WATERFOWL GARDENS TRUST
Deeping Road, Peakirk,
Peterborough PE6 7NP
Tel: (01733) 252271
20 acres of woodland, water and formal
gardens with many species of duck, goose,
swan ands flamingo, located seven miles
north of Peterborough.
SD ♿ CP ♿ E ♿ RF ♿ C 🚶
S ♿ WC 🚶 RFE ♿

CHANNEL ISLANDS

JERSEY

Largest and most southerly of the islands, set in the Bay of St. Malo, 14 miles from the French coast. Originally part of Normandy, coming under English rule when William the Conqueror invaded England. Loyal to the British Crown but has its own government and is not part of the European Community. Landscape of rugged north coast, central country lanes and southern bays.

JERSEY TOURISM
Liberation Square, St. Helier,
Jersey JE1 1BB
Tel: (01534) 500700
Fax: (01534) 500 899

BUSES/COACHES
Tantivy Blue Coaches: Tel: (01534) 722584
One 37-seater vehicle with lift, one 42-seater vehicle with proper disabled lift, one 17-seater vehicle taking folding wheelchairs.

TAXIS
Flying Dragon/Clarendon:
Tel: (01534) 722584
3 adapted vehicles.
Luxicabs: Tel: (01534) 887000
6 adapted vehicles.
Andy Tague: Tel: (01534) 758476
1 adapted vehicle.

On Jersey there are height and width restrictions on small country roads that render large vehicles impractical. It is the states that refuse licences, rather than transport companies not wanting to become disabled friendly.

FERRIES – SEE INTRODUCTION

AIRLINES – SEE INTRODUCTION

CAR PARKS
Free 4 or 2-hour disabled badge parking.

WHEELCHAIR HIRE
Available from:
Guardian Medical Supplies:
Tel: (01534) 732335   Fax: (01534) 759465
Travelsmith: Tel: (01534) 737317

GROUVILLE

Located in the south-east, joining with St. Clements to form many miles of sweeping bays. Grouville Bay is the finest on the island, reaching from Gorey harbour to La Roque Point. Many Martello towers and forts built during Napoleonic wars.

HOTEL
BEAUSITE HOTEL
Grouville Bay, Grouville JE3 9DJ
Tel: (01534) 857577
Fax: (01534) 857211
www.southernhotels.com
No. of Accessible Rooms: 3
Accessible Facilities: Lounge, Restaurant, Pool. The hotel's original granite farm buildings date back to 1636 and public rooms retain a traditional style. The remainder is modern. The property looks out onto the Royal Jersey Golf Course and the Bay of Grouville.

ATTRACTION
THE JERSEY POTTERY
Gorey Village, Grouville JE3 9EP
Tel: (01534) 851119
Fax: (01534) 856403
e-mail: jsypot@itl.net
See complex manufacturing process of hand-painted ceramics in the 600 unique lines of this commercial pottery with beautiful gardens and restaurant.
SD n/a   CP 🚻   E 🚻   RF 🚻   C 🚻
S 🚻   WC 🚻

ST. BRELADE
Parish makes up the south-western tip of island, seaside resorts in sheltered bays.

JERSEY LAVENDER
Rue Du Pont Marquet, St. Brelade JE3 8DS
Tel: (01534) 742933 Fax: (01534) 745613
admin@jerseylavender.co.uk
www.jerseylavender.co.uk
The first lavender was planted in 1983 and
now extends to approximately nine acres.
The farm exhibits the processes involved in
extracting the oil and in creating exclusive
Jersey lavender products on this working
farm. The owners took advice from the
local disabled access group when
designing the layout, but because this is a
working farm, access to some areas
without a robust pusher is a little difficult.

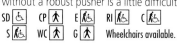
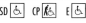 Wheelchairs available.

ST. CLEMENT
Situated just east of St. Helier with
lovely arable countryside and long
stretches of sandy beaches. This is
Jersey's smallest parish with granite
outcrop of Rocqueberg and 3m menhir
testifying to probable neolithic origin.

ATTRACTION
SAMARES MANOR GARDENS
Inner Road, St.Clement JE2 6QW
Tel: (01534) 870551 Fax: (01534) 768949
14 acres of lovely gardens, including a
Japanese garden and one of Britain's
largest herb gardens. Also a craft centre
and farm animals.

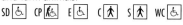

ST. HELIER
Capital of the island with paved
shopping streets and lanes, combined
with night spots, restaurants and
entertainment.

HOTEL
HOTEL DE VERE
Esplanade, St. Helier JE4 8WD
Tel: (01534) 22301
Fax: (01534) 737815
No. of Accessible Rooms: 1. Bath
Accessible Facilities: Lounge, Restaurant.

ATTRACTIONS
JERSEY MUSEUM
The Weighbridge, St. Helier JE2 3NF
Tel: (01534) 633300   Fax: (01534) 633301
Award-winning museum telling the Story
of Jersey that brings together the island's
collections in a very striking exhibition. The
art gallery offers paintings, etchings and
sculpture and a new theatre presents a
picture of Jersey's unique place in history.

MARITIME MUSEUM
New North Quay, St. Helier
Tel: (01534) 633340
Fax: (01534) 633301
Hands-on exhibits, historic objects and new
art and sculpture celebrate the relationship
of the islanders and the sea. Feel the force
of gale, float your own ships, and
experience pitch and roll of life at sea.

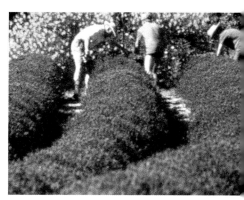

Can't you just smell the Lavender.

ST. LAWRENCE
ATTRACTION
FLYING FLOWERS
Jersey Flower Centre, St. Lawrence JE3 1GX
Tel: (01376) 575000
Fax: (01376) 575050
Home of the largest mail-order floral
company in the world. Giant glasshouses,
Flamingo Lake, Wildfowl Sanctuary,
Koi Carp reserve, exotic birds and
wildflower meadowland.

GERMAN UNDERGROUND HOSPITAL

Les Charrieres Malorey, St. Lawrence JE3 1FU
Tel: (01534) 863442   Fax: (01534) 865970
Remarkable engineering feat of the
German Occupation and an evocative
reminder of events that began in July
1940. Vast complex dug deep into a
hillside. Continuous video presentation
with memorabilia bring life of islanders at
war to life.

SD n/a   CP   E 🔲   RF 🔲   L 🔲
c 🔲   s 🔲   WC 🔲

ST. OUEN
HOTEL

MAISON DES LANDES HOTEL   🔲
St. Ouen JE3 2AA
Tel: (01534) 481683   Fax: (01534) 485327
No. of Accessible Rooms: All Accessible
Facilities: Lounge, Dining room, Indoor
Pool. Purpose-built hotel for disabled
guests and their families and fully
accessible to wheelchair users. Hoists,
wheelchairs and other equipment
available, but personal care not provided.

TRINITY

Largest parish, but one of the least
populated, a rural area with fine
granite farmhouses and picturesque
small lanes. Boulay Bay, on the north
coast, is a tranquil cove with cliff paths
through wonderful heather. Holy
Trinity Parish Church dates back to the
C12th century.

PALLOT HERITAGE STEAM MUSEUM

Rue de Bechet, Trinity JE3 5BE
Tel: (01534) 865307   Fax: (01534) 865506
Collection of displays on mechanical and
farming heritage. Host to Liberation Day
Steam Fayre early May and Steam
Threshing Fayre in autumn.

SD 🔲   CP 🔲   E 🔲   RF 🔲   C 🔲   WC 🔲

GUERNSEY

30 miles from France and 80 from the
English coast. Covering about 25 square
miles there are 20 bays and beaches,
wooded valleys, spectacular cliffs,
marshland and rolling countryside. The
islands remain part of the Duchy of
Normandy and are self-governing with
their own parliament.

DEPARTMENT OF TOURISM
PO Box 23, St. Peter Port GY1 3AN
Tel: (01481) 723552

STATES TRAFFIC COMMITTEE:
Tel: (01481) 243400
Publishes leaflet entitled "Transport and
the Disabled in Guernsey". Other leaflets
on UK and the European Union.

GUERNSEY ASSOCIATION OF PEOPLE WITH DISABILITIES
Tel: (01481) 724102/722435

BUSES
No low-floor buses on island.

TAXIS
Ace Taxis: Tel: (07781) 121180
One adapted vehicle.
Eurocab: Tel: (07781) 103615
One adapted vehicle.

WHEELCHAIR HIRE
St. John Ambulance: Tel: (01481) 729268

ATTRACTION
CASTEL
FORT HOMMET GUN CASEMATE
Fort Hommet, Castel.
Correspondence, c/o Occupation Museum,
Forest GY8 0BG
Tel: (01481) 238205
Fully restored German bunker with
original 10.5cm gun, located on Fort
Hommet headland in Vazon Bay.

SD 🔲   CP   E 🔲   C n/a   S 🔲
WC n/a

FERMAIN BAY

Close to St. Peter Port, reached by steep valley road, one of Guernsey's prettiest bays.

HOTEL
LA FAVORITA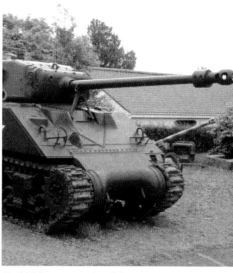
Fermain Bay GY4 6SD
Tel: (01481) 235666
Fax: (01481) 235413
www.favorita.com
No. of Accessible Rooms: 11
Accessible Facilities: Lounge, Bar, Restaurant (1st floor, via accessible lift). Originally a country house that retains its character. Set in a wooded valley leading down to Fermain Bay with fine views over the sea towards Jersey.

Forbidding example of the amazing display at the German Occupation Museum.

FOREST

Bordered by beautiful cliffs and the Bays of Petit Bot and Portlet, much of the cliff area is inaccessible to wheelchairs, but at the parish centre is the ancient church of St. Marguerite de la Foret, the patron saint of dentists, that is accessible.

ATTRACTION
GERMAN OCCUPATION MUSEUM
Forest GY8 0BG
Tel: (01481) 230205
The Channel Islands was the only British territory to be occupied by the Germans during WWII. The museum tells the story from 1940/45 through a large collection of authentic occupation items and tableaux of bunker rooms and a street. The military, occupation and civilian rooms and the prison are accessible .

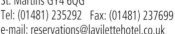

ST. MARTINS
HOTEL
LA VILLETTE HOTEL
St. Martins GY4 6QG
Tel: (01481) 235292   Fax: (01481) 237699
e-mail: reservations@lavillettehotel.co.uk

www.lavillettehotel.co.uk
No. of Accessible Rooms: 1. Bath
Accessible Facilities: Lounge, Restaurant
Attractive property surrounded by trees and lawns.

ST. PETER PORT

Capital of Guernsey, a town that has grown uphill with many of its attractive narrow streets meandering upwards. Much of the town is pedestrianised but the main High Street is cobbled.

HOTEL
ST. PIERRE PARK HOTEL
Rohais, St. Peter Port GY1 1FD
Tel: (01481) 728282   Fax: (01481) 712041
e-mail:info@stpierreparkhotel.com
www.stpierreparkhotel.com
No. of Accessible Rooms: 2. Bath
Accessible Facilities: Open plan Lounge/Bar, Restaurants (2), 1 on ground floor, one lower ground via accessible lift. Set amidst 45 acres of quiet mature parkland, this 5-star hotel is superb.

ATTRACTION
GUERNSEY MUSEUM and ART GALLERY
Candie Gardens, St. Peter Port GY1 1UG
Tel: (01481) 726518
Fax: (01481) 715177
e-mail: m.crozier@museum.gov.gg
Purpose-built to relate the history of the
island, with audio visual theatre and both
permanent art gallery and special
exhibitions February to December.

SD ⬦   CP n/a   E ⬦   RF ⬦   C ⬦
S ⬦   WC ⬦

VALE
An area of lovely sandy bays,
particularly Pembroke, offering good
access from smooth shallow slipway
at eastern end and car park adjoining
bay. Chouet Bay has a slipway to
hard sand as does Ladies Bay, but
Port Soif Bay is difficult to access.

HOTEL
PENINSULA HOTEL   ⬦
Les Dicqs, Vale GY6 8JP
Tel: (01481) 48400
Fax: (01481) 48706
www.visitguernsey.com/peninsula
No. of Accessible Rooms: 2. Bath
Accessible Facilities: Lounge, Restaurant,
Gardens. Surrounded by five acres of
gardens, located on tranquil grassy
peninsula leading to a sandy bay.

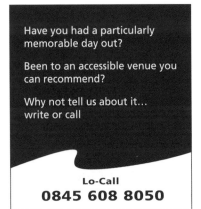

Have you had a particularly
memorable day out?

Been to an accessible venue you
can recommend?

Why not tell us about it...
write or call

Lo-Call
0845 608 8050

CHESHIRE

CHESHIRE DISABILITIES FEDERATION
Vale Royal Disability Access and
Information Service
Council House, Church Road,
Northwich CW9 5PD
Tel: (01606) 352808   Fax: (01606) 354536
Produce excellent Cheshire Welcome
Guide with attractions and
accommodation inspected by members of
the Federation and Holiday Care Service.

HALTON DISABILITY SERVICE
Unit 102 RiverWalk, Halton Lea Shopping
Centre, Runcorn, WA7 2BX
Tel: (01928) 590361

SHOPMOBILITY
Tel: (01928) 717445

ALTRINCHAM
Industrial and residential centre
surrounded by picturesque villages,
ancient churches and broad stretches
of placid water.

ATTRACTION
DUNHAM MASSEY HALL (NT)
Altrincham WA14 4SJ
Tel: (0161) 9411025
Fax: (0161) 9297508
The house, park and garden owe their
design and character mostly to the 2nd
Earl of Warrington (1675-1758). Over 30
house rooms are open and the garden
contains remnants from past layouts
including the moat, Elizabethan mount
and C18th orangery. Ancient trees outline
the avenues of the park with a 1610 water
mill, now a sawmill, with working
machinery. A motorised stair-climber has
made access to the ground floor possible
as the entrance has three steps. Park and
gardens have level easy paths, but there is
a cobbled area around the stable block
that houses a restaurant and a shop. Two
manual wheelchairs and two battery-
powered wheelchairs are available free of

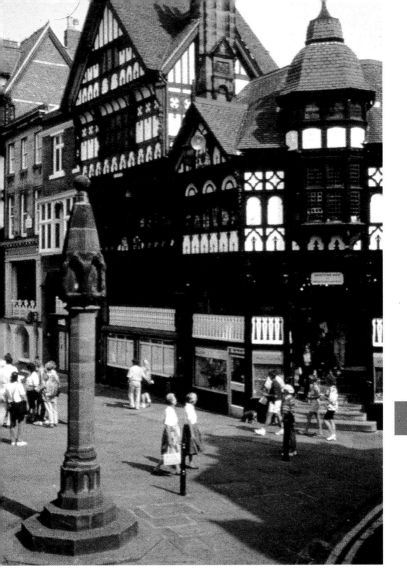

The Cross, part of Chester's unique medieval setting.

charge but must be booked in advance to ensure that support staff are available.

SD   CP   E   RF   L
C S WC G

CHESTER
Known as the black-and-white city, and famous for its half-timbered buildings, Chester's foundations are Roman as are the original forts that still surround it. There is plenty of shopping here, an historic feel, plus entertainment.

CHESTER TOURISM
Chester City Council, The Forum,
Chester CH1 2HS
Tel: (01244) 402150
Fax: (01244) 315789
www.chestertourism.com.

TOURIST INFORMATION CENTRES
Town Hall, Northgate Street, Chester
Tel: (01244) 402111   Fax: (01244) 400420
e-mail: tic@chestercc.gov.uk

Vicars Lane, Chester, CH1 1QX
Tel: (01244) 351609
Fax: (01244) 403188

Chester Railway Station, Station Road,
Chester CH1 3NT
Tel: (01244) 322220   Fax: (01244) 322211

CHESHIRE C.C. TRANSPORT CO-ORDINATION
Rivacre Business Centre, Mill Lane,
Ellesmere Port CH66 3TL
Tel: (01244) 603041 (for Chester area)
Publish "Getting There" a guide to public
transport for people with mobility
problems.

TRAVELINE
Tel: (0870) 608268

BUSES
Cheshire Traveline: Tel: (01244) 602666
Arriva: www.arriva.co.uk
First Crosville: Tel: (01244) 381461
All operate some low-floor buses.
Also operate Women's Safe Transport
Tel: (01244) 310585
Park & Ride: Tel: (01244) 602666
City-Rail link: Tel: (01244) 602666

TAXIS
Taxi Rank at Bus Station
Chester Radio Taxis: Tel: (01244) 372372
26 wheelchair-accessible vehicles.
John Morris Taxis: Tel: (01244) 851032
1 taxi with all fittings.

TRAINS
Central Trains: Assistance:
Tel: (0845) 7056027
www.centraltrains.co.uk
First North Western: Special Needs –
Tel: (0845) 6040231
Merseyrail: Special Needs –
Tel: (0151) 7022071 (minicom available)
Virgin Trains: Special Needs –
(0845) 7443366
Minicom: (0845) 7443367
Wales & West: Special Needs –
Tel: (0845) 3003005
Minicom: (0845) 7585469

CAR PARKS
Some free disabled badge parking.

SHOPMOBILITY
Kale Yards, Frodsham Street Car Park,

Chester CH1 3JH
Tel: (01244) 312626

CHESTER ACCESS OFFICER
Chester City Council
Tel: (01244) 401623

DIAL HOUSE - CHESTER
Tel/Minicom: (01244) 345655

CHESTER HOTELS
CHESTER MOAT HOUSE
Trinity Street, Chester CH1 2BD
Tel: (01244) 899988   Fax: (01244) 316118
No. of Accessible Rooms: 2
Accessible Facilities: Restaurant, Bar, gym
and pool.
Quality hotel with superb views over the
racecourse and the Welsh hills.

ABBEY COURT HOTEL
Liverpool Road, Chester CH2 1AG
Tel: (01244) 374100   Fax: (01244) 379240
www.macdonaldhotels.co.uk/abbey-court-
hotel/
No. of Accessible Rooms: Several on the
ground floor. Accessible Facilities: Lounge,
Restaurant, Bars (some steps).
Elegant porticoed hotel close to the
medieval city centre and 3 miles from the
M53.

THE CHESTER GROSVENOR
Eastgate, Chester CH1 1LT
Tel: (01244) 324024   Fax: (01244) 313246
e-mail: reservations@chestergrosvenor.co.uk
www.chestergrosvenor.co.uk
No. of Accessible Rooms: 1. Bath
Accessible Facilities: Drawing Room,
Restaurants (2). Luxurious 5-star hotel,
owned by the 6th Duke of Westminster
under the Grosvenor Estates. Located in
the city centre, adjacent to the Eastgate
Clock.

DENE HOTEL
95 Hoole Road, Chester CH2 3ND
Tel: (01244) 321165
Fax: (01244) 350277
No. of Accessible Rooms: 12. Bath
Accessible Facilities: Lounge, Restaurant
Set in its own grounds, adjacent to
Alexandra Park. 1 mile from Chester.

Tel: (01244) 335262   Fax: (01244) 335464
No. of Accessible Rooms: 7
Accessible Facilities: Lounge,Restaurant,
Pool, Sauna, Spa. 1779 manor house set
in eight acres of parklands and gardens,
two miles from Chester.

ATTRACTIONS
CHESTER CATHEDRAL
12 Abbey Square, Chester CH1 2HU
Tel: (01244) 324756   Fax: (01244) 341110
e-mail: office@chestercathedral.com
Well-preserved example of a medieval
monastic complex with all main periods of
Gothic architecture to be seen. Fine
medieval woodwork in quire stalls of 1380.

SD ♿   CP n/a   E ♿   RF ♿   C ♿
S ♿   WC ♿   RFE ♿

CHESTER VISITOR CENTRE
Vicars Lane, Chester CH1 1QX
Tel: (01244) 351609   Fax: (01244) 403188
e-mail: tic@chestercc.gov.uk
Video presentation introducing history,
main features and place of interest.

SD ♿   CP ♿   E ♿   RF ♿
C ♿   S ♿   WC ♿

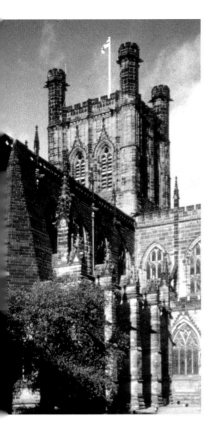

*Gothic as built, Chester's beautiful
cathedral.*

GREEN BOUGH HOTEL ♿
60 Hoole Road, Chester CH2 3NL
Tel: (01244) 326241   Fax: (01244) 326265
e-mail: luxury@greenbough.co.uk
www.greenbough.co.uk
No. of Accessible Rooms: 2
Accessible Facilities: Lounge, Dining room.
Elegant family-run hotel with homely
atmosphere in Victorian surroundings.
NB. Two steps into main entrance.

HOOLE HALL ♿
Warrington Road, Hoole, Chester CH2 3PD
Tel: (01244) 408800   Fax: (01244) 320251
No. of Accessible Rooms: 1. Roll-in
Shower. Accessible Facilities: Lounge,
Restaurant. Converted C18th manor
house set in five acres of grounds, two
miles from Chester.

ROWTON HALL HOTEL ♿
Whitchurch Road, Rowton, Chester CH3 6AD

MOULDSWORTH MOTOR MUSEUM
Smithy Lane, Mouldsworth CH3 8AR
Tel: (01928) 731781
Located six miles east of Chester and
housed in a 1937 art deco building, this is
a collection of vintage, post vintage,
classic cars, motorcycles and early bicycles.

SD ♿   CP ♿   E ♿   WC ♿

ZOOLOGICAL GARDENS
Upton-by-Chester, Chester CH2 1LH
Tel: (01244) 380280   Fax: (01244) 371274
e-mail: marketing@chesterzoo.co.uk
www.demon.co.uk/chesterzoo
The largest zoo in the UK, notable for
breeding rare and endangered species,
and an enormous variety of animals.
There is an excellent guide and map. With
the exception of waterbuses and Oakfield
WC, the zoo is accessible with long level
sections and gentle slopes. The ramps are
steep at orangutans, penguins, Europe of
the Edge Aviary, and at the Tropical Realm
and Exotic Birds sections. The overhead
railway is accessible, compartments will

take a wheelchair. A small, free fleet of four-wheel drive electric scooters is housed at the staff and pedestrian entrance at Caughall Road, not the main entrance, There are three reserved parking spaces close by, but book in advance. Adult wheelchairs are available for hire at low cost at the first-aid centre by the main entrance.

SD ♿ CP ♿ E ♿ RF ♿
C 🚶 S ♿ WC ♿

CONGLETON

Known for its cattle market. There are a few half-timbered houses remaining.

TOURIST INFORMATION CENTRE
Town Hall, High Street, Congleton CW12 1BN
Tel: (01260) 271095   Fax: (01260) 298243

BED & BREAKFAST
SANDHOLE FARM   🚶
Hulme Walfield, Congleton CW12 2JH
Tel: (01260) 224419   Fax: (01260) 224766
No. of Accessible Rooms: 2
Accessible Facilities: Lounge, Dining room.
Country farmhouse where an original L-shaped stable block has been converted.
.

ATTRACTION
LITTLE MORETON HALL (NT)
Congleton CW12 4SD
Tel: (01260) 272018
The most famous and probably the finest timber-framed moated manor house in the UK. Fine wall paintings and knot garden of particular note.

SD ♿ CP 🚶 E ♿ RF 🚶
C 🚶 S 🚶 WC ♿ RFE ♿

CREWE

Large industrial town, famous as a railway junction. Modern town centre.

HOTEL
OLD VICARAGE HOTEL   ♿
Knutsford Road, Cranage, Holmes Chapel, Crewe CW4 8EF

Tel: (01477) 532041 Fax: (01477) 535728
No. of Accessible Rooms: 1
Accessible Facilities: Lounge, Restaurant. C17th, Grade II listed building on the banks of the river Dane in the village of Cranage, Holmes Chapel. Located a mile from the M6 (J.18).

HUNTERS LODGE HOTEL   🚶
Sydney Road, Crewe CW1 1LU
Tel: (01270) 583440
No. of Accessible Rooms: 1. Bath
Accessible Facilities: Lounge, Restaurant. A rural family-run hotel, a mile from the city centre.

ATTRACTION
THE BOAT MUSEUM
South Pier Road, Ellesmere Port, CH65 4FW
Tel: (0151) 355 5017)   Fax: (0151) 355 4079
e-mail: bookings@thewaterwaytrust.org
www.boatmuseum.org.net
The history of Britain's canals brought to life in historic dock complex. Some pathways around site are cobbled and uneven. Access to the main exhibition displays and accessible route displayed on map given to all visitors. 2 manual wheelchairs available on site.

SD ♿ CP ♿ RF ♿ L ♿ C ♿
S ♿

MACCLESFIELD

Once a leading silk manufacturing town with good C18th and C19th mills remaining that contribute to the town's character. The Georgian Town Hall and the market cross, now situated in the West Park, are worth viewing. Also in the park are old iron stocks and a 30-ton boulder brought from Cumberland by ice-age glaciers. Macclesfield Forest, 5 miles east, is a tiny village on the edge of a wide stretch of wild country with crags and narrow valleys.

TOURIST INFORMATION CENTRE
Town Hall, Macclesfield SK10 1DX
Tel: (01625) 504114
Fax: (01625) 504116

SELF-CATERING
LOWER HOUSE COTTAGE
Wildboarclough, Nr. Macclesfield
SK11 0BL
Tel: (01260) 227229
No. of Accessible Units: 1. Roll-in-Shower
No. of Beds per Unit: 2 double beds but
only 1 single disabled person.
Accessible Facilities:
kitchen/sittingroom/garden.
Secluded cottage on the edge of the Peak
District. River nearby. Fishing included.

THE OLD BYRE
Pye Ash Farm, Leek Road, Bosley,
Macclesfield SK11 0PN
Tel: (01260) 273650 or (01260) 223293
No. of Accessible Units: 1. Roll-in shower.
No. of Beds per Unit: 5. Traditional
working farm on the edge of the Peak
District.

STRAWBERRY DUCK HOLIDAY
Bryher Cottage, Bullgate Lane, Bosley,
Macclesfield SK11 0PP
Tel: (01260) 223591
No. of Accessible Units: 1. Roll-in Shower
No. of Beds per Unit: 4.
Accessible Facilities: Lounge, Kitchen,
Patio.
Award-winning converted cottage close to
the Peak District National Park overlooking
Cheshire plain in the tiny village of Bosley.
Nearby there are pubs and restaurants
with wheelchair access.

ATTRACTION
JODRELL BANK SCIENCE CENTRE, PLANETARIUM and ARBORETUM
Lower Withington,
Nr. Macclesfield SK11 9DL
Tel: (01477) 571331 Fax: (01477 571695
e-mail: visitorcentre@jb.man.ac.uk
Focus of the centre is the Lovell telescope
receiving radio waves from deep space. At
the Science Centre explore the science of
Earth, energy and space and also enjoy the
Nature Experience. Divided into three
distinct categories – Exhibition Spaces,
Planetarium and Arboretum. Very
interactive and hands on.

SD   CP   E RF C n/a
S n/a WC RFE

MACCLESFIELD SILK MUSEUMS
The Heritage Centre, Roe Street,
Macclesfield SK11 6UT
Tel: (01625) 613210
Fax: (01625) 617880
e-mail: postmaster@silk-macc.u-net.com
www.silk-macclesfield.org
Three galleries display the story of silk
through AV programmes, exhibitions,
textiles, clothes and room settings.
Steep steps in front of entrance, with
access through the garden to right of
entrance. First two galleries linked by
ramp. Basement galleries accessed by
chairlift.

SD ⬚ CP ⬚ E ⬚ RF ⬚
C ⬚ S ⬚ WC ⬚ L ⬚

NANTWICH
Old market town on the River Weaver,
surrounded by rich agricultural area
producing the famous Cheshire cheese.
A fire in 1583 destroyed many original
buildings, but rebuilding gave the town
a wealth of Elizabethan structures still
standing.

TOURIST INFORMATION CENTRE
Church House, Church Walk,
Nantwich CW5 5RG
Tel: (01270) 610983   Fax: (01270) 610880

HOTELS
ROOKERY HALL
Worleston, Nantwich CW5 6DQ
Tel: (01270) 610016
Fax: (01270) 626027
www.rookeryhallhotel.com
No. of Accessible Rooms: 30. Bath
Accessible Facilities: Lounge, Restaurant.
Luxury award winning hotel set in 200
acres of countryside.

THE PEACOCK
221 Crewe Road, Nantwich CW5 6NE
Tel: (01270) 624069
Fax: (01270) 610113
No. of Accessible Rooms: 2. Bath
Accessible Facilities: Restaurant
Located .5 miles from Nantwich, good
location for Wales and the Potteries.

ATTRACTION
STAPELEY WATER GARDENS and PALMS TROPICAL OASIS
London Road, Stapeley,
Nantwich CW5 7LH
Tel: (01270) 623868   Fax: (01270) 624919
Glass pavilion of the Palm Tropical Oasis is home to exotic flowers, fish and birds, plus two-acre Water Garden centre housing, among other things, the national collection of water-lilies.

CP [&]   E [&]   C [&]   S [&]   WC [人]

NORTHWICH
Old town recently modernised. Shopping centre. Black and white houses also are modern but give the town an historic feel.

TOURIST INFORMATION CENTRE
1 The Arcade, Northwich
Tel: (01606) 353500

HOTEL
QUALITY HOTEL NORTHWICH   [人]
London Road, Northwich CW9 5HD
Tel: (01606) 44443
No. of Accessible Rooms: 2
Accessible Facilities: Lounge (ground fl.) Restaurant, Bar (1st floor, via lift)
Unique floating hotel on River Weaver

ACCESSIBLE ATTRACTIONS
ARLEY HALL AND GARDENS
Nr. Northwich CW9 6NA
Tel: (01565) 777353   Fax: (01565) 777465
The Hall, replacing a Tudor version, is Jacobean in style with fine ceilings, oak panelling and a splendid library. The gardens, that have evolved since Tudor times, are notable for a double herbaceous border laid in 1846. Ninety per cent accessible with only rootery and sundial garden inaccessible.

SD [&]   CP [&]   E [&]   RF [&]
C [人]   S [&]   WC [人]   RFE (gardens) [人]

BLAKEMERE CRAFT CENTRE
Chester Road, Sandiway,
Northwich CW8 2EB
Tel: (01606) 883261

Fax: (01606) 301495
Over 30 shops set around charming Edwardian stables. Huge selection of unusual items from antique beds to ladies fashions and handmade chocolates to fine art. Numerous craft workshops where you can watch craftsmen at work. Large Garden Centre as well as an Aquatic and Falconry Centre with birds of prey flying displays and aviaries. Children's indoor playbarn. Excellent restaurant and coffee shop.

SD [&]   CP [&]   E [&]   RF [&]   L [人]
C [&]   S [&]   WC [人]   RFE [&]

NORTON PRIORY MUSEUM and GARDENS
Tudor Road, Manor Park, Runcorn WA7 18X
Tel: (01928) 569895
Fax:(01982) 589743
e-mail: info@nortonpriory.org
www.nortonpriory.org
In this C12th home Augustinian canons, stone masons and tile makers were commissioned to decorate the priory church. The museum displays examples of their work, plus a model of the priory. 16 acres of lovely woodland gardens with contemporary sculpture trail. The mid C18th walled garden has themed areas including old roses and herbaceous borders. Sensory garden for under-fives. A truly tranquil place.

SD [&]   CP [&]   RF [&]   C [&]   S [&]
E [人] (ramped at gradient of 1:11)
WC [&]   RFE [&]

SANDBACH
Small historic town with winding streets, cobbled market place and timbered houses.

HOTEL
SAXON CROSS HOTEL   [人]
Holmes Chapel Road, Sandbach CW11 9SE
Tel: (01270) 763281
ax: (01270) 768723
No. of Accessible Rooms: 34. Bath
Accessible Facilities: Lounge, Restaurant
Modern ground-storey building situated close to the M6 motorway

STYAL

Picturesque little village with white cottages and an old mill that stands where the River Bollen flows swiftly through a deep wooded glen.

ATTRACTION
STYAL COUNTRY PARK and QUARRY (NT)
Stya, Wilmslow, Cheshire SK9 4LA
Tel: (01625) 52746 Fax: (01625) 539267
e-mail: enquiries@quarrybankmill.org.uk
www.quarrybankmill.org.uk
The Greg family gave the Styal Estate that includes the mill and mill workers' village, plus surrounding woods and farmland, to the NT in 1939, and little has changed since. In the deep valley and woodlands are fields, ponds, flowers and birds. Discover how cotton is made into cloth. Use the mill entrance and the mill kitchen for access to catering. WC is in the inner yard opposite the mill kitchen. The route for wheelchair-bound visitors includes a step-lift and runs through the heart of the mill on one level. The mini-tour is quite arduous, but ramps and seats are provided wherever possible throughout the museum. Outdoor Attractions: via Twinnies Bridge Car Park (0.25 mile from the main entrance), leading to a special wheelchair route through willow Ground Wood to the mill pool. There is no access through to the mill yard.

SD 🦽   CP 🦽   E 🦽   RF 🦽   L 🚶
C 🚶   S n/a   WC 🚶   RFE 🦽

TARPORLEY

Regular winner of Best Kept Village in Cheshire competition.

HOTELS
THE SWAN   🚶
50 High Street, Tarporley CW6 0AG
Tel: (01829) 733838   Fax: (01829) 732932
No. of Accessible Rooms: 3
Accessible Facilities: Lounge, Restaurant
C16th coaching inn in the centre of a charming Georgian village. The hotel has been home to England's oldest Hunt Club since the late 18th century.

WILD BOAR HOTEL   🚶
Whitchurch Road, Beeston,
Tarporley CW6 9NW
Tel: (01829) 260309 Fax: (01829) 261081
No. of Accessible Rooms: 10
Accessible Facilities: Lounge, Restaurant, Bar, Grounds.
C18th Tudor building with modern extensions made to integrate with original building style.

WARRINGTON

An industrial town with the locks of the Manchester Ship Canal.

HOLIDAY INN WARRINGTON   🚶
Woolston Grange Avenue, Woolston,
Warrington WA1 4PX
Tel: (01925) 838779 Fax: (01925) 838859
No. of Accessible Rooms: 1. Bath
Accessible Facilities: Lounge, Restaurant.
Modern comfortable hotel.

HANOVER INTERNATIONAL   🚶
Stretton Road, Stretton, Warrington WA4 4NS
Tel: (01925) 730706 Fax: (01925) 730740
No. of Accessible Rooms: 1. Bath
Accessible Facilities: Lounge, Restaurant.
Once the site of an old vicarage and adjacent to C19th church, set in 40 acres of grounds and situated two minutes from the M56 (J10) in a picturesque village.

BED AND BREAKFAST
TALL TREES LODGE   🚶
Tarporley Road, Lower Whitley,
Warrington WA4 4EZ
Tel: (01928) 790824 Fax: (01928) 791330
e-mail:info@talltreeslodge.co.uk
www.talltreeslodge.co.uk
No. of Accessible Rooms: 1.
Accessible Facilities: Breakfast Room.
Family-run lodge in Cheshire's heartland on the A49, south of M56 (J.10) and 10 minutes from Warrington.

ATTRACTIONS
GULLIVER'S WORLD
Warrington WA5 5YZ
Tel: (01925) 230088 Fax: (01925) 637354
Family theme park aimed at children

between three and 14 with over 40 exciting rides, All rides have at least one step.

SD ♿ CP 🚶 E 🚶 RF ♿
C ♿ S ♿ WC 🚶

WALTON HALL GARDENS
Walton Lea Road, Higher Walton,
Warrington WA4 6SN
Tel: (01925) 601617   Fax: (01925) 861868
e-mail: waltonhall@warrington.gov.uk
Located in the heart of the Mersey Forest, with mature parkland and ornamental gardens with trees and shrubs from all over the world, plus spacious lawns, picnic areas, children's zoo, heritage centre. The hall is not open to the public, but the gardens are.

SD ♿ CP ♿ E ♿ RF ♿ C ♿ S ♿
WC ♿ RFE (heritage centre, children's zoo) ♿

WIDNES
Located between Runcorn and Liverpool.

TOURIST INFORMATION CENTRE
Tel: (01928) 576776

HOTEL
EVERGLADES PARK HOTEL   ♿
Derby Road, Widnes WA8 3UJ
Tel: (0151) 4952040   Fax: (0151) 4955501
No. of Accessible Rooms: 4. Bath
Accessible Facilities: Lounge, Restaurant
Modern, private hotel in the country, a few minutes from the M62 (J7) and close to the town centre.

ATTRACTIONS
SCIENCE DISCOVERY CENTRE
Gossage Building, Mersey Road,
Widnes WA8 0DF
Tel: (0151) 4201121   Fax: (0151) 4952030
e-mail: info@catalyst.org.uk
Previous winner of the Northwest Tourism Visitor Attraction of the Year. Science and technology come alive here through a host of interactive exhibits and hands-on displays that you can tug, tease and test. Explore the impact of chemicals on everyday life through scenes from the past and multi-media programmes. There are panoramic views across the River Mersey from the roof-top observatory. The route from the car park, that has designated spaces, is along a sloping path of about 100m, with a gradient of 1:29 to the entrance. There are handrails both sides of the path. There is also close street parking available at the side of the museum. There are two wheelchairs on site, and level access to the first-floor gallery and observatory is via a glass lift.

SD ♿ CP ♿ E ♿ RF ♿
L ♿ (non-motorised chairs) C ♿
S ♿ WC ♿

SPIKE ISLAND
Mersey Road, Widnes
Tel: (0151) 4203707
Just below the Science Discovery Service with shared car parking, Spike Island was the birthplace of the British chemical industry. In late C19th it was dominated by huge factories, and a maze of railway lines crossed the Sankey Canal. By the early C20th more efficient processes made the old factories obsolete. In 1975 the land was reclaimed and Spike Island was transformed into acres of grassland, woodland and watersides. There is a ramped visitor centre alongside the Sankey Canal with exhibitions that bring to life the extraordinary history of the island. This is a lovely quiet area for watching wildlife or to sit and let the world go by.

WILMSLOW
Small town, outwardly a modern shopping centre, in the deep valley of the Bollin river.

HOTEL
DEAN BANK HOTEL   ♿
Adlington Road, Wilmslow SK9 2BT
Tel: (01625) 524268
No. of Accessible Rooms: 3. Roll-in shower. Accessible Facilities: Restaurant Family-run hotel in a countryside location, ten minutes from Manchester Airport.

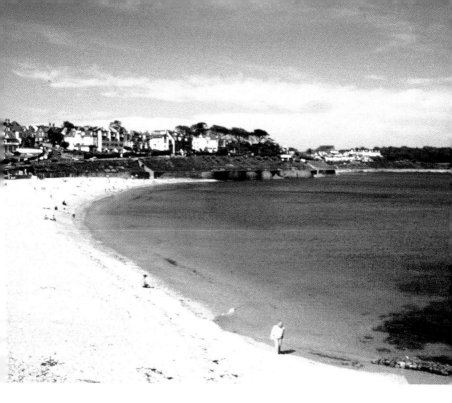

Falmouth, a beach of perfect childhood memories.

CORNWALL

CORNWALL TOURIST BOARD
Pydar House, Pydar Street, Truro TR1 1EA
Tel: (01872) 274057   Fax: (01872) 322895
e-mail: tourism@cornwallenterprise.co.uk
www.cornwalltouristboard.co.uk

DIAN (DISABILITY INFORMATION AND ADVICE NETWORK)
Poniou Way, Long Rock Industrial Estate,
Penzance, TR20 8HX
Tel: (01736) 359077
ALLDIS publish "Discover" at Marie Therese
House. Tel: (01736) 759113.

AGE CONCERN
5a Little Castle Street, Truro TR1 3DL
Tel: (01872) 223388
Provide minibuses with lifts, clamp and
ramps in Bodmin, Falmouth, Launceston,
Liskeard, Newquay, Penzance, St. Austell
and Truro.

CORNWALL FRIENDS MOBILITY CENTRE
Tel: (01872) 254920
Fax: (01872) 254921
e-mail: mobility@rcht.swest.nhs.uk
Offers breakdown service for
wheelchairs, scooters etc.

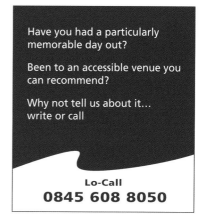

Have you had a particularly
memorable day out?

Been to an accessible venue you
can recommend?

Why not tell us about it…
write or call

Lo-Call
0845 608 8050

SPECIAL NEEDS SERVICES
Tel: (01872) 575085
Based in Falmouth, working with Tripscope. Will do anything, go anywhere, including nursing home transfer.

BUSES
TravelineSW (0870) 6082608
Truronian have one route (T1), Perranporth to The Lizard, that has raised kerbs for access by motorised wheelchairs at principal stops. This and other routes operate Easy Access buses that kneel at ordinary stops enabling wheelchairs to be pushed on board.

TRAVELINE
Information on transport in the region
Tel: (0870) 6082608

FERRIES
All local ferry operators are willing to assist passengers with difficulties, but many embarkation points are inaccessible because of steep steps, rocks, beaches etc.
Helford Passage-Helford Village: steep steps.
St Maws-Place: inaccessible. Falmouth-Flushing: steep steps. Feock-Philleigh: steep slope at low water, easier at high tide, but only from a car. Fowey-Polruan: steep steps. Fowey-Bodinnick: Car ferry. Plymouth-Mt. Edgcumbe: possible except at very low tide. Plymouth-Torpoint: car ferry. Padstow-Rock: inaccessible.

Rush hour at Looe harbour.

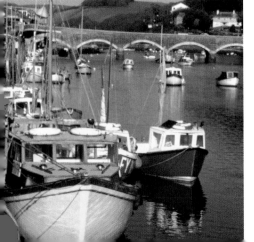

SPECIALIST OUTDOOR ACTIVITIES
CHURCHTOWN
Lanlivery, Bodmin PL30 5BT
Tel: (01208) 872148   Fax: (01208) 873377
This is Scope's accessible Adventure and outdoor education centre. Accessible residential courses for disabled persons with activities options including sailing, canoeing, orienteering, rock climbing, swimming, hands on farming.

BOSCASTLE
This is a classic beauty spot with a charming small harbour and old stone cottages. The main area of the village is in steep woods behind the harbour. It has very old houses and an unusual long, broad street that climbs straight and steeply up the hill.
A car is essential.

TOURIST INFORMATION CENTRE
Cobweb Car Park, Boscastle PL35 0HE
Tel/Fax: (01840) 250010

HOTEL
THE OLD COACH HOUSE
Tintagel Road, Boscastle PL35 0AS
Tel: (01840) 250398   Fax: (01840) 250346
info@old-coach.co.uk
www.old-coach.co.uk
No. of Accessible Rooms: 2. Roll-in shower. Accessible Facilities: Lounge. Set in a beautiful former coach house of the early 1700s, that has been now been restored and fully modernised.
NB: No dining room, breakfast is served in the conservatory.

FALMOUTH
In a beautiful setting with a large natural harbour and the most temperate climate of any British resort, Falmouth has beaches, public gardens, scattered hotels and villas lying on the south side, while in the north there are harbours and docks backed by a shopping centre and charming narrow streets.

TOURIST INFORMATION CENTRE
28 Killigrew Street, Falmouth TR11 3PN
Tel: (01326) 312300   Fax: (01326) 313457

BUSES
Truronian: Tel: (01872) 273453
Some easy-access buses.

TAXIS
Special Needs Services
(see under country heading)
Abacus Cabs: Tel: (01326) 212141
Adapted cab.
Falmouth and Penryn Radio Taxis:
Tel: (01326) 315194
3 taxis with ramps.
Kendall, DR: Tel: (01326) 316610
1 TXI.

TRAINS
Wales & West: Special Needs –
Tel: (0845) 3003005
Minicom: (0845) 7585469
Both Falmouth stations have ramps.

HOTEL
BROADMEAD HOTEL
Kimberely Park Road, Falmouth TR11 2DD
Tel: (01326) 315704   Fax: (01326) 311048
e-mail: broadmeadhotel@aol.com
No. of Accessible Rooms: 2. Bath.
Accessible Facilities: Lounge, Restaurant
Small hotel near town centre. One step at
entrance, double doors.

HELSTON
Delightful town, its most interesting
streets being the main one,
Coinagehall and Cross Streets,
boasting lovely shops and a pleasant
stroll.

HELSTON, LIZARD PENINSULA AND TIN MINING COUNTRY TOURIST INFORMATION CENTRE
79 Meneage Street, Helston TR13 8RS
Tel: (01326) 565431   Fax: (01326) 572803

ATTRACTION
FLAMBARDS VILLAGE THEME PARK
Culdrose Manor, Helston TR13 0QA

Tel: (01326) 573404   Fax: (01326) 573344
e-mail: info@flambards.co.uk
www.flambards.co.uk
Three themed attraction areas, Flambards
Victorian village, Britain in the Blitz and
Cornwall Aero park together with many
rides.

SD | CP | E | RF
S | WC | RFE

LAUNCESTON
The town stands on a hill crowned by
the ruins of its castle. The present
town is an agricultural centre with a
weekly market. It is an extremely
attractive town with narrow streets
and interesting buildings.
Outstanding among these is the St.
Mary Magdalene Church, unique
except for its C14th tower. Its outside
walls are entirely covered with
carvings.

TOURIST INFORMATION CENTRE
Market House Arcade, Market Street
Launceston PL15 8EP
Tel: (01566) 772321
Fax: (01566) 772322

SELF-CATERING
ROUNDHOUSE COTTAGE
Trenannick Cottages, Trenannick,
Warbstow, Launceston PL15 8RP
Tel/Fax: (01566) 781443
No. of Accessible Units: 1
No. of Beds per Unit: 2 + sofa bed
Accessible Facilities: Roll-in Shower,
Lounge, Kitchen/Diner, Gardens. Situated
at the end of a private drive in a south
facing hollow, the cottages are converted
from C18th farm buildings in three acres
of grounds. Roundhouse Cottage was
once the building that ground corn and
was operated by a horse walking in a
circle – hence the name. At the rear is the
main building with its own drive and
garden and a huge oak beam running
through its centre. Space is limited in the
bedroom and bathroom but the cottage
has wide doors, low work surfaces etc. -
ideal for the disabled traveller.

LISKEARD

Progressive small town, lively in atmosphere with some pleasant Georgian and Victorian architecture. Hosts the busiest livestock market in East Cornwall.

HOTEL
WHEALTOR HOTEL
Caradon Hill, Pensilia, Liskeard, PL14 5PJ
Tel: (01579) 36228
No of accessible rooms:7
Accessible Facilites: Lounge, Bar, Restaurant. Purpose built, small moorland hotel.

SELF-CATERING
Rosecraddoc Lodge
Liskeard PL14 5BU
Tel/Fax: (01579) 346768
No. of Accessible Units: 1 with bath
No of Beds per Unit: 5
Accessible Facilites: Kitchen-Living Room,Dining Room, level lawn and patio. Rosecraddoc, an area of rolling farmland,is two miles north-east of Liskeard. The modern, traditionally built bungalows are situated in gardens and woodland, once part of Rosemaddoc Manor grounds. Pets welcome.

Looe
This tourist-orientated fishing port and seaside resort becomes very overcrowded in summer, but is a delightful spot.

TOURIST INFORMATION CENTRE
The Guildhall, Fore Street, East Looe
Tel: (01503) 072262
Fax: (01503) 265426 - seasonal

SELF-CATERING
PENVITH BARN COTTAGES
St Martins by Looe, Looe PL13 1NZ
Tel: (01503) 240772
e-mail: anne@penvith.demon.co.uk
www.pilgrims.com/penvith-barns
No. of Accessible Units: 2

No of Beds per Unit: 5
Accessible Facilities: Open Plan Kitchen, Lounge, Patio, Swallow and Owl barn. Cottages have been converted from a part C16th stone barn. Facing south, they overlook open paddocks, a small copse and a field and are set in lovely unspoilt countryside. Three miles' drived from Looe.

GRANITE HENGE BUNGALOWS
Trelawne Cross, Looe PL13 2BT
Tel: (01503) 272772   Fax: (01503) 272060
No. of Accessible Units: 10. Shower
No. of Beds per Unit: 9 x 4 beds: 1 x 8 beds.
Accessible Facilities: Lounge, Dining Room, Pool. Situated on the edge of National Trust countryside, 5 minutes from Looe and Polperro. Small, privately owned holiday complex of 10 cottage style bungalows with heated pool and peaceful gardens.

BOCADDON FARM COTTAGES
Bocaddon Farm, Lanreath, Looe PL13 2PG
Tel/Fax: (01503) 220245
e-mail: alimaik@aol.com
No. of Accessible Units: 1. Roll-in Shower.
No. of Beds per Unit: 4
Accessible Facilities: Kitchen/Living Area. Stone barn conversion on 350-acre dairy farm, seven miles from Looe. Lanreath village is a quiet backwater with tea rooms, farm and country museum and shop.

ATTRACTION
LANREATH FOLK and FARM MUSEUM
Nr. Looe PL13 2NX
Tel: (01503) 220321
Hands-on exhibits reflect Cornwall's history. Facilities are limited, there is no catering, shop or WC, but this is worth a visit.

SD   CP   E

NEWQUAY
The county's most popular seaside resort. Wonderful beaches, renowned for surfing.

TOURIST INFORMATION CENTRE
Municipal Offices, Marcus Hill,
Newquay TR7 1BD
Tel: (01637) 854020
Fax: (01637) 854030
e-mail: info@newquay.co.uk

BUSES
Western Greyhound. Tel: (01637) 871871

TAXIS
Summercourt Travel: Tel: (01726) 861108

TRAINS
Virgin Trains (summer Saturdays only):
Special Needs – Tel: (0845) 7443366
Minicom: (0845) 7443367
Wales & West – Special Needs:
Tel: (0845) 3003005
Minicom: (0845) 7585469
Newquay station has a ramp.

HOTEL
CHYNOWETH LODGE HOTEL
1 Eliot Gardens, Newquay TR7 2QE
Tel: (01637) 876684
No. of Accessible Rooms: 1. Bath.
Accessible Facilities: Lounge. Small,
family-owned hotel of 9 rooms with en-
suite facilities, centrally heated in flat,
residential area near Tolcarne beach. Car
park. N.B. Non smoking.

ATTRACTION
NEWQUAY ZOO
Trenance Park, Newquay TR7 2LZ
Tel: (01637) 873342
Fax: (01637) 851318
e-mail: info@newquayzoo.co.uk
www.newquayzoo.co.uk
Preservation is a major issue here where
attractions include penguin pool, monkey,
lion and tropical houses, together with a
maze, assault course and oriental garden.

SD   CP    E   RF
C 🚶   S ♿   WC 🚶   RFE 🚶

TRERICE (NT)
Kestle Mill, Newquay TR8 4PG
Tel: (01637) 875404
Fax: (01637) 879300
Three miles from Newquay, tucked away
among narrow lanes, is this Elizabethan
manor house built in 1571 with Dutch-
style gabled façade, elaborate plaster
ceilings, fine C17th and C18th oak and
walnut furniture and oriental and English
porcelain to view. In the garden there is a
picnic area and a lawnmower museum.
Two wheelchairs are available along with a
useful map/leaflet on access.

SD ♿   CP   E   RF
C ♿   S   WC 🚶

PADSTOW
North coast fishing town with
unspoiled narrow streets converging
on its harbour.

TOURIST INFORMATION CENTRE
Red Brick Building, North Quay, Padstow
Tel: (01841) 533449
Fax: (01841) 532356
e-mail: padstowtic@visit.org.uk

SELF-CATERING
TREGINEGAR HOLIDAY BUNGALOWS ♿
St. Merryn, Nr. Padstow PL28 8PT
Tel/Fax: (01841) 521042
No. of Accessible Units: 4
No. of Beds per Unit: 4. Roll-in Shower
Accessible Facilities: Lounge, Kitchen.
Situated off the beaten track in rural
surroundings, four miles from Padstow, 12
from Newquay. Within a two-mile radius
are seven superb bays with clean sandy
beaches.

TREVORRICK FARM 🚶
St. Issey, Nr. Padstow PL27 7QH
Tel/Fax: (01841) 540574
info@trevorrick.co.uk
www.trevorrick.co.uk
No. of Accessible Units: 1. Bath
No. of Beds per Unit: 4/5
Accessible Facilities: Lounge/Diner,
Kitchen. Serendipity Cottage is a bow-
windowed cottage, one of six stone
cottages converted from old farm
buildings and arranged around a central
garden alongside an C18th farmhouse.
Situated near Camel Estuary overlooking
Petherick Creek, a haven for wildlife.
Padstow and great beaches close by.

REDRUTH

Known for its copper mining, there are traces of a major iron-age fort, hut circles and a semi-ruined castle.

ATTRACTION
CORNISH MINES AND ENGINES (NT)
Agar Road, Pool, Redruth TR15 3EB
Tel/Fax: (01209) 315027

Enormous beam engines used in tin mining industry for pumping water and lifting men and ore from workings below ground.

ST. AUSTELL

China and clay capital with pedestrian precinct of overhead walkways and plenty of modern buildings. Close to Porthpean and Kopehaven seaside spots.

TOURIST INFORMATION CENTRE
14 Church Street, Mevagissey PL26 6SP or By-Pass Service Station, Southbourne Road, St. Austell PL25 4RS
Tel/Fax: (01726) 879500

ATTRACTION
THE LOST GARDENS OF HELIGAN
Pentewan, St. Austell PL26 6EN
Tel: (01726) 845100 Fax: (01726) 845101
e-mail: info@heligan.com

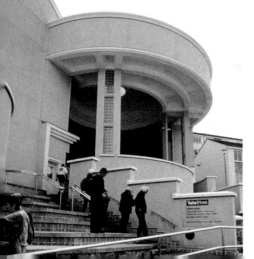

The Tate Gallery at St. Ives.

Over 80 acres of beautiful gardens and grounds including walled gardens with exotic fruit houses, kitchen, grotto, Italian and sundial gardens. Also a 22-acre sub-tropical jungle garden and 30-acre lost valley – a natural woodland. Large areas of the gardens are accessible and not to be missed. Wheelchairs available for loan.

THE EDEN PROJECT
Bodelva, St. Austell PL24 2SG
Tel: (01726) 811911
Fax: (01726) 811912
www.edenproject.com

The Eden Project is a global garden for the 21st Century, a gateway to a sustainable future and a dramatic setting in which to tell the fascinating story of mankind's dependence on plants.

This living theatre of plants and people is a vibrant reminder of our place in nature and is a living demonstration of regeneration.

In a couple of years the team transformed an exhausted clay pit into a stunning lost world reminding us of what we 'ordinary' people can do once we set our minds to it. Space age technology meets the lost world in the biggest greenhouse ever built.

Located in a 50 metre deep crater the size of 30 football pitches and beautifully sculpted to make a spectacular and unique global garden.

80% of the Eden Project is accessible to visitors with mobility difficulties. For further information please visit the website or call (01726) 811911.

ST. IVES

The shape and situation of this town is magnificent and remains mostly unspoilt. Streets are narrow and steep leading to excellent shops and museums.

TOURIST INFORMATION CENTRE
The Guildhall, Street-an-Pol, St. Ives
TR26 2DS
Tel: (01736) 796297
Fax: (01736) 798309

HOTEL
CHY-an-DOUR HOTEL ♿
Trelyon Avenue TR26 2AD
Tel: (01736) 796436   Fax: (01736) 795772
No. of Accessible Rooms: 1. Roll-in
Shower. Accessible Facilities: Lounge,
Restaurant. C19th former sea captain's
house extended to form an attractive
hotel with panoramic views of St. Ives Bay,
Porthminster beach and harbour. NB:
town centre and beaches are downhill.

ATTRACTION
TATE GALLERY ST. IVES
Porthmeor Beach, St. Ives TR26 1TG
Tel: (01736) 796226   Fax: (01736) 794480
www.tate.org.uk
The gallery, opened in June 1993,
presents modern art created in or
associated with Cornwall. It is a striking
building, full of light and intriguing
perspectives. There are no permanent
collections, displays are based on selected
works from the Tate Gallery's national
collection that also includes loans from
other public or private collections. The
gallery also presents works by
contemporary artists.
Facilities are accessible by the lift.

 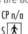 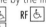

SD 👤   CP n/a   e ♿   RF 👤   I ♿
C 🚶   S 🚶   WC 🚶

TRURO
Commercial and administrative centre
of the county with a three-spired
cathedral completed in 1910.
Georgian townhouses, pedestrianised
shopping and Victoria Gardens add to
the town's ambience.

TOURIST INFORMATION CENTRE
Tel: (01872) 274555

BUSES
Truronian City Service (T5):
Tel: (01872) 273453
Regular easy access buses.

TAXIS
City Taxis: Tel: (0800) 318708
1 metrocab with ramp.

TRAINS
Virgin Trains: Special Needs –
Tel: (0845) 7443366
Minicom: (0845) 7443367
Wales & West: Special Needs –
Tel: (0845) 3003005
Minicom: (0845) 7585469

ATTRACTIONS
ROYAL CORNWALL MUSEUM
River Street, Truro TR1 2SJ
Tel: (01872) 272205   Fax: (01872) 240514
Fine displays covering Cornish history
particularly mining, including the well-known
Rashleigh mineral collection. Fine art, ceramics,
natural history and special exhibitions.

CP n/a   E 👤   RF ♿
L ♿   C 👤   S 🚶   WC ♿

TRELISSICK GARDEN (NT)
Feock, Truro TR3 6QL
Tel: (01872) 862090   Fax: (01872) 865808
A garden within a 500-acre estate of park
and farmland, particularly famous for its
large collection of hydrangeas and
rhododendrons and exotic plants, plus a
Cornish apple orchard.

CP ♿   E 👤   RF 👤   C 👤
S 👤   WC 🚶   RFE (garden) ♿

TREWITHEN GARDENS
Grampound Road, Truro TR2 4DD
Tel: (01726) 883647   Fax: (01726) 882301
e-mail: gardens@trewithen-
estate.demon.co.uk
www.trewithengardens.co.uk
Renowned 30-acre landscaped garden
with many rare trees and shrubs.

SD 👤   CP 🚶   E 👤   RF 👤
C 👤   S 🚶   WC 🚶   RFE 👤

The amazing Eden project

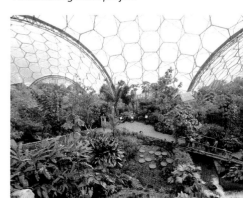

COUNTY DURHAM

An area of 861 square miles, Co. Durham is recognised as an area of outstanding natural beauty.

CO. DURHAM TOURISM
County Hall, Durham DH1 5UF
Tel: (0191) 3833698   Fax: (0191) 3833657
e-mail:tourism@durham.gov.uk
www.durham.gov.uk

NORTHUMBRIA TOURISM
www.ntb.org.uk

ACCESS DIRECTORY
Tel: (0191) 3833337.
Much information on transport services throughout County Durham available from Miss Chris Graham, The Public Transport Group, Durham City Council.

BARNARD CASTLE
Picturesque town, an excellent base for discovering the delights of Teesdale. Lovely riverside walks here, especially to Egglestone Abbey on the Yorkshire side.

TOURIST INFORMATION CENTRE
Woodleigh, Flats Road,
Barnard Castle DL12 8AA
Tel: (01833) 690909
Fax: (01833) 695320

SELF-CATERING
EAST BRISCOE FARM COTTAGES
Baldersdale, Barnard Castle DL12 9UL
Tel: (01833) 650087
e-mail: pejowi@aol.com
No. of Accessible Units: 2. Bath.
Low Barn Cottage
Studio Cottage
Situated in beautiful Teesdale, on a 14-acre Riverside estate, this 1713 farmhouse and its adjoining barns were converted in the early 90s to charming cottages. In 1998 they received the Northumbrian TB Self-Catering of the Year special award. Each cottage has access to a patio area, a shared conservatory and lawned garden. Explore the estate's fields and woods where you can. Cotherstone, two miles away, has pubs and a shop: four miles farther on is Barnard Castle, a popular market town.

ATTRACTION
THE BOWES MUSEUM
Barnard Castle DL12 8NP
Tel: (01833) 690606
Fax: (01833) 637163
French chateau-style mansion built in 1869, housing a fine collection of paintings by El Greco, Goya, Canaletto and others, plus porcelain and silver, furniture, ceramics and tapestries.

SD n/a   CP 🚶   E ♿   RF ♿   L 🚶
C 🚶   S ♿   WC 🚶   RFE ♿

BISHOP AUCKLAND
Country home of bishops of Durham since C12th with Auckland Castle, their official residence, surrounded by 800-acre Bishops' Park.

TOURIST INFORMATION CENTRE
Town Hall, Market Place,
Bishop Auckland DL14 7NP
Tel: (01388) 604922

HOTEL
REDWORTH HALL HOTEL   ♿
Redworth, County Durham DL5 6NL
Tel: (01388) 772442
Fax: (01388) 770654
No. of Accessible Rooms: 3. Accessible Facilities: Restaurants (2), Bar, Health Club (disabled chair lift into pool).
Imposing and impressive Elizabethan-style manor built around a 300-year-old great hall in 25 acres of woodland. Located a few miles south of Bishop Auckland on A6072.

CHESTER-LE-STREET
Old historic town with stone beach, a market place for surrounding areas.

HOTEL
THE OAK TREE INN   🚶
Tantobie, Stanley DH9 9RF
Tel: (01207) 235445
No. of Accessible Rooms: 1
Accessible Facilities: Lounge,
Once a manor house dating from 1700,
now carefully restored and furnished with
antiques. 25 minutes' drive from Beamish
and 20 minutes from Durham.

ATTRACTION
BEAMISH, NORTH OF ENGLAND OPEN AIR
MUSEUM
Beamish, DH9 0RG
Tel: (01207) 231811   Fax: (01207) 290933
e-mail:museum@beamish.org.uk
www.beamish.org.uk
Award-winning museum set in 300 acres
recreating northern life in early C19th and
C20th. Six main areas; The Town, Colliery
Village, Home Farm, Pockerly Manor,
Railway Station and 1825 Railway, a
replica of Stephenson's Locomotion No 1,
the world's first passenger train. Linked by
footpaths, a bus and circular tram track.
Very large open-air site with some steep
gradients, not ideal for wheelchairs, but
the museum provides a good leaflet for
visitors with mobility problems and it is
worth the effort to see it. The town is
cobbled, and co-op shops are accessible
from the street. Sweet shop/factory is
accessible from an alley on the RHS of the
shop. The garage is accessible from street.
The Sun Inn pub (no food) is accessible on
the ground floor.
Colliery Village – The pit yard surface is
crushed stone. The chapel/school is
accessible from the rear. The pit cottages
have steps, so look in the windows.
Colliery – The surface is crushed stone, the
engine shed and drift mine are accessible.
Home Farm – Not accessible, there is a
steep slope of 60m from the tram stop.
Manor – Rest stops on steep slope of
100m. Gardens and ground floor are
accessible, Old House isn't.

*One of the many attractions at the
award winning Beamish Museum*

DURHAM
One of the most visually exciting
university cities in the UK, this was
once a secure fortress against the Scots
and Danes. Towering above a loop in
the river Wear, Durham Cathedral, with
the castle close by, gives a fine sense of
Norman splendour.

TOURIST INFORMATION CENTRE
Millenium Place, Co Durham DH1 3NJ
Tel: (0191) 3843720

TRAVELINE
Tel: (0870) 6082608

BUSES
General Information: Tel: (0191) 3833337
Arriva: Tel: (0800) 085110
Super low-floor services
Stagecoach: Tel: (0191) 2761411
Super low-floor services
Go Northern: Tel: (0845) 6060260

TAXIS
Nova Travel: Tel: (01207) 270327
2 Renault Master vehicles.
Nightingale Coaches: Tel: (01207) 529729
11 vehicles with all fittings, various sizes.

TRAINS
Great North Eastern Railway: Special Needs –
Tel: (0845) 7225444
Minicom: (0191) 2330173

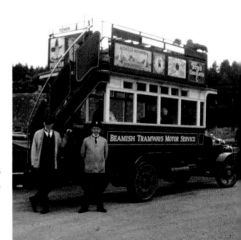

Virgin Trains: Special Needs –
Tel: (0845) 7443366
Minicom: (0845) 7443367

CAR PARKS
Free disabled badge parking in all council car parks.

HOTEL ACCOMMODATION
DURHAM MARRIOTT HOTEL ROYAL COUNTY
♿
Old Elvet, Durham DH1 3JN
Tel: (0191) 386 6821
No. of Accessible Rooms: 1. Bath
Accessible Facilities: Lounge, Restaurant
Elegant city-centre hotel overlooking River Wear, rich with antiques and paintings.

CROSSWAYS HOTEL and RESTAURANT ♿
Dunelm Road, Thornley,
Nr. Durham DH6 3HT
Tel: (01429) 821248   Fax: (01429) 820034
No. of Accessible Rooms: 1. Bath.
Accessible Facilities: Lounge, Restaurant
Family-owned and managed country hotel five miles east of Durham, originally one of 21 public houses existing during the hay-days of the mining industry. A dog track existed alongside the pub and greyhound racing remains very popular with a track about 2 miles away .

RAMSIDE HALL HOTEL and GOLF CLUB 🚶
Carrville, Durham DH1 1TD
Tel: (0191) 3865282   Fax: (0191) 3860399
e-mail: ramsidehall@easynet.co.uk
www.ramsidehall.co.uk
No. of Accessible Rooms: 2. Bath
Accessible Facilities: Lounge (three steps or portable ramp): Restaurants (three steps, portable ramp for upper and lower levels).
Charming private hotel with lovely gardens leading down to the river.

BED AND BREAKFAST
THE BRACKEN GUEST HOUSE 🚶
Bank Foot, Shincliffe, Durham DH1 2PB
Tel: (0191) 3862966   Fax: (0191) 384 5423
No. of Accessible Rooms: 1. Accessible Facilities: Restaurant.
Set in two acres of private grounds, in a rural location, a mile from Durham city centre.

WATERSIDE GUEST HOUSE 🚶
Elvet Waterside, Durham DH1 3BW
Tel: (0191) 3846660
Fax: (0191) 3846996
No. of Accessible Rooms: 2.
Accessible Facilities: Lounge, Dining room
This is a charming small property, opened since August 1997 and situated on the banks of the River Wear just a short distance from the city centre.

ATTRACTION
LIGHT INFANTRY MUSEUM and DURHAM ART GALLERY
Aykley Heads, Durham DH1 5TU
Tel: (0191) 384 2214
Fax: (0191) 386 1770
e-mail: durham.gallery@durham.gov.uk
The museum has continually changing exhibitions in the gallery and tells the Light Infantry regimental history through its collection of artefacts.

SD ♿   CP 🚶   E ♿   RF ♿   L ♿
C 🚶   S 🚶   WC 🚶   RFE 🚶

WOLSINGHAM
Entrance to some of the finest Weardale scenery, Wolsingham is built mostly of stone and boasts a beautiful parish church.

SELF-CATERING
BRADLEY BURN HOLIDAY COTTAGES 🚶
Bradley Burn Farm, Wolsingham,
Weardale DL13 3JH
Tel/Fax: (01388) 527 285
e-mail: selfcatering@bradleyburn.co.uk
www.bradleyburn.co.uk
No. of Accessible Units: 2.
No. of Beds per Unit: 2
Accessible Facilities: Stable Cottages – Lounge, Kitchen. Harvest Cottage – Open Plan Living Area. Two of the four renovated cottages overlook the pretty stream with fields and woods beyond on this family-run farm of 360 acres on the eastern edge of the north Pennines. Bradley Burn was part of a C12th settlement where Prince Bishops hunted deer each autumn. Part of the original hunting lodge at Bradley Hall still exists.

CUMBRIA

CUMBRIA TOURIST BOARD
Ashleigh, Holly Road,
Windermere LA23 2AQ
Tel: (015394) 44444
Fax: (015394) 44041
www.golakes.co.uk

CUMBRIA COUNTY COUNCIL
Public Transport Team, Citadel Chambers,
Carlisle CA3 8SG
Tel: (01228) 606060
www.cumbria.gov.uk
Produces "Getting Around Cumbria",
information on buses and trains.

ACCESSIBLE CUMBRIA
www.accessiblecumbria.co.uk

ALSTON
The highest market town in England is
now a holiday centre offering a
wonderful choice of drives around
sweeping moorland scenery.

TOURIST INFORMATION CENTRE
Alston Railway Station, Alston CA9 3JB
Tel: (01434) 381696 (Seasonal)
(see separate entry below for Railway)

BED & BREAKFAST
GREY CROFT   〔大〕
Middle Park, The Raise,
Alston CA9 3AR
Tel: (01434) 381383
enquiry@greycroft.co.uk
www.greycroft.co.uk
No. of Accessible Units: 1. Bath
No. of Beds: 1 double, 1 single
Accessible Facilities: Lounge, Dining room.
Spacious bungalow on the fringe of Raise
hamlet with open views to the south, one
mile from Alston.

ATTRACTION
SOUTH TYNEDALE RAILWAY
The Railway Station, Alston CA9 3JB
Tel: (01434) 381696

www.strpd.org.uk
Narrow-gauge railway between Alston and
Kirkhaugh along South Tyne valley.
SD 〔&〕   CP 〔大〕   E 〔&〕 (wheelchair space in carriage)
RF 〔大〕   C 〔大〕 (No provision at Alston: refreshment
vehicle at Northern Terminus Platform).
S 〔大〕   WC n/a   RFE 〔&〕

AMBLESIDE
Busy tourist centre, protected from
north and east winds by mountains,
and open to warmer air from the
south.

TOURIST INFORMATION CENTRE
Market Cross, Ambleside, LA22 9BS
Tel: (01539) 432582

SELF-CATERING
NATIONWIDE
Borrans Close, Ambleside
Book through Grooms Holidays
No. of Accessible Units: 1. Roll-in Shower
No. of Beds per Unit: 6
Accessible Facilities: Garden. Spacious
bungalow close to Lake Windermere.

ATTRACTION
ARMITT MUSEUM & LIBRARY
Rydal Road, Ambleside, LA22 9BL
Tel: (015394) 31212
Fax: (015394) 313131
e-mail: mail@armitt.com
www.armitt.com
An amazing collection of Art, Archeology,
Archives, Books, Geography and
Photography.
SD 〔&〕   CP 〔&〕   E 〔大〕   RF 〔&〕
C 〔大〕   S 〔&〕   WC 〔&〕
N.B. ENTRANCE RAMPED at 1:8, but
otherwise suitable.

BARROW-IN-FURNESS
Barrow developed from a tiny C19th
hamlet into the biggest iron and steel
centre in the world and then to a
major British shipbuilding force, all
within 40 years.

TOURIST INFORMATION CENTRE
Forum 28, Duke Street, Barrow LA14 1HU
Tel: (01229) 894 784

ACCESSIBLE ATTRACTIONS
THE DOCK MUSEUM
North Road, Barrow-in-Furness LA14 2PW
Tel: (01229) 870871
Fax: (01229) 811361
Straddling a Victorian graving dock, this museum offers exhibition gallery, film show and landscaped dock site.

SD   CP   E   RF
L   C   S   WC

BOWNESS-ON-WINDERMERE
On the shore of Lake Windermere, there is much activity centred on the lake and a winding main street with attractive shops.

LAKE DISTRICT NATIONAL PARK
Glebe Road, Bowness on
Windermere LA23 3HJ
Tel: (015394) 42895 (Seasonal)

HOTEL
THE BURNSIDE HOTEL
Bowness on Windermere LA23 3EP
Tel: (015394) 42211
Fax: (015394) 43824
No. of Accessible Rooms: 2. Roll-in Shower. Facilities: Lounge, Restaurant, Pool, Sauna, Spa. Set in mature gardens overlooking Lake Windermere and 300 metres from the Steamer Pier and village.

BURN HOW GARDEN HOUSE HOTEL
Back Belfield Road,
Bowness-on-Windermere LA23 3HH
Tel: (015394) 46226   Fax: (015394) 47000
e.mail: info@burnhow.co.uk
www.burnhow.co.uk
No. of Accessible Rooms: 4.
Accessible Facilities: Lounge, Restaurant. Charming hotel with delightful furnishings. Two minutes from Lake Windermere. Rooms for disabled guests have direct access to a rose garden and patio.

SELF-CATERING
BIRCH COTTAGE
Deloraine Holiday Homes
Helm Road,
Bowness-on-Windermere LA23 2HS
Tel: (015394) 45557
Fax: (015394) 43221
e-mail: gordon@deloraine.demon.co.uk
www.deloraine.demon.co.uk
No. of Accessible Units: 2
No. of Beds per Unit: 6. Roll-in shower
Accessible Facilities: Open plan living/dining/kitchenette. Terrace path round house with garden views. Converted and enlarged from traditional stone and slate structure, retaining timber features. Located within the grounds of an Edwardian mansion 300m above Lake Windermere in 1.5 acres of landscape.

ATTRACTIONS
WINDERMERE LAKE CRUISES
Bowness Bay Boating Division,
Bowness-on-Windermere LA23 3HQ
Tel: (015394) 43360
Fax: (015394) 40340
Cruise between Lakeside, Bowness and Ambleside on large steamers, Swan and Teal and the smaller Tern. A number of different trips are offered of about 1.5 hours' duration, including a jazz and buffet cruise in the summer. We checked the pier facilities at Bowness only, but understand that adaptive WCs are available at Lakeside and Ambleside also. Car parking is available at both these sites next to the piers.

SD   CP n/a (200m away)   E (to pier)
RF (ramped boarding onto steamers, dependent on water height, summer when water is lower, a little steep, but manageable and staff are very helpful)
C (on board),
Boatman's Café in Bowness coach/car park).
WC (on pier, on board facility not accessible)

WORLD OF BEATRIX POTTER ATTRACTION
Crag Brow,
Bowness-on-Windermere LA23 3BX
Tel/Fax: (015394) 88444
e-mail: beatrixpotter@hop-skip-jum.com
www.hop-skip-jump.com
Multi-award-winning attraction in which

to discover a magical indoor recreation of Peter Rabbit and Jemima. Where else can you call on Mrs. Tiggy-Winkle? Three-dimensional displays on Hill Top, Beatrix Potter's home and inspiration for many of the tales. A must!

The approach to the entrance is steep, but all staff have completed the Welcome All course and want to help.

SD ☑ CP n/a E ☑ RF ☑
C ☑ S ☑ WC ☑

BROUGH

Located midway between Penrith and Barnard Castle, the closest town is Appleby-in-Westmoreland.

ATTRACTION

LANCERCOST PRIORY (EH)
Brampton, Nr. Brough CA8 2HQ
Tel: (016977) 73030
Augustinian priory founded in 1166. The nave of the church has survived and is still used as the local parish church, although the chancel and priory buildings are in ruins.

SD ☑ CP ☑ E ☑ RF ☑
S ☑ WC ☑ RFE ☑

CALDBECK

Most famous village in Northern Lakes, an area of dramatic fells. Birth and burial place of John Peel.

SELF-CATERING

MONKHOUSE HILL
Sebergham, Caldbeck CA5 YHW
Tel/Fax: (016974) 76254
No. of Accessible Units: 1. Bath
No. of Beds per Unit: 2
Accessible Facilities: Open-plan Lounge/Diner/Kitchen. Lovely views across paddock from sitting area and bedroom. Mickle Rigg Cottage is one of seven delightful stone, oak-beamed cottages with panoramic views set around a courtyard of this 300-year-old farm in foothills of North Lakeland fells.

CARLISLE

Just north of Hadrian's Wall, with a small cathedral and vast amounts of Roman history. The city centre is compact, pedestrianised and accessible.

BUSES

Stagecoach Cumberland
Tel: (01228) 597222

TAXIS

A Newtown: Tel: (01228) 597222
Beeline Cabs: Tel: (01228)534440
17 vehicles of varying types
Staceys Minicoaches: Tel: (01228) 511127
Various vehicles of different sizes suitable for wheelchairs

TRAINS

First North Western: Special Needs
Tel: (0845) 6040231

CAR PARKS

Free parking for disabled badge holders in all council run car parks, some limited parking on street.

SHOPMOBILITY

Level 2, The Lanes Car Park, East Tower Street, Carlisle, CA3 8NX
Tel: (01228) 625950

ACCESSIBLE RESTROOMS

Many accessed by RADAR key, available for sale at TIC and Civic Centre, 7th Floor, Bus Station (Lowther Street), Carlisle Cathedral (separate building at the rear of the grounds), Market Hall, Old Town Hall, Railway Station, St Nicholas Toilets (Butchergate), Sands Centre, Tullie House Museum.

SELF-CATERING

ARCH VIEW
Midtodhills Farm, Roadhead, Carlisle CA6 6PF
Tel/Fax (016977) 48213
e-mail: jjames@v21mail.co.uk
www.holidaycottagescarlisle.co.uk
No. of Accessible Units: 1. Shower

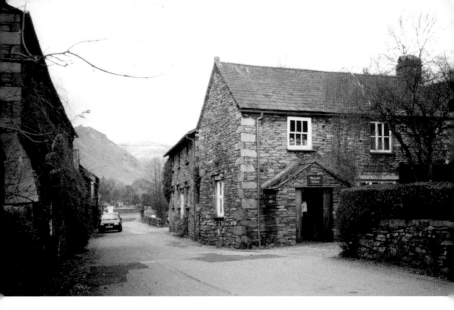

The award-winning Dove's Cottage at Grasmere. Formerly the home of Wordsworth.

No. of Beds per Unit: 2/8
Accessible Facilities: Lounge, Kitchen/Diner. Barn conversion and two cottages with lovely views on 320-acre working farm set in lovely Lyne valley near Scottish border.

GREEN VIEW LODGES

Welton, Nr. Dalston, Carlisle CA5 7ES
Tel: (016974) 76230
Fax: (016974) 76523
www.green-view-lodges.com
No. of Accessible Units: 2
No. of Beds per Unit: 6
Accessible Facilities: Open plan Lounge/Kitchen/Diner, Garden.
The site comprises traditional cottages, a converted chapel and pine lodges, of which two lodges are accessible. All properties overlook meadows. The tiny hamlet of Welton nestles in the foothills of the northern fells, three miles from the National Park with Lake Ullswater and Keswick within 30 minutes' drive.

WILDSIDE

Mealsgate, Carlisle
Tel: (01694) 371420
No. of Accessible Units: 1. Bath
No. of Beds per Unit: 6
Accessible Facilities: Lounge, Dining room. Comfortable bungalow between market towns of Wigton and Cockermouth and

four miles from the Lake District National Park boundary.

TRANQUIL OTTER

Thurstonfield, Carlisle, Cumbria CA5 6HB
Tel: (01228) 576661
Fax: (01228) 576662
info@thetranquilotter.co.uk
www.thetranquilotter.co.uk
No. of Accessible Units: 3. Roll-in showers.
No. of Beds per Unit:5/6
Accessible facilities: Lounge, Kitchen, shop on site.
2 lodges have wheelchair access sauna/whirlpool bath and log burner. One has a hot tub built into the decking outside (no hoist).
Wheelchair accessible boat for fly fishing/leisure. One mile pathway around lake and use of accessible bird hide. Chalets are on the lake shore. Tranquil surroundings with lots of nature, otters, red squirrels etc.

ATTRACTIONS
CARLISLE CATHEDRAL

Castle Street, Carlisle
(Office: 7 The Abbey, Carlisle CA3 8TZ)
Tel/Fax: (01228) 548151
Originally a Norman priory, built in 1122. Notable for its superbly decorated chancel roof and east window.

| SD n/a | CP ⟨⟩ | E ⟨⟩ | RF ⟨⟩ | C n/a |
| S ⟨⟩ | WC ⟨⟩ | RFE ⟨⟩ | | |

SPORTING VENUE
CARLISLE RACECOURSE
Durdar Road, Carlisle CA2 4TS
Booking Office: (01228) 522973
Contact booking office for up to date
details of facilites which have been
modernised.

THEATRE
THE SANDS CENTRE
The Sands, Carlisle CA1 1SQ
Admin: (01228) 625208
Fax: (01228) 625666
Booking-Box Office: (01228) 625222
CP ♿ RE ♿ ED ♿ INT ♿
WC ♿ (ground floor opposite reception desk)
AUD ♿ Standing concerts – ramp erected against far
wall for wheelchairs.
Bar/Restaurant ♿ (R. ground floor).
Note: Wheelchair spaces through main doors, on flat.

COCKERMOUTH
Home of William Wordsworth, this
bustling market town is a perfect base
for visiting the West Lakes and Fells.
Nearest train station is Workington, 8
miles away.

TOURIST INFORMATION CENTRE
The Town Hall, Market Street,
Cockermouth CA13 9NP
Tel: (01900) 822634

HOTEL
SHEPHERDS HOTEL ♿
Egremont Road, Cockermouth CA13 0QX
Tel/Fax: (01900) 822673
No. of Accessible Rooms: 1
Accessible Facilities: Restaurant, Bar, Lift to
Shop, Exhibition and Sheep Show.
Adjacent Lakeland Sheep and Wool
centre.

PHEASANT INN
Bassenthwaite Lake, Cockermouth CA13 9YE
Tel: (01768) 776234   Fax: (01768) 776002
No. of Accessible Rooms: 3 Accessible
Facilities: Lounges (3), Dining room. Bar.
Charming old coaching inn, a traditional
Cumbrian hostelry, set in lovely gardens
and woodland.

SELF-CATERING
SIMONSCALES MILL ♿
Simonscales Lane,
Cockermouth CA13 9TG
Tel: (01900) 822594
e-mail: ericlowes@simonscales.fsnet.co.uk
www.simonscales.fsnet.co.uk
No. of Accessible Units: 2. Roll-in showers
The Cottage:
No. of Beds per Unit: 4 (adjustamatic)
Accessible Facilities: Lounge, Dining room.
The Lodge:
No of beds: 6 (1 adjustamatic bed)
Accessible Facilities:
Kitchen/diner/Lounge/Large Shower room
Large decked verandah overlooking the
river. Parking adjacent to Lodge.
Fishing is from a flat river bank 30 metres
from the front door. Originally a flax and
bobbin mill, this property lies on the banks
of the River Cocker, with a private patio
overlooking the river. Just over a mile from
Cockermouth.

ATTRACTION
LAKELAND SHEEP AND WOOL CENTRE
Cumwest Visitor Centre, Egremont Road,
Cockermouth CA13 0QX
Tel/Fax: (01900) 822673
A visual show and different exhibits
introduce the life of the countryside. A
comprehensive indoor presentation
includes a face-to-face with 19 different
breeds of live sheep and surprising facts
about each breed. There is a display of
sheep dogs in the 300-seater arena.
SD ♿ CP ♿ E ♿ L ♿ C ♿
S ♿ WC 🚹 RFE ♿

GRANGE-OVER-SANDS
Seaside resort backed by wooded fells,
overlooking Morecambe Bay. Its parks
are noted for flowering shrubs,
alpines, rock and herbaceous plants.

TOURIST INFORMATION CENTRE
Victoria Hall, Main Street,
Grange-over-Sands LA11 6OT
Tel: (015395) 34026

HOTEL
NETHERWOOD HOTEL [symbol]
Lindale Road, Grange-over-Sands LA11 6ET
Tel: (015395) 32552
Fax: (015395) 34121
No. of Accessible Rooms: 1. Bath.
Accessible Facilities: Lounge, Restaurant,
Pool. C19th country residence set in 11
acres of gardens overlooking
Morecambe Bay.

GRASMERE
Famous as Wordsworth's home from
1799, the area around the village and
lake has superb scenery.

ATTRACTION
DOVE COTTAGE and THE WORDSWORTH
MUSEUM
The Wordsworth Trust, Dove Cottage,
Grasmere LA22 9SH
Tel: (015394) 35544 Fax: (015394) 35748
e-mail: enquiries@wordsworth.org.uk
www.wordsworth.org.uk
This award-winning museum displays the
trust's unique collection of manuscripts,
books and paintings, interpreting the
great poet's life and work. Dove Cottage
was Wordsworth's home from 1799-
1808. There are guided tours of the
cottage and its artefacts, all wonderfully
preserved in enchanting surroundings. The
trust has been incredibly helpful to our
researchers. NB: The cottage is accessible,
although the kitchen has a narrow door,
so retreat through Dorothy's bedroom!
Museum entrance is ramped at 1:5 and
not easily accessible.

SD [symbol] CP [symbol] E-COTTAGE [symbol] MUSEUM n/a
C [symbol] S [symbol] WC [symbol]

KENDAL
This ancient town is just outside the
Lakes, surrounded by attractive
Westmoreland fells on three sides with
many parks and open spaces.

TOURIST INFORMATION CENTRE
Town Hall, Highgate, Kendal LA9 4DL
Tel: (015395) 725758
SOUTH LAKELAND DISTRICT COUNCIL
LEISURE SERVICES DEPT.
South Lakeland House,
Lowther Street, Kendal
Tel: (015397) 33333
Fax: (015397) 40300

BED AND BREAKFAST
MITCHELLAND FARM BUNGALOW [symbol]
Crook, Nr. Kendal LA8 8LL
Tel: (015394) 47421
No. of Accessible Rooms: 1. Bath
Accessible Facilities: Lounge, Garden.
Family home shared with owners' who are
dedicated to wheelchair access (retired
nurse with holiday-care experience).
Situated on a delightful working farm
between Kendal and Bowness. There are
plans to extend the accessible
accommodation with a second purpose-
built bathroom and a self-catering unit.
Category 1 apart from two slightly narrow
doorways. Unwilling to join NAS because
there are many full and independent
wheelchair users who might be deterred
by Category 2 grading.

SELF-CATERING
BARKINBECK COTTAGE [symbol]
Barkin House, Gatebeck, Kendal LA8 0HX
Tel: (015395) 67122
e-mail:Ann@barkin.fsnet.co.uk
www.barkinbeck.co.uk
No. of Accessible Units: 1. Roll-in Shower.
No. of Beds per Unit: 1 double/2 single
Accessible Facilities: Lounge, Dining room.
Converted barn on small working farm
between Kendal and Kirby Lonsdale in
peaceful, unspoilt, open countryside.

GREENBANK [symbol]
Crosthwaite, Kendal LA8 8TD
Tel/Fax: (015395) 68598
No. of Accessible Units: 1. Shower
No. of Beds per Unit: 2
Accessible Facilities: Lounge.
Delightful old farmhouse located in
Winster valley with access to central lakes,
local limestone scars and quiet Kendal
area fells.

ATTRACTION
LEVENS HALL ESTATE GARDENS
Levens Hall, Kendal LA8 0PD
Tel: (015395) 60321
Fax: (015395) 60669
e-mail: levenshall@fsnet.co.uk
www.levenshall.co.uk
House not accessible, but the Gardens
are. Famous award-winning gardens
were laid out around 1694. The topiary,
beech hedges and colourful seasonal
bedding create an amazing impact.
There is an electric buggy available for
hire.

SD   CP   E-(Garden)   RF
C    S 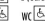   WC 🦽   RFE (Garden)

KESWICK
Major Lakeland town popular with
poets, artists and visitors. Keswick has
narrow streets and buildings of old
grey stone.

TOURIST INFORMATION CENTRE
Moot Hall, Market Square, Keswick
CA12 5HR
Tel: (01768) 772645
e-mail: information@moothall.u-net.com
www.keswick.org

KESWICK TOURISM ASSOCIATION
50 Main Street, Keswick CA12 5JS
Tel: (01768) 773607
Fax: (01768) 775738

BUSES
Stagecoach Cumberland:
Tel: (01228) 597222
Some low-floor, easy-access routes.

TRAVELINE
Tel: (0870) 6082608

HOTELS
WOODLAND COUNTRY HOUSE
Ireby, Nr. Keswick CA7 1EX
Tel: (016973) 71791
Fax: (016973) 71482
e-mail: stay@woodlandsatireby.co.uk
www.woodlandsatireby.co.uk
No. of Accessible Rooms: 3. Bath

Accessible Facilities: Lounge, Dining room,
Bar. Privately owned and managed guest
house set within delightful gardens.

DERWENTWATER HOTEL
Portinscale, Keswick CA12 5RE
Tel: (017687) 72538
Fax: (017687) 71002
e-mail: derwentwater-hotel.co.uk
www.derwentwater-hotel.co.uk
No. of Accessible Rooms: 6. Bath.
Accessible Facilities: Lounge, Dining room.
Wonderful lakeshore location in 16 acres
of conservation grounds with panoramic
views.

SELF-CATERING
CALVERT TRUST
Little Crosthwaite, Keswick
Book through Grooms Holidays or Calvert
Trust. No. of Accessible Units: 3
No. of Beds per Unit: 6, 6 and 16.
South Barn is set in two acres of
panoramic grounds at the foot of
Skiddaw peak, four miles from Keswick.
Grooms Cottage and the Coach House
form part of a listed building where
William Wordsworth once lived, located
on northern outskirts of Keswick, at the
foot of Latrigg.

ATTRACTION
MIREHOUSE HISTORIC HOUSE and GARDENS
Mirehouse, Keswick CA12 4QE
Tel/Fax: (017687) 72287
Grand C17th house with much original
furniture and portraits and works of
Francis Bacon, Carlyle and Tennyson.
Walled garden picnic area and lake where
Tennyson wrote much of Morte d'Arthur.
Four woodland adventure playgrounds for
children. Those parts of the house open
to the public are accessible to
wheelchairs. The main drive and the Bee
Garden are accessible. The garden behind
the house is reached by wheeling on the
grass close to the house. Directions for
rose garden access is given on the useful
leaflet provided.

SD 🦽   CP    E (House) 🦽
C 🦽   WC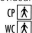

KIRKBY STEPHEN

Old picturesque market town situated on the moors with an Anglo Saxon church.

TOURIST INFORMATION CENTRE
Market Square, Kirkby Stephen CA17 4QN
Tel: (017683) 71199

HOTELS
FAT LAMB HOTEL   [♿]
Crossbank, Ravenstonedale,
Kirkby Stephen CA17 4LL
Tel: (015396) 23242
Fax: (015396) 23285
e-mail:fatlamb@cumbria.com
www.fatlamb.co.uk
No. of Accessible Rooms: 2. Bath.
Accessible Facilities: Lounge, Restaurant, Garden, Viewing point overlooking nature reserve. Lovely property dating back to the mid-1600s located midway between the Lake District and Yorkshire Dales National Parks.

BLACK SWAN HOTEL   [♿]
Ravenstonedale, Kirkby Stephen CA17 4NG
Tel: (015396) 23204   Fax: (015396) 23604
No. of Accessible Rooms: 3. Bath(1) shower (2)
Accessible Facilities: Lounges, Restaurant, Bar. This is a true country hotel built of lakeland stone in 1899 with comfortable public rooms, books and magazines and log fires. Ravenstone is a sleepy, unspoilt village with Kendal and Penrith half an hour to the west and Kirkby Stephen very close by.

SELF-CATERING
COLDBECK HOUSE   [♿]
Ravenstonedale, Kirkby Stephen
Tel/Fax: (015396) 23230
david.cannon@coldbeck.demon.co.uk
No. of Accessible Units: 1. Roll-in Shower
No. of Beds per Unit: 6
Accessible Facilities: Lounge, Dining room, garden,family pub opposite. Recently renovated self-contained wing built in 1881 attached to the owner's farmhouse that was built in early C19th.

Ravenstonedale is a small unspoilt village set at the foot of the Howgills that lie between the Lakes and the Yorkshire Dales.

NEWBY BRIDGE

Charming village on the River Leven with unusual stone bridge with arches of unequal size.

ATTRACTION
AQUARIUM OF THE LAKES
Lakeside, Newby Bridge LA12 8AS
Tel/Fax: (015395) 30153
Follow the life story of a Lakeland River from mountain top to Morecambe Bay.

SD [♿]   CP [♿]   E [♿]   RF [♿]   L [♿]
C [♿]   S [♿]   WC [♿]   RFE [♿]

PENRITH

Ancient and historic town, a touring centre for the Eden Valley. Connections with Wordsworth and his family.

TOURIST INFORMATION CENTRES
Penrith Museum, Middlegate,
Penrith CA11 7PT
Tel: (01768) 867466

GUEST HOUSE
MOSEDALE HOUSE   [♿]
Mosedale, Mungrisdale,
Penrith CA11 0XQ
Tel: (017687) 79371
mosedale@northlakes.co.uk
www.mosedalehouse.co.uk
No. of Accessible Rooms: 1. Roll-in Shower. Accessible Facilities: Lounge, Restaurant, Gardens, Path through small wood, Horse Riding, Wheelchair. Small and homely family guest house with lovely views across the Caldew valley to Bowscale fell from the lounge. From the enclosed yard there is direct access for wheelchair users to relatively quiet lanes and the riverside. Age Concern Eden Shopmobility Service base a powered scooter here that guests can book.

HOTEL
SHAP WELLS HOTEL ♿
Shap, Penrith CA10 3QU
Tel: (01931) 716628   Fax: (01931) 716377
www.shapwells.com
No. of Accessible Rooms: 2. Roll-in
Shower
Facilities: All public rooms, except Games
room. Large family owned traditional and
comfortable Victorian hotel set in 30 acres
of woodland and gardens high in the
Shap Fells. NB: the area around the hotel
is hilly.

SELF-CATERING
HOWSCALES ♿
Kirkoswald, Penrith CA10 1JG
Tel: (01768) 898666   Fax: (01768) 898710
www.eden-in-cumbria.co.uk/howscales
e-mail: liz@howscales.fsbusiness.co.uk
No. of Accessible Units: 1. Bath.
No. of Beds per Unit: 2
Accessible Facilities: Lounge, Dining room
300-year-old farm with barns and byres
converted into cottages surrounding a
central courtyard. Set in secluded open
countryside with views to the lakes and
the Pennines.

PATTERDALE HALL ESTATE 🚶
Glenridding, Penrith CA11 0PJ
Tel/Fax: (01768) 482308
e-mail: welcome@phel.co.uk
www.phel.co.uk
No. of Accessible Units: 3.
No. of Beds per Unit: 6
Accessible Facilities: Lounge/Diner,
Kitchen. Three pine lodges of 17 self-
catering properties of various types
located on a working hill farm at the
southern end of Ullswater. The estate has
wooded grounds reaching from the shores
of the lake to the lower slopes of the
Helvellyn range. Patterdale is a good base
for touring the Lakes.

ATTRACTION
RHEGED DISCOVERY CENTRE
Redhills, Penrith CA11 0DQ
Tel: (01768) 868000   Fax: (01768) 868002
e-mail: enquiries@rheged.com
www.rheged.com
In the Dark Ages, Rheged was a kingdom

of magic, myth and mystery. This new
attraction, housed in the largest earth-
covered building in the UK, celebrates the
history and mystery of Cumbria and the
Lake District with the first all-British large
format film taking viewers back in time
through centuries. There is also the huge
glass atrium of Mountain Hall with special
Cumbrian shops, plus restaurant and
coffee shops. Interior features include
babbling brooks and massive limestone
crags to ensure the visitor feels as if in the
very heart of Cumbria. Opened Easter
1999 as a millennium attraction. Full
wheelchair access to all seven levels, via
three lifts. Located close to the M6 (J40),
towards Keswick). Not to be missed!

SD ♿ CP ♿ E ♿ RF ♿ L ♿
C ♿ S ♿ WC ♿ RFE ♿

WETHERIGGS COUNTRY POTTERY
Clifton Dykes, Penrith CA10 2DH
Tel: (01768) 892733   Fax: (01768) 892722
e-mail: info@wetheriggs-pottery.co.uk
www.wetheriggs-pottery.co.uk
Working pottery since 1855, the only
steam powered country pottery in the UK.
The museum offers a history of the pottery
and an opportunity to throw a pot. All this
combines with garden and patio terracotta
to produce a fascinating day out.

SD ♿ CP ♿ E ♿ RF ♿
C ♿ S ♿ WC 🚶 RFE ♿

RAVENGLASS
Known to have one of the best
preserved Roman sites in the north.

ATTRACTION
MUNCASTER CASTLE, GARDENS AND
OWL CENTRE
Muncaster Castle, Ravenglass CA18 1RQ
Tel: (01229) 717614   Fax: (01229) 717010
e-mail: info@muncaster.co.uk
www.muncaster.co.uk
Winner of 1999 Tourism for All Award,
every effort is being made to develop the
castle into a fully accessible site. Attractions
include stunning gardens in 77 acres of
woodland, cultivated and wild areas: the
castle, family home of the Penningtons

since early C13th, and the Owl Centre, HQ of the World Owl Trust with over 180 birds. Gardens – paths paved or shale in some places, tricky with some steep slopes. Wonderful terrace views accessible from disabled parking, via old St. Michael Church and down a grass slope toward the castle.

Castle – three exterior and one interior step to the accessible ground floor. There is a ramp. Access from disabled parking is quite steep but surfaced. Wonderful views of Scarfell Pike, the highest in England. Owl Centre – 90% of aviaries are accessible via ramps and pathways. Shop, WC and catering are within the Stable Courtyard and are very accessible. An interactive Vole Maze is new, encouraging habitat awareness.

CP ♿ E ♿ RF ♿ C ♿
S ♿ WC ♿

RAVENGLASS AND ESKDALE RAILWAY
Ravenglass CA18 1SW
Tel: (01229) 717171 Fax: (01229) 717011
e-mail: rer@netcomuk.co.uk
www.ravenglass-railway.co.uk
Narrow gauge steam railway, laid down in C19th, running through beautiful countryside for seven miles.

CP ♿ SD ♿ E ♿ RF ♿
C 🚶 S ♿ WD 🚶

SEDBERGH
A hill town and busy market town, set below the slate Howgill fells, more like the Lake district than the Yorkshire dales.

TOURIST INFORMATION CENTRE
72 Main Street, Sedbergh LA10 5AD
Tel: (015396) 20125

SELF-CATERING
BAINBRIDGE COURT   ♿
Bainbridge Road, Sedbergh LA10 5BA
Tel: (015396) 21000 Fax: (015396) 21710
e-mail: nigel.close@virgin.net
No. of Accessible Units: 1. Roll-In Shower.
No. of Beds per Unit: 4. Accessible Facilities: Lounge, Dining room, Patio. Ground floor of luxury apartment block.

WINDERMERE
The largest lake in England with thickly wooded shores. Very popular tourist town, noted for its watersports and Yacht Club.

TOURIST INFORMATION CENTRE
Victoria Street, Windermere LA23 1AD
Tel: (01539) 446499

HOTEL ACCOMMODATION
HAWKSMOOR   🚶
Lake Road, Windermere LA23 2EQ
Tel: (015394) 42110
e-mail: enquiries@hawksmoor.com
www. hawksmoor.com
No. of Accessible Rooms: 3. Bath. Accessible Facilities: Dining room. Surrounded by gardens with woodland to the rear this charming guest house is situated between Windermere and Bowness-on-Windermere.

LINTHWAITE HOUSE HOTEL   🚶
Crook Road, Windermere LA23 3JA
Tel: (015394) 88600
Fax: (015394) 88601
e-mail: admin@linthwaite.com
www.linthwaite.com
No. of Accessible Rooms: 2
Accessible Facilities: Lounge, Restaurant
This privately owned, country house hotel won Hotel of the Year 1994. Set in 14 acres of gardens overlooking Lake Windermere. Great views, and reputedly fine food.

ATTRACTION
WINDERMERE STEAMBOAT MUSEUM
Rayrigg Road, Windermere LA23 1BN
Tel: (015394) 45565
Fax: (015394) 48769
e-mail: steam@insites.co.uk
www.steamboat.co.uk
Historic collection of steam and motor boats in peaceful lakeside setting. Also cruises on original Edwardian steamboats with embarkation assistance from staff. No access to steamboats for wheelchairs.

SDn/a CP ♿ E ♿ RF ♿
C ♿ S ♿ WC ♿ RFE ♿

DERBYSHIRE

DERBYSHIRE COALITION FOR INCLUSIVE LIVING
Park Road, Ripley, Derbyshire DE5 3EF
Tel: (01733) 740246
e-mail: info@dcil.org.uk
www.dcil.org.uk
A campaigning pressure group working for and on behalf of disabled people.

ASHBOURNE
Gateway to the Izaak Walton country of Dovedale, this is a small market town where little has changed since 1645.

SELF-CATERING
THE COTTAGE BY THE POND
Beechenhill Farm, Ilam, Ashbourne DE6 2BD
Tel/Fax: (01335) 310274
e-mail: beechenhill@btinternet.com
www.beechenhill.co.uk
No. of Accessible Units: 1. Roll-in Shower.
No. of Beds per Unit: 6
Accessible Facilities: Lounge/Dining room, kitchen. 92-acre working organic dairy farm located in Ilam between Dovedale and the Manifold Valley in the Peak District National Park. The cottage looks south over fields and animals.

LAKE VIEW
Yew Tree Lane, Bradley, Ashbourne DE6 1PG
Tel: (01335) 370577   Fax: (01335) 342707
e-mail:george.dutton@btopenworld.com
No. of Accessible Units: 1. Roll-in Shower
No. of Beds per Unit: 6
Accessible Facilities: Lounge, Dining room, Kitchen, Private Garden, Hydrotherapy Pool part of complex.

BAKEWELL
Small market town built almost entirely in warm, brownish stone. It lies in a sheltered valley of the Derbyshire Wye with rolling wooded hills.

ATTRACTION
CHATSWORTH
Bakewell DE45 1PP
Tel: (01246) 565300 Fax: (01246) 583536
www.chatsworth-house.co.uk
e-mail: visit@chatsworth.org
Palatial home of the Duke and Duchess of Devonshire since 1549 with a fine art collection in 26 richly furnished rooms. The garden is one of the finest in England, laid out by Capability Brown, and is famous for the work of the head gardener, Joseph Paxton in C19th. Notable for Cascade and Emperor Fountain and Angel Conner water sculpture.
THE HOUSE IS NOT ACCESSIBLE.
The garden, farmyard, shops and restaurant are accessible to a greater lesser degree as below. A useful leaflet is given out that indicates routes and their terrain. Three electric scooters and four manual wheelchairs are available free for use in the garden.

SD   CP   C   S   WC

PEAK DISTRICT NATIONAL PARK AUTHORITY
Aldern House, Baslow Road,
Bakewell DE45 1AE
Tel: (01629) 816200   Fax: (01629) 816310
The park can be divided into two parts, the Dark and White Peak. To the north and down each side lies high, desolate moor lands, named the Dark Peak for vegetation, peat and weathering of gritstone. The southern and middle, separated from the moors by shale valleys is the White Peak area. Farming, delightful villages, drystone walls, green fields and woods. The hills impose some difficulties, but worth the effort.

PLACES IN THE PARK WITH ACCESS
Bakewell (Granby Road). Large car park, level tarmac path along river, level kerbed pathway to information centre with ramped entrance. Adaptive restroom.
Curbar Gap. Popular beauty spot with small car park and paths constructed to provide reasonably level access for wheelchair users to viewpoints close to Curbar Edge and right up to Baslow Edge

with dramatic views across Derwent Valley.

Derwent. Car Park. Fairly level tarmac paths to views of Derwent Dam and Ladybower Reservoir. Adaptive restroom.

Dovedale. Car Park with fairly level road leading beside river for 0.5 mile to Stepping Stones. This road is closed to traffic at weekends and rarely used at other times. Adaptive restroom.

Dove Stone Reservoir. Circular path around entire reservoir offers moorland scenery. Large car park with tarmac gradient to level track overlooking the reservoir.

Edale. Large car park. Narrow road with slight gradient leads through village. Adaptive restroom.

Goyt Valley - Goyt's Lane. Wheelchair route along a one-mile section of former Cromford and High Peak Railway. Route winds through open moorland. Reserved car parking opposite entrance to route. Adaptive restroom.

Ernwood Reservoir. Reserved car parking near west end of dam. Ramp link to a level road alongside reservoir. Adaptive restroom.

Hathersage. No car park adjacent to street but the main village street is wide enough for parking. Adaptive restroom.

Ladybower. Reserved spaces at Heather Dene car park, plus wheelchair-accessible route. Platform for use of wheelchair anglers opposite fishery office and specially adapted boat with electric outboard.

Redmires Reservoir. Nr. Sheffield. Accessible footpath and new car park.

Tideswell Dale. Car park, firm level track

0.25 miles long to picnic site, continuing to Litton Mill where path through Water-cum-Jolly Dale can be joined. Adaptive restroom.

Tissington and High Peak Trails. Level tracks from Ashbourne and Hopton Top meeting at Parsley Hay and continuing north. Surface variable, but reasonably firm. Gradients where bridges have been removed. Bridle gates not fitted with special catches.

Water-cum-Jolly Dale. Access to level concession path through fine limestone dale. Path sometimes used by anglers with cars.

PEAK CYCLE HIRE

All centres have some or all of a range of cycles suitable for use by people with disabilities. This range includes tandems, trikes, and duet wheelchair cycles.

Mapleton Lane, Ashbourne, Derbys. DE6 2AA. Tel and Fax: (01335) 343156
Just north of town centre on Tissington Trail: a disused railway line of scenic beauty, traffic free and 13.5 miles long.

Fairholmes, Derwent, Sheffield. S30 2AQ. Tel and Fax: (01433) 651261
Off the A57 in Derwent Valley. Cycle beside historic Derwent and Ladybower reservoirs through beautiful woodland.

Parsley Hay, Buxton, Derby. SK17 0DG. Tel and Fax: (01298) 84493
At the junction of Tissington and High Peak Trails. Over 30 miles of traffic-free cycling through amazing limestone scenery.

Old Station Car Park, Waterhouses, Staffs. ST10 3EG. Tel and Fax: (0153) 308609
Located behind Crown Hotel. A 9-mile route through two super river valleys along the Manifold Track converted railway line.

Visitor Centre, Middleton-by-Wirksworth, Derbys. DE4 4LS. Tel: (01629) 823204 Fax: (01629) 825336
On the High Peak Trail near Middleton. 17.5 miles of traffic-free route with link to Tissington Trail.

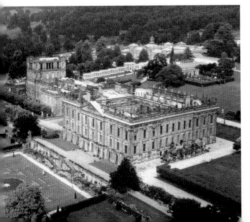

Beauty and dignity at Chatsworth, the most noble of stately houses.

Information Centre, Station Road, Hayfield,
Stockport. SK12 5ES
Tel: (01663) 746222   Fax: (01663) 741581
In Hayfield Village, 2.5 mile trail with plenty
of access to surrounding hills via
bridleways.

BUXTON

Small but rather grand town having
once been a fashionable spa. There is a
Regency crescent, restored Edwardian
theatre, museums, pump room and
pavilion with antique fairs.

HIGH PEAK TOURIST INFORMATION CENTRE

The Crescent, Buxton SK17 6BQ
Tel: (01298) 25106   Fax: (01298) 73153
e-mail: tourism@highpeak.gov.uk
www.highpeak.gov.uk

SELF-CATERING

CRESSBROOK HALL COTTAGES   [♿]
Cressbrook Hall, Cressbrook,
Nr. Buxton SK17 8SY
Tel: (01298) 871289   Fax: (01298) 871845
e-mail: stay@cressbrookhall.co.uk
www.cressbrookhall.co.uk
No. of Accessible Units: 3. Roll-in Shower.
No. of Beds per unit: 2-8
Accessible Facilities: Lounge, Dining room,
Sauna. Charming cottages within
Cressbrook Village in the Peak District,
within grounds of Cressbrook Hall.

CASTLE DONINGTON

The site of the first Norman castle, built
by Henry de Lacy, Earl of Lincoln, the
town has some lovely houses and
cottages incorporating the original
stone. Also a surprisingly attractive
power station.

HOTEL

THISTLE EAST MIDLANDS AIRPORT   [🚶]
Castle Donington DE74 2SH
Tel: (01332) 850700   Fax: (01332) 850823
No. of Accessible Rooms: 3. Bath
Accessible Facilities: Lounge, Restaurant,

Sauna. Very close to the airport, this
modern hotel is set in its own large
grounds, and has antique furnishings.

CHESTERFIELD

Known for the church's crooked spire
and its strong links with George
Stephenson, who spent his last years
at Tapton House.

HOTEL

ABBEYDALE HOTEL   [🚶]
Cross Street, Chesterfield S40 4TD
Tel: (01246) 277849   Fax: (01246) 558223
e-mail:abbeydale1ef@aol.com
www.abbeydalehotel.co.uk
No. of Accessible Rooms: 1. Shower
Accessible Facilities: Lounge, Dining
room,bar. Situated in quiet, residential
area of town, this is a family-run hotel.

SELF-CATERING

CHESTNUT and WILLOW COTTAGES   [🚶]
Priestfield Grange, Old Brampton,
Chesterfield S42 7JH
Tel: (01246) 566159
No. of Accessible Units: 2
No. of Beds per Unit: CH-3: WI-2
Accessible Facilities: CH-Lounge,
Kitchen/Diner, Patio
WI – Lounge/Diner, Kitchen, Patio and
Lawn. Secluded cottages on a farm with
surrounding grassland leading to Linacre
Reservoir and Nature Trails, close to Peak
Park, Bakewell and Chesterfield.

ATTRACTIONS

CHESTERFIELD MUSEUM AND ART
GALLERY
St. Mary's Gate, Chesterfield S41 7TD
Tel: (01246) 345727   Fax: (01246) 345720
Rich town heritage explored in different
aspects of Chesterfield's history. Local
C19th artist Joseph Syddall works are
displayed in art gallery.

| SD [♿] | CP n/a | E [♿] | RF [♿] |
| C n/a | S [♿] | WC [♿] | RFE [♿] |

EYAM HALL
Eyam, Hope Valley S32 5QW
Tel: (01433) 631976   Fax: (01433) 631603

e-mail: nicola@eyamhall.com
www.eyamhall.com
Family owned house for over 320 years
with a beautiful walled garden where
outdoor plays and concerts are performed.
Setting down point outside house is gravel
mixture, some loose. Located in the centre
of Eyam village, just off the A623, 20
minutes from Chesterfield, Bakewell and
Sheffield.

SD ♿ CP ♿ E ♿ RF ♿
C ♿ S 🚶 WC 🚶 RFE ♿

HARDWICK HALL (NT)
Doe Lea, Chesterfield DE S44 5QJ
Tel: (01246) 850430
Fax: (01246) 854200
In 1597, Bess of Hardwick, the most
powerful woman after the queen in Tudor
England, moved into this, one of the
greatest of all Elizabethan houses. Superb
collections, a glorious park, and a Tudor
herb garden.

SD ♿ CP 🚶 E ♿ RF ♿
C 🚶 S 🚶 WC 🚶
RFE - Hall and Garden ♿

DERBY
Blessed with open spaces and
interesting old houses.The most
striking building is the cathedral that
retains much from its past. Home of Sir
Henry Royce, Rolls-Royce has been
associated with Derby since 1908.

DERBY TOURISM
Assembly Rooms, Market Place, Derby
DE1 3AH
Tel: (01332) 255802
Fax: (01332) 256137

DERBY CITY COUNCIL
Roman House, Friargate, Derby DE1 1XB
Tel: (01332) 255925 Fax: (01332) 255989
Minicom: (01332) 256666
e-mail: mick.watts@derby.gov.uk
Produces Derby Access Guide for Disabled
People.

DISABILITY DIRECT
Tel: (01332) 299449

NATIONAL TRAVELINE
Tel: (0870) 608 2608

BUSES
www.derbysbus.net

TAXIS
Hackney Carriages: Tel: (01332) 757575
10 TX1s with all fittings.

TRAINS
Midland Mainline: Special Needs –
Tel: (0114) 2537654
Minicom: (0145) 7078051
Virgin Trains: Special Needs:
Tel: (0845) 7443366
Minicom: (0845) 7443367

CAR PARKS
Free three-hour disabled badge parking in
all council-owned car parks and some off-
street.

SHOPMOBILITY
The Coach Park, Derby Bus Station,
The Moreledge, Derby DE1 2AY
Tel: (01332) 200320

HOTEL
BEST WESTERN MIDLAND HOTEL 🚶
Midland Road, Derby DE1 2SQ
Tel: (01332) 345894 Fax: (01332) 293522
e-mail: sales@midland-derby.co.uk
www.midland-derby.co.uk
No. of Accessible Rooms: 88, via accessible
lift. Accessible Facilities: Lounge, Restaurant.
Quality hotel situated near the city centre,
close to the M1 (J25).

ATTRACTIONS
DERBY INDUSTRIAL MUSEUM
Silk Mill Lane, off Full Street, Derby DE1 3AR
Tel: (01332) 255308 Fax: (01332) 716670
Located in C18th silk and flour mills with
exhibits on local industries.

SD ♿ CP 🚶 E ♿ RF ♿ L ♿
S ♿ WC 🚶 RFE 🚶

DERBY MUSEUM AND ART GALLERY
The Strand, Derby DE1 1BS
Tel: (01332) 293111 Fax: (01332) 716670
Fine display of Derby porcelain and mid-
C18th painting by Joseph Wright of Derby

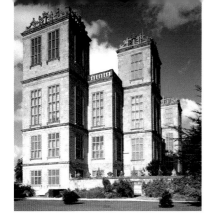

Towering Hardwick Hall.

plus many changing exhibitions.

SD ♿   CP n/a   E ♿   RF ♿   L ♿
C n/a   S 🚶   WC ♿   RFE ♿

DENBY POTTERY VISITORS CENTRE
Denby, Nr. Derby DE5 8NX
Tel: (01773) 740799   Fax: (01773) 740749
Modern complex with wide open spaces
between the Visitor Centre that houses
several shops, museum and seconds shop,
ramped at gradient of 1:19, and a cookery
demonstration area with several
wheelchair spaces. The craftsman's
workshop tour is limited to two
wheelchairs per tour. The Guided Pottery
Tour is not accessible.

SD ♿   CP ♿   E ♿   RF ♿
L ♿ Craftsman's tour on first floor.
C 🚶   S ♿   WC 🚶

THE AMERICAN ADVENTURE THEME PARK
Pit Lane, Ilkeston, Nr. Derby DE7 5SX
Tel: (01773) 531521   Fax: (01773) 716140
www.adventureworld.co.uk
Theme park based on pioneers from the
western to space in an epic story. Small
family rides allow all users to have fun so
long as restraint criteria are met. There are
also restraint consideration on Skycoaster,
Runaway Train, Niagara Rapids, Missile
and Motion Master. There is an
evacuation consideration on the Log
Flume, but a High Loading Platform for
the Twin Looper.

SD ♿   CP ♿   E ♿   RF ♿
C ♿   S ♿   WC 🚶

SPORTING VENUE
DERBY COUNTY FOOTBALL CLUB

Pride Park Stadium, Derby DE24 8XL
Disabled Liaison Officer: (01332) 667531
Full time disabled liaison officer has
ensured that the grounds are very
wheelchair friendly with 28 adapted toilets
and the front row round the ground
reserved for wheelchair users. There are
four elevated areas accessible by
wheelchair, three of which are reserved
for season ticket holders. Complies with
Part M, Building Regulations.

CP ♿   RE ♿   ED ♿   IN ♿   L ♿
WC ♿   SS ♿   B/R ♿

THEATRE
DERBY PLAYHOUSE
Eagle Centre, Derby DE1 2NF
Administration: (01332) 363271
Fax: (01332) 547200
Booking-Box Office: (01332) 363275

CP ♿   RE ♿   ED ♿   INT ♿
L ♿   WC ♿   AUD ♿   B/R ♿

MATLOCK
Riber Castle is the most famous
landmark in the Matlocks.The famous
wishing stone in Lumsdale is nearby.
Many terrific views here.

SELF-CATERING
DARWIN FOREST COUNTRY PARK
Two Dales, Matlock
Book through Grooms Holidays
No. of Accessible Units: 2
No. of Beds per Unit: 4 and 6
Accessible Facilities: Open plan lounge,
diner/kitchen.
Adapted lodges in 44 acres of woodland
and lush parkland.

MIDDLEHILLS FARM   ♿
Grange Mill, Matlock DE4 4HY
Tel/Fax: (01629) 650368
e-mail: l.lomas@btinternet.com
No. of Accessible Units: 1
No. of Beds per Unit : 2-4. Roll-in Shower
Accessible Facilities: Open plan Lounge/
kitchen/diner. Clematis Cottage is one of
three facing each other on a tarmac-
surfaced area on a small working farm five
miles from Matlock in the Peak National

Park. It is close to many interesting attractions.

ATTRACTIONS
CRICH TRAMWAY VILLAGE
Crich, Matlock DE4 5DP
Tel: (01773) 852565 Fax: (01773) 852326
www.tramway.co.uk
A vast array of indoor diversions and rides through history on vintage trams. The access Tram is a 1969 model from Berlin and is specially adapted. An extra-wide door and hydraulic lift is fitted for easy access. It carries 4 people in their wheelchairs and runs on demand, so pre-book.

SD ♿ CP ♿ E ♿ RF ♿
L ♿ C ♿ S ♿ WC 🚶

RIDGEWAY
Rural heart of the Moss Valley, south-east of Sheffield.

ACCESSIBLE ATTRACTION
RIDGEWAY COTTAGE INDUSTRIES
Main Road, Ridgeway S12 3XR
Tel: (0114) 247 3739
Set in restored and converted C17th farmhouse, visitors can watched skilled crafts people at work on modern and traditional crafts.
The Smithy: Paul Mossman Pottery:
Tel: (0114) 251158.
West Byre: Silver and Gold Jewellery:
Tel: (0114) 2477028
Courtside: Tiffany Land Stained Glass:
Tel: (0114) 2477104
East Byre: Chocolatier:
Tel: (0114) 2478626
Farmhouse Kitchen: Kent House Country Kitchen. Tel: (0114) 2473739

CP ♿ WC ♿

ROWSLEY
Located on the A6 between Bakewell and Matlock in the new Peak Village retail centre.

ATTRACTIONS
PEAK VILLAGE ESTATES
Chatsworth Road, Rowlsey DE4 2JE
Tel: (01629) 735326 Fax: (01629) 735128
e-mail: info@peakvillage.co.uk
Outlet shopping and leisure centre.

SD ♿ CP ♿ E ♿ RF ♿
C ♿ S ♿ WC 🚶

WIND IN THE WILLOWS
Peak Village, Rowsley DE4 2NP
Tel: (01629) 733433 Fax: (01629) 734850
e-mail: toad@hop-skip-jump.com
Every scene from this delightful adventure story is brought to life in a recreation of the English countryside undercover. Lighting, sound and AV techniques, and innovative and exciting displays present an animal's eye view of woods, meadow and riverbank. 4 wheelchairs available for loan.

SD ♿ CP ♿ E ♿ RF ♿
C ♿ S ♿ WC ♿ RFE ♿

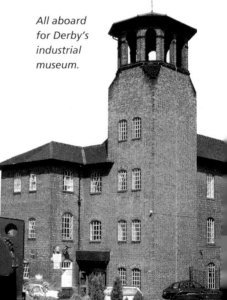

All aboard for Derby's industrial museum.

DEVONSHIRE

TOURIST OFFICE
www.devon-cc.gov.uk/tourism

DISABILITY INFORMATION SERVICE
Tel/Minicom: (01803) 552175
Fax: (01803) 556060

BARNSTAPLE
One of the oldest boroughs in Britain, the town has a fine estuary setting with a C16th arch bridge.

TOURIST INFORMATION CENTRE
36 Boutport Street, Barnstaple EX31 1RX
Tel: (01271) 375000   Fax: (01271) 374037

HOTEL
BRACKEN HOUSE
Bratton Fleming, Barnstaple EX31 4TG
Tel: (01598) 710320
No. of Accessible Rooms: 1. Bath.
Accessible Facilities: Lounge, Restaurant.
Originally an 1840 rectory, the house is now a small and intimate eight-bedroom hotel. Situated on the western edge of Exmoor and standing in eight acres of garden, woodland and paddock, including a small lake.

SELF-CATERING
CALVERT TRUST EXMOOR
Wistlandpound, Kentisbury,
Barnstaple EX31 4SJ
Tel: (01598) 763560   Fax: (01598) 763063
e-mail: exmoor@calvert-trust.org.uk
www.calvert-trust.org.uk
No. of Accessible Units: 3. Roll-in Shower
No. of Beds per Unit: 4-7.
Accessible Facilities: Dining room, TV Lounge, bar, heated indoor pool with spa and steam room. Opened in 1996 providing holidays with adventure for disabled people, their families and friends. Accommodation is in a converted farm complex. Accessible to all, set around an inner courtyard garden. Fully catering accommodation in mainly twin-bedded rooms, all with en-suite shower and wc and accessible for wheelchair users.

COUNTRY WAYS
Little Knowle Farm, High Bickerton,
Umberleigh, Nr. Barnstaple EX37 9BJ
Tel/Fax: (01769) 560503
e-mail: country-ways@virgin.net
www.country-ways.net
No. of Accessible Units: 1, roll-in shower
No. of Beds per Unit: 2-6
Converted barns hidden away on a small farm with delightful gardens and many superb views.

BRADWORTHY
Bradworthy is the northern apex of the triangle of Bradworthy, Bude and Holsworthy. Located two miles from Tamar Lakes, with National Trust Coastline and Bude's sandy beach 10 miles away.

SELF-CATERING
KIMWORTHY COTTAGES
Bradworthy EX33 7RP
No. of Accessible Units: 3
No. of Beds per Unit: Little Kimworthy 2: Wren and Jay Cottages 4 + cot.
Accessible Facilities: Open plan Lounge/Kitchen/Diner. Three lovely pine and brick cottages sharing a three-acre garden with a lawned play area, an outdoor pool and partially landscaped gardens full of shrubs and flowers.

BUDLEIGH SALTERTON
Red cliffs, large-pebbled beach leading to the mouth of the River Otter.

TOURIST INFORMATION CENTRE
Fore Street, Budleigh Salterton EX9 6NG
Tel: (01395) 445275

COLYTON
A neat, busy small town supplying a rich farm vale. Its church is remarkable for its octagonal lantern top.

SELF-CATERING
SMALLICOMBE FARM   ♿
Northleigh, Colyton EX24 6BU
Tel: (01404) 831310
Fax: (01404) 831431
www.smallicombe.com
Winner of Best Self-Catering
Accommodation in England from Holiday
Care Service in 1996. Bed and Breakfast
and evening meal available in the
farmhouse.
No. of Accessible Units: 2. Roll-in Showers
No. of Beds per Unit: 1 double and 1 twin
or 1 bunk-bed.
Accessible facilities: Lounge, Dining room,
Games room with snooker, table tennis,
skittles, darts, level concrete farmyard.
Smallicombe means narrow valley in
which the farm nestles in this unspoilt
part of Devon. Home of the prize winning
Smallicombe Herd of rare breed pigs.
Close to Honiton and the coast from
Lyme Regis to Sidmouth.

CULLOMPTON
Hemyock is situated in Blackdown
Hills, a good centre for touring
Exmoor and Dartmoor.

SELF-CATERING
HEMYOCK CASTLE   🚶
Hemyock, Cullompton EX15 3RJ
Tel: (01823) 680745
No. of Accessible Units: 1. Shower
No. of Beds per Unit: 6. Lounge has bed
settee downstairs, other bedrooms
upstairs.
Accessible Facilities: Lounge, Kitchen,
Private sitting area overlooking level
grassed area. Shared gardens mostly level.
Mow Barton is one of four holiday
cottages converted in 1993 from an open
linhay and stable block. Located in the
grounds of a medieval castle built in 1380
that surround the even older fortified
manor house.

DREWSTEIGNTON
Standing above Fingle Gorge in the
north-east of Dartmoor National Park.
Thatched cobhouses surrounded the
central square.

SELF-CATERING
CLIFFORD LODGE BARN   ♿
Clifford Bridge, Drewsteignton EX6 6QE
Tel: (01647) 24445
No. of Accessible Units: 1. Roll-in Shower
No. of Beds per Unit: 4
Accessible Facilities: Kitchen/Diner. Lift to
lounge upstairs. Garden, patio.
Barn conversion situated deep in the heart
of Upper Teign Gorge, within Dartmoor
National Park, ideal base for exploring
South Devon.

EXETER
Cathedral city dating back to Roman
times with a wealth of historical
interest and displays, combined with a
lively shopping centre and the leisurely
bank of the River Exe.

TRAVELINE
Tel: (0870) 6082608

TAXIS
Hookways Greenslades Coaches:
Tel: (01392) 469210
One 40-seater coach with lift and clamps,
available countrywide.

Exeter Hackney Carriages:
Tel: (01392) 277770
1 Metrocab with all fittings.

Ross Cabs: Tel: (07971) 169620
Seven-seater Mercedes with all fittings.

Connect 49: Tel: (01392) 491010
One Minibus with lift and ramp.

Freedom Wheels: Tel: (01392) 464206
Serving Exeter and surrounding area.

TRAINS

First Great Western: Special Needs –
Tel: (0845) 7413775

Virgin Trains: Special Needs –
(0845) 7443366
Minicom: (0845) 7443367

Wales & West: Special Needs –
Tel: (0845) 3003005
Minicom: (0845) 7585469
Exeter St. Davids station is suitable for
wheelchairs using ramp access.

SHOPMOBILITY

Deck F, King William Street Car Park,
King William Street, Exeter EX4 6PD
Tel: (01392) 494001

HOTEL

ST. ANDREWS HOTEL 　　　　　　　 ♿↑
28 Alphington Road, Exeter EX2 8HN
Tel: (01392) 276784   Fax: (01392) 250249
No. of Accessible Rooms: 1. Bath.
Accessible Facilities: Lounge, Restaurant.
Converted from a large Victorian house,
this long-established family-run hotel is
bright and spacious and located near the
city centre.

ATTRACTION

KILLERTON HOUSE AND GARDEN (NT)
Broadclyst, Nr. Exeter EX5 3LE
Tel: (01392) 881345   Fax: (01392) 883112
Rebuilt in 1778 as a comfortable family
house, home to Paulise de Bush costume
collection. Exhibition in stable courtyard,
plus hillside garden. Volunteer-driven
motorised buggies available. Wheelchairs
also available. N.B. Ground floor only
accessible.

SD ☐   CP ☐   E ☐   RF ☐
C ☐   S ☐   WC ☐   G ☐

THEATRE

NORTHCOTT THEATRE
Stocker Road, Exeter EX4 4QB
Admin: (01392) 223999
Booking-Box Office: (01392) 493493
Fax: (01392) 256835

CP ☐   RE ☐ (Queen's Drive, not Main Entrance)
ED ☐   INT ☐   WC ☐ (sited in upper foyer,
next to Queen's Drive entrance)
AUD ☐ (Wheelchair lift, 2 spaces)
B/R ☐ (Queen's Drive entrance)

101

Royal Horticulturial Society's beautiful Rosemoor Garden at Great Torrington.

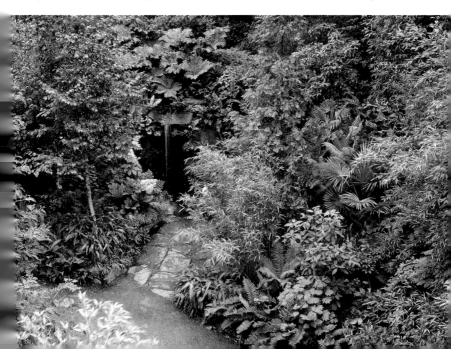

ENGLAND

GREAT TORRINGTON

Home to Dartington Crystal. Great Torrington has an interesting parish church and good views across the river Torridge towards Dartmoor from Castle Hill. The castle is no longer standing.

ATTRACTION
DARTINGTON CRYSTAL LTD
Linden Close, Torrington EX38 7AN
Tel: (01805) 626262   Fax: (01805) 626263
e-mail: enquiries@dartington.co.uk
www.dartington.co.uk
Home to the famous glass, the factory is viewed from inaccessible overhead galleries, but the Visitor Centre has an exhibition on the story of glass, demonstrations of engraving lampwork and studio glass-making.

SD 🚻 CP 🚻 E 🚻 RF 🚻 C 🚶
S 🚻 WC 🚻 RFE 🚻

ROYAL HORTICULTURAL SOCIETY ROSEMOOR GARDEN
Great Torrington EX38 8PH
Tel: (01805) 624067   Fax: (01805) 624717
40-acre site with mature planting in Lady Anne Berry's Garden and arboretum and a recent formal garden by a winding rock gorge planted with ferns and bamboos, together with herb, cottage, foliage, winter and fruit and vegetable gardens.

SD 🚻 CP 🚻 E 🚻 RF 🚻 C 🚻
S 🚻 WC 🚻 RFE 🚻

ILFRACOMBE

Holiday and retirement resort, with many public gardens.

TOURIST INFORMATION CENTRE
The Landmark Sea Front,
Ilfracombe EX34 9BX
Tel: (01271) 863001   Fax: (01271) 862586

BED AND BREAKFAST
SUNNYMEADE COUNTRY HOTEL
Dean Cross, West Down, Ilfracombe
EX34 8NT

Tel: (01271) 863668
e-mail: info @sunnymeade.co.uk
www.sunnymeade.co.uk
No. of Accessible Rooms: 2. Shower.
Accessible Facilities: Lounge, Dining room.
Charming small hotel with home cooking, surrounded by rolling green hills, in a fine location among North Devon's lovely scenery and wildlife.

IVYBRIDGE

Gateway to Dartmoor and good for exploring Erme Valley and Erme Plym trail to Plymouth.

SELF-CATERING
VENN FARM   🚻
Ugborough, Ivybridge PL21 0PE
Tel: (01364) 73240
Total No. of Accessible Units: 3. Roll-in Shower. No. of Beds per Unit: 8 + 4 + 2.
Facilities: Lounge in one unit, Dining room.
The Granary and Hams barns are built of lovely granite and overlook unspoilt countryside.

NEWTON ABBOTT

SELF-CATERING
WOODER MANOR   🚻
Widecombe-in-the-Moor,
Newton Abbot TQ13 7TR
Tel/Fax: (01364) 621391
www.woodermanor.com
No. of Accessible Units: 2
No. of Beds per Unit: 2-4. Lower Chinkwell-bath: Hameldown roll-in shower.
Accessible Facilities: Lounge/kitchen/diner.
Large shared garden. Lower Chinkwell and Lower Hameldown are two of six cottages on working family farm of 150 acres in a picturesque valley in Dartmoor National Park. Surrounded by unspoilt woodland, moors and granite tors. Widecombe village is 0.5miles along a quiet, level country lane. The famous Widecombe Fair, dating back to about 1850, still takes place annually on the second Tuesday in September.

ATTRACTION
HEDGEHOG HOSPITAL AND FARM
Prickly Ball Farm, Denbury Road,
Newton Abbot TQ12 6BZ
Tel/Fax: (01626) 362319
e-mail: hedgehog@hedgehog.org.uk
www.hedgehog.org.uk
A busy hands-on farm that also has a
hedgehog hospital, treating and returning
them to the wild. See, touch and learn
about them. This is a small farm with
undercover areas, but grassed areas are
inevitably bumpy. Advice from local Access
Team implemented. Wheelchair for hire.

SD ♿ CP ♿ E ♿ RF 🚶
C ♿ S 🚶 WC 🚶 RFE 🚶

SPORTING VENUE
NEWTON ABBOT RACECOURSE
Newton Abbot TQ12 3AF
Admin and Booking-Box Office:
(01626) 353235   Fax: (01626) 336972

CP ♿ RE ♿ ED ♿ (except Manual Door)
INT 🚶 L ♿ WC 🚶 SS ♿
B/R ♿ (Lift access)

At time of writing more facilities for
diabled access planned. Please call before
visiting to check.

OKEHAMPTON
Market town on northern boundary of
Dartmoor that prospered during the
wool period of the 18th and 19th
centuries.

BED AND BREAKFAST
WEEK FARM
Bridestowe, Okehampton EX20 4HZ
Tel: (01837) 861221
No. of Accessible Rooms: 1
Accessible Facilities: Lounge, Dining room.
C17th farmhouse surrounded by
wonderful scenery, where three
generations of the same family have
welcomed guests. Close to several local
events and attractions.

SELF-CATERING
ANGLERS UTOPIA PARADISE HOLIDAYS ♿
The Gables, Winsford, Halwill Junction,
Beaworthy EX21 5XT

Tel/Fax: (01409) 221559
No. of Accessible Units: 3. Bath.
No. of Beds per Unit: 3.
Anglers Big Wheel – 4-bedroomed villa.
Anglers Access – 2-bedroomed
villa(+shower).
Anglers Freedom – 2-bedroomed
villa(+shower).
Accessible Facilities: Fishing. Family run
venture of 12 lakes on a 70-acre estate.
Pagoda shelters available on most lakes
and purpose-built pathways to most
lakes. Suitable for non-anglers also, with
the peace and quiet of the countryside.

BLAGDON FARM COUNTRY HOLIDAYS ♿
Ashwater, Beaworthy, Nr.
Okehampton EX21 5DF
Tel: (01409) 211509   Fax: (01409) 211510
e-mail: info@blagdon-farm.co.uk
www.blagdon-farm.co.uk
No. of Accessible Units: 8. Roll-in
Showers.
No. of Beds per Unit: 6 sleep up to 6, 2
sleep up to 4.
Accessible Facilities: Open plan lounge/
diner/kitchen, balcony with patio doors.
Indoor heated pool with hoist. Licenced
bar and evening meals available. Hard
surfaced nature trails. Delightful small
development of quality bungalows built in
1995, designed to be wheelchair-friendly.
Situated on the shore of a 2.5-acre game
fishing lake in a superb rural setting, close
to the ancient port town of Holsworthy
and 10 miles from Launceston and the
beaches of Bude and Widemouth.

PAIGNTON
The town's fine features include the
red sandstone St. John's Church,
Oldway Mansion and an outstanding
zoo.

ATTRACTION
PAIGNTON ZOO ENVIRONMENTAL PARK
Totnes Road, Paignton TQ4 7EU
Tel: (01803) 697500   Fax: (01803) 523457
One of the country's largest zoos set in 75
acres of gardens where many endangered
species are nurtured, including African

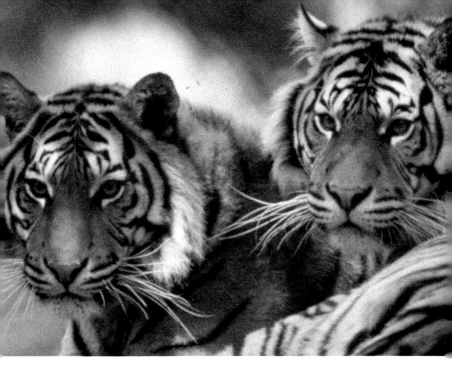

Inscrutable Paignton Zoo tigers eye up visitors.

lions and Sumatran tigers.
NB. BECAUSE OF THE NATURE OF THE
ZOO, ONE NURSE/ATTENDANT PER FIVE
DISABLED VISITORS IS REQUIRED.
It does require a fair bit of effort to wheel
around, but so long as you bear this in
mind, the facilities provide a good day out.
There is a variety of bird, lions and pandas
and of monkeys including orang-utans,
macaques and gorillas, in natural habitats.

SD ♿   CP ♿   E ♿   C ♿
S ♿   L ♿   WC ♿

Features: Access indoors to monkey and
rhino houses, the Ark, restaurant and bar.
Orang-utan and nocturnal houses have
steps to negotiate. Wheelchairs are
available free.

THE PAIGNTON AND DARTMOUTH STEAM RAILWAY

Queens Park Station, Torbay Road,
Paignton TQ4 6AF
Tel: (01803) 555872   Fax: (01803) 664313
Steam trains run along the Torbay coast to
Churston and on through the Dart estuary
to Kingswear. Wonderful scenery
throughout.

SD ♿ CP n/a (Brit. Rail next door)
E ♿ (special ramp to take wheelchairs onto the train)
RF ♿   S ♿   WC ♿   RFE ♿

PLYMOUTH

A city of distinct parts: it is well worth
while wandering through the modern
central area and the Barbican, both
offer excellent views, and Plymouth
Hoe offers one of the country's great
harbour views.

HOTELS

COPTHORNE HOTEL   ♿
Armada Way, Plymouth PL1 1AR
Tel: (01752) 224161   Fax: (01752) 670688
No. of Accessible Rooms: 1. Bath
Accessible Facilities: Lounge, Restaurant.
Located in the city centre.

NEW CONTINENTAL HOTEL   ♿
Millbay Road, Plymouth PL1 3LD
Tel: (01752) 220782   Fax: (01752) 227013
No. of Accessible Rooms: 4
Accessible Facilities: Lounge, Restaurant.
NB: The side door entrance is ramped

through the main corridor.
Privately owned Victorian hotel adjacent to the Pavilion Conference and Leisure Centre and the city centre.

NOVOTEL PLYMOUTH ⚐
Marsh Mills, Plymouth PL6 8NH
Tel: (01752) 221422   Fax: (01752) 223922
No. of Accessible Rooms: 2. Bath
Accessible Facilities: Lounge, Restaurant, Pool. Modern hotel situated on the outskirts of the town.

PLYMOUTH MOAT HOUSE ⚐
Armada Way, Plymouth PL1 2HJ
Tel: (01752) 639988   Fax: (01752) 673816
No. of Accessible Rooms: 2
Accessible Facilities: All public areas, via a lift. A modern high-rise hotel in a superb location overlooking the Hoe.

BED AND BREAKFAST
OSMOND GUEST HOUSE ⚐
42 Pier Street, West Hoe, Plymouth PL1 3BT
Tel: (01752) 229705
No. of Accessible Rooms: 2. Shower
Accessible Facilities: Dining room
Three-storey converted Edwardian house situated on Plymouth Hoe close to the sea front and main points of interest.

ATTRACTIONS
PLYMOUTH DOME
The Hoe, Plymouth PL1 2NZ
Tel: (01752) 603300   Fax: (01752) 256361
Hi-tec centre where visitors can explore an Elizabethan street, sail an epic voyage, stroll on an ocean liner, witness the Blitz.

SD ♿   CP ♿   E ⚐   RF ♿   L ♿
C ♿   S ♿   WC ⚐   RFE ⚐

THEATRE
THEATRE ROYAL
Royal Parade, Plymouth PL1 2TR
Admin: Tel: (01752) 668282
Fax: (01752) 262633
Booking-Box Office: (01752) 267222
Minicom: (01752) 600290
Fax: (01752) 252546
Complies with Part M, Building Regulations.

SD ♿   CP Nearest Public – Civic Centre
Taxi Rank: Royal Parade, outside theatre.

RE ♿   ED ♿   IN ♿   L ♿
WC ♿   Drum Foyer   AUD ⚐   B/R ♿

Route to wheelchair spaces via Door 1, wheelchair lift to stalls foyer and access via Doors 2 and 3 to stalls.

SOUTH MOLTON
Pleasant and lively small town with an attractive, mainly Georgian, square.

TOURIST INFORMATION CENTRE
1 East Street, South Molton EX36 3BU
Tel/Fax: (01769) 574122

SELF-CATERING
HAZEL COTTAGE ⚐
Bournebridge House, Meshaw,
Nr. South Molton EX36 4NL
Tel/Fax: (01884) 860134
bournebridge3@netscape.net
No. of Accessible Units: 1. Bath.
No. of Beds per Unit: 3 + cot
Accessible Facilities: Lounge, Dining room. Formerly a pig sty! Now a pretty cottage, one of three located at the head of a quiet valley in 6.5 acres amid rolling countryside.

TEIGNMOUTH
The promenade and sandy beaches border the town with family entertainment on the sea front and pier. Teignmouth has a busy working port and fishing quay.

TOURIST INFORMATION CENTRE
Tel: (01626) 215666

HOTEL
CLIFFDEN ⚐
Dawlish Road, Teignmouth TQ14 8TE
Tel: (01626) 770052   Fax: (01626) 770594
No. of Accessible Rooms: 5. Bath
Accessible Facilities: Lounge, Restaurant, Pool. This hotel is run by Action for Blind People. It is a listed Victorian building set in formal grounds of over six acres overlooking a small valley forming lovely

gardens. These give direct access to East Cliff Beach.

TIVERTON
Prosperous industrial and agricultural town on the River Exe.

TOURIST INFORMATION CENTRE
Phoenix Lane, Tiverton EX16 6LU
Tel: (01884) 255827   Fax: (01884) 257594

HOTEL
TIVERTON HOTEL
Blundells Road, Tiverton EX16 4DB
Tel: (01884) 256120   Fax: (01884) 258101
No. of Accessible Rooms: 2. Bath
Accessible Facilities: Lounge, Restaurant
This is a modern hotel on the edge of the town.

SELF-CATERING
THE BARN
Huntsham, Tiverton EX16 7NQ
Tel: (01398) 361519
No. of Accessible Units: 1. Bath
No. of Beds per Unit: 5-6.
Accessible Facilities: Lounge, Dining room, South facing courtyard with barbecue. Offers Internet short breaks, learning to discover the Net. Huntsham is a conservation hamlet: the barn is a converted stone barn.

ATTRACTIONS
KNIGHTSHAYES COURT AND GARDENS (NT)
Knightshayes, Tiverton EX16 7RQ
Tel: (01884) 254665 Fax: (01884) 243050
Begun in 1869, the rich interior combines medieval romanticism with Victorian dècor, giving rare insight into elegant countryhouse life. The gardens are notable for their water lily pool, rare shrubs and topiary.The ground floor is very spacious, ideal for wheelchairs. Two chairs are available on loan, one at the house and one at reception.

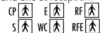

TIVERTON CASTLE
Tiverton EX16 6RP

Tel: (01884) 253200   Fax: (01884) 254200
E-mail: tiverton.castle@ukf.net
www.tivertoncastle.com
Built in 1106 and dominating the River Exe, only one original circular Norman tower remains. Grade 1 listed. Access to the building's interiors is very limited, but the inner baillie with walled garden, that is in the process of rehabilitation, is well worth a visit.

TORQUAY
The most glamorous, grandly sited and well- planned of all west country resorts with fine beaches and ambitious modern buildings.

TOURIST INFORMATION CENTRE
Vaughan Parade, Torquay TQ2 5JG
Tel: (01803) 297428   Fax: (01803) 214885
email: tourist.board@torbay.gov.uk
www.theenglishriviera.co.uk
Produces Information for Disabled People.

BUSES
TRAVELINE (0870) 6082608

TAXIS
Torbay Cab Co: Tel: (01803) 213521
Three vehicles, all with all fittings.
Torquay & Paington & Central Taxis: Tel: (01803) 616969
One TX1 with all fittings.

TRAINS
Wales and West: Special Needs –
Tel: (0845) 3003005
Minicom: (0345) 585469

Torquay station is on the flat and taxis can take wheelchairs right inside the station.

CAR PARKS
Corporate Services Dept., Civic Offices, Torquay TQ1 3DS
Tel: (01803) 201201
Free parking for visitors with mobility allowance (at the higher rate). Major

council car parks have reserved spaces:
the blue badge is recognised for on-street
parking.

WHEELCHAIR HIRE
Speedy Hire Ltd,
95 Newton Road,
Torquay TQ2 7AR
Tel: (01803) 613031

HOTELS
FAIRMOUNT HOUSE HOTEL
Herbert Road, Chelston, Torquay TQ2 6RW
Tel/Fax: (01803) 605446
No. of Accessible Rooms: 2. Bath
Accessible Facilities: Lounge, Restaurant,
Conservatory Bar. Charming small hotel,
set above Cockington Valley on south
facing hillside. Built in 1900 as a large
family home, there are mature gardens
and patios. Accessible garden level rooms
open out directly onto a paved area above
the main lawn. Accessed by a slightly
circuitous, ramped route through the side
garden. Located close to Cockington
Country Park.

FROGNEL HALL HOTEL
Higher Woodfield Road, Torquay TQ1 2LD
Tel: (01803) 298339   Fax: (01803) 215115
No. of Accessible Rooms: 2. Bath
Facilities: Lounge, Restaurant, Sauna,
Garden. Lovely adapted Victorian mansion
in two acres of peaceful private gardens
with fine views. In a quiet corner of
Torquay, but close to the harbour, sea
and town centre.

SELF-CATERING
THE CORBYN SUITES
Torbay Road, Torquay TQ2 6RH
Tel: (01803) 215595
No. of Accessible Units: 2 (Forbes and
Wallace)
No. of Beds per Unit: Forbes-2S:
Wallace-1D, 2S
Accessible Facilities: Both have
lounge/diner, kitchen. Quality suites with
classical Georgian proportions situated
within 50m of the beach and a mile from
local shops. Nearby is Torre Abbey
Mansion and Meadows.
Close to the railway station.

1 PARK ROAD
St. Marychurch, Babbacombe, Torquay
Book through Grooms Holidays
No. of Accessible Units: 1. Shower
No. of Beds per Unit: 6
Accessible Facilities: Lounge, Kitchen
This apartment is a short walk from the
pedestrianised shopping area in the
delightful seaside town of Babbacombe,
tucked into a little sandy bay.

WOOLACOMBE
Enjoy a wonderful sand and surf beach,
with the town enclosed by steep
moorland slopes rather than cliffs.

HOTEL
THE CLEEVE HOUSE HOTEL
Mortehoe, Wollacombe EX34 7ED
Tel/Fax: (01271) 870719
No. of Accessible Rooms: 1.
Roll-in Shower.
Accessible Facilities: Lounge, Restaurant.
Mortehoe is situated in an area of
outstanding natural beauty. This small
privately owned and managed hotel has
most attractive gardens and is two miles
from the beach and 100m from the
village.

YELVERTON
This old settlement has ponies
wandering all over its flat common,
and the best inland golf course in
Devon.

BED AND BREAKFAST
HEADLAND WARREN FARM
Postbridge, Yelverton PL20 6TB
Tel: (01822) 880206
No. of Accessible Rooms: 2
Accessible Facilities: Kitchen. Lounge/
Diner (on first floor, accessed by stairlift).
One of the few remaining longhouses.
These 600-year-old plus farm buildings
now consist of an original farmhouse, a
converted barn for those with disabilities,
an attached cottage and stables. Remote
but easily located 30 minutes from Exeter

off the B3212. Headland Warren is in its own 600 acres of National Park moorland in the middle of the Two Moors Way.

SELF-CATERING
MIDWAY
Book through Leigh Farm, Roborough, Plymouth PL6 7BS.
Tel: (01752) 733221
No. of Accessible Units: 1. Bath
No. of Beds per Unit: 6
Accessible Facilities: Lounge, kitchen, dining room, conservatory, garden. Large detached house, recently converted into two self-contained holiday apartments with a lovely garden. Situated in quiet crescent in sleepy village of Crapstone, a mile from Yelverton and nine from Plymouth.

ATTRACTION
BUCKLAND ABBEY (NT)
Yelverton PL20 6EY
Tel: (01822) 853607
Fax: (01822) 855448
e-mail: bucklandabbey@ntrust.org.uk
www.nationaltrust.org.uk
Originally a Cistercian Abbey, converted into a handsome home of Sir Francis Drake in 1580's. Restored buildings with exhibitions on history of the Abbey and Drake himself. Parking well marshalled with disabled spaces in separate area near Abbey.

SD ♿ CP ♿ E ♿ RF 🚶
S ♿ WC ♿

DORSET

DORCHESTER COALITION OF DISABLED PEOPLE.
Room 1, Poole Advice Centre,
54 Lagland Street, Poole BH15 1QG
Tel: (01202) 668593
Provides information throughout Dorset.

DORSET COUNTY COUNCIL
Colliton Park, Dorset
Tel: (01305) 251000
Minicom: (01305) 267933

WHEELCHAIR HIRE
Keep Able, 779 - 781 Wimborne Road,
Moordown, Bournemouth BH9 2BD37
Tel: (01202) 549121
Hire out wheelchairs.

BEAMINSTER
Set in beautiful countryside of steep hills dividing deep cuts of farmland, this is one of the most appealing towns of its size.

MAPPERTON
Mapperton, Beaminster DT8 3NR
Tel: (01308) 862645
Fax: (01308) 863348
e-mail:office@mapperton.com
www.maperton.com
Superb terraced valley garden surrounding a Jacobean manor house. Entrance through a wide gateway and archway. Wheelchair access to upper levels only. At the edge of the croquet lawn one can look down on the remainder of the gardens.

SD ♿ CP 🚶 E ♿ C ♿ S ♿
WC ♿ L ♿

BLANDFORD FORUM
Home of sculptor and painter Alfred Stevens, this is the hub of a rich farming area and has a very handsome and uniform Georgian red-brick and stone town centre.

SELF-CATERING
LUCCOMBE FARM
Milton Abbas, Blandford Forum DT11 0BE
Tel: (01258) 880558 Fax: (01258) 881384
e-mail:kayll@aol.com
www.luccombeholidays.co.uk
No. of Accessible Units: 1.Shower.
No. of Beds per Unit: 4
Accessible Facilities: Lounge, Dining room.
Pound Cottage Equestrian Centre
specialising in riding for the disabled 0.5
miles from Luccombe. 650-acre
dairy/arable working farm close to historic
thatched village of Milton Abbas. The
converted 150-year-old brick and flint-
built barns and stables house a variety of
cottage-style units, of which Old Sty has
accessible grading 3. The Cakehouse, not
graded, is considered accessible also and
has two bedrooms.

ATTRACTION
CAVALCADE OF COSTUME MUSEUM
Lime Tree House, The Plocks,
Blandford Forum DT11 7AA
Tel: (01258) 453006 Fax: (01258) 454084
Unique collection of over 500 items
exhibiting clothes and accessories from
the 1730s to the 1950s. Immediate access
to four rooms, one with a ramp 1:5, to
access three other rooms. Steward
assistance guaranteed, visitors are taken
down backwards. Off these three rooms
are four steps to another large area,
stewards carry wheelchairs.

SD   CP   E   RF
C   S   WC

BOURNEMOUTH
Wide streets, a pier, a pavilion and a
theatre. Many parks and gardens
scattered close to the town centre.
Spectacular views of the Isle of Wight
can be seen from the cliffs.

BOURNEMOUTH TOURISM AND TOURIST
INFORMATION CENTRE
Westover Road,
Bournemouth, BH1 2BU

Tel: (01202) 451702 Fax: (01202) 451743
TIC: Tel: (01202) 451700

BOURNEMOUTH BOROUGH COUNCIL
Central Office, 9 Madeira Road,
Bournemouth BH1 1QN
Tel: (01202) 458000
Publishers of Bournemouth Disabled
Visitors' Guide.

BOURNEMOUTH HELPING SERVICES
29A Alma Road, Winton
Bournemouth BH9 1AB
Tel: (01202) 536336

BRITISH RED CROSS (Bournemouth)
52 Portchester Road, Bournemouth BH8 8JY
Tel: (01202) 553433

TRAVELINE
Tel: (0870) 6082608

BUSES
Wilts and Dorset
27 The Triangle, Bournemouth
Tel: (01202) 291288
Some low-floor buses, some raised kerbs.

TAXIS
United Taxis: Tel: (01202) 556677
Three vehicles with all fittings.
Warren Cars: Tel: (01202) 555511
One minibus with all fittings as well as
adapted vehicles.

TRAINS
Connex: Customer Services:
Tel: (0870) 6030405
Fax: (0870) 6030505
Minicom: (01233) 617621
South West Trains: Special Needs –
Tel: (0845) 6050440
Minicom: (0845) 6050441
Virgin Trains: Special Needs –
(0845) 7443366
Minicom: (0845) 7443367

Bournemouth Station has a flat entry to
both sides, three orange badge spaces
(platform 2 entrance), manual entry to
ticket office (90cm wide), flexible seating,
level access to platforms and sloped

subway. Unisex WCs and buffet on platform 2 with flexible seating. Saloon cars and cabs available from the rank by platform 3, card/payphones on each platform (149cm high), no lifts, wheelchair ramps plus three wheelchairs.

CAR PARKS
Blue badge scheme operates in borough council car parks and some others.
Tel: (01202) 451365/451200

SHOPMOBILITY
Sovereign Centre Car Park, Boscombe, Bournemouth
Tel: (01202) 399700

HOTEL
CARRINGTON HOUSE HOTEL   [&]
Knyveton Road, Bournemouth BH1 3QQ
Tel: (01202) 369988 Fax: (01202) 292221
No. of Accessible Rooms: 1
Accessible Facilities: Restaurant (lift access), lounge.
Set in quiet residential area with good children's facilities.

THE CONNAUGHT HOTEL   [&]
West Hill Road, Bournemouth BH2 5PH
Tel: (01202) 298020 Fax: (01202) 298028
No. of Accessible Rooms: 4. Roll-in Shower.
Accessible Facilities: Lounge, Restaurant, Conservatory Bar, Pool, Sauna, Whirlpool, Gymnasium, Snooker Room.
Delightful hotel with a wide variety of leisure facilities located 200 metres from the town centre and the beach.

ATTRACTIONS
RUSSELL-COTES ART GALLERY AND MUSEUM
East Cliff, Bournemouth, BH1 3AA
Tel: (01202) 451800 Fax: (01202) 451851
Noted for its collection of Victorian and Edwardian paintings, plus sculpture, decorative art and furniture and modern art, all housed in East Cliff Hall, built in 1897. Catering and Shop accessed through garden entrance.

SD   CP   E [&] C [&] S
WC   L [&]

BRIDPORT
Georgian houses and a handsome arcaded town hall are of interest here.

SELF-CATERING
SHEPHERDS COTTAGE   [&]
Rudge Farm, Chilcombe, Bridport DT6 4NF
Tel: (01308) 482630 Fax: (01308) 482635
e-mail: sue@rudgefarm.co.uk
No. of Accessible Units: 1. Bath
No. of Beds per Unit: 4
Accessible Facilities: Lounge/Diner, Kitchen.
Converted old farm buildings, retaining many original features ranged round a flower decked, cobbled yard overlooking the lakes in the paddock below. The village is six miles from Bridport. A good base for exploring West Dorset, and designated as an Area of Outstanding Natural Beauty.

CONWAY HOUSE   [人]
Bettiscombe, Bridport DT6 5NT
Tel/Fax: (01308) 868313
e-mail: conway@wdi.co.uk
No. of Accessible Units: 1. Roll-in Shower
No. of Beds per Unit: 4-6
Accessible Facilities: Lounge/Dining room combined. Bungalow with lovely views.

CHARMOUTH
Jane Austen found Charmouth a nice place for "sitting in unwearied contemplation". Its hillside street is still lined with thatched houses and some Regency bow windows. The town is in one of the few gaps in the hills that break into the cliffs overlooking the sweep of Lyme Bay. Beautiful beach.

SELF-CATERING
THE POPLARS   [&]
Woodfarm Caravan Park, Axminster Road, Charmouth DT6 6BT
Tel/Fax: (01297) 560697
e-mail: holidays@woodfarm.co.uk
www.woodfarm.co.uk
No. of Accessible Units: 1. Roll-in Shower
No. of Beds per Unit: 4 + cot

Accessible Facilities: Lounge, kitchen/diner. Self-catering flat within camping and caravan park nestling in Char Valley with views over Lyme Bay. Close to the Heritage Coast and lovely villages.

DORCHESTER
Made famous by the novels of Thomas Hardy, today Dorchester is a livestock marketing and farmers' shopping centre with a large brewery and other light industries.

TOURIST INFORMATION CENTRE
Unit 11, Antelope Walk, Dorchester DT1 1BE
Tel: (01305) 267992   Fax: (01305) 266079.
Publishes "West Dorset for visitors with special needs". Includes Bridgport, West Bay, Beaminster, Lyme Regis and Sherborne.

DORCHESTER TOWN COUNCIL
North Square, Dorchester.
Tel: (01305) 266861

BUSES
First Southern National: Tel: (01305) 783645
Some low-floor, easy-access buses.
Wilts and Dorset: Tel: (01202) 673555
Some low-floor, easy-access buses.

TAXIS
Access Taxis: Tel: (01305) 768190
Two vehicles with all fittings.
Coach House Travel: Tel: (01305) 267644
Four 57-seater vehicles with all fittings.
Transport Business Unit:
Tel: (01305) 225046
Vehicles of various sizes with all fittings.

TRAINS
South West Trains: Special Needs –
Tel: (0845) 6050440
Minicom: (0845) 6050441
Wales and West: Special Needs –
Tel: (0845) 3003005
Minicom: (0845) 7585469
Dorchester South Station.
Tel: (01305) 264423.

Two disabled badge spaces, ramp from street to ticket office, wide manual door, ramp to up platform, level to down platform. Disabled ladies WC, saloon cars available at rank, card/ pay telephone, 149cm high, ramp available. Dorchester West. Unmanned. Level access to platform 1, to platform 2 via footbridge. Alternative access from Damers Road via wide steps and partly unmade path. No WCs.

CAR PARKING
Disabled badge spaces available free for first three hours. Car parks located in Dorchester Town Information Leaflet from TIC.

SELF-CATERING
THE BARN AT BAGLAKE FARM
Litton Cheney, Dorchester DT2 9AD
Tel: (01308) 482222   Fax: (01308) 482226
No. of Accessible Units: 1. Bath.
No. of Beds per Unit: 3
Accessible Facilities: Lounge, dining room. Little Cheney is along the Bride Valley, eight miles from Dorchester and within three of the sea and Chesil Beach. The Barn is one third of a thatched barn converted into a cottage.

ATTRACTIONS
ATHELHAMPTON HOUSE AND GARDENS
Dorchester DT2 7LG
Tel: (01305) 848363   Fax: (01305) 848135
e-mail: email@athelhampton.co.uk
www.althelhampton.co.uk
15th century house with many finely furnished rooms. Gardens contain the famous topiary pyramids, fountains, the River Piddle and fine flowering collections. Six ground floor rooms are accessible.

SD ⚹   CP ⚹   E ⚹   RF ⚹   C ⚹
S ⚹   WC ⚹   RFE ⚹

THE KEEP MILITARY MUSEUM
The Keep, Bridport Road, Dorchester
DT1 1RN
Tel: (01305) 264066   Fax: (01305) 250373
e-mail:keep.museum@talk21.com
www.keepmilitarymuseum.org
Located at the top of the town, the Keep was built at the 1890's and brings to life

111

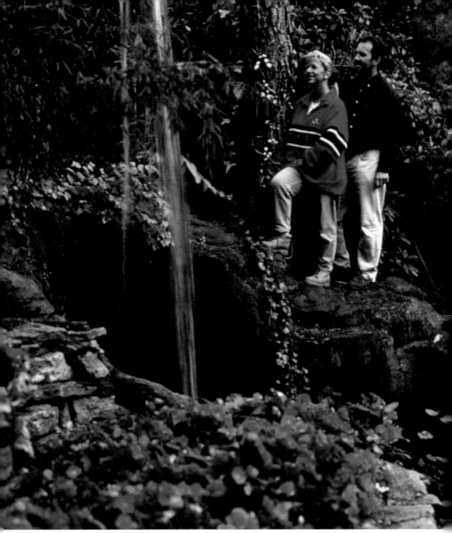

Lost in the beauty of Compton Acres Gardens.

the history of the local regiments to life with creative displays of infantry, cavalry and artillerymen and interactive displays on their social world. Delightful - an absolute find.

SD 🦽 CP 🦽 E 🦽 RF 🦽
L 🦽 S 🦽 WC 🚶 RFE 🦽

GILLINGHAM
Set in the Blackmore Vale close by the River Stour.

SELF-CATERING
TOP STALL 🦽
Factory Farm, Fifehead Magdalen,
Gillingham SP8 5RS

Tel/Fax: (01258) 820022
No. of Accessible Units: 1. Roll-in Shower
No. of Beds per Unit: 5
Accessible Facilities: Lounge, Dining room, Fishing from River Stour. Single storey cow stall conversion adjoining the farmhouse, a listed C18th former woollen and stocking factory, hence the name. Situated off the road with a garden enclosed by a stone wall, the village shops and inns of Marnhull are a mile away and Shaftesbury six.

POOLE
Tremendous natural harbour with much of its shoreline still undeveloped. Famous for its Poole Pottery.

TOURIST INFORMATION CENTRE
The Quay, Poole BH15 1HE
Tel: (01202) 253253   Fax: (01202) 684531

HOTEL
THISTLE POOLE   🚶
The Quay, Poole BH15 1HD
Tel: (01202) 666800   Fax: (01202) 684470
No. of Accessible Rooms: 1.
Accessible Facilities: Lounge, restaurant
(1st floor). Modern hotel close to Old
Poole town overlooking the lovely
natural harbour.

SELF-CATERING
ROCKLEY PARK
Poole.
Book through Grooms Holidays
No. of Accessible Units: 1. Roll-in Shower
No. of Beds per Unit: 6
Wooden forest-style chalet with views of
Poole's natural harbour close by.

SANDFORD PARK
Holton Heath, Poole
Book through Grooms Holidays
No. of Accessible Units: 1
No. of Beds per Unit: 6
Luxury pine log cabin set among
woodland in Sandford Park.

ATTRACTION
COMPTON ACRES GARDENS
Canford Cliffs, Poole, Dorset BH13 7ES
Tel: (01202) 700778   Fax: (01202) 707537
e-mail: info@comptonacres.co.uk
Gardens of 10 acres with Japanese,
Roman, Italian, water, rock and heather
gardens, plus superb bronze and marble
statuary.
SD 🦽 CP 🦽 E 🦽 RF 🦽 C- 🦽
S 🚶 (ramped at 1:11) WC 🚶 RFE-Garden 🦽

FARMER PALMER'S FARM PARK LTD
Organford, Poole
Tel: (01202) 622022   Fax: (01202) 622933
e-mail: farmerpalmers@bigfoot.co.uk
www.farmerpalmer.co.uk
The farm park operates alongside a 200-
acre working dairy farm. The park
overlooks lovely open grass fields and
forest with a wide woodland walk by the
river. Trained staff demonstrate handling

and feeding of a wide range of animals
including goats, pigs, lambs. Whatever the
weather there are undercover barns full of
activities and a milk demonstration.
SD 🦽 CP 🦽 E 🦽 RF 🦽 C 🚶
S 🚶 WC 🚶 RFE 🦽

WATERFRONT MUSEUM
4 High Street, Poole BH15 1BW
Tel: (01202) 683138   Fax: (01202) 262622
e-mail: c.fisher@poole.gov.uk
2,000 years of history displayed in C18th
warehouse. Original artefacts and
reconstructions.
SD 🦽 CP n/a E 🦽 RF 🦽 L 🦽
WC 🦽 RFE 🚶

SHAFTESBURY

Dorset's only hill-top town, to which
King Alfred gave a nunnery C880 and
an Anglo-Saxon town grew around it.
The ancient, wide, curved and cobbled
Gold Hill is probably the most
photographed street in Dorset,
although the cobbles sadly prevent
comfortable access to those in
wheelchairs.

TOURIST INFORMATION CENTRE
8 Bell Street, Shaftesbury SP7 8AE
Tel: (01747) 853514   Fax: (01747) 850593
e-mail: tourism@northdorsettis.co.uk
www.ruraldorset.com

HOTEL
THE COPPLERIDGE INN   🚶
Motcombe, Shaftesbury SP7 9HW
Tel: (01747) 851980   Fax: (01747) 851858
e-mail: thecoppleridgeinn@btinternet.com
No. of Accessible Bedrooms: All (10). Bath
Accessible Facilities: Lounge, Restaurant.
Converted C18th farmhouse set in 15
acres of meadow, woodland and gardens
overlooking Blackmore Vale. The courtyard
farm buildings have been converted into
10 bedrooms. Motcombe is two miles from
Shaftesbury.

SELF-CATERING
HARTGROVE FARM COTTAGES 🦽 🦽 🚶
Hartgrove, Shaftesbury, Dorset SP7 0JY

Tel: (01747) 811830
No. of Accessible Units: 3. Bath
No. of Beds per Unit: Each cottage sleeps 4, plus cot.
Bulbarrow Cottage (5) ♿
(Daily Mail Top 20 Holiday Cottages)
Melbury Cottage (5) ♿
(winner of Holiday Care Award)
Duncliffe Cottage(4) 🚶
Accessible Facilities: All three have wood-burning stove and small private gardens. Arrangements with nearby leisure centre for swimming, hoist access. Much of the farmyard can be accessed in a wheelchair. Outstanding family dairy farm straddling a small hill between Cranborne Chase and Blackmore Vales 1.5 miles from thatched village of Fontwell Magna. Farm buildings now converted into character cottages.

ATTRACTION
SHAFTESBURY ABBEY MUSEUM AND GARDENS
Park Walk, Shaftesbury SP7 8JR
Tel: (01747) 852910
Founded by King Alfred, this Benedictine Nunnery, was once the wealthiest in the country. It survived until the dissolution of the monasteries and the excavated remains, open during the summer, are the subject of interesting museum and garden audio-tours.

SD ♿ CP ♿ E ♿ RF 🚶
S ♿ WC 🚶

SHERBORNE
Yellowstone town with a wealth of medieval buildings and fine Abbey Church of 705.

TOURIST INFORMATION CENTRE
3 Tilton Court, Diby Road, Sherborne DT9 3NL
Tel: (01935) 815341

ATTRACTION
WORLDLIFE and LULLINGSTONE SILK FARM
Compton House, Sherborne, Dorset DT9 4QN
Tel: (01935) 474608 Fax: (01935) 429957
Elizabethan manor house, accessible except for Silk Farm on first floor. Worldlife has evolved from Worldwide Butterflies, with

displays on wildlife and environment. Butterflies fly free in a reconstruction of their natural habitat, including jungle and tropical palmhouse. Collection built up over 30 years with active breeding and hatching areas on view.

SD ♿ CP n/a E ♿ RF ♿ C ♿
S ♿ WC 🚶

SWANAGE
Cosy resort on a marvellous bay of yellow sands and white cliffs, flanked by downs grand for both walking and great views.

TOURIST INFORMATION CENTRE
The White House, Shore Road,
Swanage BH19 1LB
Tel: (01929) 422885 Fax: (01929) 423423

ATTRACTION
PUTLAKE ADVENTURE FARM
Langton Matravers, Swanage BH19 3EU
Tel: (01929) 422917
Over 50 breeds of cows, horses, pigs, goats, etc that can be touched and a farm implement collection. A delightful attraction.

SD ♿ CP ♿ E ♿ RF 🚶 C ♿
S ♿ WC 🚶

WAREHAM
Attractive small town situated on a low ridge between the Rivers Frome and Piddle. A shopping centre with friendly pubs and some light industry.

TOURIST INFORMATION CENTRE
Trinity Church, South Street,
Wareham BH20 4LU
Tel: (01929) 552740 Fax: (01929) 554491

HOTEL
KEMPS COUNTRY HOTEL 🚶
East Stoke, Nr. Wareham BH20 6AL
Tel: (01929) 462563 Fax: (01929) 405287
No. of Accessible Rooms: 6. Bath.
Accessible Facilities: Lounge, Restaurant. Victorian rectory in its own grounds facing the Purbeck Hills.

BED AND BREAKFAST
THE OLD GRANARY
West Holme Farm, Wareham BH20 6AQ
Tel: (01929) 552972   Fax: (01929) 551616
www.rural-dorset.org.uk
No. of Accessible Rooms: 1. Roll-in
Shower.
Facilities: Lounge, Dining room. Charming,
recently converted old granary with PYO
fruit, plant nursery and farm shop adjacent.

ATTRACTIONS
THE BLUE POOL
Furzebrook, Nr. Wareham BH20 5AT
Tel: (01929 551408)
Features include a designated wheelchair
route, the surface varies in both width and
surface with some gentle inclines and
declines. Allow 45 minutes to get around,
but there are numerous vantage points to
view the pool without having to complete
whole route.
The pool is surrounded by 25 acres of
heather, gorse and pine trees, interlaced
with sandy paths climbing to views of the
Purbeck Hills. Originally a clay pit, in
warmer weather the clay particles settle,
resulting in the pool showing more green
shades: in cold weather the particles rise to
the surface, making the pool look more
blue than green. The museum traces the
Furzebrook Estate industry from making
tobacco pipes to pottery.

SD ☐ CP ☐ E ☐ RF ☐ C ☐
S ☐ WC ☐

THE HERITAGE CENTRE
West Lulworth, Wareham BH20 5RQ
Tel/Fax: (01929) 400587
Video and displays on Lulworth's history
from prehistoric times to the present day.

SD n/a CP ☐ E ☐ RF ☐ S ☐
WC ☐ RFE ☐

WEYMOUTH
Pleasant sea-front, with long, tall, late
Georgian terraces backing the wide
esplanade and sandy beach.

TOURIST INFORMATION CENTRE
The King's Statue, The Esplanade,

Weymouth DT4 7AN
Tel: (01305) 785747
e-mail: tourism@weymouth.gov.uk
www.weymouth.gov.uk

HOTEL
HOTEL CENTRAL
15-17 Maiden Street, Weymouth DT4 8BB
Tel: (01305) 760700   Fax: (01305) 760300
No. of Accessible Rooms: 3. Bath.
Accessible Facilities: Lounge, Restaurant,
Lift. Located in town centre, very close to
the beach with ferry terminal and Pavilion
Theatre nearby.

ATTRACTIONS
ABBOTSBURY SWANNERY
New Barn Road, Abbotsbury,
Weymouth DT3 4JG
Tel: (01305) 871858   Fax: (01305) 871092
Voted best family attraction in Dorset 1999.
For over 600 years this colony of friendly
mute swans has made its home here,
Sheltered by Chesil Beach, this ancient site
provides protection for many nesting swans
and their broods. From the end of May you
can wander around the nests safely to see
the fluffy cygnets. An AV show about the
Swannery runs hourly. A must!

SD ☐ CP ☐ E ☐ RF ☐ C ☐ S ☐
WC ☐ (3 WCs. All Cat.1 -main toilet block between main
car park and ticket-office/shop: Restaurant: inside
Swannery).

DEEP SEA ADVENTURE
9 Custom House Quay, Old Harbour,
Weymouth DT4 8BG
Tel/Fax: (01305) 760690
Experience the Titanic Exhibition and
encounter underwater exploration and
maritime exploits both past and present.

SD ☐ CP ☐ E ☐ RF ☐ L ☐
C ☐ S ☐ WC ☐ RFE ☐

WEYMOUTH SEA LIFE PARK
Lodmoor Country Park, Lodmoor,
Weymouth DT4 7SX
Tel: (01305) 761070   Fax: (01305) 761070
Spectacular marine displays, plus tropical
jungle, blue whale splashpool and 3-D
shark academy.

CP- council owned E ☐ RF ☐ C ☐
S ☐ WC ☐ RFE ☐

WIMBORNE MINSTER

Centred on its distinctive church, dating from 1043, this small town is almost like a miniature cathedral city.

TOURIST INFORMATION CENTRE
29 High Street,
Wimborne Minster BN21 1HR
Tel: (01202) 886116   Fax: (01202) 841025

ATTRACTIONS
DORSET HEAVY HORSE CENTRE
Grains Hill, Edmondsham, Wimborne
BH21 5RJ
Tel: (01202) 824040   Fax: (01202) 821407
Many different breeds of heavy horse and miniature and Shetland ponies are on show here. There is an interesting information centre and a good display of farm implements.

SD 🚻   CP 🚶   E 🚻   RF 🚻   C 🚶
S 🚶   WC 🚶   RFE 🚻

KNOLL GARDENS AND NURSERY
Hampreston,
Nr. Wimborne BH21 7ND
Tel: (01202) 873931   Fax: (01202) 870842
Four acres of compact and mostly level gardens with herbaceous borders and water gardens. The nursery has a gravel floor with raised beds and is mostly accessible. The garden is flat and partly inclined, care is required because surfaces, widths and gradients do vary.

SD 🚻   CP 🚶   E 🚶   RF 🚻
WC 🚶   RFE 🚶

ESSEX

ESSEX TOURISM
Essex County Council, County Hall,
Chelmsford CM1 1LX
Tel: (01245) 437547   Fax: (01245) 355032
e-mail: tourism@essexcc.gov.uk
www.essexcc.gov.uk/tourism

ESSEX DISABLED PEOPLE'S ASSOCIATION
90 Broomfield Road, Chelmsford CM1 1SS
Tel: (01245) 253400   Fax: (01245) 346730
Minicom: (01245) 287177
e-mail: info@essexdpa.org
www.essexdpa.org

BILLERICAY

Here in Mayflower Hall, some of the Pilgrim Fathers met before setting sail for America in 1620. The town also has its place in history as the scene where remaining participants in the Peasants Revolt took refuge in Norsey Wood in 1381.

ATTRACTION
BARLEYLANDS FARM
Barleylands Road, Billericay CM11 2UD
Tel: (01268) 532253   Fax: (01268) 290222
e-mail: chris@barleylandfarm.co.uk
Farm museum depicting rural life in the past with an animal centre, a glass-blowing studio with a viewing gallery, and craft studios.

Time out at Knoll Gardens and nursery.

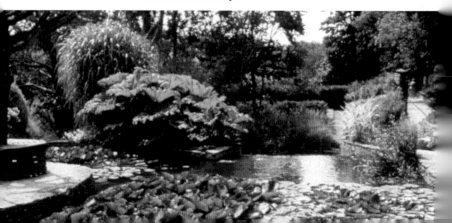

SD ⬛♿ CP ⬛♿ E ⬛♿ RF ⬛♿ C ⬛♿
S ⬛♿ WC ⬛♿

BRAINTREE
Pleasant town with several historical buildings, shops and entertainment.

TOURIST INFORMATION CENTRE
Braintree Town Hall Centre, Market Place, Braintree CM7 3YG
Tel: (01376) 550066

ATTRACTIONS
CRESSING TEMPLE
Witham Road, Cressing, Nr. Braintree
Tel: (01376) 584903 Fax: (01376) 584864
An ancient moated farmstead with two fine mediaeval timbered barns built for the Knights Templar, and a C16th walled garden.

SD ⬛♿ CP ⬛♿ E ⬛♿ RF ⬛♿ C ⬛♿
S ⬛♿ WC ⬛♿ RFE ⬛♿

CASTLE HEDINGHAM
Built on a hill overlooking the River Colne is the great castle that has given the village its name. Constructed by the de Vere family c1140.

ATTRACTION
COLNE VALLEY RAILWAY
Yeldham Road, Castle Hedingham CO9 3DZ
Tel: (01787) 461174
Award-winning station for a pleasant ride on a section of the railway of the former Colne Valley line. Incorporating a large collection of heritage railway rolling stock, steam and diesel locomotives.

SD ⬛♿ CP ⬛♿ E ⬛♿ RF ⬛♿ C-n/a
S ⬛♿ WC ⬛♿ RFE ⬛♿

CHELMSFORD
The county town of Essex is large and well-developed with a shopping complex and fine sporting facilities.

TOURIST INFORMATION CENTRE
County Hall, Market Road,
Chelmsford CM1 1GG
Tel: (01245) 283400

ATTRACTION
CHELMSFORD AND ESSEX MUSEUM
Oaklands Park, Moulsham Street,
Chelmsford CM2 9AQ
Tel: (01245) 615100 Fax: (01245) 280642
Wide range of artefacts of the town's history plus geological displays. Wheelchair access to ground floor only.

SD ⬛♿ CP ⬛♿ E ⬛♿ RF ⬛♿ S ⬛♿
WC ⬛♿ RFE ⬛♿

MOULSHAM MILL
Parkway, Chelmsford CM2 7PX
Tel: (01245) 608200 Fax: (01245) 608310
This a charming mill house the ground floor of which has been converted into a place for crafts of all kinds including lace making, wooden crafts etc. It is managed by Interact, the charity that helps those with learning difficulties back into the workplace.

SD ⬛♿ CP ⬛♿ (slight incline down to entrance)
E ⬛♿ C ⬛♿ S ⬛♿
WC ⬛♿

CHIGWELL
HOTEL
JUBILEE LODGE (Winged Fellowship)
Grange Farm, High Road,
Chigwell IG7 6DP
Tel: (020) 8501 2331
On the edge of Epping Forest with lawns and gardens galore. All rooms have en suite facilities and hoist tracking, with variable height beds. 24-hour nursing. Bar, conservatory, shop, and coffee lounge. Adaptive transport.

CHINGFORD
ATTRACTION
QUEEN ELIZABETH'S HUNTING LODGE
Ranger's Road, Epping Forest, Chingford
London E4 7QH
Tel: (0208) 529 6681
Timber-framed hunting grandstand built for Henry V111 in 1543 and then taken over after his death by Queen Elizabeth 1. The lodge is a supreme example of timber-

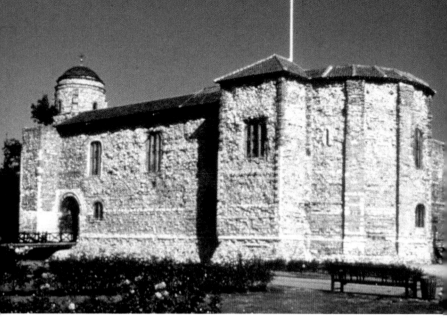

Colchester Castle, the largest ever keep built by the Normans

framed architecture at a time when English carpentry was at its peak. Exceptional carpentry set in Epping Forest with ancient oaks and fine views. Originally the upper two floors had open sides to provide panaramic views of the hunts which used to take place. Ground floor accessible to wheelchairs - wide, shallow staircase to upper floor.

SD ♿	CP ♿	E ♿	RF ♿	C ♿	
S ♿	WC 🚻	RFE ♿			

CLACTON-ON-SEA

A popular holiday resort with a pier, every possible holiday amenity and form of entertainment, and a giant scenic railway a striking feature.

TOURIST INFORMATION CENTRE
23 Pier Avenue, Clacton-on-Sea CO15 1QD
Tel: (01255) 423400

HOTEL
HERTFORD HOUSE HOTEL ♿
11 Park Way, Clacton-on-Sea CO15 1BJ
Tel/Fax: (01255) 475994
No. of Accessible Rooms: All (13)
Accessible Facilities: Lounge, dining room, bar, beach hut on sea front. Purpose-built

hotel for those with disabilities.

SELF-CATERING
GROOMSHILL
8 Holland Road, Clacton on Sea
Book through Grooms Holidays
No. of Accessible Units: 1. Roll-in Shower
No. of Beds per Unit: 7 Accessible Facilities: Comfortable bungalow tucked away on a peaceful residential street with a secluded garden. Close to local shops.

COLCHESTER

Britain's oldest recorded town was the first capital of Roman Britain. A familiar sight is undoubtedly Bourne Mill, built in 1591 and made famous in a number of paintings by John Constable.

TOURIST INFORMATION CENTRE
1 Queen Street, Colchester CO1 2PG
Tel: (01206) 282920
TAXIS
Five One Taxis: Tel: (01206) 515151
Five adapted vehicles.

TRAINS
Anglia Railways: Assistance:
Tel: (01473) 693333

Minicom: (01603) 630748 or
(0845) 6050600
Central Trains: Assistance:
Tel: (0845) 7056027
www.centraltrains.co.uk
First Great Eastern: Special Needs –
Tel: (0845) 9505050
Mincom: (0845) 9606099
Colchester station is manned most of time, although there is not 24-hour cover.

CAR PARKS
Three-hour free disabled badge spaces in council-run car parks, some off-street parking.
Tel: (01206) 282222

SHOPMOBILITY
15 Queen Street,
Colchester CO1 2PH
Tel: (01206) 505256 Fax: (01206) 500367
e-mail: info@ccvs.org

HOTEL
FORTE POSTHOUSE COLCHESTER
Abbotts Lane, Eight Ash Green,
Colchester CO6 3QL
Tel: (08704) 009020 Fax: (01206) 766577
No. of Accessible Rooms: 1
Accessible Facilities: Lounge, restaurant
Located three miles from Colchester.

ATTRACTIONS
ABBERTON RESERVOIR NATURE RESERVE
Church Road, Layer-de-la-Haye, Colchester
Tel: (01206) 738172 Fax: (01206) 738292
Essex Wildlife Trust run this conservation centre for wild duck, swans and other water birds.

SD | CP | E | RF | S
WC | RFE

BRIDGE COTTAGE (NT)
Flatford, East Bergholt, Colchester CO7 6OL
Tel: (01206) 298260 Fax: (01206) 299193
C16th cottage near Flatford Mill with John Constable exhibition, famous for paintings of this property and surrounding area. Flatford Mill is not accessible to the general public.

SD | CP | E | RF | C
S | WC | RFE

CASTLE MUSEUM
Castle Park, Colchester CO1 1JJ
Tel: (01206) 282931 Fax: (01206) 282925
This is the largest surviving Norman keep in Europe. It includes Roman displays, hands-on activities and medieval and prison displays. Discover why Colchester was chosen to be the first capital of Roman Britain.

SD | CP n/a | E | RF | L-
C | S | WC | RFE

COLCHESTER LEISURE WORLD
Cowdray Avenue, Colchester CO1 1YH
Tel: (01206) 282000 Fax: (01206) 282024

Tudor magnificence reaching skyward at Layer Marney Tower.

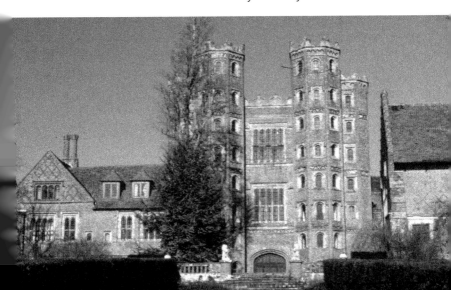

119

www.colchesterleisureworld.co.uk
Contains leisure, fitness and teaching pools, the latter two reached via a lift to the upper floor. The fitness pool has a hoist and a shower chair. In the leisure pool a carry chair is used to access the main area of the pool, apart from the flume area that is not accessible.

DISABILITY SPORT CO-ORDINATOR

CP ♿	E ♿	RF ♿	L ♿	C ♿	WC ♿

COLCHESTER ZOO

Maldon Road, Stanway, Colchester CO3 5SL
Tel: (01206) 331292   Fax: (01206) 331392
e-mail: colchester.zoo@btinternet.com
Irregular levels add to the charm but detract from accessibility. The zoo produces a good Easy Route for wheelchair users, avoiding some steeper areas, but the terrain is varied. The wide variety of animals divide in five areas – the Beginning, Aquatic Zone, Lake Lands, The Slopes and The Heights. There is some undercover viewing and outside exhibits. A good day out. Spotless WCs and good quality food.

CP ♿	E ♿	RF ♿	C ♿
SD ♿	WC ⚇	RFE ♿	

Fine example of plaster work in historic Saffron Walden.

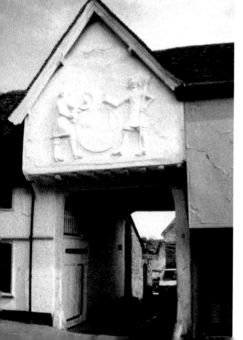

LAYER MARNEY TOWER

Nr. Colchester CO5 9US
Tel:(01206) 330784
Fax: (01206) 330884
e-mail: nicholas@layermarney.demon.co.uk
A fine example of Tudor architecture incorporating the tallest Tudor gatehouse in Britain. There is a long gallery, church, formal garden and farm. The farmyard is concrete. The farm walk is over earth and grass, requiring assistance. The upper garden is accessible with wide gravel paths, the lower garden is accessed by a steep ramp. The church has three high steps and there is no wheelchair access to the Tower.

SD ♿	CP ⚇	E ♿	RF ⚇
C ♿	S ⚇	WC ⚇	RFE ⚇

MANNINGTREE

Standing on the estuary of the River Stour. The village centre contains several Georgian and Victorian buildings of character.

SAFFRON WALDEN

Delightful historic town with a long history. Remains of an iron age fort at King Hill, evidence of Roman occupation and remains of a C12th castle. The town also hosts one of the few surviving town mazes.

TOURIST INFORMATION CENTRE

1 Market Place, Saffron Walden CB10 1HR
Tel: (01799) 510444

SELF-CATERING

WOODMORE COTTAGE   ⚇
Whitensmere Farm Cottages, Ashdown, Saffron Walden CB10 2JQ
Tel/Fax: (01799) 584244
e.mail: GFORD@lineone.net
www.holidaycottagescambridge.co.uk
No. of Accessible Units: 1
No. of Beds per Unit: 6
Accessible Facilities: Lounge, dining room. Well converted C18th farm buildings cluster around south-facing garden. Woodmore Cottage features exposed beams and log-

burning stove with its own private patio with garden furniture and barbecue.

ATTRACTION
MOLE HALL WILDLIFE PARK
Widdington, Newport,
Nr. Saffron Walden CB11 3SS
Tel: (01799) 540400
Fax: (01799) 542408
e-mail: enquiries@molehall.co.uk
www.molehall.co.uk
20 acres developed by a single family with a wide variety of animals including otters, chimpanzees and flamingos, in delightful natural surroundings. A dominant feature is the fully moated private manor house, dating back to 1280.
The deer walk and butterfly pavilion are not suitable for wheelchairs because of high stiles and gravel respectively.

SD | CP (shingle/grass) | E | RF
C | S | WC

SOUTH OCKENDON
GRANGEWATERS
Buckles Lane, South Ockendon RM15 6RS
Tel: (01708) 856422   Fax: (01708)855228
e.mail:grangewaters@thurrock.gov.uk
Small attractive country park with 26-acre lake with activities year-round.

SD | CP | E | C | S
WC | RFE-(Jetty)

STANSTEAD
Known principally for its airport designed by Sir Norman Foster, now growing rapidly with excellent links to and from London.

TRAINS
Central Trains: Assistance:
Tel: (0845) 7056027 www.centraltrains.co.uk
West Anglia Great Northern:
Special Needs – Tel: (0345) 226688
Minicom: (0345) 125988

HOTEL
LONDON STANSTEAD
Round Coppice Road,
Stansted Airport CM24 8SE
Tel: (01279) 680800   Fax: (01279) 680890

No. of Accessible Rooms: 6. Bath
Accessible Facilities: Lounge, restaurant
Quality airport hotel.

SOUTHEND-ON-SEA
Known as the holiday resort for Londoners, it has the longest pier in the world, stretching for 1.5 miles. Two funfairs offer amusement for all age groups and a wealth of day and night-time entertainment.

ATTRACTIONS
FOCAL POINT GALLERY
Southend Central Library, Victoria Avenue,
Southend-on-Sea SS2 6EX
Tel: (01702) 612621 ext. 207
Fax: (01702) 469241
e-mail: admin@focalpoint.org.uk
Photographic gallery with exhibitions of a regional, national and international nature.

SD | CP | E | RF- | L
C | S n/a | WC | RFE

SOUTHEND CENTRAL MUSEUM
Victoria Avenue, Southend-on-Sea SS2 6EW
Tel: (01702) 215130 Fax: (01702) 349806
Displays of archaeology, natural, social and local history and temporary exhibitions. Interactive discovery centre. Use side entrance that is ramped at 1:16.
SD | CP | E | RF
C n/a | S | WC n/a

SEALIFE ADVENTURE
Eastern Esplanade, Southend on Sea, SS1 2ER
Tel: (01702) 601834 Fax: (01702) 462444
e-mail: sealife@stockvale.co.uk
www.sealifeadventure.co.uk
Located at the eastern end of the seafront, busy with traffic in summer. Lots of fun with sea nursery, ray bay, rock pool, deep water and beach walk.
SD | CP | E | RF
C | S | WC
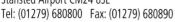
N.B. Parking owned by local council, busy without disabled spaces, but set down directly in front of the entrance. Cafe and shop can be accessed through the main entrance or from seafront itself, with single step 17cm high, 70cm long.

GLOUCESTERSHIRE

GLOUCESTER TOURISM
Herbert Warehouse, The Docks,
Gloucester GL1 2EQ
Tel: (01452) 396620   Fax: (01452) 396622

INTEGRATED TRANSPORT UNIT, Block 5,
Shire Hall, Bearland, Gloucester GL1 2TH
Tel: (01452) 425610   Fax: (01452) 426927
Timetable information and Gloucetershire
travel guides.

BOURTON-ON-THE-WATER

This is the Venice of the Cotswolds.
There are bow-arched bridges and
lovely Cotswold stone houses.

HOTEL
CHESTER HOUSE HOTEL   [人]
Victoria Street,
Bourton-on-the Water
GL54 2BG
Tel: (01451) 820266 Fax: (01451) 820471
e-mail: juliand@chesterhouse.u-net.com
www.chesterhouse.u-net.com
No. of accessible Rooms: 8
Eight ground floor rooms suitable for
wheelchairs.
Accessible Facilities: Lounge, restaurant.
Small, family-run hotel situated in
converted farm buildings of delightful
Cotswold stone with gardens.

ATTRACTIONS
BIRDLAND PARK LTD
Bourton-on-the-Water GL54 2BN
Tel: (01451) 820480   Fax: (01451) 822398
e-mail: sb.birdland@virgin.net
Set in seven acres of woodland, river
ponds and gardens, the setting is
inhabited by over 500 birds. Flamingos,
pelicans, storks, penguins, cranes, and
waterfowl can be seen, aviaries of parrots,
falcons and toucans plus tropical house
and temperate houses.

SD [&]   CP n/a   E [&]   RF [人]   C [人]
S [&]   WC [人]   RFE [&]

COTSWOLD MOTOR MUSEUM AND TOY
COLLECTION
The Old Mill, Bourton-on-the-Water GL54
2BY
Tel: (01451) 821255
Located on River Windrush in a watermill.

SD [&]   CP [&]   E [&]   S [&]
WC [人] (village WC 80m from entrance)

CHELTENHAM

Set on a sheltered ridge between the
high Cotswolds and the Severn Vale,
the town enjoys an equable climate
and is one of the finest spa towns in
Europe. There are many fine examples
of Regency architecture. Cheltenham
is notable also for its important annual
music festival and its racecourse.

TOURIST INFORMATION CENTRE
77 The Promenade, Cheltenham GL50 1PP
Tel: (01242) 522878 Fax: 01242 255848
e-mail: tic@cheltenham.gov.uk
www.visitcheltenham.gov.uk

CHELTENHAM DISABILITY ADVICE CENTRE
St. Vincents Centre, Central Cross Drive,
Cheltenham GL50 4LA
Tel: (01242) 243030
Information about disability and support
services.

DISABILITY ACTION CHELTENHAM
Equals, 287 High Street, Cheltenham GL50
3HL
Tel: (01242) 237292
Run by people with disabilities for people
with disabilities, offering support, advice
and representation.

BUSES
Stagecoach: Tel: (01242) 224853
One low-floor route with raised kerbs.

TAXIS
Starline (evenings only):
Tel: (01242) 250250
One London cab with all fittings.

Station Taxis: Tel: (01242) 573355
One FX4 with all fittings.

TRAINS
Virgin Trains: Special Needs –
Tel: (0845) 7443366
Minicom: (0845) 7443367
Wales and West: Special Needs –
Tel: (0845) 3003005
Minicom: (0845) 7585469
Cheltenham Spa station is suitable for
wheelchairs using ramp access.

HOTEL
THE PRESTBURY HOUSE HOTEL 🚶
The Burgage, Prestbury, Cheltenham
GL52 3DN
Tel: (01242) 529533   Fax: (01242) 227076
No. of Accessible Rooms: 1. Roll-in
shower
Accessible Facilities: Bar, reception area,
restaurants (two out of three), gardens.
Country manor house hotel, main house
dating back to early 1600s, typical late
William and Mary design with Georgian
wing added later. Standing in four acres
of secluded grounds, the hotel is situated
in the Burgage, an original road steeped
in English history, particularly the Civil
War. Now a quiet backwater, Prestbury is
reputed to be the most haunted village i
n England.

ATTRACTIONS
CHELTENHAM ART GALLERY AND MUSEUM
Clarence Street, Cheltenham GL50 3JT
Tel: (01242) 237431   Fax: (01242) 262334
e-mail: ArtGallery@cheltenham.gov.uk
Museum houses a fine collection relating
to William Morris' Arts and Crafts
Movement. The gallery contains Dutch
and British art from C17th onward.
Oriental Gallery has Ming dynasty pottery
and costumes, and a depiction of the true
story of local hero Edward Wilson who
joined Captain Scott on his tragic 1911
Antarctic Expedition.

SD ♿	CP ♿	E ♿	RF ♿
L ♿	C ♿	S ♿	WC ♿
RFE 🚶			

COTSWOLD HERITAGE CENTRE
Northleach, Nr. Cheltenham GL54 3JH
Tel: (01451) 860715   Fax: (01451) 860091
Museum of rural life at a time when most
people worked on the land. Hand and

craft tool displays are housed in an
C18th prison. The agricultural collection
is displayed in a purpose-built gallery
recalling Cotswold farm buildings. The
Cotswold Land and People gallery and
the Victorian kitchen in the cellar are not
accessible.

| SD n/a | CP ♿ | E ♿ | RF ♿ |
| C 🚶 | S ♿ | WC 🚶 | |

KEITH HARDINGS WORLD OF
MECHANICAL MUSIC
High Street, Northleach,
Nr. Cheltenham GL54 3ET
Tel: (01451) 860181   Fax: (01451) 861133
Living museum of the various kinds of
self-playing musical instruments,
together with unique clocks in a
workshop environment where items are
still created and clocks repaired. Set in
the joined buildings of the Oak house,
parts of which are over 300 years old
and Westwoods Grammar School that
closed in 1902.

| SD ♿ | CP 🚶 | E- ♿ | S 🚶 | WC 🚶 |

CHIPPEN CAMDEN
Charming, typical town of affluent
wool merchants of C14th and C15th
with gabled stone houses.
Surrounded by wonderful open
country, Hidecote being 4 miles
north of the town.

HIDECOTE MANOR GARDEN (NT)
Hidecote Bartram, Nr Chipping Camden,
GL55 6LR
Tel: (01386) 438333
Fax: (01386) 438817
e-mail: hidecote@nationaltrust.org.uk
www.nationaltrust.org.uk/hidecote
An absolutely delightful C20th garden,
comprising of a series of small gardens,
separated by wall, hedges and follies.
Famous for rare shrubs, trees and
herbaceous borders.   N.B. Some
pathways are difficult with steps and
slippery paths, but much of the gardens
can be enjoyed. There are two catering
units, outside cafe with level even access.
Inside restaurant, with main entrance

inaccessible, but staff will open private entrance for level both manual and electric wheelchairs availale for loan.

SD ♿ CP ♿ E ♿ RF ♿ C ♿
S ♿ WC- 🚶

CIRENCESTER

There is an elegant parish church of St. John the Baptist, appreciated at a distance when the pinnacles and embattlements, that distinguish the Cirencester skyline, can be seen.

TOURIST INFORMATION CENTRE
Corn Hall, Market Place, Cirencester GL7 2NW
Tel: (01285) 654180 Fax: (01285) 641182
www.thisisthecotswolds.co.uk

SELF-CATERING
THE COTSWOLD HOBURNE
South Cerney, Nr. Cirencester
Book through Grooms Holidays
No. of Accessible Units: 3
No. of Beds per Unit: 4
Accessible Facilities: Situated beside the lake in the Cotswold Water Park Holiday centre, close to the lovely village of Bibury.

FOREST OF DEAN

Bordered to the west by the River Wye, and to the east by the Severn, the Royal Forest of Dean is one of England's foremost primeval forests, comprising over 23,000 acres and around 20 million trees. Once famous for its huge oaks, used for almost all British Navy ships at the time of the Armada, it now boasts breathtaking scenery and many walks.

TOURIST INFORMATION CENTRE
High Street, Coleford,
Tel: 01594 812388 Fax: 01594 812267

BED AND BREAKFAST
THE FOUNTAIN INN   🚶
Fountain Way, Parkend, Nr. Lydney GL15 4JD
Tel: (01594) 562189 Fax: (01594) 564438
No. of Accessible Rooms: 1

Accessible Facilities: Dining room.
Built 200 years ago for the local mining population, now a charming pub with a garden in a delightful small village in the Royal Forest of Dean within the boundaries of the Cannop Valley Nature Reserve.

ATTRACTIONS
CLEARWELL CAVES
Nr. Coleford, Royal Forest of Dean GL16 8JR
Tel: (01594) 832535
These are ancient iron mines, you need to be adventurous because the story of iron is told in displays throughout the caves. Iron has been mined here since the Iron Age, 2,500 years ago, and continues today.

SD ♿ CP ♿ E ♿ RF 🚶 C 🚶
S ♿ WC- 🚶 RFE 🚶

DEAN FOREST RAILWAY
Norchard Railway Centre, Forest Road, Lydney GL15 4ET
Tel/Fax: (01594) 845840
e-mail: fredb@globalnet.co.uk
www.deanforestrailway.co.uk
Dean Forest Railway traces its history back to 1809, the Severn and Wye Railway preserving the last remnant of a once extensive forest railway. Steam-hauled passenger trains run from Norchard to Lydney Jcn (15 mins) but may extend northwards toward Parkend.

SD ♿ CP 🚶 at Norchard Centre only.
E- ♿ level to ramp for shop/museum, then level to station platform ramp. RF 🚶 C 🚶 S 🚶
Museum ♿ (through Shop with double doors).
WC 🚶 at Norchard Centre only.
TRAIN- ramp to adapted coach, taking 4 wheelchairs and 4 assistants. Wheelchair clamps and window views.

GLOUCESTER

The city has long been an inland port. A delightful city with some priceless C10th manuscripts, a Norman church and a fine cathedral, one of the centres of the Three Choirs Festival.

TOURIST INFORMATION CENTRE
28 Southgate Street,
Gloucester GL1 2DP

Tel: (01452) 421188   Fax: (01452) 309788
e-mail: tourism@gloucester.gov.uk
www.gloucester.gov.uk

TRAVELINE
Tel; (0870) 6082608

BUSES
Stagecoach: Tel: (01452) 523928
Gloucester City Bus – one low-floor route.

TAXIS
Andy Cars: Tel: (01452) 523000
One FX1 with all fittings.
EB Taxis: Tel: (01452) 305888
Two minibuses with all fittings.
Intacab: Tel: (01452) 527272
One minibuses with all fittings.

TRAINS
Virgin Trains: Special Needs –
Tel: (0845) 7443366
Minicom: (0845) 7443367
Wales and West: Special Needs –
Tel: (0845) 3003005
Minicom: (0845) 7585469
Gloucester station is suitable for
wheelchairs using ramp access.

SHOPMOBILITY
Hampden Way, Gloucester
Tel: (01452) 302871 Fax: (01452) 396899

HOTEL
CHELTENHAM/GLOUCESTER MOAT
HOUSE
Shurdington Road, Brockworth,
Gloucester G13 4PB
Tel: (01452) 519988   Fax: (01452) 519977
No. of Accessible Rooms: 2
Accessible Facilities: Lounge, restaurant,
pool, sauna, spa.
Modern hotel set in landscaped gardens
located just SW of the Forest of Dean
towards the Monmouth border.

MORETON-IN-MARSH
A very pleasant, prosperous-looking
town with a wide grass-verged main
street, and many C17th and C18th
houses. An old curfew bell still hangs

in its tower that overlooks the
Fosse Way.

TOURIST INFORMATION CENTRE
Cotswold District Council Office,
Moreton-in-Marsh GL56 0AZ
Tel: (01608) 650881 Fax: (01608) 651542
e-mail: tourism@cotswold.gov.uk
www.cotswolds.gov.uk

HOTEL
TREETOPS
London Road, Moreton-in-Marsh GL56 0HE
Tel/Fax: (01608) 651036
No. of Accessible Rooms: 2. Shower
Accessible Facilities: Lounge, restaurant.
Family-run guest house in 0.75 acres of
secluded garden, a short distance from
the town centre.

NAILSWORTH
Located in softly wooded South
Cotswold Hills with a mix of
architecture. C16th cottages cling to
the hillside while large C17th wool
merchants' houses present imposing
facades. Attractive Georgian houses
also can be seen.

BED AND BREAKFAST
APPLE ORCHARD HOUSE
Springhill, Nailsworth GL6 0LX
Tel: (01453) 832503   Fax: (01453) 836213
No. of Accessible Rooms: 1
Accessible Facilities: Lounge, dining room,
patio. Modern, elegant detached house in
an acre of garden with lovely views of the
Cotswold hills.

STOW-ON-THE-WOLD
The highest town in the Cotswolds,
situated where eight roads meet.

TOURIST INFORMATION CENTRE
Hollis House, The Square,
Stow-on-the-Wold GL54 1AF
Tel: (01451) 831082   Fax: (01451) 870083

ATTRACTION
COTSWOLD FARM PARK
Guiting Power,
Nr. Stow-on-the-Wold GL54 5UG
Tel: (01451) 850307   Fax: (01451) 850423
Premier UK rare breed survival centre and
a leading live animal exhibition with
demonstrations, tractor and trailer rides,
Barn houses educational interactive
displays.

SD | CP | E | RF
C | S | WC | RFE

TETBURY
A quiet small market town, developed
during the mid C17th, situated almost
on the border (01666with Wiltshire.

TOURIST INFORMATION CENTRE
33 Church Street, Tetbury GL8 8JG
Tel/Fax: (01666) 503552
e-mail: tourism@tetbury.com
www.tetbury.com

HOTEL
HUNTERS HALL
Kingscote, Nr. Tetbury GL8 8XZ
Tel: (01453) 860393   Fax: (01453) 860707
No. of Accessible Rooms: 1. Roll-in shower
Accessible Facilities: Lounge, restaurant.
Country hotel.

ATTRACTIONS
CHAVENAGE HOUSE
Chavenage, Nr. Tetbury GL8 8XP
Tel: (01666) 502329   Fax: (01666) 836778
e-mail: info@chavenage.com
www.chavenage.com
Historic Elizabethan house of 1576,
during the Civil War (1641-49). Contains
fine tapestries, stained glass windows and
furniture.

SD | CP | E | RF | WC

WESTONBIRT ARBORETUM
Tetbury GL8 8QS
Tel: (01666) 880220   Fax: (01666) 880559
www.forestry.gov.uk
Over 18,000 trees from all over the world
have been planted here from 1829 to the
present day, producing 600 acres of
landscaped Cotswold countryside. There
are 17 miles of waymarked trails where
you will be accompanied by birds, badgers
and deer. Particularly notable for
rhododendrons, azaleas, magnolias and
the wild flowers of Silk Wood that can be
seen from March to June, and for the
autumn colour spectacular from late
September to early November.

SD | CP | E | RF
C | S | WC | RFE

New England in the fall? No, just a blaze of colour at Westonbirt Arboretum.

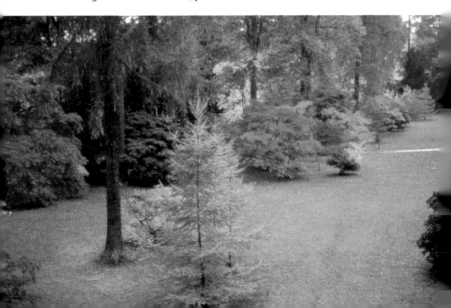

HAMPSHIRE

HAMPSHIRE CENTRE FOR INDEPENDENT LIVING
4 Plantation Way, Whitehill,
Borden G035 9HD
Tel: (01420) 474261

ALRESFORD
THE WATERCRESS LINE
Station Offices, Arlesford S)24 9JG
Tel: (01962) 73381   Fax: (01962) 735448
e-mail: info@watercressline.co.uk
www.watercressline.co.uk
Hampshire's only preserved steam railway, running between Alresford and Alton with new Goods Shed Visitor Centre Museum. The railway came here in 1865 and assisted the developing watercress industry, allowing access to London markets. Watercress is still a significant local industry. The station is delightful, manned by volunteers, with hanging baskets and utterly nostalgic. Boarding the train is by BR ramp with slight incline.
SD 🦽 CP 🦽 E 🦽 RF 🦽 S 🦽
WC 🚹

BASINGSTOKE
Although not a beautiful town, the modern development here is very interesting.

TOURIST INFORMATION CENTRE
Willis Museum, Old Town Hall, Market Place, Basingstoke RG21 7QD
Tel: (01256) 817681   Fax: (01256) 356231
e-mail: leisure.services@basingstoke.gov.uk
www.hampshire-information.co.uk

HOTEL
AUDLEYS WOOD THISTLE HOTEL   🚹
Alton Road, Basingstoke RG25 2JT
Tel: (01256) 817555   Fax: (01256) 817500
e-mail: audleys.wood@thistle.co.uk
No. of Accessible Rooms: 1
Accessible Facilities: Lounge, restaurant
C19th. mansion with preserved original features, set in seven acres of landscaped gardens and lightly wooded grounds on the edge of the Hampshire Downs. Located on the A339. Two miles from M3 (J6).

HANOVER INTERNATIONAL HOTEL
& CLUB   🚹
Nately Scures, Hook RG27 9JS
Tel: (01256) 764161   Fax: (01256) 768341
No. of Accessible Rooms: 6
Accessible Facilities: Lounge, restaurants (2), cocktail bar. Originally a private country residence, now an elegant country retreat located on the main A30 London road, but set well back. Set in 4.5 acres and surrounded by mature woodland.

BEAULIEU
BEAULIEU: NATIONAL MOTOR MUSEUM
Beaulieu, Nr Brockenhurst SO42 7ZN
Tel: (01590) 612345
Fax: (01590) 612624
e-mail: info@beaulieu.co.uk
www.beaulieu.co.uk
World's largest collection of historic vehicles and motoring memorabilia, including Donald Campbell's "Bluebird" of 1964. Lift access between floors through the replica of a 1930's country garage. The C16th house is a long walk (or push!) on firm tarmac, but leading to a difficult gravel drive immediately outside the house. House entrance 90cm and two rooms accessible, remainder down several steps.
SD 🦽   CP 🦽 E 🦽 RF 🦽
S 🦽   c 🦽 WC 🚹 L 🚹

FORDINGBRIDGE
A medieval bridge, much restored and widened, crosses the Avon here, giving the town its name. Set NW of the New Forest, the views are spectacular with outdoor pursuits popular.

SELF CATERING
SANDY BALLS HOLIDAY CENTRE   🦽
Godshill, Fordingbridge SP6 2JZ
Tel: (01425) 653042 Fax: (01425) 653067
www.sandy-balls.co.uk
No. of Accessible Lodges: 3
No. of beds per lodge: 5
Accessible Facilities: Open plan

lounge/kitchen. One lodge has wheel-in shower, others have bath. Site facilities accessed by level tarmac, including indoor pool with hoist, and gently ramped outdoor pool. Adaptive changing room, pizza restaurant and pub, and shop. A number of adapted WCs with RADAR key available from reception. Winner of England for Excellence 1998 Caravan Holiday Park of the Year and David Bellamy Gold Award. Bordered by the Avon and set in 120 acres of woods and parkland in the New Forest area.

ATTRACTION
ROCKBOURNE ROMAN VILLA
Rockbourne, Fordingbridge SP6 3PG
Tel: (01725) 518541
On the site of the remains of a 40-room Roman village, this on-site museum displays many artefacts found during its excavation.

SD [♿]   CP [♿]   E [♿]   RF [♿]   S [♿]
WC [♿]   RFE [♿]

GOSPORT
Famous for its yacht and boat building, many of the buildings were destroyed in a C19th fire, but those remaining are still pretty.

BED AND BREAKFAST
WEST WIND GUEST HOUSE   [♿]
197 Portsmouth Road, Lee on the Solent, Gosport PO13 9AA
Tel: (0239) 2552550   Fax: (0239) 2554657
e-mail: maggie@west-wind.co.uk
www.west-wind.co.uk
No. of Accessible Rooms: 1. Accessible Facilities: Dining room, beach access by ramped slipway (gradient 1:20). Situated 50m from the beach. A one-mile promenade is fully accessible to wheelchair users.

LIPHOOK
Beautifully situated in the shadow of the downs, this is a charming village with a pond, pretty cottages and a famous late C17th posting inn.

ATTRACTION
HOLLYCOMBE STEAM COLLECTION
Iron Hill, Liphook GU30 7LP
Tel: (01428) 724900   Fax: (01428) 723682
Relive the days of the traditional fairground. The main attractions are fairground rides and railways. Wheelchair passengers can be accommodated on some, but not all, of these. Gardens are accessible but paths can be steep.

SD [♿]   CP [♿]   E [♿]   RF [♿]   C [♿]
S [♿]   WC [♿]   RFE [♿]

LYMINGTON
Pleasant town on the edge of the New Forest. Bright cottages and attractive Georgian and C19th houses in a broad high street.

TOURIST INFORMATION CENTRE
St. Barb Museum, New Street, Lymington SO41 9BH
Tel/Fax: (01590) 672422

BED AND BREAKFAST
OUR BENCH   [♿]
Lodge Road, Pennington, Lymington SO41 8HH
Tel/Fax: (01590) 673141
e-mail: ourbench@newforest.demon.co.uk
No. of Accessible Rooms: 1
Accessible Facilities: Dining room, pool, sauna, Jacuzzi. Holders of ETB England for Excellence award in Tourism for All Categories, 1997. Large bungalow in 0.3 of an acre of garden in quiet village two miles from the New Forest. Evening meals are an optional extra.

ATTRACTION
BRAXTON GARDENS
Lynmore Lane,
Milford on Sea, Lymington SO41 0TX
Tel: (01590) 642008
Lovely walled garden and courtyard designed around red brick barns of an original Victorian farmyard. Fine selection of unusual herbs, alpines and shrubs.

SD [♿]   CP [♿]   E [♿]   RF [♿]   C [♿]
S [♿]   WC n/a

NEW MILTON

Small town, close to New Forest.
Lowland heath and mixed forestation.

BED AND BREAKFAST
ST. URSULA
30 Hobart Road, New Milton BH25 6EG
Tel: (01425) 613515
No. of Accessible Rooms: 1
Accessible Facilities: Lounge, dining room.
Located two miles from the New Forest.

SELF-CATERING
NAISH HOLIDAY VILLAGE
New Milton
Book through Grooms Holidays
No. of Accessible Units: 3
No. of Beds per Unit: 4
Accessible Facilities: Paved patio. Timbered
chalets in the New Forest with fine views
across the Solent to the Needles and the
Isle of Wight.

PETERSFIELD

Set in a wide valley, there are many
elegant Georgian buildings in this
market and agricultural town.

ATTRACTION
UPPARK (NT)
South Harting, Petersfield GU31 5QR
Tel: (01730) 825415
Fax: (01730) 825873
e-mail: uppark@ntrust.org.uk
Elegant late C17th house high on the
South Downs with fine views. The mid
C18th interior has been fully restored after
a disastrous fire in 1989. The house
contains a collection of grand tour
paintings, fine ceramics and furniture.
Evocative servants' rooms where H G Wells
spent part of his youth. NB: Entrance ramp
gradient 1:11. The lift only goes down to
the basement.

SD CP E RF 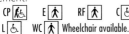 C
S L WC Wheelchair available.

PORTSMOUTH

In naval terms the history of
Portsmouth has long been important.
Home to Charles Dickens and to Jones
Hanway, inventor of the umbrella,
Portsmouth as a town grew by itself,
rather than to plan. Many modern
buildings and plenty of entertainment.

TOURIST INFORMATION CENTRE
Clarence Esplanade, Southsea,
PO5 3PB (mail address)
Tel: (0239) 2826722   Fax: (0239) 2827519
e-mail: tic@portsmouthcc.gov.uk
www.visitportsmouth.co.uk
www.portsmouth.co.uk

PORTSMOUTH HARBOUR TOURISM
102 Commercial Road, Portsmouth PO1 1EJ
Tel: (023) 92 838382   Fax: (023) 92 730116
e-mail: phammond@portsmouthcc.gov.uk
www.portsmouthand.co.uk

HOTEL
HILTON NATIONAL PORTSMOUTH
Eastern Road, Farlington, Portsmouth   PO6
1UN
Tel: (023) 92 219111   Fax: (023) 92 210762
No. of Accessible Rooms: 2. Bath
Accessible Facilities: Lounge (split level
area with steps to raised section),
restaurant (split level ramped to lower
section), pool, sauna and steam room
(accessible with assistance).Modern hotel
situated on the A2020 at the junction of
the A27(M) and 1.5 miles from the A3(M)
from London. 4.5 miles from city centre.

ATTRACTIONS
FLAGSHIP PORTSMOUTH
Building 1/7 College Road, HM Naval Base,
Portsmouth PO1 3LJ
Tel: (023) 92 870999   Fax: (023) 92 29525
www.flagship.org.uk
This is a working naval base so visitors with
restricted mobility should be accompanied.
After setting down, car parking is at the
Victory Gate 600/800m from the visitor
centre. There is disabled badge parking in
4/5 spaces outside the centre. Wheelchairs
are available from the visitor centre, Mary

Rose, HMS Warrior 1860 and Royal Naval Museum. We recommend the special access route map.

HMS Victory
Tel: (023) 92 722351
Lord Nelson's famous flagship at Trafalgar, and the world's most outstanding example of maritime restoration. The tour involves fairly steep steps. A video tour is provided on the lower gundeck.

SD ♿ CP n/a E ♿ RF ♿
C ♿ S ♿ WC ♿

HMS Warrior 1860
Tel: (023) 92 291379
World's first iron-hulled armoured warship that spanned the periods of wood, iron, sail and steam. Four decks are connected by steep steps but there is alternative access to two decks. A ramp gives access to the upper deck although tides may make the gradient steeper. A stairlift from the upper to the main gun deck requires a transfer from wheelchair to lift with staff assistance.

SD ♿ CP n/a E ♿ RF ♿ L ♿
C ♿ S ♿ WC ♿

Mary Rose Museum
Tel: (023) 92 812931
Amazingly preserved in the Solent for 437 years, the Mary Rose, Henry VIII's warship, was raised in 1982. A short audio-visual presentation is followed by a themed display on the many artefacts recovered, including weapons, clothing and pewterware. An absolute must! Fully accessible.

SD ♿ CP n/a E ♿ RF ♿
C ♿ S- ♿ WC ♿

Royal Naval Museum
Tel: (023) 92 727562
Devoted to the Navy's history. Relics of Lord Nelson, artefacts, model ships and a wide range of displays. Ramps in all buildings. Little inaccessible to wheelchair users.

SD ♿ CP n/a E ♿ RF ♿ L ♿
C ♿ S ♿ WC ♿

SOUTHSEA MODEL VILLAGE
Lumps Fort, Eastney, Esplanade, Southsea,
Portsmouth PO4 9RU
Tel: (023) 92 294706
1/12th scale models of over 40 buildings plus G scale miniature garden railway, toy museum and gardens watercourse.

SD ♿ CP 🚶 E ♿ RF ♿
C ♿ WC n/a

RINGWOOD
Situated by the River Avon, just outside the New Forest, but with heath and woodland close at hand. Houses here date from all periods, many with lovely thatched roofs.

TOURIST INFORMATION CENTRE
The Furlong, Ringwood BH24 1AZ
Tel/Fax: (01425) 470896

ATTRACTION
MOORS VALLEY COUNTRY PARK
Horton Road, Ashley Heath,
Nr. Ringwood BH24 2ET
Tel: (01425) 470721
Fax: (01425) 471656
email: mvalley@eastdorset.gov.uk
www.moors-valley.co.uk
Trails and a lake, with fishing from west bank with a platform for wheelchair users. A comprehensive map of trails is available, only the Tree-Top Trail appears inaccessible, but a companion is advised for all trails.

SD ♿ CP ♿ E ♿ RF ♿
C ♿ S ♿ WC 🚶 RFE ♿

For visitors in a wheelchair or those that have difficulty walking, a pedal-powered Tandem chair is available.

SOUTHAMPTON
Situated on a peninsula with the River Test to the south and west of the city. Heavy devastation during WWII has led to many new buildings, although some fascinating houses have remained.

TOURIST INFORMATION CENTRE
9 Civic Centre Road, Southampton SO14 7JP
Tel: (023) 8083 3333 Fax: (023) 8083 3381

BUSES
First Southampton: Tel: (023) 80 224854
Some low-floor routes
Solent Blue Line: Tel: (023) 80 223224
Stagecoach: Tel: (01256) 464501
Passenger Transport Group:
Tel: (01962) 845614
Publishers of Connections, bus and
train timetables.

TAXIS
Cabmobility: Tel: (023) 80 899291
Three adapted vehicles.
Radio Taxis: Tel: (023) 80 666666
Four adapted vehicles.
Streamline Taxis: Tel: (023) 80 223355
One adapted vehicle.

TRAINS
Connex: Customer Services:
Tel: (0870) 6030405
Fax: (0870) 6030505
Minicom: (01233) 617621
Southwest Trains: Special Needs –
Tel: (0845) 6050440
Minicom: (0845) 6050441
www.swtrains.co.uk
Virgin Trains: Special Needs –
(0845) 7443366
Minicom: (0845) 7443367
Wales and West: Special Needs –
(0845) 3003005
Minicom: (0845) 7585469
Southampton Parkway (airport) station.
Level access, but ensure you arrive at the
correct side of the station for direction of
travel. Six disabled badge spaces; level
access via automatic door to ticket office;
adapted WC in station building; accessible
taxis can be ordered on request; standard
height pay/card phones; ramp; two
wheelchairs available.
Southampton Central Station. Level access
both sides; no disabled badge spaces in
long-term car park; accessible automatic
doors to ticket office; lift to all platforms;
unisex adapted WCs on platforms 1 and 4;
standard height pay/card phones; ramps;
wheelchairs on each platform.

CAR PARKS
Contact local services:
Tel: (023) 80 832539

SHOPMOBILITY
7 Castle Way, Southampton SO14 2BX
Tel/Fax: (023) 80 631263
Minicom: (023) 80 228291
HOTELS
NETLEY WATERSIDE HOUSE
(Winged Fellowship)
Abbey Hill, Netley Abbey,
Southampton SO31 5FA
Tel: (023) 80 453 686
On the shores of Southampton Water,
minutes away from local shops. Well
placed for visits to Portsmouth Dockyard,
Stonehenge etc. Large number of nurses
and care assistants. Lounge, bar, shop,
craft area. Garden sun house. Garden
viewing platform over the water.
Adaptive transport.

HILTON SOUTHAMPTON   〖👤〗
Bracken Place, Chilworth,
Southampton SO16 3RB
Tel: (023) 80 702700   Fax: (023) 80 767233
No. of Accessible Rooms: 1. Bath.
Accessible Facilities: Lounge, restaurant,
pool, sauna. Bright and modern hotel
north of the city at the junction of the
M3/A33.

ATTRACTION
EXBURY GARDENS
Exbury, Nr. Southampton SO45 1AZ
Tel: (023) 80 891203   Fax: (023) 80 899940
200 acres of landscaped woodland with
fine flowering shrub collections, ponds,
rock gardens. In the summer the garden
of 53 acres is ideal for picnics.

SD 〖♿〗   CP 〖♿〗   E 〖♿〗   RF 〖♿〗

C 〖♿〗 S 〖♿〗   WC 〖👤〗   RFE 〖♿〗

SOUTHAMPTON FOOTBALL CLUB
The Dell, Milton Road,
Southampton SO15 2XH
Admin: (023) 80 220505
The disabled enclosure is situated by the
corner flag/players' entrance, at the
Milton Road end. Experienced,
designated stewards are stationed in
enclosure.
**CP – NO PARKING AVAILABLE but Disabled badge holders
are usually allowed to park on the road close to the
disabled enclosure.**

RE 🕴 (steep slope)
WC 🕴 (near entrance to disabled supporters' area)
B/R 🕴 (steward available to obtain for you)

WINCHESTER

Important in Roman times, this became England's capital under the Anglo-Saxons: William the Conqueror kept Winchester as the capital and as late as the C17th, Charles II planned to build a palace here. The focal points are the C19th High Street and Guildhall, and there are many small alleyways with houses of all centuries.

TOURIST INFORMATION CENTRE
Guildhall, The Broadway, Winchester
SO23 9LJ
Tel: (01962) 840500   Fax: (01962) 850348
e-mail: tourism@winchester.gov.uk
www.winchester.gov.uk

WINCHESTER GROUP FOR DISABLED PEOPLE
Disability Advice Office,
The Winchester Centre, 68 St Georges Street,
Winchester, Hampshire, SO23 8AH
Tel: (01962) 840600 (Disability Advice Line)
Tel: (01962) 848013 (Office)
Fax: (01962) 848029

TRAVELINE: (0870) 6082608

Winchester Cathedral.

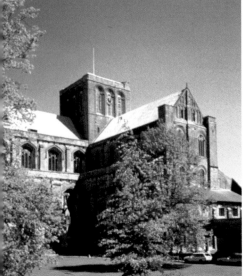

BUSES
Stagecoach Hampshire Bus:
Tel: (01256) 464501

TAXIS
Wessex Cars: Tel: (01962) 877749
Five adapted vehicles.
Wintax: Tel: (01962) 866208
Two adapted vehicles.
Hackney Carriages: Ranks at The Broadway, Silver Hill and the station.
20 adapted vehicles.

TRAINS
South West Trains. Special Needs –
Tel: (0845) 6050440
Minicom: (0845) 6050441
www.swtrains.co.uk

Winchester Station
Some disabled badge spaces; level entry to ticket office via automatic door; stairmate in operation, disabled WC on platform 2, taxi rank; standard height pay/card phones; wheelchair ramp.

CAR PARK
Free parking for disabled badge holders in all city car parks and use of residents' parking.
Tel: (01962) 848346

SHOPMOBILITY
Upper Parking Level, Brooks Car Park, Winchester SP23 8QY
Tel: (01962) 842626   Fax: (01962) 854844

HOTEL
WINCHESTER MOAT HOUSE 🕴
Worthy Lane, Winchester SO23 7AB
Tel: (01962) 709988   Fax: (01962) 840862
No. of Accessible Rooms: 1
Accessible Facilities: Lounge, bar, restaurant. Located on the edge of the city in a quiet residential area.

MARWELL HOTEL 🕴
Thompsons Lane, Colden Common,
Nr. Winchester SO21 1JY
Tel: (01962) 777681   Fax: (01962) 777625
Email: info@marwellhotel.co.uk
www.marwellhotel.co.uk
No. of Accessible Rooms: 4

Accessible Facilities: Lounge/bar, restaurant.
Delightful safari and colonial-style hotel, with airy glass and timber walkways, set in wooded grounds. Located six miles from Winchester and opposite to Marwell Zoological Park.

BED AND BREAKFAST
SHAWLANDS
46 Kilham Lane, Winchester SO22 5QD
Tel/Fax: (01962) 861166
e-mail:kathy@pollshaw.u-net.com
No. of Accessible Rooms: 1
Accessible Facilities: Lounge, dining room.
Guest house located in a quiet lane overlooking fields, 1.5 miles from Winchester city centre. Near the M3 (J11).

ATTRACTIONS
MARWELL ZOOLOGICAL PARK,
Colden Common, Marwell SO21 1JH
Tel: (01962) 777407   Fax: (01962) 777511
e-mail: marwell@marwell.org.uk
www.marwell.org.uk
Over 150 species from Siberian tigers to tamarins, from rhino to meerkat. Highlights include penguin world with underwater viewing, Encounter Village for pet and farm animals, Tropical World for a rainforest experience and aviaries for rare owls.

CP   E   RF   C
S   WC   RFE

WINCHESTER CATHEDRAL
The Close, Winchester SO23 9LS
Tel: (01962) 857200   Fax: (01962) 857201
e-mail:cathedral.office@winchester-cathedral.org.uk
www.winchester-cathedral.org.uk
Founded in 1079, this is the longest medieval church in England. It is rightly world-famous famous for its 12th-century illuminated Winchester Bible and its black marble font. Many kings lie here as do Jane Austen and Izaak Walton. An absolute must.

SD   CP n/a   E   RF
C   S   WC   RFE

HEREFORD AND WORCESTERSHIRE

HEREFORDSHIRE TOURISM
Education Centre, Blackfriars Street, Hereford HR4 9HS
Tel: (01432) 277286   Fax: (01432) 266156

WORCESTERSHIRE TOURISM
www.valenet.com

OUTDOOR ACTIVITIES
THE BRUCE WAKE CHARITABLE TRUST
Ayston, Oakham LE15 9AE
Tel: (01572) 822183
Berthed at Upton Marina on the River Severn, 10 miles south of Worcester, the narrow boat Charlotte is designed for a wheelchair user and an accompanying family of up to eight passengers. Includes hydraulic lifts, ceiling hoist, shower wheelchair, wide access ramp, fingertip control panel. One and two-week cruises available on River Severn, River Avon and Staffs. & Worcs. canal.

GLOUCESTERSHIRE DISABLED AFLOAT RIVERS TRUST (DART)
Diocesan Office, 4 College Green, GL1 2LR
Tel: (01452) 410022
Specially built river boat designed to provide residential facilities for disabled persons. Moored at Upton-on-Severn, the Dart cruises the rivers Severn and Avon and the Gloucester/Sharpness canal passing through beautiful countryside and the historic towns of Tewkesbury, Gloucester, Worcester, Evesham and Stratford-on-Avon. Accommodation for 12 persons including five wheelchairs. Fully accessible with lift and adapted WCs, shower and galley.N.B. Administration due to move to marina in early 2003 but it will be possible to get referral number using above.

ABBERLEY
Thriving village with good shops, pub and hotel. Eleven miles from Worcester.

133

SELF-CATERING
OLD YATES COTTAGES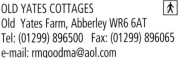
Old Yates Farm, Abberley WR6 6AT
Tel: (01299) 896500   Fax: (01299) 896065
e-mail: rmgoodma@aol.com
www.oldyatesfarm.co.uk
No. of Accessible Units: 1. Bath
No. of Beds per Unit: 2
Beagle and Bassett Cottages can be linked together and have commanding views towards the Teme Valley. On a farm growing grass and cereal crops built 100 years ago to house the squire's hounds. Now converted, you'll certainly not feel in the dog-house!

BROMSGROVE
Situated in the Lickey Hills, surrounded by lush orchard country, Bromsgrove is an ancient and sizeable market town. The church, surrounded by yew trees planted in 1790, has fascinating early C18th tombstones.

HOTEL
HILTON BROMSGROVE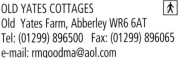
Birmingham Road, Bromsgrove B61 0JB
Tel: (0121) 4477888   Fax: (0121) 4477273
No. of Accessible Rooms: 2. Bath
Accessible Facilities: Lounge, bar, restaurant, health club (pool, sauna, spa). Quality hotel with extremely spacious reception area and extra large rooms. Located close to the M5 and M42 and several attractions.

BROMYARD
Surrounded by orchards and hop fields.

ATTRACTION
LOWER BROCKHAMPTON/BROCKHAMPTON ESTATE (NT)
Bringsty, Nr. Bromyard WR6 5UH
Tel: (01885) 482077
www.nationaltrust.org.uk/brockhampton
e-mail:brockhampton@ntrust.org.uk
Late C14th medieval moated manor house. The hall, screens, parlour and garden are accessible. Along the Access for All trail in the Brockhampton woodlands majestic oaks, ash trees and conifers abound as do all types of wildlife. The trail passes Lawn Pool, a glade with benches and picnic tables and there is a series of sculptures depicting the history of the estate and the area. An excellent leaflet is available about the trail.

SD ☒ CP ☒ E ☒ RF ☒ WC ☒ RFE ☒

EVESHAM
This is an important market town and the centre of the fruit-growing area of the Vale of Evesham. There are tree-lined walks and lawns along the banks of the Avon, many quality houses and old inns including the late C15th restored Booth Hall with fine timberwork. Part of the town's original medieval wall stands in Bridge Street.

HOTEL
BEST WESTERN
NORTHWICK ARMS HOTEL
Waterside, Evesham WR11 6BT
Tel: (01386) 40322
No. of Accessible Rooms: 1. Bath
Accessible Facilities: Restaurant
Privately owned, attractive hotel, close to the town centre.

HAY-ON-WYE
At the northern end of the Brecon Beacons, this sleepy town is synonymous with books and bookshops as the site of the best-known literary festival in England. Held in the last week of May, the atmosphere is incredible.

TOURIST INFORMATION CENTRE
Oxford Road, Haye-on-Wye HR3 5DG
Tel: (01497) 820144   Fax: (01497) 820015

HEREFORD
Situated on a level plain bounded in the distance by low-lying hills. The Wye

runs through the southern part of the town, under a medieval bridge. This is a cathedral city and an important agricultural centre. Many interesting buildings date from C4th.

TOURIST INFORMATION CENTRE
1 King Street, Hereford HR4 9BW
Tel: (01432) 268430   Fax: (01432) 342662

HEREFORD PUBLIC TRANSPORT
Tel: (01432) 260948

BUSES
Sargent Brothers: Tel: (01544) 230481
Operates access bus in city centre.
County Busline: Tel: (0345) 125436
Timetables and phone numbers of all local operators available.
Stagecoach Red & White:
Tel: (01633) 485118

TAXIS
Ace Taxis: Tel: (01432) 343399
Four adapted vehicles.
Blue Line Taxis: Tel: (01432) 263000
Two adapted vehicle.
Hereford Taxis: Tel: (01432) 343343
Two adapted vehicles.

TRAINS
Wales and West: Special Needs –
Tel: (0845) 3003005
Minicom: (0845) 7585469
Hereford station is suitable for wheelchairs using ramp access.

DISABILITY ADVICE LINE
DIAL
Coningsby St, Hereford, HR1 2DY
Tel: (01432) 277770

SHOPMOBILITY
Maylord Orchards, Hereford
Tel: (01432) 342166

HOTEL
STARTING GATE BEEFEATER
&TRAVEL INN
Holmer Road, Holmer, Hereford HR4 9RS
Tel: (01432) 274853   Fax: (01432) 343003

Take the A49 Leominster road, the inn is 0.5 miles past the Hereford Leisure Centre.

ATTRACTION
HEREFORD CIDER MUSEUM TRUST
21 Ryelands Street, Hereford HR4 0LW
Tel: (01432) 354207
Explore the story of traditional cider-making with reconstructed cider farmhouse and Champagne Cider cellars and sample!

| SD | CP | E | RF |
| S | WC | RFE | |

KIDDERMINSTER
Lying on the Stour, the town is known for its carpet manufacturing. There is pleasant wooded countryside to the NW of the town and in the centre there is a late medieval red sandstone church.

135

Try not to sample too much of the produce at the Hereford Cider Museum.

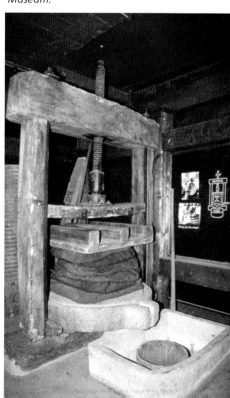

HOTEL
THE GRANARY HOTEL and
RESTAURANT
Heath Lane, Shenstone,
Kidderminster DY10 4BS
Tel: (01562) 777535   Fax: (01562) 777722
No. of Accessible Rooms: 1. Bath
Accessible Facilities: Lounge, restaurant.
Small, family-run hotel with views across
fields to Great Witley and Abberley Hills.

ATTRACTION
WORCESTERSHIRE COUNTY MUSEUM
Hartlebury Castle, Hartlebury,
Nr. Kidderminster DY11 7XZ
Tel: (01299) 250416   Fax: (01299) 251890
e-mail: museum@worcestershire.gov.uk
Hartlebury Castle was home to the
Bishops of Worcester for over 1000 years.
In the former servants' quarters in the
north wing, there are permanent
exhibitions showing past lives of the
county's inhabitants from Roman times to
the present day.

SD [♿]   CP [♿]   E [♿]   RF [♿]
C [♿]   S [♿]   WC [♿]   RFE [♿]

LEOMINSTER
Set among pastureland, hop fields and
orchards in countryside watered by
three streams, Leominster has many
medieval, Tudor and Georgian houses
and is also rich in early English
domestic architecture.

TOURIST INFORMATION CENTRE
1 Corn Square, Leominster HR6 8LR

Tel: (01568) 616460   Fax: (01568) 615546

ATTRACTION
BERRINGTON HALL (NT)
Leominster HR6 0DW
Tel: (01568) 615721   Fax: (01568) 613263
e-mail: berrington@ntrust.org.uk
An C18th Henry Holland-built house set in
parkland designed by Capability Brown.
Enquire about parking at the ticket office
which is approximately 200m from the
house cars with disabled drivers or
passengers may drive up to the courtyard
of the house. Paths are mostly suitable for
wheelchair users. There is a stair climber in
the house but it must be booked in
advance to ensure that trained staff are on
duty. There are 2 wheelchairs available at
the house and one self-drive single-seater.
These must be booked in advance. N.B.
The house can be congested at busy
periods please telephone before visiting.

SD [♿]   CP [♿]   E [♿]   WC [♿]   RFE [♿]

MALVERN
The town has a continental flavour,
being terraced on its hillside site. There
are many interesting buildings and
artefacts in the church dating mostly
from the C15th.

MALVERN HILLS TOURISM and LEISURE
SERVICES
Rockliffe House, 40 Church Street,
Gt. Malvern WR14 2AZ
Tel: (01684) 862 411   Fax: (01684) 862 441
Publishes a useful guide to disabled access

Caperbility Brown's grounds at Berrington Hall.

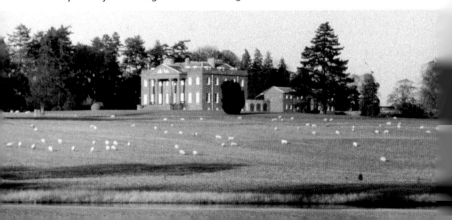

to places of interest and beauty.

MALVERN TOURIST INFORMATION CENTRE
21 Church Street, Malvern WR14 2AA
Tel: (01684) 892 289   Fax: (01684) 892 872

SELF-CATERING
CIDAR MILL COTTAGE
Mutlows Farm Cottages, Drake Street,
Welland, Nr. Malvern WR13 6LP
Tel/Fax: (01684) 310878
No. of Accessible Units: 1. Bath
No. of Beds per Unit: 3
Accessible Facilities: Lounge/diner, kitchen.
Private courtyard patio with raised flower/
herb garden and furniture.
An old cow byre and a cider store have
been converted into a spacious single-
storey detached cottage. At the foot of the
Malvern Hills three miles from Upton, the
farm has acres of ancient orchards with
wild flowers.

ATTRACTION
GREAT MALVERN PRIORY
6 Church Street,
Malvern WR14 2AY
Tel/Fax: (01684) 561020
Norman priory church, built 22 years after
the Conquest and famous for its stained
glass, of which original jewelled fragments
remain in the east window, also for
hundreds of detailed wall tiles made
between 1453/6. Two rows of original
dark oak monastic choir stalls, dating from
C15th, also survived the Dissolution.

SD   CP   E   RF
S   WC   RFE

ROSS-ON-WYE
Modest market town set on a red
sandstone cliff above a lovely sweep of
the Wye.

TOURIST INFORMATION CENTRE
Edde Cross Street, Ross-on-Wye HR9 7BZ
Tel: (01989) 562768   Fax: (01989) 565057

HOTEL
MERTON HOUSE HOTEL
Edde Cross Street, Ross-on-Wye HR9 7BZ
Tel: (01989) 563252   Fax: (01989) 763505

e-mail: mertonhouse@clara.co.uk
No. of Accessible Rooms: 13. Roll-in
shower.
Accessible Facilities: Lounge, dining room.
Located on the edge of town, this
beautiful Georgian house has been
adapted as a holiday hotel for disabled
people. Glorious views across to the Welsh
mountains.

WORCESTER

Built on both sides of the Severn, today the
principal part of the city is on the eastern
bank. Famous for its superb cathedral,
Royal Worcester porcelain and the
Guildhall.

TOURIST INFORMATION CENTRE
The Guildhall, High Street,
Worcester WR1 2EY
Tel: (01905) 726311   Fax: (01905) 722481

**CITY OF WORCESTER COMMUNITY
SERVICES**
Orchard House, Farrier Street,
Worcester WR1 3BW
Tel: (01905) 722306   Fax: (01905) 722350
www.cityofworcester.gov.uk

DIAL South Worcestershire
54 Friary Walk, Crowngate Centre,
Worcester WR1 3LE
Tel: (01905) 27790   Fax: (01905) 612692
Minicom: (01905) 22191
dial.worcs@wyenet.co.uk

MOBILITY HIRE
13 Droitwich Road, Worcester WR3 7LG
Tel: (0800) 592436
Wide range of wheelchairs and scooters for
hire, nationwide.

TRAVELINE (0870) 6082608

TAXIS
Associated Blue Star Taxis:
Tel: (01905) 610022
Two adapted vehicles.
Central Taxis: Tel: (01905) 22292
15 adapted vehicles.

Crown Radio Taxis: Tel: (01905) 357788
Two adapted vehicles.
Knights Radio Taxis: Tel: (01905) 820827
One adapted vehicle.

TRAINS
Wales and West: Special Needs –
Tel: (0345) 125625
Minicom: (0345) 585469
Worcester Foregate and Shrub Hill are
suitable for wheelchairs using ramp access.

CAR PARKS
Free three-hour disabled badge parking in
some council-owned car parks, some on-
street parking. A map is available from
DIAL.

SHOPMOBILITY
Crowngate Shopping Centre, Worcester
Tel: (01905) 610523

HOTEL
FOWNES HOTEL
City Walls Road, Worcester WR1 2AP
Tel: (01905) 613151   Fax: (01905) 23742
No. of Accessible Rooms: 1
Accessible Facilities: Lounge, restaurant
Former Victorian glove factory converted
into an interesting-looking, modern hotel
in the city centre.

SELF-CATERING
HIDELOW LODGE
Hidelow House, Acton Green,
Acton Beauchamp, Worcester WR6 5AH
Tel: (01886) 884547   Fax: (01886) 884060
e.mail: smoothrides@hidelow.co.uk
www.hidelow.co.uk
No. of Accessible Units: 1 - 4/6 1 - 2
Both with roll-in showers.
Accessible Facilities: Lounge,
kitchen,private garden.
Newly refurbished detached stone
building, set in grounds of small secluded
country house with lovely views.

ATTRACTIONS
THE COMMANDERY CIVIL WAR CENTRE
Sidburgh, Worcester WR1 2HU
Tel: (01905) 355071
NB. We have included this museum
because it is unique, but beyond the

entrance and the shop, there is a heavily
cobbled path to the museum. This was the
Royalist headquarters at the Battle of
Worcester in 1651. The museum tells the
turbulent story of the English Civil War
with scenes, models and interactive
displays. Originally a monastic hospital, it
was bought privately by the wealthy Wylde
family after the Dissolution. From 1900-
1975 the building housed a printing
factory until purchased by the local council
and restored. This is the only museum in
England dedicated to the Civil War and, if
the cobblestones can be managed, it is
well worth a visit. At weekends activities
such as re-enactments, historical crafts,
etc. take place in the charming garden.

SD CP E RF- Cobblestones
C S WC

THE MUSEUM OF WORCESTER PORCELAIN
Severn Street, Worcester WR1 2NE
Tel: (01905) 23221   Fax: (01905) 617807
The first Worcester porcelain,
manufactured here in 1751, specialised in
tableware and ornamental vases in
distinctive vivid colours. The museum has a
Georgian Gallery including vignettes of
dining scenes, and shop fronts that show
the collections in an historical context. The
Victorian Gallery offers a contrast to the
C18th displays as design and the social
history of the Victorian era unfolds. There
is an extensive shop and factory seconds
shop, plus demonstrations. Much to see,
do – and buy!

SD CP E RF L
C S WC

WORCESTER CATHEDRAL
The Chapter of Worcester, 10A College
Green, Worcester WR1 2LH
Tel: (01905) 21004   Fax: (01905) 611139
Dominated by a fine C14th. tower, much of
the cathedral belongs to this period,
although the See was founded in 650 and
there have been previous buildings on this
site. Among notable things to see are the
monumental effigy of King John; the
C16th. Prince Arthur's chantry, built by
Henry VII for his son who died at Ludlow in
1502; fine misericords and works by famous
sculptors. There are superb glass windows

and a modern altar hanging, in the colours of the liturgical year, representing the cathedral's pinnacles as reflected in the river Severn. Although the quire is on a higher level than the nave, it can be entered using a different entrance door. A ramped access (gradient:1:19) to the cloisters is clearly marked. The crypt, lady chapel, library and tower are not accessible.

SD 🚹 CP n/a E- 🚹 RF 🚹 C 🚹
S 🚹 WC 🚹

SPETCHLEY PARK GARDEN
Spetchley Park, Worcester WR5 1RS
Tel: (01905) 345213
Located three miles east of the city, this 100-acre deer park and 30-acre garden contains a large collection of trees and shrubs, many rare or unusual.

SD 🚹 CP 🚹 E 🚹 RF- 🚹
C 🚹 RFE 🚹

SPORTING VENUE
WORCESTER RACECOURSE
Pitchcroft, Worcester WR1 3EJ
Admin & Booking-Box Office: (01905) 25364
Fax: (01905) 617563
Complies with Part M, Building Regulations.

CP 🚹 RE 🚹 ED 🚹 (except manual door)
INT 🚹 L 🚹
WC 🚹 (Gents, ground floor, Ladies, first floor)
SS 🚹 (Lift access) Designated viewing platform by track at the winning post route through the grandstand main entrance and by lift to the first floor B/R 🚹

THEATRE
WORCESTER SWAN THEATRE
The Moors, Worcester WR1 3EP
Admin: (01905) 726969
Fax: (01905) 723738
Booking-Box Office: (01905) 27322

SD 🚹 CP 🚹 Public CP – Pitchcroft car park, rear of theatre, access via sloping road.
Taxi rank – city centre, payphone on the premises.
RE 🚹 ED 🚹 INT 🚹
WC 🚹 (access via double doors adjacent to auditorium
AUD 🚹 B/R 🚹
Add. Notes: Route to wheelchair spaces position 'A' on level through Aud. doors to Row A: position 'B' as above and across front of seating in Row A to far end of Row A. Transfer seating into wide seat at either end of Row A.

HERTFORDSHIRE

HERTFORDSHIRE ACTION ON DISABILITY
The Woodside Centre, The Commons, Welwyn Garden City AL7 4DD
Tel: 01707 324581
Fax: 01707 371297
e-mail: information@hadnet.co.uk
www.hadnet.com
The association runs an Easier Living Centre of useful equipment with help and advice, together with general information and counselling services. They offer a wheelchair-accessible transport service, driving school for both lessons and assessments. They produce a series of ten holiday fact sheets for accessible holidays as well as having a purpose-built hotel in Clacton. There is a counselling service for people with disabilities, their carers and families.

HERTS AND DISTRICT ADD/ADHD SUPPORT
23 Foxglove Bank, Royston SG8 9TH
Tel: (01763) 242782
e-mail: petershr@aol.com

Transport Service: Tel: (01707) 375159
Fax: (01707) 371297

NATIONAL TRAVELINE
(0870) 6082608

HERTFORDSHIRE TRAVEL LINE
Tel: (0345) 244344

BROXBOURNE
PARADISE WILDLIFE PARK
White Stubbs Lane, Broxbourne EN10 7QA
Tel: (01992) 470490
Fax: (01992) 440525
Touch and feed the paddock animals including zebras and camels and meet lion cubs in this family-run leisure park, complete with paddling pool.

Parking and approach 🚹 E 🚹 C 🚹
S 🚹 WC 🚹

HATFIELD

Divided into the old and the new, the latter an industrialised area, the former retaining its historic character with half-timbered C16th houses and Georgian properties.

ATTRACTION

HATFIELD HOUSE and GARDEN
Hatfield AL9 5NQ
Tel: (01707) 262823   Fax: (01707) 287033
Jacobean house built by Robert Cecil, the 1st Earl of Salisbury in 1611. The state rooms are rich in world-famous paintings. There are superb examples of Jacobean craftsmanship throughout. NB. A special entrance for wheelchair users is via a long pathway and electronic doors. The end of the path is rather cobbled and bumpy.

SD CP E RF L

C S WC G

HEMEL HEMPSTEAD

Developed market town with attractive stretches along the river Gade.

REACH OUT PROJECTS CANAL BOATS
Diocesan Education Centre, Hall Grove,

Welwyn Garden City AL7 4PJ.
Tel: (01707) 335968
Fax: (01707) 373089
e-mail: stalbansdys@enterprise.net
Reach out projects include Enable holidays for a weekend or a few days that provide resource for young people of all abilities. Narrow and wide-beam boats are moored on the Grand Union Canal and are available for self-steer hire or skippered.

ST. ALBANS

This beautiful and ancient city was one of the most important Roman towns. It has an historic city centre with narrow, twisting and hilly streets and several coaching inns and houses of medieval construction.

TOURIST INFORMATION CENTRE

Town Hall, Market Place, St. Albans
Tel: (01727) 864511
Fax: (01727) 863533
e-mail:tic@stalbans.gov.uk
www.stalbans.gov.uk

ST. ALBANS CITY AND DISTRICT COUNCIL

St. Peter's Street, St. Albans AL1 3JE
Tel: (01727) 866100

Dinner is served. The state rooms at Hatfield House.

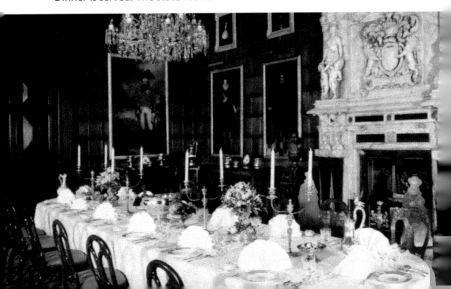

NATIONAL TRAVELINE
(0870) 6082608

TAXIS
Goldline Taxis: Tel: (01727) 840000
Four adapted vehicles.
Arena Taxis: Tel: (01727) 844844
One adapted vehicle.

TRAINS
Thameslink: Special Needs –
Tel: (0207) 6206333
Minicom: (0207) 6205561

HOTEL
HERTFORDSHIRE MOAT HOUSE
London Road, Markyate,
Nr. St. Albans AL3 8HH
Tel: (01582) 449988 Fax: (01582) 842282
No. of Accessible Rooms: 140
Accessible Facilities: Restaurant, lounge
Re-opened in January 2000, convenient for
the M1 but with pleasant rural outlook.

ATTRACTION
THE GARDENS OF THE ROSE
Chiswell Green Lane, St. Albans AL2 3NR
Tel: (01727) 850462   Fax: (01727) 850362
e-mail: mail@rnrs. org.uk
Gardens of the Royal National Rose Society
with over 30,000 plants in 1,650 different
varieties, including old-fashioned and
modern roses and roses of the future. This
is the International Trial Ground for new
roses.

SD 🧑‍🦽   CP 🧑‍🦽   E 🧑‍🦽   RF 🧑‍🦽
C 🧑‍🦽   S 🧑   WC 🧑   G 🧑‍🦽

ROMAN THEATRE
Gorhambury Drive, St. Michaels,
St. Albans AL3 6AH
Tel: (01727) 835035
Built about AD160 and excavated in 1935,
this semi-circular theatre is unique. about
60m across it held 2,000 spectators. Entry
is free for disabled visitors.

SD 🧑‍🦽   CP 🧑   E 🧑‍🦽   S 🧑   RFE 🧑‍🦽

VERULAMIUM MUSEUM
St. Michaels Street, St. Albans AL3 4SW
Tel: (01727) 819339 Fax: (01727) 859919
A museum of everyday life in Roman
Britain, it stands on the site of

Verulamium, one of the most important
cities in Roman Britain. Excavated objects
range from mosaics to everyday pottery
and metalwork.

SD 🧑‍🦽   CP 🧑‍🦽   E 🧑‍🦽   L 🧑‍🦽
S 🧑‍🦽   WC 🧑‍🦽   RFE 🧑‍🦽

BOWMANS OPEN FARM
Coursers Road, London Colney,
St. Albans AL2 1BB
Tel: (01727) 822106   Fax: (01727) 826406
Farm trail past paddocks of pigs, cattle
and sheep and a working farmyard. Pets
Corner; tractor rides in an Adventure
Playground; watch cows being milked;
see hawks and falcons in the falconry
area; the wildlife on the lake and visit an
Indoor touching Barn.

SD 🧑‍🦽   CP 🧑‍🦽   E 🧑‍🦽   RF 🧑‍🦽   S
🧑‍🦽
WC 🧑   RFE- Barns 🧑‍🦽   Paddocks 🧑

De HAVILLAND HERITAGE and MOSQUITO AIRCRAFT MUSEUM
PO Box 107, Salisbury Hall, London Colney,
St. Albans AL2 1EX   Tel: (01727) 822051
This is the oldest aviation museum in
Britain. It opened in 1959 on uneven, but
accessible land with 20 types of de
Havilland aircraft with hands-on
experience and working displays. The
Mosquito was made of a light but strong
balsa wood sandwich. Timber was used
during the war because it was easier to
obtain than metal and so furniture
factories were able to build aircraft.

SD 🧑‍🦽   CP 🧑   E 🧑‍🦽   RF 🧑
C 🧑   WC 🧑   RFE 🧑

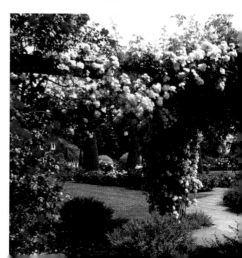

The Garden of the Roses.

THEATRE

MALTINGS ART THEATRE
The Maltings, St. Albans AL1 3HL
Tel: (01727) 844222   Fax: (01727) 836616
CP ♿   RE ♿   ED ♿ INT – Box Office
Counter 🚶   widths ♿   L 🚶   AUD ♿
B/R ♿

STEVENAGE

There are both old and new towns, the latter, spacious, modern and well-planned and the old retaining its charm and historical interest with many old cottages and houses now turned into shops.

STEVENAGE SHOP MOBILITY

15 Queensway, Stevenage
Tel: (01438) 350300

WATFORD

Hertfordshire's largest town with a long, narrow high street leading to the River Colne that skirts the hills on which the town stands. C16th and C18th houses are still to be found, although the town is much modernised.

ATTRACTION

WATFORD MUSEUM
194 High Street, Watford WD1 2HG
Tel/fax: (01923) 232297

A Watford Football Club display includes Elton John associations, historic printing presses, a reconstructed Victorian bar, and a collection of paintings and sculpture.
SD ♿   CP ♿   E ♿   RF ♿
L ♿   C n/a   S ♿   WC 🚶

WELWYN

Small old town with much charm: many of the houses are Georgian and the river Mimram runs through the village.

ATTRACTION

SHAW'S CORNER (NT)
Ayot St. Lawrence, Nr. Welwyn AL6 9BX
Tel/Fax: (01438) 820307

An Edwardian villa and home of playwright George Bernard Shaw. Presented much the way he left it to the NT. The ground floor (study, drawing room, dining room, kitchen) is level with wide doors. Outside, access to the garden is via the front door, down a ramp and through a side gate. Gravel paths and grassy slopes lead to the lawns.
CP ♿   E 🚶   WC 🚶   G 🚶

Port Erin, Isle of Man.

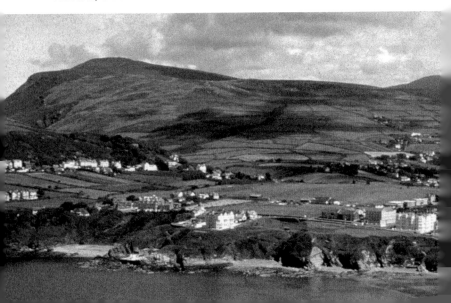

ISLE OF MAN

ISLE OF MAN TOURISM
Sea Terminal Building, Douglas IM1 2RG
Tel: (01624) 686 766 Fax: (01624) 627 443
e-mail: tourism@gov.im
www.gov.im/tourism

MANX FOUNDATION FOR THE PHYSICALLY DISABLED
Marsham Court Day Centre, Victoria Avenue, Douglas IM2 4AW
Tel: (01624) 628926 Fax: (01624) 670821

BALLAUGH
This is a large expanse of marshland in north of the island.

ATTRACTION
CURRAGHS WILDLIFE PARK
Ballaugh
Tel: (01624) 897323 Fax: (01624) 897327
A wide range of species of animals and birds in natural settings with large walk-through enclosures. Located midway between Kirkmichael and Ramsey.

SD   CP   E   RF
C S WC

DOUGLAS
Rather grand Victorian resort and the island's capital, with sweeping promenade, hotels, attractive quayside and yacht haven, entertainment and activities.

HOTEL
SEFTON HOTEL
Harris Promenade, Douglas IM1 2RW
Tel: (01624) 645500
Fax: (01624) 676004
www.seftonhotel.co.im
No. of Accessible Rooms: 3. Bath
Accessible Facilities: Lounge, restaurants (2), pool, sauna, whirlpool. Located on the promenade next to the Gaiety Theatre, with a wide range of facilities.

ATTRACTION
MANX MUSEUM AND NATIONAL TRUST
Douglas IM1 3LY
Tel: (01624) 648000 Fax: (01624) 648001
The Story of Man with a film portrayal of Manx history combined with gallery displays. NB: Entrance is stepped at 7.5cm from the pavement.

SD CP E RF
L C S WC

SELF-CATERING
KIONSLIEU FARM COTTAGES
Kionslieu Farm, Higher Foxdale IM4 3HB
Tel/Fax: (01624) 801349
No. of Accessible Units: 1 (Cottage No. 5). Bath. No. of Beds per Unit: 4
Accessible Facilities: Open plan kitchen/diner, sitting room. Combination of newly built and renovated farm buildings in a rural location about 10 minutes' drive from Douglas. Cottage 5 has been created from a former dairy and is by a wooded area.

SANTON
HOTEL
MOUNT MURRAY HOTEL
AND COUNTRY CLUB
Santon IM4 2HT
Tel: (01624) 661111 Fax: (01624) 661116
e-mail: mountmurray@advsys.net
www.mountmurray.com
No. of Accessible Rooms: 8. Bath
Accessible Facilities: Lounge, restaurants, not all tables in bistro are accessible.
Sports hall, driving range.
Modern hotel in 200 acres overlooking the island's newest golf course with an extensive leisure complex.

143

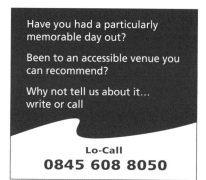
Have you had a particularly memorable day out?

Been to an accessible venue you can recommend?

Why not tell us about it… write or call

Lo-Call
0845 608 8050

ISLES OF SCILLY

An Area of Outstanding Beauty, an
archipelago of granite islands and
outcrops, five of which are inhabited,
concentrated mainly on St. Mary's. The
islands are famous for bird life and seals,
particularly on the more remote spots.
There is a flourishing flower industry,
notably narcissi, with about 30 million
blooms harvested from October to March
and shipped worldwide. The Gulf Stream
ensures the Scillies enjoy the mildest UK
climate, although Atlantic winds mean
considerable rainfall.

ST. MARY'S
The largest island with nine miles of
coastline. Hugh Town has most
amenities, including the famous
Mermaid pub.

TOURIST INFORMATION CENTRE
Hugh Street, Hugh Town, St. Mary's TR21 0LL
Tel: (01720) 422536
Fax: (01720) 423782
e-mail: tic@scilly.gov.co.uk

TAXIS
No taxis are licensed on the islands, The
matter is in the hands of solicitors!

FERRIES
Isles of Scilly Travel Centre
Tel: (01736) 362009
e-mail: sales@islesofscilly-travel.co.uk
www.ios-travel.co.uk
Foot passengers only, wheelchairs carried
as cargo.

SELF-CATERING
ALTAMIRA FLATS
Porthlow Farm, St. Mary's TR21 0NF
Tel: (01720) 422636
No. of Accessible Units: 1
No. of Beds per Unit: 4
Accessible Facilities: Kitchen, lounge/diner.
Close to Porth Loo Beach and under a mile
to Hugh Town.

ISLE OF WIGHT

ISLE OF WIGHT TOURISM
Westridge Centre, Brading Road,
Ryde PO33 1QS
Tel: (01983) 823873
e-mail: post@isle-of-wight-tourism.gov.uk
www.isle-of-wight-tourism.gov.uk

DIAL Isle of Wight
Riverside Centre, The Quay, Newport
PO30 2QR
Tel: (01983) 522823

TRAVELINE
Tel: (0870) 6082608

TAXIS
Norman Bakers Taxis: Tel: (01983) 403545
One adapted vehicles.

TRAINS
Island Line: Tel: (01983) 812591
Accessible for wheelchairs, ring in advance.

FERRIES
Red Funnel, a car ferry from Southampton,
and Wightlink, a passenger ferry from
Portsmouth and Lymington. See under
Ferries in the Introduction.

ALUM BAY
Home to amazing multi-coloured cliffs
and the Needles.

ATTRACTION
NEEDLES PLEASURE PARK
Alum Bay PO39 0JD
Tel: (01983) 752401   Fax: (01983) 755260
Family attraction with rides and
entertainment plus a chairlift to the beach
to see the unique coloured sands.

BINSTEAD
Village two miles west of Ryde.

ATTRACTION
BRICKFIELDS HORSECOUNTRY

Newnham Road, Binstead PO33 3TH
Tel: (01983) 566801 Fax: (01983) 562649
e-mail: brickfields@binsteadiow
www.brickfield.net

Shire horses, miniature ponies, heritage
and carriage collections. Most is outside
over several acres, flat and unobstructed,
except where ramped for bar/restaurant.
The restaurant ramp gradient is 1:5.

SD ☒ CP ☒ E ☒ C n/a
S ☒ WC ☒ RFE ☒

BRADING

One of the oldest towns on the island,
and an ancient port with the remains
of an extensive Roman villa built
AD300 and a C12th parish church.

ATTRACTION
OASIS
Carpenters Road, Brading PO36 0QA
Tel: (01983) 613760 Fax: (01983) 615335
World of indoor living with a delightful
range of arts and crafts shops.

SD n/a CP ☒ E ☒ RF ☒
C ☒ S ☒ WC ☒

COWES

Located on the northern tip of the
island. Linked with sailing and
boatbuilding and a mecca for
yachtsmen, particularly during the
international festival of Cowes Week
during the first week of August.

TOURIST INFORMATION CENTRE
9 The Arcade, Cowes PO31 7AR
Tel: (01983) 813818   Fax: (01983) 280078

SELF-CATERING
NEW STABLE COTTAGE ☒
Little Thorness Farm, Nr. Cowes PO31 8NG
Tel: (01983) 297863
No. of Accessible Units: 1. Bath
No. of Beds per Unit: 2
Accessible Facilities: Dining room.
The cottage is central to the working farm
here. In summer the beach is accessible by
car for accompanied wheelchair users.

ATTRACTIONS
ISLE OF WIGHT MODEL RAILWAYS
The Parade, Cowes PO31 7QJ
Tel/Fax: (01983) 280111

Not just a model railway layout, but a view
of the world in miniature. A large diorama
gives a picture of the English countryside as
many different toy and model trains from
the turn of the century onwards run. A
delightful experience. Changes of level are
by ramps at 1:18 and the exhibition can be
seen from all view points.

SD n/a CP ☒ E ☒ RFE ☒

OSBORNE HOUSE
York Avenue, East Cowes PO32 6JY
Tel: (01983) 200022
Fax: (01983) 281380

Designed by Prince Albert, and built
between 1845/48 to resemble an Italian
villa. This was Queen Victoria's favourite
home. It is untouched, the state and family
apartments are open to the public and the
grounds are full of English trees, a
miniature fort and a Swiss cottage.
NB: The car park is 300m. from house and
so is inaccessible.

SD ☒ CP n/a E ☒ RF ☒
C ☒ S ☒ WC ☒

NEWPORT

The island's capital was originally an
inland port, located in the centre of the
island with some attractive old quays.

TOURIST INFORMATION CENTRE
The Car Park, South Street,
Newport PO30 1JU
Tel: (01983) 525450 Fax: (01983) 822929

ATTRACTIONS
CARISBROOKE CASTLE (E.H.)
Carisbrooke, Newport PO30 1XY
Tel: (01983) 529130 Fax: (01983) 528632

This is the only medieval castle on the
island. It has Elizabethan and Jacobean
additions, and Charles I was a prisoner
here in 1647. NB. Entrance ramped at a
gradient of 1:11

SD ☒ CP n/a E   RF ☒ C ☒
S ☒ WC

GUILDHALL MUSEUM
High Street, Newport PO30 1TY
Tel: (01983) 823366 Fax: (01983) 823841
Explore the island's history in this new museum using touch-screen computer technology, hands-on exhibits, microscopes, quizzes and games.

SD [♿]   CP n/a E [♿]   RF [♿]
S [♿]   WC [♿]

RYDE
The Island's largest town with six miles of sandy beaches stretching from west of the pier through to Springvale, and excellent leisure facilities.

TOURIST INFORMATION CENTRE
81-83 Union Street, Ryde PO33 2LW
Tel: (01983) 562905   Fax: (01983) 567610

BED AND BREAKFAST
SEAWARD GUEST HOUSE   [♿]
14-16 George Street, Ryde PO33 2EW
Tel/Fax: (01983) 563168
No. of Accessible Rooms: 1. Shower Accessible Facilities: Dining room on first floor (no lift) but meals can be served in rooms. Located very close to all the major transport and entertainment centres plus shopping, cafes and restaurants.

ATTRACTIONS
L.A.BOWL
The Pavilion, The Esplanade, Ryde PO33 2EL
Tel: (01983) 617070   Fax: (01983) 611581
www.labowl.co.uk

This family entertainment centre incorporates tenpin bowling, a children's indoor adventure play area and restaurants. The centre is open plan, on one level with a shallow ramp to the bowling lanes. Special equipment allows wheelchair users to enjoy bowling, including specially designed launching chutes and small ramps to gain access to the approaches (a small step of 5cm).

SD [♿]   CP [♿]   E [♿]   RF [♿]
C [♿]   WC [♿]

WALTZING WATERS
Westridge, Brading Road, Ryde PO33 1QS
Tel/Fax: (01983) 811333
An elaborate and exciting water, light and music production with thousands of dazzling patterns of moving water synchronised with music.

SD [♿]   CP [♿]   E [♿]   RF [♿]
S [♿]   WC [♿]   RFE [♿]

SANDOWN
A holiday resort bay with a fine sandy beach and a pier packed with amusements.

TOURIST INFORMATION CENTRE
High Street, Sandown, PO36 8DA
Tel: (01983) 403886   Fax: (01983) 406482

SELF-CATERING
BARN COTTAGE   [♿]
Knighton Barn, Newchurch,
Sandown PO36 0NT

Carisbrooke Castle. The enforced home of Charles I – for a while.

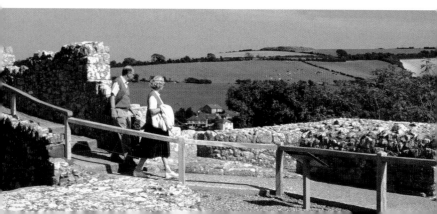

Tel/Fax: (01983) 865349
No. of Accessible Units: 1. Bath
No. of Beds per Unit: 4,
Accessible Facilities: Living/dining room, kitchen. Lovely area between Ryde and Newchurch to the south of the Downs. Cottage at end of C17th listed barn with large garden.

ATTRACTIONS
FRONT LINE AND AVIATION MUSEUM
Sandown Airport, Sandown PO36 0JP
Tel: (01983) 404448
90 years of aviation history from Louis Bleriot's flight across the Channel in 1909, and the Red Baron's triplane, to the jet age, displayed in two hangars.
SD 🚹 CP 🚹 E 🚹 (entrance from rear car park direct into hangers, opened when required).
RF 🚹 C- 🚹 S 🚹 WC 🚹 RFE 🚹

AMAZON WORLD
Watery Lane, Newchurch,
Nr. Sandown PO36 0LX
Tel: (01983) 867122
Fax: (01983) 868560
Over 200 different species of rare and exotic animals, birds, reptiles and insects set in a natural jungle environment that recreates the story of the rainforest.
SD 🚹 CP 🚹 E 🚹 RF 🚹 C 🚹
S 🚹 WC 🚹 RFE 🚹

SHANKLIN
A popular family resort, Shanklin offers a sandy beach, safe bathing and entertainment, and a charming older village with a collection of lovely thatched cottages, antique shops and fragrant gardens.

TOURIST INFORMATION CENTRE
67 High Street, Shanklin PO38 6JJ
Tel: (01983) 862942   Fax: (01983) 863047

TOTLAND BAY
Quiet sandy beach with pier, promenade and restaurant in the west of the Island.

HOTEL
COUNTRY GARDEN 🚹
Church Hill, Totland Bay PO39 0ET
Tel/Fax: (01983) 754521
No. of Accessible Rooms: 4
Accessible Facilities: Lounge, restaurant. Charming small hotel in lovely grounds.

VENTNOR
Mediterranean in ambience and style, this Victorian spa town is built on terraces that climb steeply towards St. Boniface Down where there are superb views across the bay.

TOURIST INFORMATION CENTRE
34 High Street, Ventnor PO38 1RZ
Tel: (01983) 853625   Fax: (01983) 856232

ATTRACTION
BLACKGANG CHINE FANTASY PARK
Glackgang, Nr. Ventnor,
Isle of Wight.   PO38 2HN
Tel: (01983) 730330
Fax: (01983) 731267
Set in 40 acres of cliff-top gardens. Rides and attractions include Maritime World, a Pirate Ship, a wild west town, dinosaurs, troublesome goblins and a sawmill.
SD 🚹 CP 🚹 E 🚹 RF 🚹 C 🚹
S 🚹 WC- 🚹 RFE 🚹

ISLE OF WIGHT
OWL AND FALCONRY CENTRE
Appledurcombe House, Wroxall,
Nr. Ventnor PO38 3EW
Tel: (01983) 852484
Baroque elegance is evident in this partly restored building aided by Capability Brown ornamental gardens and 11 acres of grounds containing the Falconry Centre. The house is surrounded by level flagstones and there is good access inside with no more than a couple of steps. The cellars are not accessible. Impacted gravel paths in the grounds are difficult for wheelchairs. Cars with disabled visitors should report to the shop from where they can proceed to the house. Assistance is available in

Falconry Centre if requested.

SD ♿ CP 🚶 E- 🚶 RF ♿ C ♿
S ♿ WC 🚶 RFE 🚶

RARE BREEDS AND WATERFOWL PARK
Undercliff Drive (A3055),
St. Lawrence,
Ventnor PO38 1UW
Tel: (01983) 852582
75% ACCESSIBLE BUT TELEPHONE IN
ADVANCE. There are 35 acres of park.
One of largest survival collections with
over 40 rare breeds of cattle, deer, sheep,
pigs, ponies, miniature horses, llamas, owls
and other species. Natural streams, ponds
and lakes house waterfowl and poultry:
lovely picnic areas and aviaries. Separate
entrance from lower car park avoids some
of the worst gradients. The key to this
entrance is available on request from the
main entrance.

SD ♿ CP 🚶 E ♿ RF ♿ C ♿
S ♿ WC 🚶 RFE ♿

YARMOUTH
Not an over-populated area with
rolling countryside and breathtaking
views, Yarmouth is the main town in
West Wight with a pretty harbour and
a castle built by Henry VIII.

TOURIST INFORMATION CENTRE
The Quay, Yarmouth PO41 4PQ
Tel: (01983) 760015
Fax: (01983) 761047

ATTRACTION
FORT VICTORIA MODEL RAILWAY
Fort Victoria, Westhill Lane,
Yarmouth PO41 0RR
Tel: (01983) 761553
This is the largest and most advanced
model railway layout in Britain. Both the
Model Railway and Maritime Museum here
are accessible. The Boathouse Cafe,
Planetarium, Aquarium and Country Park
are not accessible.

SD ♿ CP 🚶 E- ♿ RF ♿
C n/a S ♿ WC 🚶 RFE ♿

KENT

NATIONAL TRAVELINE
Tel: (0870) 6082608 PUBLIC TRANSPORT

ASHFORD
A changing market town, once a major
rail works and now an embarkation
point for Eurostar services to France
and Belgium. The town holds a regular
cattle auction, one of the oldest of its
kind in the country. The largest factory
shop outlet in Europe is near the
station.

TOURIST INFORMATION CENTRE
18 The Churchyard, Ashford TN23 1QG
Tel: (01233) 629165   Fax: (01233) 639166

ATTRACTIONS
BEECH COURT GARDENS
Challock, Nr. Ashford TN25 4DJ
Tel: (01233) 740735   Fax: (01233) 740842
Unbordered woodland garden where the
discovery of Roman artefacts suggests the
site is ancient. Developed to harmonise
with the seasons and produce interest and
colour throughout the year.

SD ♿ CP 🚶 E ♿ RF ♿
C 🚶 S 🚶 WC 🚶 G ♿

SOUTH OF ENGLAND RARE BREEDS CENTRE
Woodchurch, Ashford TN26 3RJ
Tel: (01233) 861493   Fax: (01233) 861457
The farm is owned and run by Canterbury
Oast Trust, a charity providing homes,
training and supported work experience
for learning and physically disabled adults.
All staff are experienced in understanding
the needs of disabled people. The farm is
home to many rare British farm breeds
with plenty of hands-on experience. There
is also a plant centre.

SD ♿ CP ♿ E ♿ RF ♿ C ♿
S ♿ WC 🚶

RFE- Outdoor open farm with park surfaces varying in
quality and construction. Most is accessible, although some
is bumpy. Paths vary from brick and concrete to dirt and
grass. Woodland inaccessible.

BEXLEY/BEXLEYHEATH
HOTELS
BEXLEY HEATH MARRIOTT
1 Broadway, Bexleyheath DS6 7JZ
Tel: (020) 8298 1000   Fax: (020) 8298 1234
No. of Accessible Rooms: 2. Bath
Accessible Facilities: Lounge, restaurant,
disabled lift for access to Leisure Club and
hoist into pool, bar.

FORTE POSTHOUSE BEXLEY
Black Prince Interchange, Southwold Road,
Bexley DA5 1ND
Tel: (0870) 4009006   Fax: (01322) 526113
No. of Accessible Rooms: 1
Accessible Facilities: Lounge, restaurant,
lift. A mile from Bexleyheath town centre,
this is convenient for visitors to Greenwich,
Leeds Castle and the Thames Barrier and is
35 minutes by train to central London.

BIRCHINGTON
ATTRACTION
QUEX HOUSE and GARDENS and POWELL-
COTTON MUSEUM
Quex Park, Birchington CT7 0BH
Tel: (01843) 842168   Fax: (01843) 846661
Built as a Regency gentleman's country
residence with oriental and period
furniture on display, the museum has eight
galleries with an amazing variety of items
and the walled gardens have been
returned to their Victorian splendour.

Features. Museum floors are level except between galleries
2 and 3 where there is a mobile ramp. Ramped also
between the museum and the house. Gardens have
tarmaced drives.

CANTERBURY
A beautiful and picturesque city, most
famous for its cathedral to which
Chaucer's pilgrims and many others
came to visit the shrine of Thomas à
Becket, murdered here in the C12th.
The city is the centre of Christianity in
England. Half the city's medieval walls,
dating back to the C13th and C14th,
stand. St. Martin's is probably the
oldest church in England still in use.

CANTERBURY, HERNE BAY AND
WHITSTABLE TOURISM
c/o Canterbury City Council, Military Road,
Canterbury CT1 4YW
Tel: (01227) 763763   Fax; (01227) 763727
web: www.canterbury.gov.uk

TOURIST INFORMATION CENTRES
34 St. Margaret's Street, Canterbury CT1 2TG
Tel: (01227) 766567   Fax: (01227) 459840

Coach Car Park, Kingsmead, Canterbury
Tel: (01227) 451096

BUSES
Stagecoach East Kent: Tel: (01227) 472082
No low-floor buses in Canterbury
Kent County Council Transport Services:
Tel: (01622) 605022/605098

TAXIS
Cabco: Tel: (01227) 455455
11 adapted vehicles.
Lynx Taxis: Tel: (01227) 464232
Eight adapted vehicles.
Procab: Tel: (01227) 478338
Five adapted vehicles.
TRAINS
Connex South Eastern: Customer Services:
Tel: (0870) 6030405   Fax: (0870) 6030505

CAR PARKS
The city centre is pedestrianised. Disabled
badge holder parking in Watling Street;
behind Woolworth's in Canterbury Lane;
behind the Library in Orange Street
(specifically for O.B.H.)

HOTEL
EXPRESS BY HOLIDAY INN
Upper Harbledown,
Canterbury CT2 9HX
Tel: (01227) 865000   Fax: (01227) 865100
No. of Accessible Rooms: 5
Accessible Facilities: Lounge, restaurant.
Modern business-style property located on
A2, four miles east of the city centre.

ATTRACTIONS
ASH COOMBE VINEYARD
Coombe Lane, Ash, Canterbury
Tel: (01304) 813396
Small family-owned vineyard with grass

path. WC facility within the family home. Experience with PHAB groups.

SD ♿ CP ♿ E ♿ RF ♿
S ♿ WC 🚶 RFE 🚶

CANTERBURY CATHEDRAL
The Precincts, Canterbury CT1 2EH
Tel: (01227) 762862
Fax: (01227) 865222
e-mail: visits@canterbury-cathedral.org
Mother church of the Anglican community, dominating the city. A centre of pilgrimage for many centuries, the Shrine of Thomas à Beckett is a main attraction. The treasures of the shrine were carried off during the Dissolution and of the original cathedral nothing remains, but there is a great deal to see and much of its medieval design, including fine stained glass and central Bell Harry Tower remain. The C15th nave is high, narrow and awe-inspiring. Only one English king, Henry IV, is buried here, lying beside his queen, Joan of Navarre in Trinity Chapel. Access is by the NW door, lift into the quire. The crypt is ramped at 1:7, and together with Corona and Martyrdom are not accessible.

SD ♿ CP 🚶 E RF ♿ L ♿ Cn/a
S 🚶 WC 🚶

CANTERBURY TALES VISITOR ATTRACTION
St. Margarets Street, Canterbury CT1 2TG
Tel: (01227) 454888 Fax: (01227) 765584
Fine reconstruction of the C14th world of Chaucer's famous pilgrims as they journey from the Tabard Inn, London towards the shrine of St. Thomas à Becket at Canterbury Cathedral. Medieval streets, houses and markets, together with Becket's shrine.
SD/CP n/a Nearest parking in Watling Street.

E ♿ RF ♿ L ♿ C ♿
S ♿ WC 🚶 RFE ♿

HOWLETTS WILD ANIMAL PARK
Bekesbourne, Canterbury CT4 5EL
Tel: (01303) 264647 Fax: (01303) 264944
Home to a famous breeding colony of captive lowland gorillas, African elephants, tigers, lemurs, deer, antelope, snow leopards and more in natural style surroundings.

SD ♿ CP ♿ E ♿ RF ♿ C ♿
S ♿ WC 🚶

PARSONAGE FARM RURAL HERITAGE CENTRE
North Elham, Canterbury CT4 6UY
Tel: (01303) 840766 Fax: (01303) 840183
Family-run for over 100 years, this working farm in situated in heart of the Elham valley on the north Downs. Part of the farmhouse dates from medieval times. Explore 600 years of history following trails around the farm with old and rare animal breeds. Plants, butterflies typical of the area. There is a little museum in the farmhouse and visitors can browse around the barns.

SD ♿ CP ♿ E ♿ RF 🚶
C ♿ S ♿ WC 🚶

ST. AUGUSTINES ABBEY (EH)
Longport, Canterbury CT1 1TF
Tel/Fax: (01227) 767345
Explore the abbey founded in 598 by St. Augustine after he was sent by Pope Gregory from Rome to convert pagan King Ethelbert of Kent. The abbey served for 1,000 years until the Dissolution. This is one of the most important religious sites in England. Remarkable artefacts have been uncovered during archaeological digs on the site.
A Batterican is available free of charge. Nearest parking is at the corner of Longport and Lower Chantry Lane.

E ♿ RF ♿ S ♿ WC ♿ RFE ♿
SD/CP n/a

WINGHAM WILDLIFE PARK
Rusham Road, Wingham, Canterbury CT3 1JL
Tel: (01227) 720836 Fax: (01227) 722452
Delightful park with a variety of purpose-built environments, including walk-through orchard aviary, pet village, landscaped lakes and exhibition room.

SD ♿ CP ♿ E ♿ RF ♿ C ♿
S ♿ WC 🚶 RFE ♿

THEATRE
MARLOWE THEATRE
The Friars, Canterbury
Tel: (01227) 787787
A side entrance is ramped. Bell for quick access through the door. There is a platform to the booking office.

CHATHAM

A busy commercial town where Charles Dickens spent some of his boyhood. The gates to the docklands are worth seeing, and there are good parks and gardens.

ATTRACTION
ROYAL ENGINEERS MUSEUM OF MILITARY ENGINEERING
Brompton Barracks, Chatham ME4 4UG
Tel: (01634) 406397   Fax: (01634) 822371
e-mail: remuseum.rhgre@gtnet.gov.uk
Government designation as museum with outstanding collection. Displays of equipment, working models, costumes and curios from around the world.
SD   CP   E   C
S   WC

DOVER

Famous for its castle begun in 1168 and used as a military base until the 1980s, its white cliffs and as a major Channel port.

TOURIST INFORMATION CENTRE
Townwall Street, Dover CT17 1JR
Tel: (01304) 205108   Fax: (01304) 225498

HOTEL
THE PLOUGH TRAVEL INN
Folkestone Road, Dover CT15 7AB
Tel: (01304) 213339
No. of Accessible Rooms: 4
Accessible Facilities: Lounge, restaurant.
Located on the B2011 between Dover and Folkestone.

ATTRACTIONS
DOVER CASTLE
Castle Hill Road, Dover CT16 1HU
Tel: (01304) 211067
Fax: (01304) 214739
Standing on a high hill, dominating the town and harbour, the castle was a military headquarters until the 1960s.
Today much of its 2,000 year history can be experienced by visitors. Its underground tunnel system that was a command centre where many important decisions of WWII were made, is now open to the public.
SD   CP   E   C
S   WC   F

DOVER OLD TOWN GAOL
Biggin Street, Dover CT16 1DL
Tel: (01304) 202723   Fax: (01304) 201200
AV and talking TV heads take visitors back to Victorian England to experience the horrors of life behind bars. Reconstructed courtroom, exercise yard and cells.
SD   CP   E   S

Dover Castle. The first view of England for many would-be invaders.

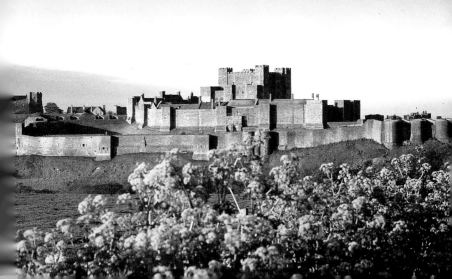

FAVERSHAM

ATTRACTION

FARMING WORLD
Nash Court, Boughton,
Faversham ME13 9SW
Tel: (01227) 751144   Fax: (01795) 520813
e-mail: farmingworld@freeserve.co.uk
Traditional farm animals, rare breeds, heavy
horses, farming bygones in the shape of
machinery and methods and seasonal fruit
are part of this charming attraction.

SD ♿   CP ♿   E ♿   RF ♿   C ♿
S ♿   WC ♿   RFE ♿

FOLKESTONE

A popular seaside resort with Victorian
hotels and guest houses on the front.
Old buildings are towards the harbour
with some fine paths in and around
the town with extensive views of the
white cliffs.

TOURIST INFORMATION CENTRE

Harbour Street, Folkestone CT20 1QN
Tel: (01303) 258594   Fax: (01303) 259754
Covers The Garden Coast of Folkestone,
Hythe and Romney Marsh.

HOTEL

GARDEN LODGE   🚶
324 Canterbury Road, Densole,
Folkestone CT18 7BB
Tel: (01303) 893147   Fax: (01303)894581
e.mail: stay@garden-lodge.com
No. of Accessible Rooms: 1
Accessible Facilities: Lounge, restaurant,
indoor pool with four steps.   Award
winning guest house and restaurant with
pets' corner, barbecue and patios. Three
miles from Folkestone and 12 from
Canterbury.

GILLINGHAM

Prehistoric and Roman traces have
been found in this modern town.

ATTRACTION

ROYAL ENGINEERS MUSEUM
Prince Arthur Road, Gillingham ME4 4UG

Tel: (01634) 406397   Fax: (01634) 822371
Displays of equipment, working models,
and a costume and curio collection.

SD ♿   CP ♿   E ♿   RF 🚶
C 🚶   S ♿   WC 🚶

LYDD

Noted for the pinnacled tower of its
parish church of the 13 and 15th
centuries.

ATTRACTION

DUNGENESS RSPB NATURE RESERVE
Boulderwall Farm, Dungeness Road
Lydd TN29 9PN
Tel: (01797) 320588   Fax: (01797) 321962
This is a coastal reserve of over 2,000
acres of shingle beach and flooded pits,
famous for rare migrants and permanent
species. The two-mile nature trail can be
traversed by wheelchair, although the
shingle surfaces may prove difficult. Four
of five bird-watching hides have low
windows for wheelchair visitors, and may
be reached by car on request.

SD ♿   CP ♿   E ♿   RF ♿
C 🚶   S 🚶   WC 🚶   RFE ♿

MAIDSTONE

County town with many C14th
buildings, parks and gardens all
worth visiting.

TOURIST INFORMATION CENTRE

The Gatehouse, The Old Palace Gardens,
Mill Street, Maidstone ME15 6YE
Tel: (01622) 602169   Fax: (01622) 673581

SELF-CATERING

COURTLODGE COTTAGES
West Peckham, Maidstone ME18 5JN
Tel/Fax: (01622) 812529
Two accessible cottages:
STAPLE COTTAGE   ♿
No. of Accessible Units: 1. Bath
No. of Beds per Unit: 6
Accessible Facilities: Lounge, dining room.
LIME TREE COTTAGE
No. of Accessible Units: 1. Bath

No. of Beds per Unit: 3
Accessible Features: lounge, dining room.
In a quiet village with little traffic, both
cottages are full of character and many
original features. A pub with food that
welcomes wheelchair users is 50m away
on a hard surface.

ATTRACTIONS

BEARSTED VINEYARD
24 Caring Lane, Bearsted,
Maidstone ME14 4NJ
Tel/Fax: (01622) 736974
e-mail: enquiries@bearstedwines.co.uk
www.bearstedwines.co.uk
Produces award-winning English wines
from fresh grapes grown in the open.
White, red and rose wines are made in the
on-site winery.

SD ♿ CP ♿ Entrance ♿ C n/a Shop ♿
Wine is sold to callers from the house. Groups are given
tastings at the winery and can buy wine there.
WC ♿ Features ♿ . Winery is level except for one
small area.

LEEDS CASTLE
Maidstone ME17 1PL
Tel: (01622) 765400 Fax: (01622) 735616
e-mail: enquiries@leeds-castle.co.uk
www.leeds-castle.co.uk
Located on two small islands in the middle
of an encircling lake, this most English of
castles was the home of the manor of the
Saxon royal family in the C9th. The castle
has been a Norman stronghold, a royal
residence for six of England's medieval
queens and a palace for Henry VII. Now
restored, it offers collections of paintings,
furnishings and tapestries. In the 500-acre
park are woodlands, lakes, waterfalls, and
gardens. There is an accessible route that
includes a Stannah Stair Lift between the
Heraldry Room and a corridor to main
visitor route. The castle provides a comprehensive leaflet for visitors with disabilities.
The entrance is ramped at gradient of 1:8
with a threshold of 20cm. Well worth the
effort. Free wheelchair loan available.

SD ♿ CP ♿ E- (ramped at l:8)
RF ♿ L--Wheelchair lift. C ♿
S 🚶 WC 🚶

MUSEUM OF KENT LIFE – COBTREE
Lock Lane, Sandling, Maidstone ME14 3AU
Tel: (01622) 763936 Fax: (01622) 662024
e-mail: enquiries@museum-kentlife.co.uk
www.museum-kentlife.co.uk
Open-air working farm and social history

153

Leeds Castle is stunning for all visitors.

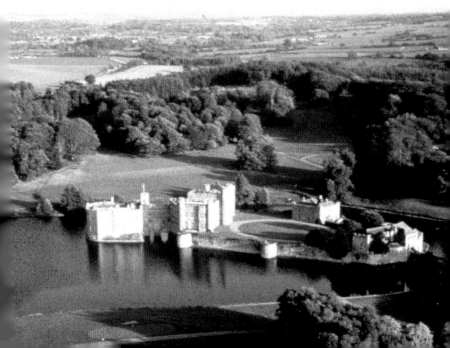

museum of 50 acres with many farm. There are historic buildings which house period displays. Interactive activites for children. Three large picnic areas and calandar of weekend events throughout the year. Other attractions include herb, hop and vegetable gardens.

SD ♿ CP ♿ E ♿ RF ♿
C ♿ S ♿ WC 🚹 RFE ♿

NEW ROMNEY

One of the original Cinque Ports although now a mile from the sea. The church, once lapped by the sea, has fine stained-glass windows and is in the Norman style.

TOURIST INFORMATION CENTRE
(Summer months only)
Magpies, Church Approach,
New Romney TN28 8QT
Tel: (01797) 364044   Fax: (01797) 364194

ATTRACTION
ROMNEY, HYTHE AND DYMCHURCH RAILWAY
New Romney TN28 8PL
Tel: (01797) 362353   Fax: (01797) 363591
e-mail: RHDR@dels.demon.co.uk
A mainline railway built for a millionaire racing driver in the 1920s with all locomotives and carriages one third full size. It runs from Hythe, via Dymchurch, St. Mary's Bay and New Romney to fishermen's cottages at Dungeness.
TRAIN – 1 disabled coach taking three wheelchairs and four helpers. Coach has on-board ramps, panoramic windows and large sliding doors.
  NB. ADVANCE NOTICE REQUIRED.

SD ♿ CP ♿ E ♿ C 🚹
S 🚹 WC ♿

RAMSGATE

Refined seaside resort and working port with Channel access to France/Belgium. Victorian redbrick houses on the cliff top have sweeping roads down to the seafront.

TOURIST INFORMATION CENTRE
Queen Street, Ramsgate CT11 8HA
Tel: (01853) 591086

ATTRACTION
SPITFIRE and HURRICANE MEMORIAL BUILDING
The Airfield, Manston Road,
Ramsgate CT12 5DF
Tel: (01849) 821940
Situated on the site of one the very few surviving airfields that participated in the Battle of Britain. This was the closest airfield to the enemy coast and bore the brunt of Luftwaffe attacks in 1940. Fine examples of these two WWII fighter aircraft, now written in the folklore of Britain, are permanently housed here.

SD ♿ CP ♿ E ♿ RF ♿
C ♿ S ♿ WC 🚹 RFE ♿

SANDWICH

Delightful old town with lovely walls. Pleasant paths along the river Stour and an old moat.

TOURIST INFORMATION SERVICE
Guildhall, Sandwich CT13 9AH
Tel/Fax: (01303) 613565

SELF-CATERING
THE OLD DAIRY ♿
Updown Park Farm, Eastry, Nr. Sandwich
Bookings through Mrs. J. R. Montgomery,
Little Brooksend Farm,
Birchington Kent CT7 0JW
No. of Accessible Units: 2
No. of Beds per Unit: 4-6: 7
Accessible Facilities: Kitchen/lounge.
2 holiday homes set in 30 acres of secluded parkland, approached via private roadway.

SEVENOAKS

Located 25 miles from London. Seven oaks were originally planted in 1902, but sadly all but one were lost in the 1987 hurricane. Access point for Knole.

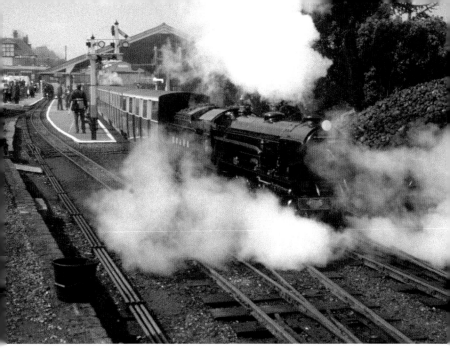

Letting of steam at the Romney Hythe and Dymchurch Railway.

ATTRACTIONS

EMMETTS GARDEN (NT)
Ide Hill, Sevenoaks TN14 6BA
Tel: (01732) 750367   Fax: (01732) 868193
Standing on one of highest spots in Kent
with fine views over the unspoilt Weald,
this charming garden was laid out in the
late C19th with exotic and rare trees and
shrubs. There are formal, rock, south and
north gardens, a bluebell bank and
woodlands that surrounds the garden.

SD [♿]   CP [♿]   E [♿]   RF [♿]
C [♿]   S [♿]   WC [♿]   G [♿]

SEVENOAKS WILDFOWL RESERVE
Bradbourne Vale Road, Sevenoaks TN13 3DH
Tel: (01732) 456407
First example in Britain of a gravel-pit being
developed for nature conservation. 135
acres of equal proportions of water and
land. Ponds and reedbeds combine with
woodland. There is access to visitor centre,
except one first-floor display, and three
bird-watching hides. 50% of the nature
trail is accessible by car.

SD [♿]   CP [♿]   E [♿]   RF [♿]
C [♿]   S [♿]   WC [♿]   RFE [♿]

SITTINGBOURNE
Situated in the Medway and Maritime
area, between Whitstable and
Chatham.

BED AND BREAKFAST

PALACE FARMHOUSE   [♿]
Chequers Hill, Doddington,
Sittingbourne ME9 0AU
Tel: (01795) 886820
No. of Accessible Rooms: 1.
Accessible Facilities: Lounge, dining room
Early Victorian farmhouse set in orchards
on the edge of the village of Doddington.

ATTRACTION

THE DOLPHIN SAILING BARGE MUSEUM
Crown Quay Lane, Sittingbourne
Tel: (01795) 423215
History of the Thames sailing barge with
large display of tools, models, plans and
photographs. Inlet alongside the museum
usually contains at least one vessel
brought to the yard for restoration,
including the Cambria, launched in 1906.

She was the last vessel in the UK to carry commercial cargo under sail. Shipwright's shop, forge and barge are on the level: The sail loft is up a flight of stairs.

SD [♿] CP [♿] E [♿] RF [♿]
S [♿] WC [🚶] RFE [♿]

STAPLEHURST
ATTRACTION
BRATTLE FARM MUSEUM
Brattle Farm,
Staplehurst TN12 0HE
Tel: (015980) 891222
Privately owned, unique country collection dealing with agricultural bygones, showing country life, skills and tools from rural trades and crafts of the past two centuries. Housed in old cowsheds and oast house of the farm. NB. By appointment only. The first floor is not accessible.

SD [♿] CP   E [♿] RF [♿]
S   WC [🚶] RF

TENTERDEN
A charming town, its high street lined with shops and houses still retaining their original facades from Elizabethan to Georgian times. Many antique shops.

HOTEL
LITTLE SILVER COUNTRY HOTEL [🚶]
Ashford Road, St. Michaels,
Tenterden TN30 6SP
Tel: (01233) 850321 Fax: (01233) 850647
e-mail: enquiries@little-silver.co.uk
www.little-silver.co.uk
No. of Accessible Rooms: 3. Bath
Accessible Facilities: Lounge, restaurant. Charming country house hotel with a personal touch. Victorian style conservatory and delightful gardens.

TUNBRIDGE WELLS
Forest until discovered in 1606, this is a tranquil country town with much charm and taste in its architecture, parks and gardens.

TOURIST INFORMATION CENTRE
The Old Fish Market, The Pantiles,
Tunbridge Wells TN2 5TN
Tel: (01892) 515675
Fax: (01892) 534660
Produces Access in Tunbridge Wells.

BUSES
Arriva Kent and Sussex: Tel: (01634) 281100
Some low-floor routes.

TAXIS
Goodfellows Taxis (Paddock Wood):
Tel: (01892) 837799
Five adapted vehicles.
Kent and Sussex Cars: Tel: (01892) 513377
Three adapted vehicles.

TRAINS
Connex South Eastern: Customer Services:
Tel: (0870) 6030405   Fax: (0870) 6030505
Minicom: (01233) 617621

CAR PARKS
Free disabled badge parking in all borough council car parks.

SHOPMOBILITY
Lower Mall, Royal Victoria Place.
Tel: (01892) 544355

HOTELS
THE SPA HOTEL [🚶]
Mount Ephraim,
Royal Tunbridge Wells   TN4 8XJ
Tel: (01892) 520331
Fax: (01892) 510575
e-mail: info@spahotel.co.uk
www.spahotel.co.uk/
No. of Accessible Rooms: 1. Bath
Accessible Facilities: Lounge, restaurant, pool, sauna, gardens. Built in 1766 this is a family owned hotel set in 15 acres of fine gardens overlooking the town.

RAMADA JARVIS TUNBRIDGE WELLS [♿]
8 Tonbridge Road, Pembury,
Tunbridge Wells TN2 4QL
Tel: (01892) 823567   Fax: (01892) 823931
No. of Accessible Rooms: 2. Bath
Accessible Facilities: Lounge, restaurant, steam and beauty rooms.
Quality modern hotel on the east of town.

ATTRACTIONS
TUNBRIDGE WELLS MUSEUM AND GALLERY
Civic Centre, Mount Pleasant,
Royal Tunbridge Wells TN1 1JN
Tel: (01892) 526121   Fax: (01892) 534227
Museum displays local and natural history,
archaeology and agricultural artefacts: the
art gallery has changing exhibitions.
SD ♿ CP ♿ E ♿ L ♿ Thyssen Stairlift
S ♿

SISSINGHURST CASTLE GARDEN
Sissinghurst, Cranbrook TN17 2AB
Tel: (01580) 715330   Fax: (01580) 713911
Transformed by Vita Sackville-West and
Harold Nicholson in the 1920s into one of
the finest gardens in the country. Each
area is planted with colour or seasonal
theme, notably White and Cottage
Gardens. Located 12 miles east of town.
SD ♿   CP ♿   E ♿   RF ♿   C ♿
S ♿   WC ♿   G ♿

BEWL WATER
Lamberhurst, Tunbridge Wells TN3 8JH
Tel: (01892) 890661   Fax: (01892) 890232
Largest area of inland water in the south
east, with 21kms of shore line to explore.
SD ♿   CP ♿   E ♿   C ♿
S ♿   WC ♿   RFE ♿

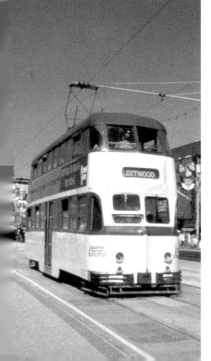

LANCASHIRE

WEST LANCS DISABILITY HELPLINE
Skelmersdale Library, Skelmersdale
Tel: (01695) 51819

**GENERAL INFORMATION ON ALL
TRANSPORT**
Tel: (0870) 6082608
Minicom: (01257) 241693

WARRINGTON DISABLED LIVING CENTRE
Beaufort Street, Warrington
Tel: (01925) 240064

SPECIALIST OUTDOOR ACTIVITIES
NEW HORIZONS
Bookings: 2 Fishers Bridge, Hayfield, High
Peak SK22 2JZ
Tel: (01663) 742796)
Information: 6 Sunfield, Romiley,
Stockport SK6 6BH
Tel: (0161) 440 8082
www. newhorizons.org.uk
Canal boat trips and cruises designed for
disabled people navigated by skipper and
volunteer crew. The narrow boat is fully
accessible with boarding ramp and lift, fully
accessible WC, raised open viewing deck at
front. The Cheshire Canal Ring serves
Manchester as a vast water pleasure
ground, and New Horizons is based in
Marple, 11 miles SE of Manchester's city
centre.

ACCRINGTON
Originally an East Lancashire Mill town,
now without the chimneys or the
smoke.

LANCASHIRE'S HILL COUNTRY TOURISM
Freepost NWW8077, Accrington BB5 0ZZ
Tel: (01254) 380678   Fax: (01254) 380600
e-mail: lhc@hyndburnbc.gov.uk

Blackpool tram and the famous tower.

TOURIST INFORMATION CENTRE
Town Hall, Blackburn Road,
Accrington BB5 1LA
Tel: (01254) 386807   Fax: (01254) 380291

ATTRACTION
OSWALDTWISTLE MILLS
Moscow Hill, Collier Street, Oswaldtwistle,
Accrington BB5 3HL
Tel: (01254) 871025   Fax: (01254) 770790
A family attraction, set within one of the
very few remaining Victorian mills still
producing cotton fabric and owned by the
same family since 1847. Start in the
handloom weaver's cottage of 1700 and
learn about the Industrial Revolution. Also
includes reconstructed Victorian factory
yard, craft workshops, traditional sweet
factory, gardens and wildfowl preserve. An
excellent day out.

SD 🧑‍🦽   CP 🧑‍🦽   E 🧍   C 🧍
S 🧍   WC 🧍   RF 🧍

Nab Lane, Blackburn BB2 1LN
Tel: (01254) 511111   Fax: (01254) 268801
Tropical water park with shipwreck slide,
hot tub, alien encounter, white knuckle
ride, and disabled sessions.

SD 🧑‍🦽   CP 🧑‍🦽   E 🧑‍🦽   RF 🧑‍🦽   L 🧑‍🦽
C 🧑‍🦽   WC 🧍

SPORTING VENUE
BLACKBURN ROVERS FOOTBALL AND
ATHLETIC PLC
Ewood Park, Blackburn BB2 4JF
Tel: (01254) 698888   Fax: (01254) 671042
Ticket Office: (01254) 671666
Minicom: (01254) 668008
Facility complies with Part M, Building
Regulations.

CP 🧑‍🦽   RE 🧑‍🦽   ED 🧑‍🦽   INT 🧍
L 🧑‍🦽   WC 🧑‍🦽   (20 units located in all stands)
SS 🧑‍🦽   From designated entrance gate on level,
unobstructed route to designated spaces at ground floor
level.   B/R – Lift Access.

BLACKBURN
Deeply involved in the Industrial
Revolution, this old mill town has, in
recent years, seen much development
and re-planning.

TOURIST INFORMATION CENTRE
King George Hall, Northgate,
Blackburn BB2 1AA
Tel: (01254) 53277   Fax: (01254) 683536

BED AND BREAKFAST
MYTTON FOLD HOTEL AND GOLF
 COMPLEX
Whalley Road, Langho, Blackburn BB6 8AB
Tel: (01254) 240662   Fax: (01254) 248119
e-mail: reception@myttonfold.co.uk
www.myttonfold.co.uk
No. of Accessible Rooms: 3
Accessible Facilities: Lounge, restaurant,
gardens. Independent hotel run by third-
generation family at the gateway to Ribble
Valley. Lovely gardens from where to enjoy
views of Pendle Hill, guardian of C17th
secrets of the famous Pendle witches.

ATTRACTION
WAVES WATER FUN CENTRE

BLACKPOOL
An extremely popular holiday resort
stretching along the Lancashire coast,
with every conceivable form of
entertainment. Its landmark tower
offers an outstanding view. Trams run
along the promenade and its famous
Christmas illuminations are spectacular,
as is its Pleasure Beach.

TOURIST INFORMATION CENTRES
1 Clifton Street, Blackpool FY1 1LY
Tel: (01253) 478222/477477
Fax: (01253) 478210
e-mail: blackpool.tourism@dial.pipex.com
Publishes Special Needs Guide to
Blackpool.
Blackpool Pleasure Beach, Unit 11,
Ocean Boulevard, Blackpool FY4 1PL
Tel: (01253) 403223
Fax: (01253) 408718

BLACKPOOL TRANSPORT
Tel: (01253) 473001
General information for Blackpool.

BUSES
Easy Access Handy Bus: Tel: (01253) 473000

TAXIS
Blacktax: Tel: (0585) 175321 (mobile),
(07930) 578401 (mobile)
'C' Cabs: Tel: (01253) 62201
10 adapted vehicles.
Radio Cabs: Tel: (01253) 293222
Four adapted vehicles.

TRAINS
First North Western: Special Needs:
Tel: (0845) 6040231
Arriva Trains: Special Needs:
Tel: (0845) 6008008
Virgin Trains: Special Needs:
Tel: (0845) 7443366
Minicom: (0845) 7443367

CAR PARKS
Municipal surface car parks – three hours
free disabled badge parking, thereafter
normal rates apply.
Tel: (01253) 291091

SHOPMOBILITY
52 Clifton Street, Blackpool FY1 1JP
Tel: (01253) 476451

HOTELS
BOND HOTEL   ♿
120 Bond Street, South Shore,
Blackpool FY4 1HG
Tel: (01253) 341218   Fax: (01253) 394952
No. of Accessible Rooms: 19. Roll-in
Shower
Accessible Facilities: Lounge, dining room,
bar, sun roof. Award winning hotel for
able-bodied and disabled guests. Located
close to the promenade, Pleasure Beach
and Sandcastle Leisure Complex. The Lido
Swimming Pool that is equipped for
disabled visitors is also close by.

SHELLARD HOTEL   ♿
18-20 Dean Street, South Shore,
Blackpool FY4 1AU
Tel/Fax: (01253) 342679
No. of Accessible Rooms: 10. Roll-in
Shower
Accessible Facilities: Lounge, restaurant,
bar. Both disabled and able-bodied guests
are welcome here in a hotel very close to
the Pleasure Beach, Sandcastle Leisure
Centre and Granada Studios.

ATTRACTIONS
BLACKPOOL PLEASURE BEACH ARENA
Ocean Boulevard, Blackpool FY4 1EZ
Tel: (01253) 341033   Fax: (01253) 405467
Over 145 rides and attractions, plus
spectacular shows. The Accessibility Guide
Book is comprehensive and worth
obtaining from the number above. For full
details of catering and shopping facilities,
plus rides, check the guide.

SD ♿   CP ♿   E ♿   WC ♿

BLACKPOOL ZOO
East Park Drive, Blackpool FY3 8PP
Tel: (01253) 765027   Fax: (01253) 798884
Wheelchair access throughout on tarmac
paths with no major slopes or gradients .
32-acre park, its population divided into
weather-orientated regions from tropical
forest and hot grasslands and desert
through to winter regions, water world,
farming and domestic exhibits.

SD ♿   CP ♿   E ♿   RF ♿   C ♿
S ♿   WC ♿   RFE ♿

BURNLEY
TOURIST INFORMATION CENTRE
Burnley Mechanics, Manchester Road,
Burnley BB11 1JA
Tel: (01282) 455485
Fax: (01282) 457428

ATTRACTION
TOWNELEY HALL ART GALLERY AND MUSEUMS
Burnley BB11 3RQ
Tel: (01282) 424213
Fax: (01282) 436138
Home of the Townley family from C14th
until 1902, offering a glimpse of how the
family lived. Original period rooms include
the Elizabethan long gallery and Regency
rooms, Victorian kitchen together with
fine glass, ceramic and oak furniture
collections. The Museum of Local Crafts
and Industries tells the story of the
inhabitants at home and at work.
Together with the Natural History Centre,
this is a wonderful day out.
NB. Accessible entrance at rear by request.

SD ♿   CP ♿   E ♿   RF ♿   L ♿

C ♿   S ♿   WC ♿   RFE ♿

CARNFORTH

LEIGHTON MOSS RSPB NATURE RESERVE

Myers Farm, silverdale, Carnforth LA5 0SW
Tel: (01524) 7011601
Fax: (01524) 701413
e-mail: leighton-moss@rspb.org.uk
www.rspb.org.uk

Largest remaining reedbeds in NW England attracting a wide range of wildlife including marsh harriers, roe and red deer. 5 miles of trails, bird feeding station to Lillian's hide, to Jackson's hide to Griesdale hide all accessible with sloped gradient of no more then 1:15. Public hide accessed via shallow 1:40 ramp with specially adapted wheelchair places at left of hide.

N.B. Restaurant is accessed via lift

CLITHEROE

A very old Ribble Valley town with pleasant country atmosphere and lovely walks. The C12th. castle, set on limestone crag, is a dominant landmark and much of its grounds are part of a recreational area.

TOURIST INFORMATION CENTRE

12-14 Market Place, Clitheroe BB7 2DA
Tel: (01200) 425566   Fax: (01200) 426339

SELF-CATERING

HIGHER GILLS FARM
Rimington, Clitheroe BB7 4DA
Tel: (01200) 445370
e-mail: pilko@highergills.co.uk
www.highergills.co.uk
No. of Accessible Units: 1. Bath/shower.
No. of Beds per Unit: 3 – 4
Accessible Facilities: Lounge, dining room, kitchen, patio and lawn. Working farm with sheep and cows with two apartments.
Situated at the foot of Pendle Hills, offering fine views of western Yorkshire Dales and Trough of Bowland.

LANCASTER

Surrounded by superb moorland where Lancashire and Yorkshire meet, the history of the town dates back 7.5 centuries, some buildings still survive from this period.

TOURIST INFORMATION CENTRE

29 Castle Hill, Lancaster LA1 1YN
Tel: (01524) 32878
Fax: (01524) 847472
www.lancaster.gov.uk

LANCASTER CITY COUNCIL

Tel: (01524) 582000
Minicom: (01524) 582175/582875
Produces Lancaster, Morecambe and District Access Guide.

DISC (Disablement Information Support Centre)
Trinity Community Centre,
Middle Street, Lancaster LA1 1JZ
Tel: (01524) 34411/32660
e-mail: disc@lancasterdisc.free-on-line.co.uk
People with disabilities providing information and support for others.

BUSES

Lune Valley Transport: Tel: (01524) 844944
Operate a semi-scheduled service, but need 48hrs' notice.
Stagecoach: Tel: (01772) 886633

TAXIS

Beatstream: Tel: (01524) 32090
Five adapted vehicles.
D & C Taxis: Tel: (01524) 69824
One adapted vehicle.
Westgate Taxis: Tel: (01524) 412781

TRAINS

First North Western: Special Needs:
Tel: (0845) 6040231
Virgin Trains: Special Needs:
Tel: (0845) 7443366
Minicom: (0845) 7443367

HOTELS

LANCASTER HOUSE HOTEL

Green Lane, Ellel, Lancaster LA1 4GJ
Tel: (01524) 844822
Fax: (01524) 844766
e-mail: lanchouse@elh.co.uk
No. of Accessible Rooms: 4
Accessible Facilities: Lounge, restaurant, limited access because on split levels with pillars. Pre-book for accessible area, bar. Prestigious property located close to the city, and three minutes from the M6.

THURNHAM MILL HOTEL
Thurnham, Lancaster LA2 0BD
Tel: (01524) 752852
Fax: (01524) 752477
No. of Accessible Rooms: 4. Bath
Accessible Facilities: Lounge, restaurant
Historic C16th converted mill beside a canal, close to the remote Forest of Bowland with high moorland and fine views over the Flyde Coast and Lune Valley. For nearly 100 years the mill was driven by canal water, whereas most mills are driven by rivers.

ATTRACTIONS
LANCASTER MARITIME MUSEUM
Custom House, St. George's Quay, Lancaster LA1 1RB
Tel: (01524) 64637
Fax: (01524) 841692
Discover Lancaster's seafaring history spanning 2,000 years from Roman harbour to major C18th port for the West Indies. This waterfront museum occupies the historic Custom House of 1764 with modern displays, reconstructions, sound effects and even authentic smells!

 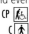

PETER SCOTT GALLERY
Lancaster University, Lancaster LA1 4YH
Tel: (01524) 593057   Fax: (01524) 592603
e-mail: m.p.gavagan@lancaster.ac.uk
Although not as accessible as we would wish, this gallery houses the University's fine art collection including contemporary British artists from the St. Ives School such as Barbara Hepworth, and examples of Inuit, African ands far eastern art and ceramics.

   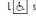 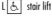 stair lift

WILLIAMSON PARK AND BUTTERFLY HOUSE
Aston Memorial Williamson Park, Lancaster LA1 1NX
Tel: (01524) 33318
Fax: (01524) 848338
e-mail: office@williamsonpark.com
See the colourful world of the butterfly.

LYTHAM ST. ANNES
Some half-timbered buildings mingle pleasantly with peaceful parks and gardens. Known for its championship golf course.

TOURIST INFORMATION CENTRE
290 Clifton Drive South, Lytham FY8 1LH
Tel: (01253) 725610   Fax: (01253) 713754

HOTEL
CHADWICK HOTEL
South Promenade,
Lytham St. Annes FY8 1NP
Tel: (01253) 720061
Fax: (01253) 714455
No. of Accessible Rooms: 12 (1 is Cat.1)
Accessible Facilities: Lounge, restaurant. Family owned and managed since 1947. Sea front position overlooking the Ribble Estuary and the Irish Sea.

MORECAMBE
Originally an ancient fishing village and now a popular holiday resort.

TOURIST INFORMATION CENTRE
Old Station Buildings, Marine Road Central, Morecambe LA4 4DBA
Tel: (01524) 582808   Fax: (01524) 582663

SELF-CATERING
MORECAMBE BAY BUNGALOW
6 Marine Drive, Hest Bank, Morecambe LA4
Tel: 0800 0180586
No. of Accessible Units: 1
No. of Beds per Unit: 2
Accessible Facilities: Lounge, kitchen.

ORMSKIRK

Located a few miles inland of the north-east coast, south of Southport, long associated with the Stanley family, Earls of Derby from Knowsley Hall.

HOTEL
BEAUFORT HOTEL 🚶
High Lane, Burscough, Ormskirk L40 7SN
Tel: (01704) 892665
Fax: (01704) 895135
e-mail: info@beaufort.co.uk.com
www.Beaufort.uk.co
No. of Accessible Rooms: 1
Accessible Facilities: Lounge, restaurant, bar. Smart, modern, commercial hotel ideally situated to explore Ormskirk's fascinating traditional market or take a trip to Liverpool's historic Albert Dock.

ATTRACTION
THE WILDFOWL and WETLANDS TRUST – MARTIN MERE
Burscough, Nr. Ormskirk L40 0TA
Tel: (01704) 895181
Fax: (01704) 892343
e-mail: carl.lamb@wwt.org.uk
376 acres of wetlands with swan, flamingo, African, Siberian and Australasian goose and oriental and North and South American species. Special leaflet, Access the Wild Side, is very helpful.

SD ♿ CP ♿ E ♿ RF ♿ C ♿
S ♿ WC ♿ RFE ♿ 6 wheelchairs available.

PRESTON

Site of the Battle of Preston in 1648 and centre of the Industrial Revolution in the C18th, today the city is the legal, commercial and administrative capital of the county. Surrounded by breathtaking countryside.

TOURIST INFORMATION CENTRE
Guildhall Arcade,
Lancaster Road,
Preston PR1 1HT
Tel: (01772) 253731

HOTEL
THE GIBBON BRIDGE HOTEL 🚶
Chipping, Preston PR3 2TQ
Tel: (01995) 61456
Fax: (01995) 61277
No. of Accessible Rooms: 2, Roll-in shower
Accessible Facilities: Lounge, dining room. Country hotel set in the Forest of Bowland.

ATTRACTIONS
ASTLEY HALL MUSEUM and ART GALLERY
Astley Park, off Hallgate,
Chorley, Nr. Preston PR7 1NP
Tel: (01257) 515555
Fax: (01257) 515556
400-year-old Grade 1 listed building with much original furniture and decoration. Ground floor accessible but Art Gallery on first floor, with changing exhibitions is NOT ACCESSIBLE. Video guide to upper floors and exhibitions is available.

SD ♿ CP 🚶 E ♿
RF 🚶 S ♿ WC 🚶

CAMELOT THEME PARK and
RARE BREEDS FARM
Charnock Richard, Chorley,
Preston PR7 5LP
Tel: (01257) 453044   Fax: (01527) 452320
Over 100 rides, shows and attractions on Arthurian theme, including Merlin's Magic Show and live jousting tournament plus petting area in Rare Breeds Farm.

SD ♿ CP ♿ E ♿ RF ♿
C ♿ S ♿ WC 🚶 RFE ♿

LONGTON BRICKCROFT NATURE RESERVE
off Liverpool Road, Longton,
Preston PR4 5YY
Tel: (01772 611497)
Covering over 11 hectares this is a wetland reserve in two distinct areas – the southern area set aside for recreation such as fishing and picnics. The northern area is established as a nature reserve with wildlife conservation the main priority. Good range of semi-natural habitats supporting an extensive number of birds, mammals, insects, wild flowers and pond life. The visitor centre contains informative environmental displays. NB: No shop/ catering facility on site.

CP 🚶   E 🚶   WC 🚶   RFE ♿

LEICESTERSHIRE AND RUTLAND

MOSAIC
The Guild Hall, Colton Street,
Leicester LE1 1QB
Tel: (0116) 2515565   Fax: (0116) 2519969
Minicom: (0116) 2511009

BRITISH RED CROSS
Leicestershire and Rutland Branch
244 London Road, Leicester LE2 1RN
Tel: (0116) 2705087

HINCKLEY

HOTEL
HANOVER INTERNATIONAL HOTEL
A5 Watling Street, Hinckley LE10 3JA
Tel: (01455) 631122   Fax: (01455) 630030
www.hanover-international.com
No. of Accessible Rooms: 8
Accessible Facilities: Lounge, restaurant,
bar. Extremely modern large hotel with
lovely lake running alongside, seconds
from the M69 (J1).

BED AND BREAKFAST
WOODSIDE FARM GUESTHOUSE
Ashby Road, Stapleton, Nr. Hinckley LE9 8JF
Tel: (01455) 291929   Fax: (01455) 292626
No. of Accessible Rooms: 1. Bath
Accessible Facilities: Lounge, dining
room. Country guest house five miles
from Hinkley.

LEICESTER
Largely modern city dating back over
2,000 years with Celtish and Roman
history. The castle, built in 1088, has
a beautiful church, St. Mary de
Castro, with a superb 700-year-
old font.

TOURIST INFORMATION CENTRE
Dicsover Leicester
7-9 Every Street, Town Hall Square,
Leicester LE1 6AG

Tel: (0906) 2941113*
*All calls will be charged at 25p per minute
premium rate and will be answered
between the hours, Mon - Fri 8am -
10.30pm and Sat and Sun 8am - 8pm.
e-mail:info@discoverleicester.com
www.discoverleicester.com

BUSES
Access Bus: Tel: (0116) 2657311/2657248
Single decker following timetabled route,
but will stop on request.

TAXIS
Colemans of Leicester:
Tel: (0116) 2856126/2912317
Variety of adapted vehicles.
Kings Taxis: Tel: (0116) 2425260
Three adapted vehicles - please book in
advance.
Gold Line Cabs: Tel: (0116) 2731110

TRAINS
Central Trains: Assistance:
Tel: (0845) 7056027
www.centraltrains.co.uk
Midland Mainline: Special Needs:
Tel: (0114) 2537654
Minicom: (0845) 7078051

SHOPMOBILITY
Haymarket Shop,
Charles Bus Station:
Tel: (0116) 2532596

HOTELS
THE RED COW
Hinckley Road, Leicester Forest East LE3 3PG
Tel: (0116) 2387878   Fax: (0116) 2386539
No. of Accessible Rooms: 1
Accessible Facilities: restaurant
An historic inn with a thatched roof and ivy
covered frontage, recently refurbished. 31
rooms and an attractive garden. Located
close to the M1/M69 junction at Leicester.

FIELD HEAD HOTEL
Markfield Lane, Markfield,
Leicester LE67 9PS
Tel: (01530) 245454   Fax: (01530) 243740
No. of Accessible Rooms: 1. Bath
Accessible Facilities: Lounge, restaurant.
Built from local stone and in the style of its

163

original farmhouse building of 1672. Situated on the edge of Charnwood Forest, eight miles from Leicester.

ATTRACTIONS
LEICESTERSHIRE
NATIONAL SPACE SCIENCE CENTRE
Exploration Drive, Leicester LE4 5NS
Tel: (0870) 60 77223   Fax: (0116) 258 2100
e-mail: info@spacecentre.co.uk
www.nssc.co.uk

Unique and exciting education and leisure facility based on space science. The National Space Centre is the UK's largest attraction dedicated to space science and astronomy. Five differently themed galleries, with amazing space rockets, satellites and capsules, take part in hundreds of inter-active activities and experience the latest in audio-visual equipment. The Centre is located just off the A6, two miles north of Leicester city Centre midway between Leicester's inner and outerring roads. Brown signs will direct from the arterial routes around Leicester.

SD 🦽   CP 🦽   E 🦽   RF 🦽   L 🦽
C 🦽   S 🦽   WC 🦽   RFE 🦽 (Tower)

LOUGHBOROUGH
Second largest town in the county with a Thursday market that began in 1206. Known for its university, and so is lively, with plenty of shops and entertainment.

HOTEL
QUALITY HOTEL 🚶
New Ashby Road, Loughborough LE11 4EX
Tel: (01509) 211800   Fax: (01509) 211868
e-mail: admin@gb613.u-net.com
www.choicehotelseurope.com

No. of Accessible Rooms: 2. Bath and shower.
Accessible Facilities: Lounge, restaurant and bar.
Located five minutes from the M1 (J23), between Leicester and Nottingham, a good base for touring the Peak District. In the other direction are Burghley House

and the lovely Georgian town of Stamford.

MARKET BOSWORTH
Village with lovely thatched cottages, a red brick and white stone hall of the English renaissance period and a Tudor grammar school where Samuel Johnson taught as second master.

BED AND BREAKFAST
BOSWORTH FIRS 🚶
Bosworth Road,
Market Bosworth CV13 0DW
Tel: (01455) 290727

No. of Accessible Rooms: 1
Accessible Facilities: Lounge, dining room.
Small, chalet-style dorma bungalow in pleasant, rural location surrounded front and back by fields, a mile from town.

ATTRACTION
BOSWORTH BATTLEFIELD VISITOR CENTRE
Sutton Cheney CV13 0AD
Tel: (01455) 290429   Fax: (01455) 292841

Historic site of the Battle of Bosworth Field where in 1485 King Richard III lost his crown and his life to the future Henry VII. Discover the sights, sound and smells of long ago in the Exhibition and Film Theatre plus 1.75 mile Battle Trail with illustrated boards detailing each stage of the battle. A useful map of the Battle Trail is available. It is a circular route, one small section has a gradient of 1:8. This is avoidable if you take the same route to and from King Richard's Field via Ambion Wood and Henry's Lines. Battle re-enactments held annually, ring for dates.

SD 🦽   CP 🦽   E 🦽   RF 🚶   C 🚶
S 🚶   WC 🚶   RFE 🚶 Battle Trail, garden

MARKET HARBOROUGH
On Northamptonshire border, created by Henry II especially to be a market. Historically important as HQ of Royalist army on the eve of the defeat at the Battle of Naseby in 1645.

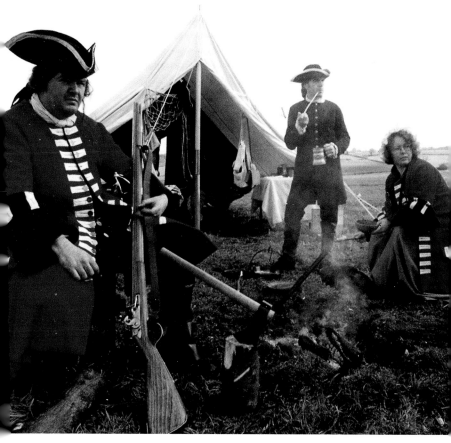

Re-enactment groups at The Bosworth Battlefield Visitor Centre.

TOURIST INFORMATION CENTRE
Adam & Eve Street,
Market Harborough LE16 7AG
Tel: (01858) 821270   Fax: (01858) 821144

HOTEL
HOTHORPE HALL   ♿
Theddingworth LE17 6QX
Tel: (01858) 880257   Fax: (01858) 880979
No. of Accessible Rooms: 9. Roll-in shower.
Accessible Facilities: Lounge, restaurant,
lift. Primarily a Christian conference centre
that also takes families and groups for
holidays. Large country house in 12 acres
of ground located between the M1 (J20)
and Market Harborough.

OADBY
Peaceful village and suburb of
Leicester, three miles from the city
centre.

REGAL HERMITAGE HOTEL   🚶
Wigston Road, Oadby LE2 5QE
Tel: (0116) 2569955   Fax: (0116) 2720559
www.corushotels.com
No. of Accessible Rooms: 1. Bath
Accessible Facilities: Lounge, bar.
Originally a private house, now an
attractive red-brick modern hotel.

ATTRACTIONS
FARMWORLD
Stoughton Farm Park, Gartree Road,
Oadby LE2 2FB
Tel: (0116) 2710355
Fax: (0116) 2713211
www.farmworld.co.uk
A farm park with rare breeds, shire horses, modern milking parlour, chicken hatchery. Lots of opportunities to touch and feel the animals. Adventure playground, woodland walks.

SD   CP   E   RF   C
S   WC   RFE

UNIVERSITY OF LEICESTER BOTANIC GARDENS
Beaumont Hall, Stoughton Drive South,
Oadby LE2 2NA
Tel: (0116) 2717725
The grounds of four houses, not open to the public, make up the grounds of this 16-acre garden. A wide variety of plants in many different settings. The garden is on a south-facing slope with gravel paths throughout. The herb, limestone and sunken gardens and east lawn of the hall are inaccessible.

SD   CP

OAKHAM
Home of the infamous Titus Oates, this is a pleasant town with an old Butter Cross in the market place.

ATTRACTION
OAKHAM CASTLE
Market Place, Oakham
All enquiries to Rutland Co. Museum,
Catmos Street,
Oakham LE15 6HW
Tel: (01572) 758 440
e-mail: museum@rutland.gov.uk
C12th fortified manor house with superb Norman Great hall which has a range of C12 figure sculptures.

SD  CP E

LINCOLNSHIRE

NORTH LINCOLNSHIRE TOURISM TEAM
Church Square House, PO Box 42,
Scunthorpe, DN15 6XQ
Tel: (01724) 297350   Fax: (01724) 297426
www.northlinks.gov.uk/tourism
www.barton-net.org

SOUTH WEST LINCOLNSHIRE
Guildhall Arts Centre, St. Peter's Hill,
Grantham NG31 6PZ
Tel: (01476) 590191   Fax: (01476) 591810
www.guildhallartscentre.com
210 seat theatre, ballroom which can hold up to 200 people, gallery/exhibition space, several small studios, coffee house, Tourist information centre and cyber cafe.
Access to the Guildhall Arts Centre is flat and via double dooors. There is a slight ramped area within the building which allows for access to the venue's lift. Spaces for wheelchair users at all performances. Spaces available on auditorium balconies but on limited number of performances spaces only available at front of auditorium.

LINCS. ASSOCIATION OF PEOPLE WITH DISABILITIES
Beech House, Witham Park,
Waterside South, Lincoln LN5 7JH
Tel: (01522) 806622   Fax: (01522) 806626
e-mail: stella.tuplin@lapd.org.uk

LINCOLNSHIRE COUNTY COUNCIL
City Hall, Lincoln LN1 1DN
Tel: (01522) 552222
Fax: (01522) 516050
Minicom: (01522) 552055

BARTON
www.barton-net.org
Unspoilt market town on the edge of the Lincolnshire wolds. This is North Lincolnshire at its best, where rolling chalk wolds meet the wide Humber estuary and a rich maritime history blends with colourful street festivals. Web site offers complete overview.

BRIGG

Small brick town on the river Ancholme. The mill at nearby Wrawbry is the last working post mill in the north of England.

ATTRACTION
ELSHAM HALL COUNTRY AND WILDLIFE PARK
Elsham, Nr. Brigg DN20 0QZ
Tel: (01652) 688698
Fax: (01652) 688240
Miniature zoo and children's farmyard; garden and design centre; craft and exhibition centres; carp feeding jetty; wild butterfly garden walkway; arboretum and woodland garden, children's animal farm, falconry and conservation centre.

SD [♿] CP [♿] E [♿] S [♿]
WC [♿] RFE [♿]

CLEETHORPES

Family resort, famous for miles of golden sands, lovely parks and peaceful gardens. Has one of England's few remaining piers, now totally refurbished.

ATTRACTION
HUMBER ESTUARY DISCOVERY CENTRE
Lakeside, Kings Road,
Cleethorpes DN35 0AG
Tel: (01472) 323232
Fax: (01472) 323233
Combination of aquarium displays with a state-of-the-art exhibition.

SD [♿] CP [♿] E [♿] RF [♿] L [♿]
C [♿] S [♿] WC [♿] RFE [♿]

GAINSBOROUGH

Britain's most inland port with an attractive shopping centre and a fine Georgian parish church.

SELF-CATERING
BLACK SWAN GUEST HOUSE [♿]
21 High Street, Marton,
Gainsborough DN21 5AH
Tel/Fax: (01427) 718878
e-mail: info@blackswan-marton.co.uk
No. of Accessible Units: 1. Roll-in Shower
No. of Beds per Unit: 2
Accessible Facilities: Open plan sleeping/living/dining/kitchenette, plus lounge in guest house. Originally part of an C18th coaching inn, believed to have provided accommodation to Oliver Cromwell during the Battle of Gainsborough in 1643. This complex of farm buildings offers one accessible unit from several around an attractive courtyard.

ATTRACTION
GAINSBOROUGH OLD HALL (EH)
Parnell Street, Gainsborough DN21 2NB
Tel: (01427) 612669   Fax: (01427) 612779
e-mail: cumminsh@lincolnshire.gov.uk
One of best preserved medieval manor houses in Britain, built by Sir Thomas Burgh c1460. Little has changed architecturally in this timber-framed building with its characteristic striped appearance. At its centre is the Great Hall where Richard III

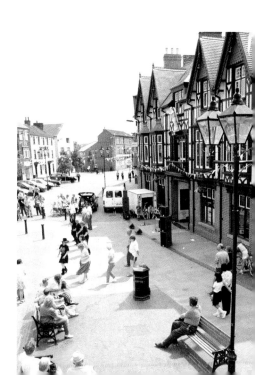

Brigg Market Place.

and Henry VIII once banqueted. The original medieval kitchens remain unchanged and the room settings provide historic impressions. NB. The ground floor only is accessible. Experience the upper floor through an interactive AV presentation in the shop.
Access to Radar key.

SD ⬤ CP n/a (nearest 200m with designated parking).
E ⬤ RF ⬤ C ⬤ S ⬤ WC n/a

GRANTHAM

Interesting red brick and stone town with a high steepled parish church. Once an important staging post on the Great North Road, now famous because Lady Thatcher was born here, and because Sir Isaac Newton was born at nearby Woolsthorpe Manor.

HOTELS
KINGS HOTEL
130 North Parade, Grantham NG31 8AU
Tel/Fax: (01476) 590800
No. of Accessible Rooms: 3. Bath
Accessible Facilities: Lounge, restaurant. Originally a Victorian gentleman's residence now well refurbished, this small, privately owned hotel is on the main northern route out of Grantham to the A1.

GRANTHAM MARRIOTT
Swingbridge Road, Grantham NG31 7XT
Tel: (01476) 593000   Fax: (01476) 592592
No. of Accessible Rooms: 2. Bath
Accessible Facilities: Lounge, restaurant, pool (three steps). Opened in 1992, this quality courtyard-style hotel is just off the A1 near Grantham. Actively promotes its disabled facilities.

GRIMSBY

Surrounded by beautiful countryside with easy access to miles of sandy beaches, Grimsby is famous for its fishing industry.

ATTRACTION
NATIONAL FISHING HERITAGE CENTRE

Alexandra Dock, Grimsby DN31 1UZ
Tel: (01472) 323345   Fax: (01472) 323355
Fascinating history of the British fishing industry through Grimsby's vision. Experience life at sea on a trawler, hearing, smelling and touching recreated environments.

SD ⬤ CP ⬤ E ⬤ RF ⬤ L ⬤
C ⬤ S ⬤ WC ⬤ RFE ⬤

LINCOLN

Few cathedrals are as awe inspiring as Lincoln's, dominating the skyline here at the top, or upper part of the city. And following the heritage trail around uphill Lincoln is a good way of discovering the city's history. The trail does need a good pusher, but the streets between the accessible attractions below are a delight. Downhill offers a medieval high bridge with half-timbered buildings and a river cruise.

TOURIST INFORMATION CENTRES
9 Castle Hill, Lincoln LN1 3AA
Tel: (01522) 873700/873703

The Cornhill, Lincoln LN5 7HB
Tel: (01522) 873703

DIAL-A-RIDE AND SHOPMOBILITY
TEL: (01522) 514477

TRAVELINE
(0870) 6082608

TAXIS
Bob's Taxis: Tel: (01522) 688151
One adapted vehicle.

TRAINS
Central Trains: Assistance:
Tel: (0121) 654 1200
www.centraltrains.co.uk
Arriva: Special Needs:
Tel: (0845) 6008008

CAR PARKS
Free disabled badge spaces in all council-owned car parks and some on-street parking, map available from TIC.

SHOPMOBILITY
Tentercroft Street Car Park.

HOTEL
DAMON MOTEL [🚶]
997 Doddington Road, Lincoln LN6 3SE
Tel: (01522) 887733
Fax: (01522) 887734
No. of Accessible Rooms: 3. Bath
Accessible Facilities: Lounge, restaurant.
Purpose-built, quality motel on Lincoln
by-pass in the south-west area of the city.

MOOR LODGE HOTEL [🚶]
Sleaford Road, Branston, Lincoln LN4 1HU
Tel: (01522) 791366
Fax: (01522) 794389
No. of Accessible Rooms: 3. Bath
Accessible Facilities: Lounge, restaurant.
Michelin-recommended country hotel in a
village three miles south of Lincoln.

ATTRACTIONS
HARTSHOLME COUNTRY PARK
Skellingthorpe Road, Lincoln LN6 0EY
Tel/Fax: (01522) 873577
100 acres of heath, lawns and woodland
surrounding a large lake. Educational
visitor centre, aviary and nature trails - fun
and informative activities for all ages.
SD-[♿] CP[🚶] E[🚶] RF[♿]
C[🚶] WC[🚶]

LINCOLN CATHEDRAL
Minster Yard, Lincoln LN2 1PX
Tel: (01522) 544544
www.lincolncathedral.com
This is the third largest cathedral in
England after York and St. Paul's. It was
rebuilt in 1192 in the Early English style,
enduring today, although much is Gothic,
from the C13th and C14th. The vast
interior is reached through the arch of
Exchequergate at the front. Attractive
features include the magnificent open
nave, St. Hugh's choir, the angel choir and
the beautiful stained glass windows, the
wooden-roofed cloisters and the ten-sided
chapter house.
NB: Enter at the west front Entrance where
the external ramp is 1:7, the internal is
1:15. Good pusher needed. The chapter
house entrance from inside the cloister is
1:26. The entrance to the choir north is
1:8, and from the nave to the choir aisle is
1:13. A motorised wheelchair is available.
SD[♿] CP n/a E n/a RF[🚶]
C[🚶] S[🚶] WC[🚶]

LINCOLN CASTLE
Castle Hill, Lincoln LN1 3AA
Tel: (01522) 511068 Fax: (01522) 512150
One of the first great castles built by
William the Conqueror, this was begun in
1068. For 900 years the castle has been
used as a court and a prison. Many original
features still stand, although the wall walks
are not accessible. A major highlight is the
ten-year Magna Carta exhibition that is
now in its eighth year. This document,
almost 800 years old, one of four surviving
originals sealed by King John at
Runnymede in 1215, is housed within the
exhibition. Originally every county had its
own copy. To see the real thing is an
overwhelming experience.
NB: Use Eastgate car park and entrance.
CP[♿] E[♿] RFE[♿] C[♿]
S[🚶] WC[♿] G[♿]

MUSEUM OF LINCOLNSHIRE LIFE
Burton Road, Lincoln LN1 3LY
Tel: (01522) 528448 Fax: (01522) 521264
Award-winning social history museum
housed in extensive barracks built for Royal
North Lincoln Militia in 1857. Varied
displays depict many aspects of
Lincolnshire life including the schoolroom,
chapel, wagon and wheelwright's
workshop among many others.
A delightful museum.
SD[♿] CP[♿] E[♿] RF[♿]
C[🚶] S[♿] WC[🚶]

USHER GALLERY
Lindum Road, Lincoln LN2 1NN
Tel: (01522) 527980 Fax: (01522) 560165
Lincolnshire's main visual arts venue with
a permanent collections of C20th work by
L S Lowry, John Piper and Walter Sickert.
These are combined with fine porcelain
and jewellery in excellent collection.
SD[♿]   CP[🚶]   E[♿] (via street level entrance
intercom to reception, then lifts to ground and first floors)
RF[♿] L[♿] C[♿] S[🚶] WC[🚶]

RAF DIGBY SECTOR OPERATIONS ROOM MUSEUM

RAF Digby, Lincoln LN4 3LH
Tel: (01526) 327592   Fax: (01526) 327560

Just outside Sleaford, beneath a mound, is an operations room restored and refurbished to represent it as it was during WWII. RAF stations like Digby were in the front line during the war when teenage airmen took to the skies in Hurricanes, Spitfires and Lancasters. The museum was founded to commemorate their bravery.

SD CP E RF WC

MARKET RASEN

Traditional small market town with Georgian and Victorian buildings, and original shop fronts.

MININGSBY

A small village off the beaten track surrounded by quiet country lanes.

SELF-CATERING ACCOMMODATION

STAMFORD FARM HOUSE
Miningsby PE22 7NW
Tel: (01507) 588 682

No. of Accessible Units: 1. Roll-in shower
No. of Beds per Unit: 1S/1D
Accessible Facilities: Lounge, dining room, kitchen. Victorian farmhouse in village between Lincoln and Spilsbury.

SCUNTHORPE

Garden town that has evolved from five small villages in line with the development of the steel industry. Fine parklands.

ATTRACTION

NORMANBY HALL COUNTRY PARK
Normanby, Nr. Scunthorpe DN15 9HU
Tel: (01724) 720588
Fax: (01724) 721248

Sadly the hall is not accessible, it has four steps, but the remainder is good with a very pro-active principal keeper. There is a delightful Victorian walled garden, specialising in period varieties of fruit, vegetables and flowers with wide gravel, paving paths and small, fascinating museum exhibits on the life of gardeners. A farming museum with exhibits on rural trades and crafts is also accessible by a newly installed lift to the first floor. 300 acres of parkland surrounding the hall include lovely trails, impressive main lawns outside the hall and duck ponds and a deer park. A perfect place to unwind.

SD CP E RF
C S WC (at car park)
L (farming museum) G

The splendid walled garden at Normamby Hall Country Park.

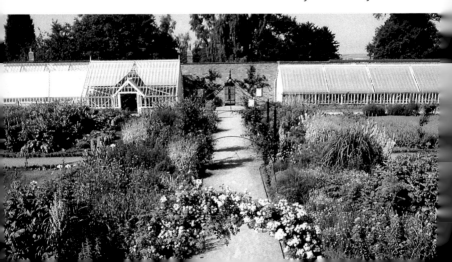

SKEGNESS

Family seaside resort with six miles of sandy beaches and many attractions.

HOTEL
THE CHATSWORTH HOTEL
North Parade, Skegness PE25 2UB
Tel: (01754) 761417   Fax: (01754) 761173
e-mail: Altipper@chatsworthskegness.com
www.chatsworthskegness.com
No. of Accessible Rooms: 1. Bath
Accessible Facilities: Lounge, restaurant, chair lift.
Situated in a good position on the seafront a few minutes walk away from all the major attractions - Marine Zoo, Bowling Greens, Amusement Park, Embassy Centre and Theatres.

SELF-CATERING
KINGS CHALET PARK
Trunch Lane, Chapel-St-Leonards, Skegness.
Book through Grooms Holidays
No. of Accessible Units: 1
No. of Beds per Unit: 8
Accessible Facilities: Kitchen/diner, lounge. Chalet overlooking lush green lawns in a chalet park a few minutes away from a picturesque village and close to Skegness on the east Lincolnshire coast.

ATTRACTIONS
CHURCH FARM MUSEUM
Church Road South, Skegness PE25 2HF
Tel: (01754) 766658
Fax: (01754) 898243
e-mail: walker@lincolnshire.gov.uk
Stroll into a bygone era in a period furnished farmhouse, traditional farm buildings, a thatched cottage with nurtured flower beds.

SD 🔻 CP 🚶 E 🔻 RF 🔻
C 🚶 S 🚶 WC 🔻

SKEGNESS NATURELAND SEAL SANCTUARY
North Parade, Skegness PE25 1DB
Tel/Fax: (01754) 764345
Known for its seal rescue centre, rearing and returning abandoned seal pups to their natural environment . Also an aquarium, pets' corner, floral palace and tropical house. The tropical house is the only inaccessible area.

SD 🔻 E 🔻 RF 🔻 C 🔻
S 🔻 WC 🔻

SPALDING

A peaceful town at the centre of the flower industry. Georgian terraces front the tree-lined river Welland with many buildings showing a Dutch influence.

TOURIST INFORMATION CENTRE
Ayscoughfee Hall, Churchgate,
Spalding PE11 2RA
Tel: (01775) 725458

ATTRACTION
THE BUTTERFLY and WILDLIFE PARK
Long Sutton, Spalding PE12 9LE
Tel: (01406) 363833   Fax: (01406) 363182
Utterly captivating attraction of 12 acres that includes superb tropical house where hundreds of butterflies enchant in natural surroundings of pathways, bridges and pools. In the famous Ant Room see leaf-cutting ants at work and visit the Insecteria. Bird of prey exhibits include an American bald eagle, a trained vulture and charming owls, including the Barn and Tawny species. There is a lovely café with a picnic area. Wheelchairs available. Owned and run by charming couple, this is a must.

SD 🔻 CP 🔻 E 🔻 RF 🔻
C 🔻 S 🔻 WC 🔻 RFE 🔻

STAMFORD

The town still retains its medieval street pattern of narrow passageways and cobbled streets opening out into spacious squares. Superb historical architecture remains, most of the town is devoid of C20th or Victorian buildings. The water meadows are right in the centre of the town.

HOTEL
GARDEN HOUSE HOTEL
St. Martins, Stamford PE9 2LP
Tel: (01780) 763359   Fax: (01780) 763339

No. of Accessible Rooms: 4. Bath
Accessible Facilities: Lounge, restaurant
Part of this charming house dates back to
1796 and has changed little. It is now a 20-
bedroomed hotel with an acre of
beautiful gardens.

ATTRACTION
BURGHLEY HOUSE
Stamford PE9 3JY
Tel: (01780) 752451   Fax: (01780) 480125
e-mail: info@burghley.co.uk
www.burghley.co.uk
Built between 1565/87 by William Cecil,
Elizabeth I's trusted adviser, this remains
his descendants' family home and contains
a fine collection of C17th Italian paintings,
a Breughel and a Gainsborough, wood-
carvings by Grinling Gibbons and Japanese
ceramics. A new sculpture garden and a
Capability Brown park complement the
house. The first-floor state rooms are
accessed by a Stannah chairlift, so there is
limited access to this and the restaurant.
SD 🚫   CP 🚫   E 🚫   C 🚶
S 🚶   WC 🚶

LIVERPOOL AND MERSEYSIDE

A fishing village that grew into one of the
world's largest ports, trading in slaves,
freight and emigration until the middle of
this century, Liverpool's legacy is manifest
is some fine buildings, two cathedrals and
the city's mercantile history that is well
displayed in museums. The rejuvenation of
the Albert Docks and the Beatles
connections ensure there is some life in the
old dog yet.

TOURIST INFORMATION CENTRES
Merseyside Welcome Centre, Clayton Square
Shopping Centre, Liverpool L1 1QR
Tel: (0151) 7093631
Fax: (0151) 7080204
Atlantic Pavilion, Albert Dock,
Liverpool L3 4AE
Tel: (0151) 7088854   Fax: (0151) 7093350

BUSES
Merseytravel, 24 Hatton Garden,
Liverpool L3 1AN
Tel: (0151) 2367676
Produces an Access Guide.

TAXIS
City Council: Tel: (0151) 2273911
1,400 taxis, most able to carry wheelchairs.
There are ranks all over city including at
Lime Street station.

TRAINS
Central Trains: Assistance:
Tel: (0845) 7056027
www.centraltrains.co.uk
First North Western: Special Needs:
Tel: (0845) 6040231
Merseyrail: Special Needs:
Tel: (0151) 7022071 (minicom available)
Arriva: Special Needs:
Tel: (0845) 6008008
Virgin Trains: Special Needs:
Tel: (0845) 7443366
Minicom: (0845) 7443367
Wales and West: Special Needs:
Tel: (0845) 3003005
Minicom: (0845) 7585469
Portable ramps are available at Liverpool
Moorfields and Southport Stations.

CAR PARKS
Disabled badge holders may park on-street
or in Pay & Display parks free of charge
with no time limit.

SHOPMOBILITY
48a Clayton Square, Liverpool L11 0QR
Tel: (0151) 7089993   Fax: (0151) 7080775

HOTELS
LIVERPOOL MOAT HOUSE   🚶
Paradise Street, Liverpool L1 8JD
Tel: (0845) 60 60 611
No. of Accessible Rooms: 1. Bath
Accessible Facilities: Restaurant
Large, modern and centrally located hotel
close to Albert Dock and Tate Gallery with
fine views across the Mersey.
TRAVEL INN LIVERPOOL WEST DERBY   🚶
The Stag & Rainbow Beefeater, Queens Drive
West Derby, Liverpool L13 0DL
Tel: (0151) 2284724   Fax: (0151) 2207610

www.travelinn.co.uk
No. of Accessible Rooms: 4
Accessible Facilities: Restaurant
A508, left past the Esso Garage, travelling towards Bootle on the NE side of the city.

ATTRACTIONS

CROXTETH HALL AND COUNTRY PARK
Croxteth Hall Lane, Liverpool L12 0HB
Tel: (0151) 2285311   Fax: (0151) 2282817
Former home of the Earls of Sefton, the rooms are furnished in Edwardian period pieces. The grounds contain a Victorian walled garden, a collection of rare-breed animals.

SD 🚽   CP 🚶♿   E 🚶   RF 🚶♿
C ♿   S ♿   WC 🚶
RFE-Building, Garden ♿

LIVERPOOL FOOTBALL CLUB MUSEUM AND TOUR CENTRE
Anfield Road, Liverpool L4 0TH
Tel: (0151) 2606677   Fax: (0151) 264 0149
The museum is accessible, the tour is not. For grounds see sporting venue below.

SD ♿   CP 🚶♿   E ♿   L 🚶♿   S 🚶
WC 🚶   RFE 🚶

MERSEYSIDE MARITIME MUSEUM
Albert Dock, Liverpool L3 4AQ
Tel: (0151) 4784507   Fax: (0151) 4784590

History of the great port of Liverpool, its ships and its people. Titanic and Lusitania exhibits and others on emigration to the new world. Visit the Transatlantic Slavery Gallery to learn of the origins of slavery and its legacy. Pass through a reconstruction of a slave ship. Lifeline galleries display WWII exhibits. The HM Customs & Excise National Museum is located within this museum, where you can enter a world of secret cargoes, concealment and smuggling.

SD ♿   CP 🚶♿   E ♿   RF ♿
L 🚶♿   C ♿   S ♿   WC 🚶

METROPOLITAN CATHEDRAL OF CHRIST THE KING
Mount Pleasant, Liverpool L3 5TQ
Tel: (0151) 7099222   Fax: (0151) 7087274
e-mail: met.cathedral@cwcom.net
Modern Roman Catholic cathedral, consecrated in 1967. Renowned for glass designs by John Piper.

SD ♿   CP 🚶♿   E ♿ (disabled entrance accessed via underground car park)   RF ♿
L ♿   S 🚶♿   WC 🚶   RFE ♿

MUSEUM OF LIVERPOOL LIFE
Pierhead, Liverpool L3 1PZ
Tel: (0151) 4784063
Mersey culture, Liverpool's sporting life and industrial development, trade union and

The modern Metropolitan Cathedral of Christ the King, Liverpool.

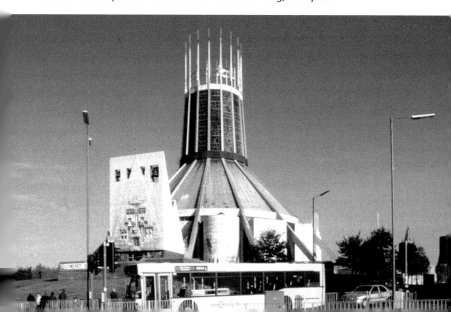

women's suffrage displays and a local perspective on the 1981 Toxteth Riots.

SD ♿ CP ♿ E ♿ RF ♿ S ♿
WC ♿

SPEKE HALL (NT)
The Walk, Speke, Liverpool L24 1XD
Tel: (0151) 4277231
Fax: (0151) 4279860
Famous half-timbered house, built in 1490. The interior is of many periods, Victorian, Jacobean, Tudor. Delightful restored garden.

SD ♿ CP ♿ E ♿ C ⚦
S ⚦ WC ⚦ RFE ♿

TATE GALLERY LIVERPOOL
Albert Dock, Liverpool L3 4BB
Tel: (0151) 7093223
Fax: (0151) 7093122
e-mail: liverpool.info@tate.org.uk
Fine examples of the national collection of C20th art from private and public collections.

SD ♿ CP n/a E ♿ L ♿
C ♿ S ♿ WC ♿

WALKER ART GALLERY
William Brown Street,
Liverpool L3 8EL
Tel: (0151) 4784199
Fax: (0151) 4784190
Superb collection of European paintings and sculpture, plus temporary exhibitions throughout the year. Adjacent to the main entrance is an adapted door that opens electronically. It is operated by pressing a large button 85cm off the floor. Pay and Display car parking is in William Brown St, 50m from the gallery.

SD ♿ CP ⚦ E ♿ RF ♿
L ♿ C ♿ S ♿ WC ♿

SPORTING VENUE
LIVERPOOL FOOTBALL CLUB
Anfield Road, Liverpool L4 0TH
Admin: Tel: (0151) 2632361
Fax: (0151) 2608813
Booking: General: (0151) 2608680
CC: (0151) 2635727 Fax: (0151) 2611415
Complies with Part M, Building Regulations.

CP ♿ (for annual pass holders only.)
P ⚦ (public parking at nearby Anfield Comprehensive School, Utting Avenue) RE ♿
ED ♿ (except non-automatic)
INT ♿ L ♿
WC ♿ (16 adapted throughout stadium)
SS ♿ 82 designated positions through dedicated entrance door for wheelchair and helpers only.
B/R ♿

THEATRE/CONCERT HALL
PHILARMONIC HALL
Hope Street, Liverpool L1 9BP
Admin: (0151) 2102895
Fax: (0151) 2102902
Booking-Box Office: (0151) 7093789
Complies with Part M, Building Regulations.

SD ♿ CP ♿ Public CP-Caledonia Street
Nearest taxi rank is outside the main entrance
RE ♿ ED ♿ INT ♿ L ♿
WC ♿ (rear of auditorium next to lift)
AUD ♿ B/R ♿
Lift from foyer to rear stalls, slight incline to box seats, slight decline to stalls.

MERSEYSIDE

LIVERPOOL-MERSEY TOURISM
5th Floor, Cunard Building, Pier Head,
Liverpool L3 1ET
Tel: (0151) 2272727
Fax: (0151) 2272325
info@merseyside.org.uk
www.merseyside.org.uk

LIVERPOOL ASSOCIATION OF DISABLED PEOPLE
Lime Court Centre, Upper Baker Street,
Liverpool L6 1NB
Tel: (0151) 2638366

DISABLEMENT RESOURCE UNIT
c/o Local Solutions,
Mount Vernon Green, Hall Lane,
Liverpool
Tel: (0151) 7090990

MERSEY VOLUNTEER BUREAU
35 Lime Street, Liverpool
Tel: (0151) 7071113

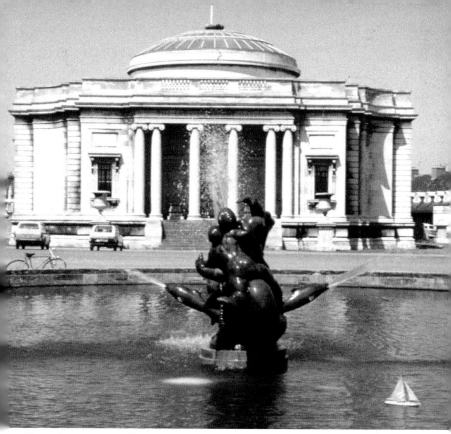

The Lady Lever Art Gallery at the wonderfully eclectic Port Sunlight, Liverpool.

WIRRAL ASSOCIATION FOR DISABILITY
Shopmobility Centre, 5 St. John Street, Birkenhead
Tel: (0151) 6476162

WHEELCHAIR REPAIRS
Mobility Shop
143 Thomas Lane, Broadgreen, Liverpool L14 5NT
Tel: (0151) 220 7080

BIRKENHEAD
Situated near the head of the Wirral peninsula. Considerable residential and shopping development in recent years.

SPORTS/LEISURE
EUROPA POOLS
Conway Street, Birkenhead, Wirral L41 6RN
Tel: (0151) 6474182 Fax: (0151) 6474178

SD ♿ CP ♿ E ♿ RF ♿ L ♿
C ♿ S ♿ WC ♿ RFE ♿

PORT SUNLIGHT
A garden village on Liverpool's outskirts created in 1888 by industrialist William Hesketh Lever for his soap factory employees.

ATTRACTION
LADY LEVER ART GALLERY
Port Sunlight Village, Bebington CH62 5EQ
Tel: (0151) 4784136 Fax: (0151) 4784140
Collection of mainly C18th and C19th paintings, ceramics, furniture and sculpture, and is notable for pre-Raphaelite pictures.

SD ♿ CP ♿ E ♿ RF ♿ L ♿
C 🚶 S ♿ WC ♿

SOUTHPORT

Pleasant resort, notable for Lord Street, a boulevard lined with elegant shops running parallel to the coast for 1.5 miles.

TOURIST BOARD

SOUTHPORT TOURIST INFORMATION CENTRE
112 Lord Street, Southport PR8 1NY
Tel: (01704) 533333
Fax: (01704) 500175
e-mail: info@visitsouthport.com
www.visitsouthport.com

ACCESSIBLE TOILETS

The RADAR National Key Scheme. Keys obtainable from the Tourist Information Centre, 112 Lord Street, at the corner with Eastbank Street. Available at the Floral Hall, Promenade Central, Princes Park, Hill Street, Market Street and Queen Anne St.

ACCESSIBLE PARKING

On-street disabled parking available in Chapel Street and both sides of Lord Street.

ACCESSIBLE TAXIS

YELLOW TOP CABS
Tel: (01704) 531 000
Three specially adapted taxis to accommodate wheelchairs.

WHEELCHAIR HIRE

BRADLEYS CHEMIST
34 Shakespeare Street, Southport
Tel: (01704) 532326

HOTELS

SANDPIPERS (Winged Fellowship)
Fairway, Southport PR9 0LA
Tel: (01704) 538388   Fax: (01704) 549764
No. of Accessible Rooms: All (24). Roll-in Shower
Accessible Facilities: Lounge, restaurant, bar, grounds, including sun deck.
A holiday centre for those with physical disabilities. Located on sand dunes on the edge of the town's Marine Lake with easy beach access .

THE ROYAL CLIFTON HOTEL (BEST WESTERN)

The Promenade, Southport PR8 1RB
Tel: (01704) 533771   Fax: (01704) 500657
No. of Accessible Rooms: 3. Bath
Accessible Facilities: Lounge, restaurant
Quality hotel in front of Lord Street.

BED AND BREAKFAST

SANDY BROOK FARM
Wyke Cop Road, Scarisbrick,
Southport PR8 5LR
Tel: (01704) 880337
No. of Accessible Rooms: 1. Bath
Accessible Facilities: Lounge, dining room.
Converted farm building on a small arable farm 3.5 miles from Southport.

SELF-CATERING

SANDY BROOK FARM
As above. The Dairy
No. of Accessible Units: 1. Roll-in shower.
No. of Beds per Unit: 2/4
Accessible Facilities: Open plan lounge/dining/kitchen. C18th barn converted into five holiday apartments, The Dairy being specially designed. Many of the barn's original features have been retained.

ATTRACTION

SOUTHPORT ZOO AND CONSERVATION TRUST
Princes Park, Southport PR8 1RX
Tel: (01704) 538102/548894
Fax: (01704) 538102
Family-owned zoo with a varied collection of animals living in family groups. The emphasis is on breeding.

SD	CP	E	RF
C	S	WC	RFE

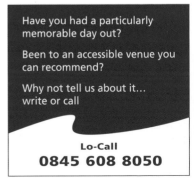

Have you had a particularly memorable day out?

Been to an accessible venue you can recommend?

Why not tell us about it... write or call

Lo-Call
0845 608 8050

LONDON (GREATER)

CENTRAL INNER LONDON POSTAL CODES:
E1, E2, E9, EC1, EC2, EC3, EC4, N1, NW1, NW8, SW1, SW3, SW5, SW7, SW10, SE1, SE11, SE17, WC1, WC2, W1, W2, W6, W8, W9, W10, W11, W14.
GREATER LONDON – ALL OTHER CODES:

GREATER LONDON ASSOCIATION OF DISABLED PEOPLE (GLAD)
336 Brixton Road, London SW9 7AA
Tel: (020) 7346 5800

LONDON TOURIST BOARD AND CONVENTION BUREAU
Glen House, Stag Place, London SW1E 5LT
Tel: (020) 7932 2000   Fax: (020) 7932 0222
www.londontown.com

CITY OF LONDON SOCIAL SERVICES DEPARTMENT
Access Officer, Milton Court, Moor Lane, London, EC2Y 9BL
Tel: (020) 7332 1995   Fax: (020) 7332 3398

TAXIS
Computer Cab, Taxis House,
7 Woodfield Road, London W9 2BA
Tel: (020) 7286 6070
London Taxi company with a number of accessible vehicles.

TRAINS
Central Trains: Assistance:
Tel: (0845) 7056027
www.centraltrains.co.uk
Chiltern Railways: Mobility Impaired:
Tel: (01296) 332113/4
www.chilternrailways.co.uk
Connex: Customer Services:
Tel: (0870) 6030405
Fax: (0870) 6030505
Minicom: (01233) 617621
First Great Eastern: Special Needs:
Tel: (0845) 9505050
Minicom: (0845) 9606099
First Great Western: Special Needs:
Tel: (0845) 7413775
Great North Eastern Railway:

Special Needs: Tel: (0845) 7225444
Minicom: (0191) 2330173
London Transport: Special Needs:
Tel/Minicom: (01702) 357640
Midland Mainline: Special Needs:
Tel: (0114) 2537654
Minicom: (0845) 7078051
Silverlink: Special Needs:
Tel: (01923) 207818   Fax: (01923) 207023
Minicom: (01923) 256430
Thameslink: Special Needs:
Tel: (020) 7620 6333
Minicom: (020) 7620 5561
Stationlink bus:
Tel: (0207) 9183312
Virgin Trains: Special Needs:
(0845) 7443366
Minicom: (0845) 7443367
Wales and West: Special Needs:
Tel: (0845) 3003005
Minicom: (0845) 7585469
West Anglia Great Northern:
Special Needs (0345) 226688
Minicom: (0345) 125988

CITY PARKING
Parking Services, City Engineer's Dept.
2 White Lyon Court, Barbican,
London, EC2Y 8PS
Tel: (020) 7332 1548   Fax: (020) 7332 1557
Because of the pressure on parking, the national Disabled Badge Scheme does not apply in central London, including the City of London. There is, however, 150 specific parking provisions for visitors within the square mile for those with disabilities. Streets with designated bays for disabled badge holders are:
Aldermanbury, America Square, Bartholomew Close, Basinghall Street, Bridewell Place, Bury Street, Carmelite Street, Cloak Lane, Coleman Street, Creechurch Lane, Crosswall, Crutched Friars, Deans Court,Devonshire Square, Dowgate Hill, Eastcheap, Eldon Street, Farringdon Street, Fetter Lane, Finsbury Circus, Fore Street, Furnival Street, Godliman Street, Gravel Lane, Gt. Tower Street, Gt. Winchester Street, Gresham Street, Gutter Lane, Harrow Place, High Timber Street, Houndsditch, Jewry Street, John Carpenter Street, Laurence Poutney Hill, Little Britain, Little New Street, Little

Trinity Lane, Liverpool Street, Lloyds Avenue, Lower Thames Street, Tower, Mark Lane, Middlesex Street, Mincing Lane, Minories, Monument Street, Moor Lane, Mumford Court, Muscovy Street, New Fetter Lane, Noble Street, Old Jewry, Pepys Street, Plumtree Court, Queen Victoria Street, Salisbury Court, Savage Gardens, Seething Lane, Shoe Lane, Silk Street/Barbican, Snow Hill, St. Andrews Hill, St. Bride Street, St. Mary at Hill, Staining Lane, Temple Avenue, Thavies Inn, Trump Street, Tudor Street,Watergate, Watling Street, West Smithfield, Whitefriars Street, Wood Street.Apply in writing to parking services above for permission to park while in the City.

WHEELCHAIR-ACCESSIBLE WCS

With RADAR key:
West Smithfield, opposite St. Bartholomew's Hospital.
St. Paul's Churchyard, between the coach park and New Change. Fenchurch BR Station, take the lift to the first floor. City Thameslink BR Station, Ludgate Hill, through the ticket barrier on the ground floor. Liverpool Street BR Station, in the ticket office.
Other wheelchair accessible public toilets Barbican Centre. Pit floor (level 2), Mezzanine (only during performances),

The London Eye.

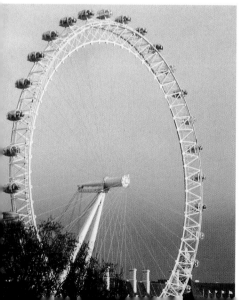

Library floor (level 2), Conference floor (level 4), Stalls floor (level 1).
Guildhall. Ground and 4th floors of north block, 2nd floor of west wing.
Museum of London. level 4.
Exchange Square, Broadgate. Ring the bell at the entrance to request entry.
Tower Hill. In Tower Place, unisex.
Tower of London. Behind the Jewel House.

MUSEUM AND GALLERIES DISABILITY ASSOCIATION - MAGDA

C/o Saffron Walden Museum, Museum Street, Saffron Walden, Essex CB10 1JL
Tel: (01799) 522836   Fax: (01799) 510333
Promotes access to museums for visitors with disabilities.

HOTELS

COPTHORNE TARA

Scarsdale Place,
off Kensington High Street W8 5SR
Tel: (020) 7937 7211   Fax: (020) 7937 7100
No. of Accessible Rooms: 10
Accessible Facilities: Lounge, restaurant
Large hotel in a residential area off Kensington High Street with a smart atmosphere. Highly recommended for visitors with mobility difficulties.

THISTLE MARBLE ARCH

Bryanston Street W1A 4UR
Tel: (020) 7629 8040   Fax: (020) 7499 7792
No. of Accessible Rooms: 10. Roll-in Shower. Accessible Facilities: Lounge, restaurant. The award-winning rooms for disabled guests are among the very best. Situated in the heart of the West End, where Park lane meets Oxford Street.

THE BONNINGTON IN BLOOMSBURY

Southampton Row WC1B 4BH
Tel: (020) 7242 2828   Fax: (020) 7831 9170
No. of Accessible Rooms: 4. Bath
Accessible Facilities: Lounge, restaurant, lift. Late Edwardian hotel with good access to central London theatreland.

COLUMBIA HOTEL

95-99 Lancaster Gate W2 3NS
Tel: (020) 7402 0021
Fax: (020) 7706 4691

No. of Accessible Rooms: 1. Bath
Accessible Facilities: Lounge, restaurant
Originally five large Victorian town houses.
Located a mile from Marble Arch on the
north side of Hyde Park, overlooking the
park and Kensington Gardens. Lively
Queensway with ethnic restaurants, cafes
and multi-storey shopping is very close.
The hotel supplied considerable detail on
its accessible room and has a pro-active
and positive policy.

THE BARBICAN THISTLE HOTEL
120 Central Street, Clerkenwell,
London EC1V 8DS
Tel: (020) 7251 1565   Fax; (020) 7253 1005
No. of Accessible Rooms: 1
Accessible Facilities: Open plan on ground
floor. On the edge of the City of London.

THE FORUM HOTEL
97 Cromwell Road SW7 4DN
Tel: (020) 7370 5757   Fax: (020) 7373 1448
No. of Accessible Rooms: 2
Accessible Facilities: Lounge, restaurant
London's tallest hotel with rooms offering
panoramic views over the capital.

THE SELFRIDGE THISTLE HOTEL
Orchard Street, London W1G 0JS
Tel: (020) 7408 2080   Fax; (020) 7409 2295
No. of Accessible Rooms: 1
Accessible Facilities: Lounge, restaurant on
the 1st floor, accessed by a lift. Elegant
hotel located behind Selfridges department
store in heart of the West End.

LONDON HILTON
22 Park Lane W1Y 4BE
Tel: (020) 7493 8000   Fax: (020) 7208 4142
No. of Accessible Rooms: 3. Roll-in
Shower.
Accessible Facilities: Lounge, restaurants
(except Trader Vics), lift. Well-established
property, always buzzing with activity, with
sweeping views of Hyde Park.

NOVOTEL LONDON WATERLOO
113 Lambeth Road SE1 7LS
Tel: (020) 7793 1010
Fax: (020) 7793 0202
No. of Accessible Rooms: 10. Roll-in
Shower. Accessible Facilities: Lounge,

restaurant, fitness area. Close to Waterloo
International Station.

TOWER THISTLE HOTEL
St. Katherine's Way E1 9LD
Tel: (020) 7481 2575   Fax: (020) 7488 4106
e-mail: Tower.BusinessCentre@Thistle.co.uk
No. of Accessible Rooms: 3. Roll-in Shower
Accessible Facilities: Lounge, restaurants
(2), two on the ground floor, one via an
accessible lift.
Situated next to Tower Bridge and the
Tower of London, the hotel is in unique
location overlooking St. Katherine's Dock
with yachts, shops, walkways and bridges.

WESTLAND HOTEL
154 Bayswater Road W2 4HP
Tel: (020) 7229 9191   Fax: (020) 7727 1054
No. of Accessible Rooms: 3. Bath
Accessible Facilities: Lounge, restaurant.
Located directly opposite Kensington
Palace, five minutes from Whitleys
Shopping Centre.

THE BERNERS HOTEL
Berners Street W1A 3BB
Tel: (020) 7666 2000   Fax: (020) 7666 2001
e-mail: berners@berners.co.uk
www.thebernershotel.co.uk
No. of Accessible Rooms: 6. Bath
Accessible Facilities: Lounge, dining room,
lift. Relatively small but gracious property
with personal ambience. In a very central
location behind Oxford Street, between
Oxford Circus and Tottenham Court Road.

THE DORCHESTER
Park Lane W1A 2HJ
Tel: (020) 7629 8888   Fax: (020) 7409 0114
No. of Accessible Rooms: 2. Bath
Accessible Facilities: Lounge, restaurants
(4), lift, sauna and spa, (three steps,
landing, two steps).
Renowned Mayfair hotel facing Hyde Park.

ATTRACTIONS
BRITISH AIRWAYS LONDON EYE
Jubilee Gardens, County Hall, SE1 1GZ
Tel: Bookings: (0870) 5000 600
Groups: (0870) 4003 005
www.ba-londoneye.com
Largest observation wheel in the world at

450ft high. Overhanging the Thames on the South Bank between Westminster and Hungerford Bridges. 32 capsules carrying passengers on a 35 minute journey taking in some of the best London views, spanning 25 miles. NB. Set down in Belvedere Road, with entrance via Jubilee Gardens – distance 70m. The Wheel – wheelchairs are limited to one per capsule and a maximum of four per revolution. The wheel is stopped with a special ramp coming down to make entrance level to each capsule.

SD [♿]   P N/A   E [♿]   RF [♿]
C [♿]   S [♿]   WC [♿]

BETHNAL GREEN MUSEUM OF CHILDHOOD
Cambridge Heath Road, London E2 9PA
Tel: (020) 8980 5200   Fax: (020) 8983 5225
Parking Access-Tel: (020) 8983 5205
www.vam.ac.uk

One of the largest toy collections in the world, a branch of the Victoria and Albert Museum. Children's interests and experiences also are explored through their playthings, clothes and furniture. Most of the toys are in the lower galleries and on the upper gallery follow the path from Birth and Infancy through Early Years to Breaking Away. A charming museum for adults and children alike. Telephone in advance. Park at the rear entrance in Victoria Park Square, where a small curb cut leads directly to the new lift, and to the ground, first and upper floors. Base to ground is always controlled by a staff member, first and upper floors lift access. From first to ground apart from the lift there is also a ramp with a gradient of 1:12.

SD n/a   CP 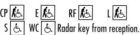   E   RF   L [♿]
C [♿]   S [♿]   WC [♿]   Radar key from reception.

BRITISH MUSEUM
Great Russell Street, London WC1B 3DG
Tel: (020) 7323 8599   Fax: (020) 7323 8616
e-mail: info@british-museum.ac.uk
www.british-museum.ac.uk
Recorded information for disabled visitors:
Tel: (020) 7637 7384
Minicom: (020) 7323 8920
Founded in 1753, this is the oldest museum in the world. Collections include prehistoric and Roman Britain, medieval, renaissance and modern objects, ancient Egyptian, western, Asian, Greek, Roman and oriental art. Highlights include the Elgin Marbles, Lindow Man, Egyptian mummies and the Lindisfarne Gospels. The Great Court will open in November 2000 and access will be disrupted until then. The main foyer is noisy and crowded while the Great Court is being built. Ultimately there will be two lifts with independent access located on left hand side of the main entrance, close to disabled parking, and one assisted lift on the right hand side of entrance. Access to the upper floors from the main entrance is by a stair lift next to the restaurant. The north lift, from the Montague Place entrance, allows access to the Japanese galleries, the prints and drawing gallery, the Arts of Korea exhibition, and the Hotung oriental gallery. Level access from this section to the rest of the museum is on Level 3. The Great Court will house a centre for education, galleries, exhibition space and a restaurant. Complimentary wheelchairs are available at both entrances.

CP [♿] MUST ADVISE WELL IN ADVANCE – TEL. AS ABOVE
E [♿]   RF [♿]   L [♿]   S [♿]   WC [♿]

BANKSIDE GALLERY
48 Hopton Street SE1 9JH
Tel: (020) 7928 7521
Fax: (020) 7928 2820
e-mail: re&rws@bankside-gallery.demon.co.uk

Home of the Royal Watercolour Society and Royal Society of Painter-Printmakers with changing contemporary exhibitions.

SD [♿]   CP n/a   E [🚶]   RF [♿]   S [♿]
WC n/a

BUCKINGHAM PALACE
1. THE STATE ROOMS
The Visitor Office, Buckingham Palace, SW1A 1AA
Tel: (020) 7839 1377   Fax: (020) 7930 9625
Ticket Office: (020) 7321 2233 credit card bookings.
e-mail: information@royalcollection.org.uk
www.royal.gov.uk

Buckingham Palace is again welcoming visitors to the summer opening, and a chance to see the memorable State Rooms with their treasures. Here you are caught up in the echoes of history. Characters from Britain's past appear about to step out of the paintings in the long Portrait Gallery. Beauty and colour everywhere turns your head and eye for a lingering look at silk-lined walls, exquisite furniture, sculptures, fabled ornaments and the diamond-dazzle of chandeliers. Disabled access is excellent, so too is the disabled toilet. Alongside a privileged parking spot. a stair rider is manipulated in the hands of well-practised staff. From there a lift takes you to the sweep of the majestic west-facing rooms overlooking lawns and lake. Entry for designated parking is at North Centre Gate. Electric chairs are not allowed inside, but six wheelchairs are available for loan. The wheelchair access route uses a vertical lift. NB. PRE-BOOKING ESSENTIAL.

SD ♿ CP – Vehicles with a disabled driver or passenger may apply for permission to park right inside the Palace grounds. It is essential that you phone the Special Access Officer (020 7839 1377) or write to Royal Collection Enterprises, The Visitor Office, Buckingham Palace, London SW1A 1AA   E- ♿ Stair rider L ♿ (Stair lift)   S ♿   wc ♿

2. THE ROYAL MEWS

The monarch's magnificent gilded state carriages and coaches, including the unique Gold State Coach, are housed here together with their horses and state liveries. Accessible with fully accessible WC. Open all year, on Monday, Tuesday, Wednesday, and Thursday.

3. QUEEN'S GALLERY

Major restoration completed in spring 2000. All facilities advised as accessible, but pre-check.

CABINET WAR ROOMS
Clive Steps, King Charles Street SW1A 2AQ
Tel: (020) 7930 6961   Fax: (020) 7839 5897
www.iwm.org.uk
Rooms used by Winston Churchill and his chiefs of staff during WWII.

SD ♿   CP n/a   E ♿   L ♿
C n/a
S 🚶   WC 🚶

CHELSEA PHYSIC GARDEN
66 Royal Hospital Road SW3 4HS
Tel: (020) 7352 5646
Fax: (020) 7376 3910
Founded in 1673 by the Society of Apothecaries, this is one of Europe's oldest botanic gardens. Its 3.5 acres contain a garden showing the history of medicinal plants and an ethnobotanical garden of world medicines: There is also a very old rock garden (1773), and many rare and tender plants including the largest outdoor olive tree in Britain.

SD ♿   CP ♿   E 🚶   C 🚶
S 🚶   WC 🚶   G 🚶

COMMONWEALTH INSTITUTE AND EXPERIENCE
Kensington High Street, London W8 6NQ
Tel: (020) 7603 4535   Fax: (020) 7602 7374
e-mail: cburkitt@commonwealth.org.uk
A museum dedicated to exploring the diverse history and culture of over 40 Commonwealth countries with an amazing range of displays and exhibits. Truly fascinating.

SD ♿   CP ♿   E ♿   RF ♿   L ♿   WC 🚶

CRAFT COUNCIL GALLERY
44 Pentonville Road, London N1 9BY
Tel: (020) 7806 2542
Fax: (020) 7837 0858
e-mail: crafts@craftscouncil.org.uk
www.craftscouncil.org.uk
Within a neo-classical facade this gallery contains fine collections of contemporary British crafts plus changing temporary displays.

SD n/a   CP ♿   E ♿   L ♿   C ♿
S 🚶   RFE ♿ Gallery.

DESIGN MUSEUM
Shad Thames, London SE1 2YD
Tel: (020) 7403 6933
Fax: (020) 7378 6540
A museum devoted to design for mass production. A first floor gallery is dedicated to Modern Britain 1929/29, with both historical and artistic exhibits. The second floor collections illustrate modern design in its social and economic context. A shop and café are on the ground floor. Galleries are accessed only by an attended lift.

SD ♿ | CP n/a | E ♿ | RF ♿ | L ♿
C ♿ | S ♿ | WC 🚹 | RFE ♿

THE GEFFRYE MUSEUM
Kingsland Road, London E2 8EA
Tel: (020) 7739 9893   Fax: (020) 7729 5647
e-mail: info@geffrye-museum.org.uk
www.geffrye-museum.org.uk
Set in the former almshouses of the Ironmonger's Company, a delightful C18th building with attractive gardens and mature trees. The museum presents the changing style of the domestic interior, a walk through time from the C17th, past the refined splendour of the Georgian period and high style of the Victorians, to C20th modernity seen through a 1930s flat, a mid-century room in the contemporary style, and a late C20th living space in a converted warehouse.

SD ♿   CP-0 (2 disabled badge bays outside the main entrance),   E ♿ (through small gate to L of main entrance in Kingsland Road)   RF ♿   L ♿
C ♿   S ♿   WC 🚹   RFE n/a (Gardens)

THE GUILDHALL
PO Box 270, Aldermanbury,
London EC2P 2EJ
Tel: (020) 7 332 1462
www.cityoflondon.gov.uk
Home to the Corporation of London, Guildhall has been the seat of municipal government since the C12th and its ancient walls have twice survived catastrophic fire, in 1666 in the Great Fire of London, and in 1940 during the Blitz. This is a Grade 1 listed building and a rare example of medieval architecture. The Great Hall is the setting for ceremonial and civic occasions. Recent events of significance have included 1995 VE Day celebrations and the bestowing of the Honorary freedom of the City on Nelson Mandela in July 1996. There is a high-level security check. Access to the Great Hall is by a back entrance between the hall and the catering department, ramped and then level. The new library and art gallery building connected to the old library avoids stairs.

SD ♿ (Roadside onto pavement and into Guildhall Yard, always free)   E ♿   RF ♿   S 🚹
WC ♿   RFE ♿

HAYWARD GALLERY
Belvedere Road, South Bank Centre,
London SE1 8XX
Tel: (020) 7928 3144
Fax: (020) 7921 0830
Modern, concrete venue for large art exhibitions of classical and contemporary work with the accent on modern British art. NB: Ramps here can be steep but there is always a guard on duty who will help.

SD ♿   CP ♿   E ♿   RF ♿   L ♿
C 🚹   S ♿   WC 🚹

HOUSES OF PARLIAMENT
Palace of Westminster, London SW1A 0AA
Tel: Serjeant at Arms: (020) 7219 3050
Fax: (020) 7799 2178
Rebuilt in the 1830s after a disastrous fire, this Gothic-style building is 310m long, covers eight acres and includes 1,100 apartments along two miles of passages. Telephone Black Rod's Office or Serjeant at Arms' Office WELL IN ADVANCE. Dispensation entrance is from Black Rod's Garden using the sovereign's lift in the House of Lords up to the Principal Floor, then following the normal line of route until returning to the Member's Lobby in the House of Commons. There is space for four wheelchairs at the back of the Strangers Gallery where visitors listen to debates. Access to the gallery is by No 1 lift from the Principal Floor. There is a comprehensive leaflet for those with mobility problems.

SD ♿   CP n/a   E ♿   S ♿   WC n/a

IMPERIAL WAR MUSEUM
Lambeth Road SE1 6HZ
Tel: (020) 7416 5000
Fax: (020) 7416 5374
e-mail: mail@iwm.org.uk
www.iwm.org.uk
Display of modern warfare plus exhibits relating to the social effect of C20th wars and period art, films and photographs. First and Second World War exhibitions, and the Blitz Experience. Galleries on all four levels are accessible.

SD n/a   CP ♿   RF ♿   L ♿
C 🚹   S 🚹   WC 🚹

KENSINGTON PALACE STATE APARTMENTS and ROYAL CEREMONIAL DRESS COLLECTION

Kensington Gardens, London W8 4PX
Tel: (020) 7937 9561   Fax: (020) 7376 0198
www.hrp.org.uk
Displays of court uniforms and protocol from c1760, including dresses of the present royal family. NB: There is no vehicular access or disabled parking in the Orangery Gardens. ADVANCE BOOKING ON THE ABOVE NUMBER IS ESSENTIAL. The Royal Ceremonial Dress Collection is on the Garden Floor.
NB: There is no access to state apartments.

SD   CP n/a   E   C
S   WC 🚹   RFE 🦽

LONDON AQUARIUM

County Hall, Riverside Building, Westminster Bridge SE1 7PB
Tel: (020) 7967 8000 Fax: (020) 7967 8029
A voyage of discovery through the waters of the world with hundreds of live specimens in superb underwater scenes, aided by touchtanks and educational, inter-active displays. Car parking is available in Jubilee Gardens or at the Shell Building. There is a pathway past the BA Eye along a wide walkway on the south bank of the Thames.
Two floors are accessed by lift with disabled WC on both. The wheelchair/pushchair route is well signed throughout from the lift exit on each floor. There is a shallow exit ramp. The Ray Touchpool is too high to touch but the Sea Shore Touchpool at 64cm high, is accessible.

SD N/A   CP 🦽   E 🦽   RF 🦽   L 🦽
S 🦽   WC 🦽   RFE 🦽

LONDON CANAL MUSEUM

12-13 New Wharf Road N1 9RT
Tel: (020) 7713 0836
e-mail: martins@dircon.co.uk
www.charitynet.org/
Here is the story of London's canal development, particularly of Regent's Canal with exhibits on vessels, people and trade, notably the import of ice from Norway, all housed in a former ice warehouse and stables.

On two floors, the majority of the ground floor gallery is accessible. The first floor is accessed via stairs, but as part of the historic fabric, there is a ramp designed for horses! This can be used to assist wheelchair users who must have two fit and strong people to assist. A very positive attitude everywhere.

SD 🦽   CP 🚹   E 🦽   C n/a
S 🦽   WC 🦽

LONDON DUNGEON

28-34 Tooley Street SE1 2SZ
Tel: (020) 7403 7221   Fax: (020) 7378 1529
Historic death, torture and witchcraft brought vividly to life in sights and sounds. Some passageways are quite narrow and dark. A companion is recommended.

SD 🦽   CP n/a   E 🦽   RF 🦽   C 🦽
S 🦽   WC 🦽   RFE 🦽

LONDON PLANETARIUM

Marylebone Road NW1 5LR
Tel: (020) 7487 0200   Fax: (020) 7465 0862
www.london-planetarium.com
Two inter-active space zones, plus 30-minute Planetary Quest star show under the green dome – educational and fascinating.

SD 🦽   CP n/a   E 🦽   RF 🦽   L 🦽
C n/a   S 🦽   WC 🚹   RFE 🚹

LONDON TRANSPORT MUSEUM

Covent Garden Piazza, London WC2E 7BB
Tel: (020) 7379 6344   Fax: (020) 7565 7254
e-mail: contact@ltmuseum.co.uk
www.ltmuseum.co.uk
The story of travel since 1800 told through wonderful displays of old trams, buses, the Tube and posters. Hands-on fun with buses and train simulators and working models. A must!

SD 🦽   CP n/a   E 🦽   RF 🦽   L 🦽
C 🦽   S 🦽   WC 🚹

LONDON ZOO

Regent's Park, NW1 4RY
Tel: (020) 7449 6551   Fax: (020) 7449 6579
Houses 8,000 species of animals, insects, reptiles and fish. Captive breeding programmes include the rare Asiatic lion and black rhinos. There is also a Children's Zoo and activities. The zoo grounds are

level except at the entrances/exits to two tunnels leading from one area to another. These are steeper than 1:10 and are about 15-20m long. There is level or short-ramped access into the animal houses except at the Aquarium that has three steps, but volunteers assist via a side, level door. The Moonlight World is not accessible: and there's a steep ramp to the elephant house.

SD ♿ CP n/a E ♿ RF ♿ C 🚶
S 🚶 WC 🚶 RFE ♿ 🚶

MADAME TUSSAUD'S
Marylebone Road NW1 5LR
Tel: (020) 7935 6861 Fax: (020) 7465 0862
This world-famous waxwork collection, where visitors can mix with the famous and notorious, includes a re-vamped Chamber of Horrors. NB. All areas are accessible except Superstars and the continuous Dark Ride. Entrance is via a ticket-holders entrance in Marylebone Road. Wheelchair visitors are limited to three at any one time so phoning in advance is strongly recommended. Catering has a steep ramp and help is needed from staff.
The shop is accessed by a stair lift, operated by staff, that takes a wheelchair.

The very Gothic,
Natural History Museum.

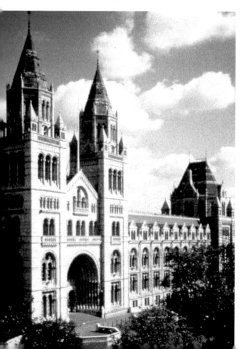

SD ♿ CP n/a E ♿ RF ♿
C 🚶
S 🚶 WC ♿ L ♿

NATIONAL GALLERY
Trafalgar Square
London WC2N 5DN
Tel: (020) 7747 2885 Fax: (020) 7747 2423
e-mail: information@ng-london.org.uk
One of the country's great galleries, the neo-classical building houses paintings from all the great periods of western European art from 1260-1900. The Sainsbury Wing, opened in 1991, contains early renaissance works from 1260-1510. Level entrance is gained from both the Sainsbury Wing and the Orange Street entrances, though the former is specifically accessible. The SW lift accesses all five levels of the wing, including the main floor from which there is a direct, level and very wide corridor joining the remaining wings of the gallery. All gallery rooms are very spacious with ample room to view. There is one disabled parking space at the Orange Street entrance that should be booked in advance. Wheelchairs are available here also and throughout the gallery. The WCs are Radar operated, a key is obtainable from the warder on each floor. The gallery provides detailed information on access, which is very useful.

SD ♿ CP ♿ E ♿ RF ♿
L ♿ C ♿ S ♿ WC 🚶

NATIONAL PORTRAIT GALLERY
St. Martin's Place, London WC2H OHE
Tel: (020) 7306 0055 Fax: (020) 7306 0056
www.npg.org.uk
British history seen through portraits of the famous and infamous from the medieval period to present day.
Undergoing extensive rebuilding work as part of the NPG 2000 Masterplan Millennium project. The needs of disabled visitors are under discussion. Telephone for further information.

NATURAL HISTORY MUSEUM
Cromwell Road, SW7 5BD
Tel: (020) 7938 9123 Fax: (020) 7938 9066
www.nhm.ac.uk

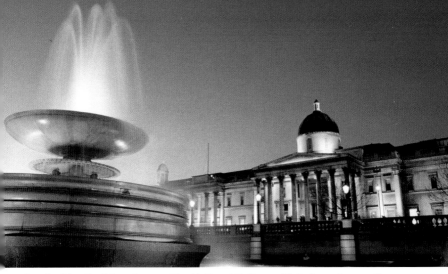

Overlooking Trafalgar Square, The National Gallery with its imposing portico.

Covering four acres, this superb nature museum includes the new Earth Gallery. Wheelchair entrance is at the Earth Gallery Exhibition Road by the Museum car park, reserve a space in advance. There is unreservable on-street disabled badge parking, or general parking. The entrance is through glass swing doors. A lift takes you to the mezzanine level WC. All areas are linked by lifts or ramps (some steep). The Earth Sculpture is accessed by escalator but the Earth Lab exhibit is not accessible. Galleries are linked on the ground floor through Waterhouse Way, through the main entrance with the famous dinosaurs and onwards. The gallery shop and bookshop, the gallery restaurant and the Waterhouse Coffee Bar are all on this access route.

SD ♿ CP ♿ E ♿ RF ♿ L ♿
C ♿ & ♿ S ♿ WC ♿ RFE ♿

ROYAL ACADEMY OF ARTS
Burlington House, Piccadilly,
London W1V 0DS
Tel: (020) 7300 8000   Fax: (020) 7300 8001
Founded in 1768, Britain's oldest fine arts institution is known for its permanent and important temporary art exhibitions. Famous among permanent sculpture is the Michaelangelo relief of the Madonna and Child outside the Seckler Galleries. WARNING: ACCESS ONLY IN ELECTRIC WHEELCHAIR. GALLERIES ACCESSED BY LIFT AND STANNAH STAIR LIFT.

SD n/a   CP ♿   E ♿ (electric/ramped at 1:5 - 1:10)
RF ♿   L ♿   C ♿ (main restaurant ramped at 1:10, courtyard cafe level)   S ♿ (lift access)
WC ♿ (would be 1, but positioned adjacent to gents, and constant traffic makes access difficult)

ST. BRIDE'S CHURCH
Fleet Street, London EC47 8AU
Tel: (020) 7353 1301   Fax: (020) 7583 0239
e-mail: info@stbrides.com
This famous Wren church, just off Fleet Street, is a traditional venue for memorials to journalists. Wall plaques commemorate them and printers. Its wonderful octagonal spire, added to the church in 1703, has been a model for tiered wedding cakes since. Bombed in 1940, the interior has been fully restored.

SD ♿   CP n/a   E ♿ (Fleet St. entrance, 4/5 steps, use Salisbury Court level entrance.
RF 🚶   S ♿

ST. GILES and ST. LUKE CRIPPLEGATE
c/o St. Giles Rectory, 4 The Postern,
Wood Street, London EC2Y 8BJ
Tel/Fax: (020) 7638 1997
e-mail: stgiles@globalnet.co.uk
www.users.globalnet.co.uk
Only the tower survives from the original St Giles of 1550, now the parish church for the Barbican. Oliver Cromwell was married here and John Milton is buried here.

SD ♿   CP 🚶   E ♿   RF ♿   WC ♿

ST. JAMES, PICCADILLY
197 Piccadilly, London W1V 0LL
Tel: (020) 7734 4511 Fax: (020) 7734 7449
A major Wren church, built in 1684 and
bombed in 1940, it retains its essential
features, tall arched windows, an ornate
C17th Grinling Gibbons screen behind
the altar, carvings above the organ and
his marble font. William Blake and Pitt
the Elder were baptised here. A busy
urban church welcoming all.

SD n/a   CP [🚶]   E [♿]
C [🚶] Franchise adjacent.
RFE [♿] Church itself.

ST. KATHERINE'S DOCK
Taylor Woodrow Property Co. Ltd
International House,
1 St. Katherine's Way, London E1 9TW
Tel: (020) 7488 0555 Fax: (020) 7481 4515
e-mail: mark.heran@taywood.co.uk
Since the C10th St. Katherine's Dock has
played an important part in the life of
London. During WWII the docks suffered
appalling damage and although
commerce continued here, container
shipping became too massive for the old
docks, which were closed in 1968, the
other docks also closing by 1983. It has
now been completely renovated and is
one of the city's most successful and
attractive commercial, residential and
entertainment facilities. The yacht basin
buzzes with activity of cafes, restaurants,
shops and the continual throb of shipping.
Set down in St. Katherine's Way, a small
left hand side turning onto a service road.
An NCP car park is 100m. Further on, but
here is no designated parking. All areas are
connected by wide, planked or
pavemented pathways, with only the
bridge dividing the central and eastern
basins being rather narrow and
inaccessible.

SD [♿]   CP [♿]   E [♿]   C [♿]
S [♿]   WC [♿] Radar Key

ST. MARTIN-IN-THE-FIELDS
Trafalgar Square, London WC2N 4JJ
Tel: (020) 7930 0089 Fax: (020) 7839 5163
The present church is the fourth to stand
on this site. Completed in 1726 by James
Gibbs, the fine facade was a new style,
with its huge Corinthian columns, a great
tower and graceful steeple, topped with a
gilt crown. Notable in the interior are
delicate Italian scrolls and cherubs on the
ceiling, but it is the essential being of
St.Martin's, a church in the middle of a

The Tower of London.

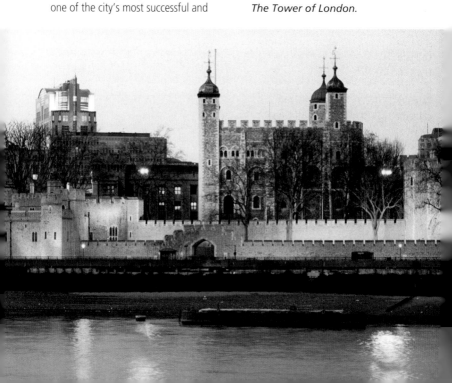

lively city, which emanates. The church is indeed in-the-fields, working with all who fall outside the social net of urban life, with a busy Social Care Unit attending to the homeless or less fortunate. There are free lunchtime concerts several days each week. The crypt, with cafe and brass rubbing centre is, unfortunately, not accessible. Set down in Adelaide Street, level onto pavement and go through a small market with large, level flagstones, to a ramp at a side entrance.

SD♿ CP n/a E♿ RF♿ WC🚶

ST. PAUL'S CATHEDRAL
Ludgate Hill, London EC4
Tel: (020) 7236 4128

The present St. Paul's, designed by Sir Christopher Wren, and built between 1675 and 1710, is the fifth cathedral to stand on the hill that dominates the ancient City of London. Built in the shape of a cross, with one of the largest cathedral domes in the world, its sheer scale and grandeur are quite overwhelming. Europe's largest crypt contains the tombs of the Duke of Wellington, Nelson and Wren and also houses a cafe, refectory, shop and WC facilities. The Whispering Gallery, quire and American Memorial Chapel in the apse behind the high altar, are not accessible. Disabled access is on the south transept, a short walk through the churchyard from Ludgate Hill. An accessible lift connects the crypt and the main floor, alternately there is a stair lift. There is an NCP car park in Paternoster Row, to the west of the cathedral, but no designated parking spaces, and the surface is cobbled.

SD♿ CP n/a E♿ RF♿ L♿ WC♿ C♿ S♿

SCIENCE MUSEUM
Exhibition Road, South Kensington, London
Tel: (020) 7938 9841 Fax: (020) 7938 9804
e-mail: control@nmsi.ac.uk
www.nmsi.ac.uk

Seven floors of items taken from every area of experimental science. Power, Space and Transport; Space Gallery; Launch Pad; Food for Thought; Challenge of Materials; Science and Art of Medicine; Navigation and Surveying; and Land Transport to name a few. An absolute must.

SD♿ CP n/a E♿ RF♿ L🚶 C🚶 S🚶 WC🚶

THE SERPENTINE GALLERY
Kensington Gardens, London W2 3XA
Tel: (020) 7402 6075 Fax: (020) 7402 4103
www.serpentinegallery.org

Temporary exhibitions of contemporary painting and sculpture in a former tea pavilion built in 1912. Located in SE corner of Kensington Gardens.

SD♿ CP n/a E♿ RF♿ S♿ WC♿

TATE GALLERY
Millbank, London SW1P 4RG
Tel: (020) 7887 8000 Fax: (020) 7887 8007
e-mail: information@tate.org.uk

National Collection of British art from C16th to present day in a family of Tates including Bankside, Liverpool and St. Ives. Millbank includes the Turner Bequest, Hogarth, Constable, Spencer and much controversial contemporary art. Not to be missed. NB: An accessible entrance is on Clore Street. A comprehensive access guide is available.

SD♿ CP♿ E♿ L♿ C♿ S♿ WC🚶

TOWER OF LONDON
Tower Hill, London EC3N 4AB
Tel: (020) 7709 0765
www.hrp.org.uk

Probably the most famous castle in the world, and an amazing example of Norman military architecture. Frequently used as a state prison, two of Henry VIII's wives were executed here and during both world wars German prisoners were housed here. Yeoman Warders or Beefeaters are keepers of The Tower. They are welcoming while also protecting the Crown Jewels. NB: Set down/parking is at the WEST GATE. Wheelchair access is very limited, only the Jewel House is really accessible, but an excellent access guide is available. General:

SD♿ P♿ E♿ RF♿ C♿ S n/a WC🚶 L n/a RFE♿

Jewel House: E♿ S♿
Education Centre: E♿ RF♿
Chapel: E🚶

VICTORIA & ALBERT MUSEUM
Cromwell Road SW7 2RL
Tel: (020) 7942 2000   Fax: (020) 7942 2524
e-mail: postmaster@vam.ac.uk
www.vam.ac.uk

Probably the world's finest museum of decorative arts with several miles of galleries of ancient and modern displays, including the national collection of John Constable, plus special exhibitions. The wheelchair entrance is on Exhibition Road, opposite the Natural History museum with non-reservable disabled badge parking spaces on the road. WC access is by ramp. Steep temporary ramps lead to some galleries and galleries 2-7, 40a, 43, 11-117 are not wheelchair accessible.

SD 🚹   CP 🚶   E 🚹   L 🚹
C 🚹   S 🚹   WC 🚹   RFE 🚹

WESLEY'S CHAPEL, HOUSE AND MUSEUM
49 City Road, London EC1Y 1AU
Tel: (020) 7253 2262   Fax: (020) 7608 3825

John Wesley (1703-91), founder of Methodism, built this chapel as his London base. Built in 1779, it is one of London's undiscovered jewels. The museum houses a fine collection of Wesleyan ceramics and Methodist paintings. The whole building has a calm, welcoming ambience. The chapel and museum are accessible, the house is not.

SD 🚹   E 🚹   RF 🚹   L 🚹
C 🚹   S 🚹   WC 🚹

SUTTON HOUSE (NT)
2 and 4 Homerton High Street, London E9 6JQ
Tel: (020) 8986 2264   Fax: (020) 8533 0556
e-mail: tshrbd@smtp.ntrust.org.uk

In the City's East End, a rare example of a Tudor red-brick house, built in 1535 for Henry VIII with C18th alterations and later additions. Many early details are displayed, plus an exhibition on the history of the house and a multi-media presentation of local archive material. There are changing shows of contemporary arts and sculpture. Only the ground floor is accessible.

SD 🚹   CP n/a   E 🚹   RF 🚹
C 🚹   S 🚹   WC 🚶

WESTMINSTER ABBEY
Dean's Yard, London SW1P 3PA

Tel: (020) 7222 7100   Fax: (020) 7233 2072
e-mail: press@westminster-abbey.org
www.westminster-abbey.org

Consecrated in 1065, although the present building was improved by Henry III in the C13th. The Abbey has been the setting for every coronation since 1066 and has the tallest Gothic nave in Britain. The royal families of England and many famous people are buried here, including Chaucer and others in Poets Corner. The Abbey produces a useful access leaflet. The entrance, through the North Door, has a small step, but is ramped. Cloisters are accessible via Dean's Yard. Little Cloister with a C17th fountain court is accessible. The College Garden, open on specific days, is accessible. The Lady Chapel, Queen Elizabeth and Queen Mary Chapels, Chapter House, Library and Pyx Chamber are not accessible. Disabled parking is in Dean's Yard by permit only and must be applied for in advance. The nearest adapted WC is in the nearby Queen Elizabeth II Conference Centre.

SD n/a   CP 🚹   E 🚹   RF 🚶   C n/a
S 🚶   WC n/a

WHITECHAPEL ART GALLERY
80-82 Whitechapel High Street,
London E1 7QX
Tel: (020) 7522 7888   Fax: (020) 7377 1685

An art nouveau facade leads into light, spacious galleries of contemporary art. Frequent exhibitions reflect local community cultural origins. David Hockney had his first exhibition here. The shop and gallery are on the ground floor: the café and upper galleries are accessed by lift.

SD 🚹   CP 🚹   E 🚹   RF 🚹
L 🚹 (goods lift, attended)   C 🚹   WC 🚶
S 🚹   RFE 🚹

EAST OF THE CENTRE

GREENWICH

GREENWICH TOURISM
151 Powis Street, Woolwich SE18 6JL
Tel: (020) 8855 6130
Fax: (020) 8317 2822

188

GREENWICH ASSOCIATION OF DISABLED PEOPLE (GAD)
Centre for Independent Living, Christchurch Forum, Trafalgar Road, London SE10 9QE
Tel: (020) 8305 2221
One of pioneering organisations of the independent-living movement. Runs training courses for disabled people wishing to live independently.

ATTRACTIONS
CUTTY SARK CLIPPER SHIP
King William Walk, Greenwich SE10 9HT
(020) 8858 3445 Fax: (020) 8853 3589
e-mail: info@cuttysark.org.uk
Built in 1869, this was the fastest of all the tea clippers. Now preserved in a dry dock, dominating the riverside at Greenwich, with exhibitions and a video telling its story.
SD/A & CP – work in progress, check
E ♿ C n/a S n/a WC n/a
RFE – Access to Tween deck only.

NATIONAL MARITIME MUSEUM
Greenwich, London SE10 9NF
Tel: (020) 8312 6603 Fax: (020) 8312 6521
e-mail: rscates@nmm.ac.uk
www.nmm.ac.uk
The story of Britain and the sea, including exhibitions on the C20th, sea power and, of course, on Nelson.
SD ♿ CP ♿ E ♿ RF ♿
L ♿ C ♿ S ♿ WC 🚹

ROYAL OBSERVATORY GREENWICH
Greenwich Park, Greenwich, London SE10 9NF
Tel: (020) 8858 4422 Fax: (020) 83126632
e-mail: bookings@nmm.ac.uk
www.nmm.ac.uk
The meridian (0 degrees longitude) dividing earth's eastern and western hemispheres, passes through here and in 1884 Greenwich Mean Time was established. The original building, Flamsteed House, was designed by Sir Christopher Wren, and was the government observatory from 1675 until 1948 when London lights became too strong and astronomers moved to Sussex. Access to the facilities is level, but is over a cobbled courtyard and paving slab. Wheelchair access to Royal Observatory is limited to courtyard, part of Meridian Building and shop. Flamsteed House entrance has five steps.
SD ♿ CP ♿ E ♿ S 🚹 WC ♿

NORTHWEST OF THE CENTRE

HENDON

ROYAL AIR FORCE MUSEUM
Grahame Park Way, Hendon, London NW9 5LL
Tel: (020) 8204 2266 Fax: (020) 8200 1751
e-mail: richard.tweed@rafmuseum.org.uk
Fine range of aeroplanes and extensive galleries tell the story of flight through the ages and its impact on transport and communication. The excellent Battle of Britain experience includes Tornado flight simulator and touch-and-try Jet Provost.
SD ♿ CP ♿ E ♿ RF ♿ L ♿
C ♿ S ♿ WC ♿ RFE ♿

SOUTH OF THE CENTRE

CROYDON
This is a bustling borough that has grown incredibly fast with numerous tall modern buildings. Good, traffic-free shopping precinct. Good access to centre of the town.

TOURIST INFORMATION CENTRE
Katherine Street, Croydon, Surrey CR9 1ET
Tel: (020) 8253 1009

HOTEL
HILTON NATIONAL CROYDON 🚹
101 Waddon Way, Purley Way, Croydon CR9 4HH
Tel: (020) 8680 3000 Fax: (020) 8681 6171
No. of Accessible Rooms: 2. Bath
Accessible Facilities: Lounge, restaurant, pool, sauna, whirlpool. A modern hotel located on the A23.

THEATRE
FAIRFIELD HALLS
Park Lane, Croydon CR9 1DG
Tel: (020) 8681 0821   Fax: (020) 8760 0835
Box Office: (020) 8688 9291
Complies with Part M, Building Regulations
- Y

SD ♿   CP ♿ (book in advance) Nearest taxi
rank – taxi telephone on premises.   RE ♿
ED ♿   INT ♿   L ♿   WC ♿⚹
AUD ♿   B/R ♿ (foyer coffee shop)
Lift to 2nd floor Concert Hall.
Lift to ground floor Aschcroft Theatre.

MORDEN

ATTRACTION
MORDEN HALL PARK (NT)
Morden Hall Road, Morden, Surrey SM4 5JD
Tel: (020) 8648 1845   Fax: (020) 8687 0094
A green oasis in this London suburb, this
former deer park with waterways, hay
meadows and old estate buildings, has
craft workshops and a newly restored rose
garden. An excellent information sheet and
map for visitors in wheelchairs is provided.
And wheelchairs available.

SD ♿   CP ⚹   E ♿   RF ♿
C ♿   S- ♿   WC ⚹

SOUTHWEST OF THE CENTRE

HAMPTON WICK

ATTRACTION
HAMPTON COURT PALACE
Hampton Wick, Nr. Kingston-upon-Thames,
Surrey KT8 9AU
Tel: (020) 8781 9500   Fax: (020) 8781 5362
Started in early C16th by Cardinal Wolsey,
extended by Henry VIII himself and in
1690s, by William and Mary who employed
Sir Christopher Wren. His influence
particularly noticeable in the Baroque
landscaped gardens. As a historic Royal
Palace, Hampton Court bears witness to all
kings and queens of England from Henry
VIII to Elizabeth II. The Great Hall, Tudor
Court, Clock and Fountain Courts and

Queen's Gallery are among notable areas
of the Palace. NB: For parking in main
Entrance (West Front), please notify in
advance. There are cobbled stones in both
Tudor courtyards. All rooms with incline
have ramps. Lift access to all State
Apartments. Electrical and mechanical
chairs available at West Front entrance,
where electric buggies also available for
gardens. 3 of 4 shops accessible - kitchen
shop is not.

SD ♿   CP ♿   E ♿   RF ♿   C ♿
S ♿   L ♿   WC ♿   G ♿

WEST OF THE CENTRE

BRENTFORD

ATTRACTION
KEW BRIDGE STEAM MUSEUM
Green Dragon Lane, Brentford,
Middlesex TW8 0EN
Tel: (020) 8568 4757
Fax: (020) 8569 9978
Housed in C19th Pumping Station, a fine
collection of water pumping machinery.
Many engines in steam every weekend,
including the largest working beam engine
in the world – the Cornish grand Junction
90. In the Water for Life Gallery learn
about water supply in London from Roman
times to the Thames Water Ring Main (you
can walk through a slice of it) and about
life and disease in the sewers. Also a
waterworks railway.

SD ♿   CP ⚹   E ♿   RF ♿
L ♿   C ⚹   S ♿   WC ♿

CHISWICK

ATTRACTION
HOGARTH'S HOUSE
Hogarth Lane, Great West Road, Chiswick,
London W4 2QN
Tel: (020) 8994 6757
Very small Georgian house, home of
William Hogarth, with fine permanent
display of artist's famous black and white
engravings. Ground floor rooms accessible

upper rooms are not. Curator happy to bring a particular picture downstairs.

SD n/a   CP [♿]   E [♿]   S [♿]   WC [♿]

LONDON HEATHROW AIRPORT

TRAINS
Heathrow Express: Disabled Assistance:
Tel: (020) 7313 1041

HOTEL
NOVOTEL HEATHROW   [♿]
Cherry Lane, West Drayton, Middlesex
UB7 9HB
Tel: (01895) 431431   Fax: (01895) 431221
No. of Accessible Rooms: 5. Bath
Accessible Facilities: Lounge, restaurant,
Pool. Located four miles from Airport at
M4 (J4) with shuttle bus service to/from
the airport.

RICHMOND
Situated on a delightful stretch of the
River Thames, a mile upstream from
Kew, rich in parks and gardens.
Richmond Park, once the hunting
ground of Charles I, is Europe's largest
city park, famous for its deer.

ATTRACTIONS
ROYAL BOTANIC GARDENS, KEW
Richmond TW9 3AB
Tel: (020) 8940 1171   Fax: (020) 8332 5197
Grows more species in its 300 acre site
than any other garden in the world.
Experience the magnificent glasshouses
displaying a wide range of plants from the
rainforest to the desert.

SD [♿]   CP [♿]   E [♿]   RF [♿]   C [♿]
S [♿]   WC [♿]

RFE [♿]   Entire site has level tarmac paths.
Kew operates a 'Discovery' mobility bus for groups with
special needs with space for two permanent wheelchair
users. Must pre-book.

CONCERT HALLS
ROYAL ALBERT HALL
Kensington Gore, London SW7 2AP
Tel: (020) 7589 3203   Fax: (020) 7823 7725
e-mail: admin@royalalberthall.com

Huge concert hall, a London landmark,
modelled on the Roman amphitheatre and
completed in 1871. Famous as home of
the Proms concerts, but also used for major
boxing matches and other events. NB: Use
the West Car Park, almost completely
designated for disabled users. Entrance
ramped at 1:16.

SD [♿]   CP [♿]   E [♿]   RF [♿]   L [♿]
C [♿]   S n/a   WC [♿]

ROYAL FESTIVAL HALL
Belvedere Road, South Bank Centre,
London SE1 8XX
Tel: (020) 7921 0926
Fax: (020) 7921 0607
e-mail: customer@rfh.org.uk
First major public building in London after
WWII, a major concert venue, with
sweeping staircases leading up from foyer.

SD [♿]   CP [♿]   E [♿]   RF [♿]   L [♿]
C [♿]   S [♿]   WC [♿]   RFE [♿]

WIGMORE HALL
36 Wigmore Street, London W1H 0BP
Tel: (020) 7486 1907   Fax: (020) 7224 3800
Box Office: Tel: (020) 7935 2141
Fax: (020) 7935 3344
Complies Part M, Building Regulations.
NB. Nearest Public car park, NCP Cavendish
Square and Marylebone Lane.
Access straight in from foyer to rear of
auditorium to wheelchair spaces.

SD [♿]   CP [♿]   E [♿]   RF [♿]
L [♿]   WC [♿]   C [♿]

THEATRES. FOR FULL DETAILS CONTACT
ARTSLINE – LONDON'S LEADING CHARITY
FOR INFORMATION ON DISABLED ACCESS TO
ALL ARTS VENUES.
ARTSLINE
54 Chalton Street, London NW1 1HS
Tel/Minicom: (020) 7388 2227
Fax: (020) 7388 2653
e-mail: artsline@dircon.co.uk
www.dircon.co.uk/artsline
All listed offer designated seats and
accessible WC facilities.
All require an able-bodied companion.

ADELPHI
The Strand WC2E 7NA
Tel: Ticketmaster: (020) 7344 0055

BARBICAN THEATRE
Barbican Centre, Silk Street EC2Y 8DS
Tel: (020) 7638 8891
Minicom: (020) 7382 7297
Fax: (020) 7382 7270

CAMBRIDGE THEATRE
Earlham Street WC2 9HU
Box Office through Stoll Moss:
Tel: (020) 7494 5470   Fax: (020) 7494 5147

COLISEUM
St. Martin's Lane EC2N 9HU
Tel: (020) 7632 8300
Minicom: (020) 7836 7666

CRITERION
Piccadilly Circus W1V 9LB
Tel: (020) 7839 8811

DRURY LANE
Theatre Royal, Catherine Street WC2B 5JF
Tel: Stoll Moss (020) 7494 5470
Fax: (020) 7494 5154

HER MAJESTY'S
Haymarket SW1 4QR
Tel: Stoll Moss: (020) 7494 5470
Fax: (020) 7494 5154

LONDON PALLADIUM
Argyll Street W1V 1AD
Tel: Stoll Moss: (020) 7494 5470
Fax: (020) 7494 5154

LYCEUM
Wellington Street WC2E 7DA
Tel: (020) 7420 8112   Fax: (020) 7240 4346
LYRIC
Shaftesbury Avenue W1V 7HA
Tel: Stoll Moss: (020) 7494 5470
Fax: (020) 7494 5154

NATIONAL THEATRE
South Bank SE1 9PX
Three auditoria housed in one building.
Tel: (020) 7928 2252
Minicom: (020) 7928 1963
Information Desk: (020) 7633 0880

OLD VIC
Waterloo Road SE1 8NB
Tel: (020) 7928 7616   Fax: (020) 7928 3608

OPEN AIR
Inner Circle, Regent's Park NW1 4NP
Tel: (020) 7486 2431   Fax: (020) 7487 4562

The original Dome, the Royal Albert Hall.

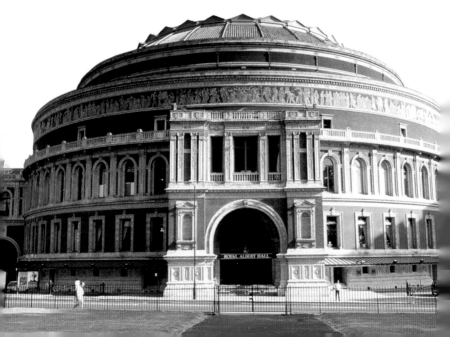

PALACE
Shaftesbury Avenue W1V 8AY
Tel: (020) 7434 0909
Fax: (020) 7734 6157

PHOENIX
Charing Cross Road WC2H 0JP
Tel: (020) 7465 0211
Fax: (020) 7465 0212

THE PLAYERS' THEATRE
The Arches, Villiers Street,
Strand WC2N 6NG
Booking: (020) 7839 1136
Fax: (020) 7839 8067
e-mail: THEPLAYERS@aol.com
Not covered by Artsline.
Access: Cars drop passengers at entrance
to Arches in Villiers Street (40m. on flat).
Taxis can also be called to this spot. Route
to Entrance is level: Main entrance
accessible, although with manual door:
Interior doors 75cm wide and corridors
120cm: Adapted unisex WC on entrance
level (Access to three dispersed designated
wheelchair spaces with companion spaces
adjacent, through front entrance. Level
access Restaurant and Bar.

THE PLAYHOUSE
Northumberland Avenue WC2N 5DE
Tel: (020) 7839 4401
Fax: (020) 7839 1195

PRINCE EDWARD
Old Compton Street W1V 6HS
Tel: (020) 7447 5400

ROYAL COURT THEATRE DOWNSTAIRS
(Duke of York's)
St. Martin's Lane WC2N 9HN
Tel: (020) 7565 5000
Fax: (020) 7565 5001

SAVOY
The Strand WC2R 0ET
Tel: (020) 7836 8888

VICTORIA PALACE
Victoria Street SW1E 5EA
Tel: (020) 7834 1317

SPORTING VENUES

ARSENAL FOOTBALL CLUB
Arsenal Stadium, Highbury, London N5 1BU
Tel: (020) 7704 4000   Fax: (020) 7704 4001
www.arsenal.co.uk
Booking: as above.
CP 🚶 (Elwood Street)   RE ♿   ED ♿   INT ♿
L ♿   WC ♿ (10 units in various locations)
SS ♿ (Direct access to enclosure)   B/R 🚶

ALL ENGLAND LAWN TENNIS AND CROQUET CLUB (WIMBLEDON)
Church Road, Wimbledon, London SW19 5AE
Tel: (020) 8944 1066   Fax: (020) 8947 8752
Booking: Only by public Ballot
Facility complies with Part M, Building
Regulations. 'Wheelchair Users Guide to
the Championships' brochure available.
Wheelchair spaces: Centre & No. 1 Courts – ticket holders
only. Courts 6, 13, 14, 15, 18, 19 – unreserved space.
CP ♿   RE ♿   ED (On-the-day sales) ♿
L ♿   WC ♿ (5 units)   SS 🚶   B/R 🚶

WEST HAM UNITED FOOTBALL CLUB
Boleyn Ground, Green Street, Upton Park,
Plaistow, London E13 9az
Admin. & Box Office: Tel: (020) 8548 2748
Fax: (020) 8548 2758
www.westhamunited.co.uk
Complies with Part M, Building Regulations
CP ♿   RE ♿   ED ♿ (except door non-
automatic)   INT ♿   L ♿   WC ♿
SS ♿ (5 separate wheelchair locations)   B/R 🚶

WIMBLEDON FOOTBALL CLUB
Selhurst Park Stadium, South Norwood,
London SE25 6PY
Tel: (020) 8771 2233   Fax: (020) 8768 0641
Booking: Tel: (020) 8777 8841
Fax: (020) 8653 4708
Tailor made area, Holmesdale Stand with
steward on duty.
CP ♿   ED ♿   WC 🚶 (2 sites within disabled area)
SS ♿   B/R ♿

193

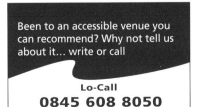

Been to an accessible venue you
can recommend? Why not tell us
about it... write or call

Lo-Call
0845 608 8050

MANCHESTER (GREATER)

GREATER MANCHESTER COALITION OF DISABLED PEOPLE (GMCDP)
Aked Close, Ardwick, Manchester, M12 4AN
Tel: (0161) 273 5154

GREATER MANCHESTER CENTRE FOR VOLUNTARY ORGANISATIONS
St.Thomas Centre, Ardwick Green North,
Manchester M12 6FZ
Tel: (0161) 2771000

BOLTON
Fine industrial heritage and Victorian architecture situated in the lee of the West Pennine Moors, with excellent shopping, large selection of mill shops and diverse range of attractions.

TOURIST INFORMATION CENTRE
Town Hall, Victoria Square, Bolton BL1 1RU
Tel: (01204) 334400 Fax: (01204) 398101
www.explore.destinationmanchester.com

HOTEL
BOLTON MOAT HOUSE
1 Higher Bridge Street, Bolton BL1 2EW
Tel: (01204) 879988 Fax: (01204) 380777
No. of Accessible Rooms: 2
Accessible Facilities: Lounge, Restaurant, Lift, Pool, Sauna, Spa. Premier hotel set within former church in heart of town centre. Promotes welcome to wheelchair users travelling independently.

MANCHESTER
Fast becoming one of the UK's most dynamic cities with a rich combination of arts, entertainment, heritage, leisure activities and shopping.

TOURIST INFORMATION CENTRE
Town Hall Extension, Lloyd Street,
Manchester M60 2LA
Tel: (0161) 234 3157 Fax: (0161) 236 9900

COMMUNITY RESOURCES DEPARTMENT,
9 Portland Street, Piccadilly Gardens,
Manchester M60 1HX
Tel: (0161) 242 6243
Produces comprehensive Rough Guide for people with disabilities, covering Central Greater Manchester and surrounding area.

BUSES
GMPTE enquiry line: Tel: (0161) 2287811 - (textphone available)
Some low-floor buses.
Metrolink: tel: (0161) 2052000
Fully accessible trams and every stop is wheelchair accessible.

TAXIS
Taxi Licensing officer: Tel: (0161) 2344956
Mantax: Tel: (0161) 2303333
702 adapted vehicles.

TRAINS
First North Western: Special Needs:
Tel: (0845) 6040231
Virgin Trains: Special Needs:
Tel: (0845) 7443366
Minicom: (0845) 7443367
Wales & West: Special Needs:
Tel: (0845) 3003005
Minicom: (0845) 7585469
Piccadilly Station: Tel: (0345) 697275
Victoria Station: (0845) 6040231

CAR PARKS
Free unlimited parking in pay and display car parks:
Tel: (0161) 234 4039

SHOPMOBILITY
Unit 129, Market Way, Upper Mall, Arndale Centre, Manchester M4 2EA
Tel: (0161) 839 4060   Fax: (0161) 839 5110

HOTELS
COPTHORNE MANCHESTER
Clippers Quay, Salford Quays,
Manchester M5 2XP
Tel: (0161) 873 7321 Fax: (0161) 873 7318
No. of Accessible Rooms: 1. Bath
Accessible Facilities: Lounge, Restaurant. Modern hotel with fine waterfront location in unique setting of Salford Quays.

RENAISSANCE MANCHESTER
Blackfriars Street, Manchester M3 2EQ
Tel: (0161) 835 2555 Fax: (0161) 833 0731
No. of Accessible Rooms: 2. Bath
Accessible Facilities: Lounge, Restaurant,
Bar. Quality city centre hotel, modern and
bright with large bedrooms.

**LE MERIDIEN VICTORIA & ALBERT
HOTEL**
Water Street, Manchester M3 4JQ
Tel: (0161) 832 1188 Fax: (0161) 834 2484
No. of Accessible Rooms: 2. Bath
Accessible Facilities: Lounge, Restaurant.
Listed building of mellowed brickwork and
exposed beams, standing on banks of River
Irwell.

NOVOTEL MANCHESTER WEST
Worsley Brow, Worlsey, Manchester
M28 2YA
Tel: (0161) 799 3535 Fax: (0161) 703 8207
No. of Accessible Rooms: 2. Bath
Accessible Facilities: Lounge, Restaurant,
Pool. Modern hotel located west of city
near M62.

**RADISSON SAS HOTEL
MANCHESTER AIRPORT**
Chicago Avenue, Manchester M90 3RA
Tel: (0161) 490 5000 Fax: (0161) 490 5095
www.radisson.com/manchester
No. of Accessible Rooms: 18. Roll-in
Shower. Accessible Facilities: Lounge,
Restaurant. Situated between Terminals 1
and 2 and the railway station and directly
connected to these by a Skylink walkway.

CROWNE PLAZA THE MIDLAND
Peter Street, Manchester M60 2DS
Tel: (0161) 236 3333 Fax: (0161) 9324100
No. of Accessible Rooms: 1. Bath
Accessible Facilities: Lounge (ramped),
Restaurants (2 of 3 -Nico's not accessible),
Health Centre (Pool-2 steps).
Large, quality hotel of grand Edwardian
architecture, built in 1903, in city centre.
Venue of first meeting between Messrs
Rolls and Royce in 1904.

JURYS MANCHESTER INN
56 Great Bridgewater Street,
Manchester M1 5LE

Tel: (0161) 9538888 Fax: (0161) 9539090
e-mail: enquiry@jurys.com
www.jurys.com
City centre location

**MANCHESTER AIRPORT
MOATHOUSE**
Altrincham Road, Wilmslow SK9 4LR
Tel: (01625) 889988 Fax: (01625) 531876
No. of Accessible Rooms: 2
Accessible Facilities: Lounge, Restaurant.
Conveniently situated for the Airport
and M6.

THISTLE MANCHESTER
Portland Street, Manchester M1 6DP
Tel: (0161) 2283400 Fax: (0161) 2286347
e-mail: sales.manchester@thistle.co.uk
No. of Accessible Rooms: 1. Roll-in
shower
Accessible Facilities: Lounge, Restaurant
Quality hotel in central location

ATTRACTIONS
GREATER MANCHESTER
THE LOWRY
The Lowry Centre, West Pavilion, Harbour
City, Manchester M5 2BH
Tel: (0161) 955 2032   Fax: (0161) 955 2021
e-mail: info@thelowry.org.uk
www.thelowry.com
Waterfront complex in Salford Quays with
1650 seat Lyric theatre, gallery to present
works by L S Lowry, children's hands-on
gallery, national industrial centre for
virtual reality. There are 3 manual and 1
motorised wheelschairs available for free
hire. These can be booked through the
Box Office on 0161 876 2000. There are
13 designated parking spaces but visitors
are advised to inform the booking office
of their requirements when booking
theatre tickets to ensure all seating
requirements are met.

MUSEUM OF TRANSPORT
Boyle Street, Cheetham, Manchester M8 8UL
Tel/Fax: (0161) 2052122
Travel through the ages here with over 70
buses and other vehicles from the city's past.

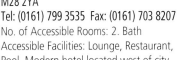

THE PUMP HOUSE:
PEOPLE'S HISTORY MUSEUM

The Pump House, Bridge Street,
Manchester M3 3ER
Tel: (0161) 839 6061
Fax: (0161) 839 6027

The Museum houses the galleries of the
National Museum of Labour History, and
tells the story of the ordinary people of
Britain and how they organised together to
change society. Displays and
reconstructions recreate day to day lives.

SD 🚶 CP 🚶 E 🚶 C ♿
S ♿ WC 🚶 L ♿

TRAFFORD ECOLOGY PARK

Lake Road, Trafford Park,
Manchester M17 1TU
Tel: (0161) 873 7182 Fax: (0161) 876 0523

SD ♿ CP 🚶♿ E ♿ C & S n/a WC 🚶

50% of the park is grass covered making
chair movement difficult in places.

Sensory Garden ♿   Picnic Area 🚶
Bird Hide 🚶♿   Bee observation Hide ♿
Ponds 🚶

MANCHESTER CITY ART GALLERY

Mosley Street, Manchester M2 3JL
Tell: (0161) 234 1456 Fax: (0161) 236 7369

New gallery is fully accesible with ramps
throughout and lifts to all floors.

THEATRE
MANCHESTER OPERA HOUSE

Quay Street, Manchester M3 3HP
Tel: (0161) 8341787   Fax: (0161) 834 5243

SD 🚶
CP 🚶 Nearest Public CP: Haldman Street
Nearest Taxi Rank: Byron Street.
RE ♿   ED 🚶♿
INT 🚶 Box Office Counter widths 🚶
WC 🚶   AUD ♿

STOCKPORT

Originally a market centre with its own
bridge across the River Mersey in the
C13th, it developed during the
Industrial Revolution. There are mills,
great chimneys and a fine C19th
railway viaduct.

The Manchester Opera House. Built when cotton was king.

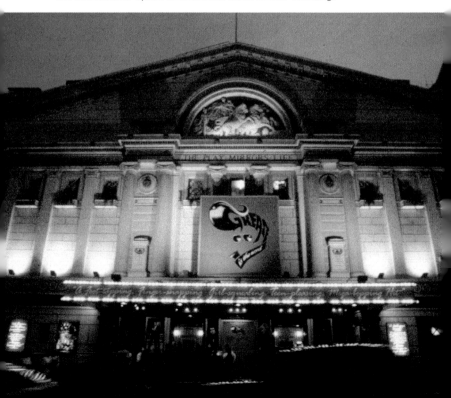

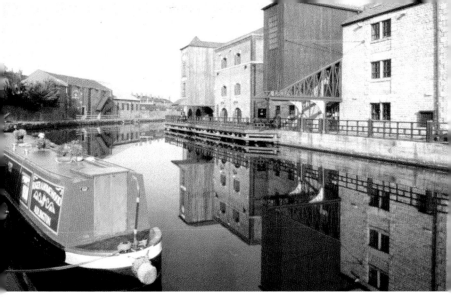

Wigan Pier on the Leeds & Liverpool Canal.

TOURIST INFORMATION CENTRE
Graylaw House, Chestergate,
Stockport SK1 1NH
Tel: (0161) 4743320/3321
Fax: (0161) 4296348

BUSES
GMPTE: Tel: (0161) 2287811
All information on local bus &
train services.

TAXIS
Rank at railway station
1919 Taxis: Tel: (0161) 4941919
1 adapted minibus
Metro Taxis: Tel: (0161) 4773633
6 adapted vehicles
Teletaxis: tel: (0161) 4804864
50 adapted vehicles including minibuses
with tail lifts.

TRAINS
First North Western: Special Needs:
Tel: (0845) 6040231
Wales & West: Special Needs:
Tel: (0845) 3003005
Minicom: (0845) 7585469

CAR PARKS
Disabled badge parking provided both on-
and-off-street.
Tel: (0161) 480 4949

SHOPMOBLITY
Level 2, Merseyway Car Park,
Stockport SK1 1PD
Tel: (0161) 6661100   Fax: (0161) 6661101

HOTELS
THE SAXON HOLME
230 Wellington Road North, Stockport SK4 2QN
Tel: (0161) 432 2335   Fax: (0161) 431 8076
No. of Accessible Rooms: 29. Shower
Family owned hotel on outskirts of town
within easy reach of the Peak District,
North Wales, Lakes and Yorkshire Dales
(close to Chatsworth, Styal and Lyme Hall)

COUNTY HOTEL
Bramhall Lane, South Bramhall,
Stockport SK7 2EB
Tel: (0161) 4559988   Fax: (0161) 4408071
No. of Accessible Rooms: 1
Accessible Facilities: Lounge, Restaurant.
Modern and comfortable property located
in village of Bramhall, a few miles from
Stockport, in pleasant countryside.

WIGAN
Interesting blend of picturesque
countryside and hidden villages, award
winning shopping centres and some
heritage and culture. Originally
important for its coal production.

TOURIST INFORMATION CENTRE
Trencherfield Mill, Wallgate,
Wigan WN3 4EL
Tel/Fax: (01942) 825677

HOTEL
WIGAN/STANDISH MOAT HOUSE 🚹
Almond Brook Road, Standish,
Nr. Wigan WN6 0SR
Tel: (01257) 499988
Fax: (01257) 427327
No. of Accessible Rooms: 2. Bath
Accessible Facilities: Reception, Lounge,
Restaurant, Bar (2 steps)
Modern, light and airy property within
easy reach of Manchester and Blackpool.

ATTRACTION
WIGAN PIER 'The Way we Were' MUSEUM
Wallgate, Wigan WN3 4EU
Tel: (01942) 323666
Fax: (01942) 322031
Recreation of Lancashire life at the turn
of the century through series of set and
exhibits. On 3 floors with passenger lift. 8
wheelchairs available. The Engine Room
in Trencherfield Mill houses world's
largest original mill steam engine is
accessed by lift. Waterbuses around the
Pier complex offer wheelchair lifts on
'Emma' and 'Netta' but with Pier
wheelchairs only. Canal-side towpaths
are not accessible. Useful Access leaflet.
SD 🚽 CP 👨‍🦽 E 🚽 RF 🚽 L 👨‍🦽
WC 🚹

WIGAN PIER 'Museum of Memories'
Address as above.
Opened in May 1999, this is a visual
journey through Wigan's social history
from Victorian times to present day. Recreation of shops and evocative displays,
all aspects of daily life are explored.
SD n/a CP 🚽 E 🚽 RF 🚹 C 🚹
S 🚽 WC 🚹

WIGAN COUNTRYSIDE SERVICES
1-3 Worlsey Terrace, Standish Gate, Wigan
Tel: (01942) 828906
Accessible countryside.
Pennington Flash. Tel: (01942) 605253
Turn of the century mining subsidence
and flooding now developed in park with
180 acre lake focal point surrounded by
wetland, attracting many bird species.
Ramped bird hides placed around well-
maintained circular footpath. Paths are
double width for wheelchair access, but in
some parts a pusher needed.
Very accessible.

Leeds-Liverpool Canal
Tel: (01942) 242239
Part of Wigan's industrial heritage, the
canal and locks provide varied scenery.
Blocked paved stretches provide good
surfaces although some gradients around
the locks need pusher. Top Lock at New
Springs well worth a visit.
Assistance required in places.

The Three Sisters
Tel: (01942) 720453
Reclaimed from 3 huge colliery tips, this
recreation area offers family fun.
Accessible footpath encircling lake.
Very accessible.

NORFOLK

NORFOLK DISABILITY INFORMATION SERVICE
The Vauxhall Centre, Johnson Place,
Vauxhall Street, Norwich NR2 2SA
Tel: (01603) 763295
Fax: (01603) 610632
e-mail: heather.davy.socs@norfolk.gov.uk
NDIS newsletter published regularly.

CASTLE ACRE
Conservation village 4 miles north of
Swaffham. Straddled by ancient
Roman road, the Peddlars Way, with
C15th church, the village has two EH
sites: ruins of C11th castle built by son
in law of William the Conqueror, and
remains of C12th Cluniac priory. Full
of Restaurants, pubs, antique and
craft shops.

SELF-CATERING
CHERRY TREE COTTAGE
Wellington House, Back Lane, Castle Acre,
Kings Lynn PE32 2AR
Tel/Fax: (01760) 755000
e-mail: boswell@paston.co.uk
No of Accessible Units: 1. Roll-in Shower
No. of Beds per Unit: 6 but disabled
access room is a single.
Accessible Facilities: Lounge, Dining Room,
Kitchen. One of a pair of traditional
Norfolk brick and flint cottages of C19th
on the periphery of the village.

CROMER
Victorian seaside town, once a
renowned port with the tower of St.
Peter & St. Paul standing 55m tall.

TOURIST INFORMATION CENTRE
Cromer Bus Station, Prince of Wales Road,
Cromer NR27 9HS
Tel: (01263) 512497

HOTEL
ROMAN CAMP INN
Holt Road, Aylmerton, Nr. Cromer NR11 5QD
Tel: (01263) 838291   Fax: (01263) 837071
www.romancampinn.co.uk
No. of Accessible Rooms: 2. Shower
Accessible Facilities: Lounge, Conservatory
Restaurant, Landscaped Gardens.
Fine old fashioned rural inn atmosphere,
with lovely gardens, located between
Sheringham and Cromer, close to Norfolk's
highest point, Beacon Hill.

DEREHAM
Busy market town originally established
as a religious community by the
daughter of a Saxon king. It has a
Grade II listed windmill and a quaint
local history museum housed in the
C16th Bishop Bonner's cottages.

SELF-CATERING
MOOR FARM STABLE COTTAGES
Moor Farm, Foxley, Dereham NR20 4QN
Tel/Fax: (01362) 688523

www.moorfarmcottages.com
e-mail: moorfarm@aol.com
No. of Accessible Units: 2. Shower
No. of Beds per Unit: 2
Accessible Facilities: Lounge, Dining Room,
kitchen, 2 , of 7 converted stable cottages
a courtyard. Situated on a working farm in
village between Fakenham and Dereham.

ATTRACTION
NORFOLK RURAL LIFE MUSEUM
Gressenhall Hall, Dereham NR20 4DR
Tel: (01362) 860563
200 years of Norfolk's rural history with
displays which include a typical farm
labourer's home at the turn of the century,
a working farm with machinery used
before the age of the tractor and farm trail
and woodland.

SD	CP	E	RF
C	S	L	WC
			RFE

DISS

ATTRACTION
BRESSINGHAM STEAM MUSEUM TRUST & GARDENS
Bressingham, Diss IP22 2AB
Tel: (01379) 687386   Fax: (01379) 686907
Gardens: The steam trains run through 2.5
miles of Europe's largest hardy plant
nursery. The Dell Garden has wonderful
species of perennials and alpines: Foggy
Bottom has panoramas, pathways, trees
and shrubs. Trains: Entrance and area for
40m beyond are level: thereafter the site
sits on gentle gradient of 1:55. The
features of the site include 3 ramps: 1) over
level crossing, avoidable by path around
outside of adjacent building): 2) Ramp to
another level crossing of 1:20: 3) Ramp up
from same level crossing of 1:10. Ramps 2
and 3 lead to the gardens. Level crossings
themselves are smooth. The Nursery
Railway, the main railway feature, has
specially converted carriage to carry
wheelchairs and boarding is via a wide and
level gangplank. The miniature Garden
railway is not accessible. All the railways
can be watched easily from almost
anywhere on the site.

SD	CP	E	RF
C	S	WC	RFE

FAKENHAM

Thriving market town in lovely countryside. Famous for one of finest National Hunt courses in the country.

TOURIST INFORMATION CENTRE
Red Lion House, Market Place, Fakenham
Tel: (01328) 851981

SPORTING VENUE
FAKENHAM RACEOURSE
Fakenham NR21 7NY
Admin & Booking-Box Office:
(01328) 862388   Fax: (01328) 855908

CP [♿]   RE [♿]   ED [♿]   INT [♿]
WC [♿]   B/R [♿]

GREAT YARMOUTH

Situated where three Rivers, the Bure, Waveney and Yare, converge to find their way into the North Sea, this watery surrounding gives the town a character similar to that of Dutch and Flemish cities. Busy harbour, market town and popular seaside resort.

HOTELS
HORSE & GROOM MOTEL   [♿]
Main Road, Rollesby, Gt. Yarmouth
NR29 5ER
Tel: (01493) 740624   Fax: (01493) 740022
No. of Accessible Rooms: 1. Bath
Accessible Facilities: Restaurant.
Located 6 miles from Gt. Yarmouth.

BURLINGTON & PALM COURT HOTELS   [♿]
North Drive, Great Yarmouth NR30 1EG
Tel: (01493) 844568   Fax: (01493) 331848
No. of Accessible Rooms: 5. Bath
Accessible Facilities: Lounge, Restaurant, Pool (3 steps). Family owned and managed adjacent hotels facing the seafront.

ATTRACTION
THRIGBY HALL WILDLIFE GARDENS
Thrigby, Great Yarmouth NR29 3DR
Fax: (01493) 368256   Tel: (01493) 369477
e-mail: mail@thrigbyhall.co.uk
www.thrigbyhall.co.uk

Home to the animals of Asia. Tropical bird house, blue willow-patterned garden, tree walk and summerhouse. Jungle swamp hall has underwater viewing of crocodiles.

SD [♿]   CP [♿]   E [♿]   RF [♿]   C [♿]
S [♿]   WC [♿]   RFE [♿]

HOLT

Site of the famous Greshams School, founded in 1555, the town has pleasant buildings.

TOURIST INFORMATION CENTRE
3 Pound House, Market Place, Holt
Tel: (01263) 713100

HOTEL
THE PHEASANT HOTEL   [♿]
The Coast Road, Kelling, Nr. Holt NR25 7EG
Tel: (01263) 588382   Fax: (01263) 588101
e-mail: stay@hotel-pheasant.co.uk
www.hotel-pheasant.co.uk
No. of Accessible Rooms: 5. Bath
Accessible Facilities: Lounge, Restaurant.
Attractive country hotel situated on the coast road in a delightful setting, midway between Blakeney and Sheringham.

ATTRACTION
THE MUCKLEBURGH COLLECTION
Weybourne Military Camp, Weybourne,
Holt NR25 7EG
Tel: (01263) 588210
Fax: (01263) 588425
www.muckleburgh.co.uk
The UK's largest privately owned collection of large military collection with 3000 exhibits including restored tanks and artillery of WWII, Falklands and Gulf War equipment and model displays and dioramas, and much more.

SD [♿]   CP [♿]   E [♿]   RF [♿]
C [♿]   S [♿]   WC [♿]

HORNING

Well-known Broadland centre on River Bure, with picturesque cottages and attractive glimpses of the River from the main street.

SELF-CATERING
LADY LODGE
HORNING LODGES 1, 2 & 3
KINGS LINE CRUISES
Ferry Road, Horning, Norwich NR12 8PT
Tel/Fax: (01692) 630297
e-mail: kingline@norfolk-broads.co.uk
www.norfolk-broads.co.uk
No. of Accessible Units: 5
Lady Lodge facilities: wheel in access/roll-in shower/lateral transfer to toilet/1:12 ramp to building. One double and 2 single.
Horning 1 & 2:
Facilities: Roll-in shower/no lateral transfer/extra wide doors/1:15 ramps (1) one double, 2 singles (2) 4 singles, 1 double.
Horning 3:
Facilities: Extra wide door, 1:15 ramp,lateral transfer to toilet,separate roll-in shower, four singles, 1 double.
Eagle Cottage:
Facilities: Extra wide doors, 3 accessible toilets, 1 roll-in shower, five single, 2 double.
N.B. Majority of beds are extra large.
Family owned and operated cottages on Norfolk Broads. Superb location with frontage on the River Bure, about 10 miles from Norwich.
A new all electric day boat is available for hire with electric hoist, accommodating 11 people including three wheelchairs.

HORSEY
Only a barrier of sand dunes separates this Broad from the North Sea, and the seepage of seawater makes this the most brackish of all the Norfolk Broads. As a result, bird and insect life is particularly interesting.

HUNSTANTON
Facing into the Wash, on the west coast of Norfolk, there is a vast shingle and sand beach backed by cliffs. Much of the town is Victorian, built simultaneously with the railway line.

TOURIST INFORMATION CENTRE
Green, Hunstanton PE36 6BQ
Tel: (01485) 532610

HOTEL
GOLDEN LION HOTEL
The Green, Hunstanton PE36 6BQ
Tel: (01485) 532688 Fax: (01485) 535310
No. of Accessible Rooms: 3. Shower
Accessible Facilities: Lounge, Restaurant
Hunstanton's oldest building, constructed in 1846 of red brick and recently refurbished, is the hub of much of Hunstanton's social activity.

ATTRACTION
NORFOLK LAVENDER
Caley Mill, Heacham, Nr. Hunstanton
PE31 7JE
Tel: (01485) 570384
Fax: (01485) 571176
e-mail: admin@norfolk-lavender.co.uk
Caley Mill, originally a water mill for grinding corn, and now set in the Lavender Gardens, which hold the National Collection of Lavenders. Each of the 50 variety or species has its own bed. Also Herb Garden, Fragrant Meadow Garden and Plant Centre.

| SD | ♿ | CP | ♿ | E | ♿ | RF | ♿ |
| C | ♿ | S | 🚶 | WC | 🚶 | RFE | ♿ |

KING'S LYNN
Originally a walled city of considerable importance, much of the wall remains in this busy town, seaport and agricultural centre.

TOURIST INFORMATION CENTRE
The Custom House, Purfleet Quay, Kings Lynn PE30 1HP
Tel: (01553) 763044

HOTEL
FFOLKES ARMS HOTEL
Lynn Road, Hillington, King's Lynn PE31 6BJ
Tel: (01485) 600210 Fax: (01485) 601196
No. of Accessible Rooms: 10. Roll-in Shower
Accessible Facilities: Lounge, Restaurant.
Constructed over 300 years ago, the hotel

201

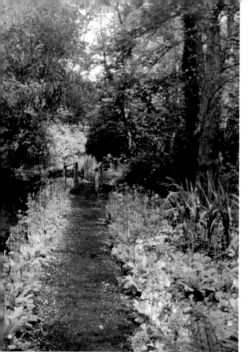

*Fairhaven Woodland and
Water Gardens.*

became well known as a coaching inn, and has been completely modernised without losing any of its original charm. Located 6 miles from nearest town or railway station.

SELF-CATERING
PARK COTTAGE
Narford Road, Narborough,
King's Lynn PE32 1HZ
Tel: (01760) 337220
No. of Accessible Units: 1
Accessible Facilities: garden
Peaceful Bungalow in 3 acres of garden and woodland in village near town.

NORTH WALSHAM
Located between Cromer and Great Yarmouth.

TOURIST INFORMATION CENTRE
Brentnall House, 32 Vicarage Street,
North Walsham NR28 9DQ
Tel: (01692) 407509

SELF-CATERING
DAIRY FARM COTTAGES
Manor Farm, Dilham,
North Walsham NR28 9PZ
Tel: (01692) 536883
Fax: (01692) 536723
e-mail: JAPdilman@farmline.com
No. of Accessible Units: 2
No. of Beds per Unit: 4. Roll-in Shower
Accessible Facilities: Kitchen/Living area combined. 2 of 6 cottages converted from farm buildings, facing south across large grassed area. Each has a patio. Small traditional farm in peaceful rural setting, surrounded by woodland. Dilham is in the heart of the Norfolk Broads, 5 miles from North Walsham.

NORWICH
The capital of Norfolk, a beautiful city developed by a large double bend in the River Wensum and within its medieval walls. Its lack of industrialisation and geographical position have help to preserve many of the city's older buildings, with Colman's mustard the only large industrial company here. It is hilly and the Saxon street layout is disorientating but the landmarks of Cathedral and Norman castle stand out.

TOURIST INFORMATION CENTRE
The Forum, Millenium Plain, Norwich
NR2 1TF
Tel: (01603) 727927 Fax: (01603) 765389
e-mail: tourism@norwich.gov.uk
www.norwich.gov.uk

NORWICH ACCESS GROUP
34 Neville Street
Norwich
NR2 2PR
Tel/Fax: (01603) 413485

BUSES
Bus Information Centre: Tel: (0500) 626116
Publishes information on services and park & ride.

TAXIS
Rank at station
Express Taxis: Tel: (01603) 767626
20 adapted vehicles.

TRAINS
Anglia Railways: Assistance:
Tel: (01473) 693333
Minicom: (0845) 6050600

CAR PARKS
Car Park services: Tel: (01603) 212420

SHOPMOBILITY
2 Castle Mall, Norwich NR1 3DD
Tel: (01603) 766430

WHEELCHAIR HIRE
New Life: Tel: (01603) 623200
Sells and services wheelchairs.

HOTELS
ASHWELLTHORPE HALL HOTEL ♿
Ashwellthorpe, Norwich NR16 1EX
Tel: (01508) 489324 Fax: (01508) 488409
No. of Accessible Rooms: 6. Roll-in Shower
Accessible Facilities: Lounge, Restaurant,
Games & TV Rooms. 8 miles south of
Norwich, an Elizabethan manor house set
in 11 acres of easily accessible grounds.
Fully accessible and equipped for disabled
people, whilst maintaining hotel ambience
and suitable for non-disabled guests also.

THE BEECHES HOTEL ♿
2-6 Earlham Road, Norwich NR2 3DB
Tel: (01603) 621167 Fax: (01603) 620151
e-mail: reception@beeches.co.uk
No. of Accessible Rooms: 5 doubles, 1
twin, 3 singles with ground floor access.
Accessible Facilities: Lounge, Bar,Dining
Room. Set in a 3-acre garden 0.5 mile
from city centre.

THE OLD RECTORY 🚶
North Walsham Road, Crostwick,
Norwich NR12 7BG
Tel: (01603) 738513 Fax: (01603) 738712
No. of Accessible Rooms: 1.Bath
Accessible Facilities: Lounge, Restaurant,
Bar, Garden, Outdoor Pool.
Original building dates back to mid 18thC
to which 13 lovely rooms have been
added. Located 4 miles north of Norwich.

SELF-CATERING
THE HIDEAWAY 🚶
c/o Heath Bungalow, Woodbastwick Road,
Blofield Heath, Nr. Norwich NR15 4AB
Tel: (01603) 715052
No. of Accessible Units: 1. Shower
No. of Beds per Unit: 1
Accessible Facilities: Lounge, Dining
Room, Kitchen. Holiday flat adjoining
owner's home, in village about 7 miles
east of city centre on A27.

ATTRACTIONS
SAINSBURY CENTRE FOR VISUAL ARTS
University of East Anglia, Norwich NR4 7TJ
Tel: (01603) 593199
Fax: (01603) 259401
e-mail: scva.@uea.ac.uk
European art of 19th and 20thCs on
display together with African tribal
sculpture and North American and pre-
Colombian art. Antiquities from Egypt,
Asia and Europe also on show.

SD ♿   CP ♿   E ♿   RF ♿
L ♿   C 🚶   S ♿
WC ♿ (horizontal support rail 57cm from seat
centre.)
RFE ♿

THE FAIRHAVEN WOODLAND & WATER GARDEN
School Road, South Walsham,
Nr. Norwich NR13 6DZ
Tel/Fax: (01603) 270449
e-mail: fairhavengardens@norfolkbroads.com
www.norfolkbroads.com/fairhaven
Delightful gardens with splendid array of
shrubs and plants leading to private
Broad with boat trips. I visited in late
spring when rhododendrons and
candelabra primulas at their finest.
Extensive walks with wide paths are
grassy and solid earth. River launch
cruises around south Walsham Broads
from May till end of August. Although
boat staff happy to assist in swinging
from chair onboard, there is a ramp over
the 2 steps and handrail, ramp height
adjusted to tide and sufficient space
inside. There is a year round programme
of outdoor events, please telephone the
above number for details.

CP ♿   E - Direct access from CP
RF ♿   C ♿   S 🚶   WC 🚶
RFE ♿   BOAT ♿

FELBRIGG HALL (NT)
Felbrigg, Norwich NR11 8PR
Tel: (01263) 837444 Fax: 01263 837032
Fine C17th house with outstanding library and Grand Tour paintings. Restored walled garden with small orchard. Park of fine trees.

SD   CP   E   RF
C   S   WC

SANDRINGHAM

Famous for Sandringham House, residence of the Royal Family. The estates are extensive and include several parishes and farms, woodlands and other agricultural activities.

HOTEL
PARK HOUSE
Sandringham, PE35 6EH
Tel: (01485) 543000 Fax: (01485) 540663
No. of Accessible Rooms: All 16
Accessible Facilities: Lounge, Dining Room, Grounds (terraced patio, raised flower beds, wheelchair paths leading through trees), Outdoor Pool with hoist (May-Sept). Adapted Vehicles for area visits to places of interest. Birthplace and childhood home of the late Diana, Princess of Wales, this impressive Victorian country house is set in its own grounds amidst the trees and parkland of the Sandringham Royal Estate. Leased from Her Majesty the Queen by Leonard Cheshire, a leading disability care charity, and converted in a unique purpose-built

Royal retreat of Sandringham House.

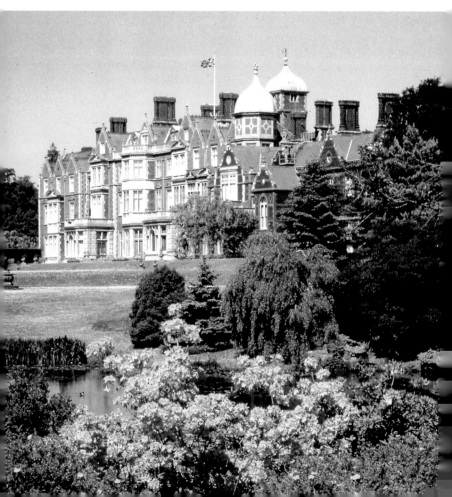

hotel for people with disabilities and their companions or carers.

ATTRACTION
SANDRINGHAM HOUSE, GROUNDS & MUSEUM
Estate office, Sandringham PE35 6EN
Tel: (01553) 772675
Fax: (01485) 541571
Norfolk country retreat of HM the Queen. The imposing house was built in 1870 and all main rooms used by the Royal Family are open to the public. The 60 acres of grounds are full of shrubs, trees and flowers and the museum contains exhibits of memorabilia of the Royal Family.

CP   E   RF   C
S   WC   RFE

SWAFFHAM
Elegant town, once a fashionable centre for the Norfolk gentry in the C18th. Today the triangular market place with its 'market cross' retains a number of fine Georgian houses.

TOURIST INFORMATION CENTRE
Market Place, Swaffham
Tel: (01760) 722255

BED & BREAKFAST
CORFIELD HOUSE
Sporle, Nr. Swaffham PE32 2EA
Tel: (01760) 723636
e-mail: corfieldhouse@virgin.net
www.corfieldhouse.co.uk
No. of Accessible Rooms: 1
Accessible Facilities: Lounge, Dining Room. Family run guest house in peaceful village of Sporle. Accessible room overlooks half-acre of gardens and open fields.

GLEBE BUNGALOW
8a Princes Street, Swaffham PE37 7BP
Tel: (01760) 722764
No. of Accessible Rooms: 3. Bath
Accessible Facilities: Dining Room, Garden, Patio. Situated on northern edge of the market town of Swaffham, a comfortable home.

SELF-CATERING
HALL BARN COTTAGES
Old Hall Lane, Beachamwell,
Nr. Swaffham PE37 8BG
Tel: (01366) 328794
No. of Accessible Units: 1
Accessible Facilities:
1 of 5 architect designed cottages created from C17th barn. Set in five acres of grounds, each cottage has its own terrace and shares a lovely walled garden. Cowslip Cottage has levelled and ramped access and stairlift to first floor.

THETFORD
Small market town on River Thet, centrally placed at the junction of eight main roads. Its most famous citizen was Thomas Paine, author of The Rights of Man written in 1791. A town full of interesting streets and buildings.

TOURIST INFORMATION CENTRE
Ancient House Museum,
21 White Hart Street, Thetford
Tel: (01842) 752599

HOTEL
POUND GREEN HOTEL
Pound Green Lane, Shipdham,
Thetford IP25 7LS
Tel: (01362) 820940
Fax: (01562) 821253
e-mail: poundgreen@aol.com
www.poundgreen.co.uk
No. of Accessible Rooms: 5. Bath
Accessible Facilities: Lounge, Restaurant. Recently refurbished, attractive property set in 1 acre of own grounds in peaceful village.

BED & BREAKFAST
JUNIPERS
18 South Street, Hockwold,
Nr. Thetford OP26 4JG
Tel: (01842) 827370
No. of Accessible Rooms: 1
Accessible Facilities: Dining Room
Spacious bungalow in walled half-acre garden in quiet village location.

UPPER SHERINGHAM

A village built on the hillside above the coastal strips. All Saints Church is mainly perpendicular with a fine C15th screen and overhang.

TOURIST INFORMATION CENTRE

Railway Approach, off Station Road, Sheringham NR26 8RA
Tel: (01263) 824329

BED & BREAKFAST

THE BAY LEAF GUEST HOUSE
10 Saint Peters Road, Sheringham NR26 8QY
Tel: (01263) 823779   Fax: (01263) 820041
No. of Accessible Rooms: 2
Accessible Facilities: Dining room
Delightful Victorian B & B in central location for amenities and seafront.

ATTRACTION

SHERINGHAM PARK (NT)
Upper Sheringham NR26 8TB
Tel/Fax: (01263) 823778
Woodland park of over 700 acres SW of the town designed by Humphry Repton, particularly notable for rhododendrons and azaleas in late spring. Stunning views of coast and countryside from viewing towers.
SD ☐   CP ☐   E ☐   RF ☐
C- Outside kiosk   WC ☐
RFE ☐ boarded walkway from car park to viewpoints.
Self-drive vehicle and wheelchair available on request when staff on duty in car park.

WALTON HIGHWAY

4 miles SW of Wisbech and 9 miles SW of King's Lynn, with much to do in the area.

BED & BREAKFAST/SELF-CATERING

STRATTON FARM B & B: Q S/C: W
West Drove North, Walton Highway
PE14 7DP
Tel: (01945) 880162
B & B: No. of Accessible Rooms: 1. Bath
Accessible Facilities: Lounge, Dining Room
S/C: No. of Accessible Units: 1. Bath

No. of Beds per Unit: 4
Accessible Facilities: Open Plan Kitchen/Diner, Lounge. Spacious farm bungalow and self-catering unit (Carysfort) set amidst 22 acres of grassland, grazed by Beef Shorthorn cattle. There is a lake.

WROXHAM

Busy yachting centre which has grown up on either side of River Bure. Wroxham Broad, although quite small, is very popular.

SELF-CATERING

BROOMHILL
Station Road, Hoverton, Wroxham
Book through Grooms Holidays
No. of Accessible Units: 2. Roll-in Shower
No. of Beds per Units: 8
Accessible Facilities: communal Garden. Quality apartments set in quiet village of Hoveton on Wroxham Broad, close to shops.

ATTRACTION

THE SARAH ROSE II
Book through Grooms Holidays
21m. long wide Beam Barge providing day trips or cruising holidays on the Norfolk Broads. She sleeps 8, has a hoist on board and shower with chair. Qualified Dept. of Transport Boat Master on board at all times. There are 2 lifts.

WYMONDHAM

A busy market town lying on the main London/Norwich road, subject to quite heavy traffic. Fine Abbey Church of St. Mary & St. Thomas of Canterbury. There are also several timbered houses and fascinating local inns.

ATTRACTION

WYMONDHAM HERITAGE MUSEUM
10 The Bridewell, Norwich Road,
Wymondham NR18 0NS
Tel: (01953) 600205

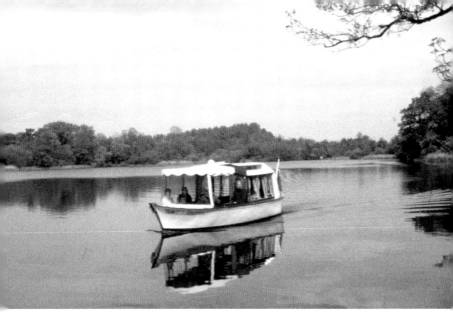

Messing around in boats on the Norfolk Broads.

The Bridwell was built in 1785 as a model prison after John Howard's instigation of the Prison Reform Acts 1782/85. This Museum tells the story of this historic building from original Elizabethan foundation to its "reformed" prison in 1785 and beyond. Also travel through Wymondham's growth. Excavation in rear garden is not accessible, but viewable from its edge.

SD   CP n/a   E   RF
C   S   WC

NORTHAMPTONSHIRE

NORTHAMPTONSHIRE COUNCIL FOR THE DISABLED PEOPLE
13 Hazlewood Road, Northampton NN1 1LG
Tel: (01604) 624088   Fax: (01604) 605124

KETTERING
An industrial town set in lovely countryside: of architectural interest are the Victorian and Edwardian buildings centred around the church, reached by narrow, twisting high street and large market place.

ATTRACTION
ALFRED EAST ART GALLERY
Sheep Street, Kettering NN16 0AN
Tel: (01536) 534381   Fax: (01536) 534370
Fine arts, crafts and photography in changing temporary exhibitions. Entrance to the Gallery is via the Library. Both are ground floor buildings connected by a corridor. Visitors can park by the Library front door and go directly in, although the road (tarmac) does slope slightly.

SD   CP    E

NORTHAMPTON
Large town merging into countryside with several interesting Victorian and Georgian buildings and probably the largest market square in England.

BUSES
Gas Bus: Tel: (01604) 751431
Some low floor buses.

TAXIS
Take 6 Taxis: Tel: (01604) 764678
2 adapted vehicles
Mayfair Taxis: Tel: (01604) 638888
12 adapted vehicles including minibus
Door to Door: Tel: (01604) 466669

TRAINS
Connex South Central & South Eastern:
Customer Services:
Tel: (0870) 6030405
Fax: (0870) 6030505 Minicom: (01233) 617621
www.connex.co.uk

CAR PARKS
Disabled badge holders park free up to 4 hours in short stay parks, all day in long term parks.
Tel: (01604) 238515

HOTEL ACCOMODATION
NORTHAMPTON MOAT HOUSE 　　🚶
Silver Street, Northampton NN1 2TA
Tel: (01604) 739988
Fax: (01604) 230614
No. of Accessible Rooms: 2
Accessible Facilities: Lounge, Restaurant
City centre hotel with smart public areas.

NORTHAMPTON MARRIOTT 　　🚶
Eagle Drive, Northampton NN4 7HW
Tel: (01604) 768700
Fax: (01604) 769011
No. of Accessible Rooms: 2. Bath
Accessible Facilities: Lounge, Restaurant.
Modern hotel on the edge of town.

THEATRE
THE ROYAL THEATRE
Guildhall Road, Northampton NN1 1EA
Admin: (01604) 638343
Fax (01604) 602408
Booking-Box Office: (01604) 632533
Minicom/Fax: (01604) 233095
Leaflet available on access.
　SD 🦽　CP 🚶 Nearest Public CP at St. Johns.
Nearest Taxi Rank: 200m.
　RE 🦽　ED 🚶　INT 🚶　WC 🚶
AUD 🦽　　B/R unknown
Stalls accessed by ramp into Royalties CafÈ-Bar and into Stalls.

NORTHANTS THEATRE, Derngate,
Northampton
Tel: (01604) 626222
Fax: (01604) 250901
Box Office: (01604) 624811
N.B. Book disabled spaces when making booking.

NORTHUMBERLAND

HADRIAN'S WALL TOURISM PARTNERSHIP
14b Gilesgate,Hexham NE46 3NJ
Tel: (01434) 602505
Fax: (01434) 601267
e-mail: info@hadrians-wall.org
www.hadrians-wall.org

ALNWICK
Narrow streets, cobblestones and passageways, sturdy grey buildings and monuments. Situated on the River Aln, there is also a fine castle, outwardly barely changed since the C14th.

TOURIST INFORMATION CENTRE
2 The Shambles, Alnwick NE66 1TN
Tel: (01665) 510665

SELF-CATERING
CRASTER PINE LODGES 　　🦽
9 West End, Craster, Alnwick NE66 3TS
Tel/Fax: (01665) 576286
No. of Accessible Units: 1. Roll-in Shower.
No. of Beds per Unit: 6
Accessible Facilities: Open plan Lounge/Kitchen. Located on edge of small village of Craster, near picturesque harbour.

VILLAGE FARM 　　🚶
Town Foot Farm, Shilbottle, Alnwick NE66 2XR
Tel/Fax: (01665) 575591
e-mail: crissy@villagefarm.demon.co.uk
www.villagefarm.demon.co.uk
No. of Accessible Units: 4
No. of Beds per Unit: 6/7
Accessible Facilities: all open plan Lounge/Kitchen/Diner.
Coquet Lodge: Danish chalet.
Pantile Cottage: old stone farm building.
Cedar & Pine Chalets: 4 of 8 units around C17th farmhouse with Scandinavian chalets and cosy cottages. 3 miles from Alnwick between A1 and Northumbrian coast.

BAMBURGH

No castle could look more imposing than Banburgh, a magnificent red sandstone mass, a startling sight from all approaches. The road takes motorists directly under its walls on the land side, whilst on the other it towers over the sea from a 50m precipice. The village itself is tiny, very close to two fine sandy beaches.

SELF-CATERING
POINT COTTAGES 🚶
39 The Wynding, Bamburgh NE69 7DD
Tel: (0191) 266 2800
Fax: (0191) 215 1630
No. of Accessible Units: 1
No. of Beds per Unit: 2 - 5
Accessible Facilities: Living Room, Open-plan Kitchenette. Shared Garden. Cluster of cottages in superb location at the end of the Wynding, next to a lovely golf course. Adjacent to, and overlooking sandy beaches with views to Lindisfarne and Bamburgh Castle.

BERWICK-UPON-TWEED

Originally Berwick was one of the 4 ancient Scots royal burghs, the largest town in Scotland and its greatest seaport. From 1296 it changed hands 14 times during 3 centuries of Anglo-Scots warfare. The only town in GB whose walls (Elizabethan) remain intact. At 8pm the curfew stills rings a reminder of the times when the town gates were securely locked at night.

TOURIST INFORMATION CENTRE
106 Marygate, Berwick upon Tweed
TD15 1BN
Tel: (01289) 330733

BED & BREAKFAST
MEADOW HILL GUEST HOUSE CAT2
Duns Road, Berwick-upon-Tweed TD15 1UB
Tel/Fax: (01289) 306325
e-mail: barryandhazel@meadow-hill.co.uk
www.meadow-hill.co.uk

No. of Accessible Rooms: 2.
Roll-in Shower
Accessible Facilities: Lounge, Dining Room. Approximately 170 yrs old, the house is situated on the edge of town at the foot of Halidon hill-site of the battle of 1333 when Edward lll took Berwick and re-drew the English/Scots border. Wonderful views of the River Tweed, to the east Berwick and across the coast to Lindisfarne and south to the Cheviots.

CORNHILL-ON-TWEED

HOTEL
THE COACH HOUSE ♿
Crookham, Cornhill-on-Tweed TD12 4TD
Tel: (01890) 820293
Fax: (01890) 820284
No. of Accessible Rooms: 3. Roll-in Shower
Accessible Facilities: Lounge, Dining Room. Warm stone building around an ancient courtyard.

GREENHEAD

SELF-CATERING
HOLMEAD FARM ♿
Hadrian's Wall, Greenhead,
Nr. Carlisle CA8 7HY
Tel: (016977) 47402
www.bandbhadrianswall.com
No. of Accessible Units: 1
No. of Beds per Unit: 4
Accessible Facilities: Open plan Lounge/Kitchen
On Hadrian's Wall, near Haltwhistle.

HEXHAM

Good base for exploring Hadrian's Wall, this is an attractive market town with a fine C11th Abbey.

TOURIST INFORMATION CENTRE
The Manor Office, Hallgate,
Hexham NE46 1XD
Tel: (01434) 605225

SELF-CATERING
CONHEATH COTTAGE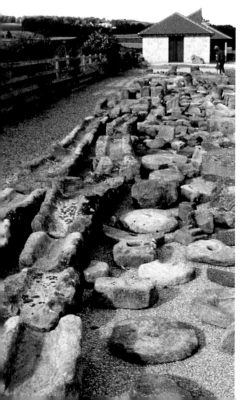
Blakelaw Farm, Bellingham,
Hexham NE48 2EF
Tel/Fax: (01434) 220250
No. of Accessible Units: 1. Bath
No. of Beds per Unit: 5
Accessible Facilities: Living room,
Kitchen/Diner, walled garden with
barbecue and furniture. Lovely stone semi-
detached holiday cottage in the North Tyne
Valley, 1.5 miles from Bellingham. Bed-
rooms are upstairs, accessed by stair lift.

GIBBS HILL FARM COTTAGES
Once Brewed, Bardon Mill,
Hexham NE47 7AP
Tel/Fax: (01434) 344030
No. of Accessible Units: 1
No. of Beds per Unit: 2
Stone cottages on working organic family
farm near Hadrian's Wall. Fine views and 5
minutes from main Roman sites.

Corbridge Roman archaeology site.

ATTRACTIONS
CHESTERS ROMAN FORT (EH)
Chollerford, Humshaugh,
Hexham NE46 4EP
Tel: (01434) 681379
Remains of a Fort built for 500
cavalrymen including 5 gateways,
barracks and fine military bath house.

SD | CP | E | RF 3
WC | RFE

CORBRIDGE ROMAN SITE (EH)
Corbridge NE45 5NT
Tel: (01434) 632349
Archaeological site with uneven loose
surfaces-access is limited. The Museum
is accessible. Wheelchair available.
Extensive remains include 2 large
granaries, strongroom, fountain house
and aqueduct.

SD | CP | E | RF | S
WC

KELSO
Situated in the Tweed Valley at
junction of Rivers Tweed and Teviot,
originally famous for its Abbey of
1128, now in poor state of ruin.
Attractive Square with neo-classical
town hall and 18th and 19thC pastel
buildings.

KELSO RACES
Office: 18-20 Glendale Road, Wooler NE71
6DW
Admin & Booking-Box Office: (01668)
281611 Fax: (01668) 281113
Facility complies with Part M, Building
Regulations

CP | RE | ED
WC (2 units, one in each enclosure)
SS | B/R

MORPETH
Attractive town in a U-shaped bend
of the River Wansbeck with plentiful
trees and parks. Gateway to the
moors, hills and coast of
Northumberland.

TOURIST INFORMATION CENTRE
The Chantry, Bridge Street,
Morpeth NE61 1PD
Tel: (01670) 500700

HOTELS
LINDEN HALL HOTEL & HEALTH SPA
Longhorsley, Morpeth NE65 8XF
Tel: (01670) 500001
Fax: (01670) 788544
No. of Accessible Rooms: 1. Roll-in shower.
Accessible Facilities: Lounge, Restaurant
Grade II listed Georgian country house
hotel set in 450 acres of private park and
woodland. Much of the interior has been
restored since it was built in 1812.

WHITTON FARMHOUSE HOTEL
Whitton, Rothbury, Morpeth NE65 7RL
Tel/Fax: (01669) 620811
No. of Accessible Rooms:1. Bath
Accessible Facilities: Lounge, Restaurant,
Bar. Built in 1829 in traditional
Northumbrian style, farmhouse and
buildings converted to charming small
hotel located on the edge of the
Northumberland National Park, overlooking
Coquet Valley.

THE SWAN
Choppington, Nr. Morpeth NE62 5TG
Tel: (01670) 826060
No. of Accessible Rooms: 1. Bath
Accessible Facilities: Restaurant,
Conservatory.

SELF-CATERING
DENE HOUSE FARM COTTAGES
Dene House Farm, Longframlington ,
Morpeth NE65 8EE
Tel: (01665) 570549
No. of Accessible Units: 4. Roll-in Shower
No. of Beds per Unit: 4
Accessible Facilities: Open plan
Lounge/Kitchen. (Only 1 kitchen
accessible). 4 cottages a mile from the
village designed for disabled access. It has
a new leisure facility. The swimming pool
is equipped with a hoist. There is also
tennis, golf driving range, gym, archery,
beauty therapy, holistic therapy, hairdresser
and physiotherapy. Previous Holiday Care
Award winner.

OAK & ELM COTTAGES
Beacon Hill Farm, Longhorsley,
Morpeth NE65 8QW
Tel/Fax: (01670) 788372
e-mail: alun@beacon-hill.demon.co
www.beacon-hill.demon.co.uk
No. of Accessible Units: 2. Bath, Shower.
No. of Beds per Unit: 1D 7 1T
Accessible Facilities: Open Plan Kitchen &
Lounge. Beacon Hill is a 350 acre farm
deep in unspoilt countryside between
Cheviot Hills and Northumbrian
coastline. There are 10 stone cottages
with gardens.

ATTRACTION
THE WHITEHOUSE FARM CENTRE
North Whitehouse Farm, Morpeth
Tel: (01670) 789998
Fax: (01670) 789113
www.whitehousefarmcentre.co.uk
A good day out for adults and children -
learn how a farm works, see guinea pigs,
rabbits, chicks, ducks and exotic animals.

SD | CP | E | RF
C | S | WC | RFE

PONTELAND
Located just NW of Newcastle
Airport, a small village.

ATTRACTION
BELSAY HALL, CASTLE & GARDENS (EH)
Belsay, Nr. Ponteland NE20 0DX
Tel: (01661) 881636
Fax: (01661) 881043
Neo-classical Regency hall which is
unfurnished. 30 acres of landscaped
gardens and C14th Castle. Long walk to
Castle through delightful woodland, with
some wheelchair adjusted paths, but
worth it even although Greek Revival Hall
and ground floor areas only are
accessible. Visited on damp June
morning, paths of fairly firm gravel.
Wheelchairs are available for free hire but
book in advance if there is an event on or
bank holiday.

SD | CP | E | RF
C | S | WC | RFE

211

PRUDHOE

Occupying a bank of the River Tyne, consisting mainly of long terraces of houses on steep river bank. Prudhoe Castle is situated on a wooded spur overlooking river. There is a legend that Prudhoe is connected to Bywell Castle – situated several miles away – by a special underground passage.

SPORTS/LEISURE/TOURIST INFORMATION CENTRE
PRUDHOE WATERWORLD
Front Street, Prudhoe NE42 5DQ
Tel: (01661) 833144
Fax: (01661) 833885
Lovely leisure pool. On Wednesday evenings there is "Be Able Disabled" session in the pool.

SD 🦽   CP 🦽   E 🦽   RF 🚶
C 🚶   S 🚶   RFE – Pool – Direct access via
Shower Chair into water via beach area.
WC – Dryside 🚶   Wetside 🦽

WARKWORTH

Village set in the loop of the River Coquet, a famous castle at its head. Used by Harry Hotspur, hero of the Battle of Otterbun in 1402, by Great Earl of Warwick in 1462 as a base to attack the Borders castles. The area has wonderful beaches and landscapes - northwards to Holy Island and the Farne Islands and to the west the Rolling Hills.

HOTEL
WARKWORTH HOUSE   🦽
16 Bridge Street, Warkworth NE65 0XB
Tel: (01665) 711276
Fax: (01665) 713323
No. of Accessible Rooms: 2. Roll-in Shower. Accessible Facilities: Lounge, Restaurant.
This hotel carries a specific brochure and map of its disabled ground floor rooms.
Built in 1830 and family owned, it is located in the village centre.

NOTTINGHAMSHIRE

EDWINDSTOW

Lying at the edge of spacious common, leading to Birklands and Bilhagh, two of the most beautiful parts of Sherwood Forest. Also close to Warsop on the River Maun, in whose church Robin Hood and Maid Marian are said to have been married.

ATTRACTION
SHERWOOD FOREST COUNTRY PARK & VISITOR CENTRE
Edwinstow NG21 9HN
Tel/Fax: (01623) 823202
View over 450 acres of Robin Hood's original forest with waymarked paths, including the famous Major Oak. VC shows exhibition on Robin Hood

SD 🦽   CP 🦽   E 🦽   RF 🦽 (Visitor Centre)
C 🦽   S 🦽   WC 🦽
RFE 🦽 (Major Oak-Robin Hood hiding place)

MANSFIELD

TOURIST INFORMATION CENTRE
Old Town Hall, Market Place,
Mansfield NG18 1HX
Tel: (01623) 427770

ATTRACTION
MANSFIELD MUSEUM & ART GALLERY
Leeming Street, Mansfield NG18 1NG
Tel: (01623) 463088
Fax: (01523) 412922
3 permanent galleries tell Mansfield's story through displays of natural, industrial and social history with examples of fine and decorative arts of local significance. Also temporary exhibitions.

SD 🦽   CP n/a   E 🦽   RF 🦽
L 🚶   C n/a   S 🚶   WC 🚶

NOTTINGHAM

Famous for its association with Robin Hood, C13th. outlaw, and for lace and (Boots has its HQ here) pharmacy, plus Luddites (pre-Union strikers). The Old Market Square remains the centre of the city, with the Lace Market close by. In 1840s the city introduced machined lace clothing and industry boomed until the end of WWI. There are Georgian and neo-classical buildings and Victorian warehouses.

TOURIST INFORMATION CENTRES
1-4 Smithy Row, Nottingham NG1 2BY
Tel: (0115) 9155330

County Hall, West Bridgford,
Nottingham NG2 7QP
Tel: (0115) 9773558   Fax: (0115) 9773886

BUSES
Nottingham City Transport:
Tel: (0115) 9503665
Some low floors, some raised kerbs
Park & Ride: Tel: (0115) 9240000 -
accessible to folding chairs.

TAXIS
City Cabs: Tel: (0115) 9701701
120 adapted vehicles
Royal Cabs: Tel: (0115) 9608608
123 adapted vehicles

TRAINS
Midland Mainline: Special Needs:
Tel: (0114) 2537654
Minicom: (0845) 7078051
Robin Hood Line Assisted Travel Line: Tel: (0345) 056027
All trains carry ramps, but cannot take all powered wheelchairs because of limited space.

CAR PARKS
Disabled badge spaces free for first 4 hours, thereafter chargeable - also some on-street parking.
Tel: (0115) 9158282

SHOPMOBILITY
Victoria Centre, off Woodborough Road,
Broad Marsh Centre, Nottingham.
Tel: (0115) 9153888
Fax: (0115) 9155377
e-mail:
building.control@nottinghamcity.gov.uk

HOTELS
SKYLARKS (Winged Fellowship)
Adbolton Lane, West Bridgford,
Nottingham NG2 5AU
Tel: (0115) 9820962   Fax: (0115) 9824920
No. of Accessible Rooms: 31. Roll-in Shower.
Accessible Facilities: Lounge, Dining Room, Bar, Indoor Pool, Rose Garden, Ornamental Pond. Purpose- built holiday accommodation located at city's edge, an ideal starting point for trips to Nottinghamshire and beyond.

HOLIDAY INN
Castle Marina Park, Nottingham NG7 1GX
Tel: (0115) 9935000   Fax: (0115) 9934000
No. of Accessible Rooms: 3 Deluxe, 22 others.
Accessible Facilities: Lounge, Restaurant. Award winning hotel near the castle on the new Marina.

THE NOTTINGHAM GATEWAY HOTEL
Nuthall Road, Nottingham NG8 6AZ
Tel: (0115) 9794949   Fax: (0115) 9794744
No. of Accessible Rooms: 5. Bath
Accessible Facilities: Lounge, Restaurant
Modern hotel located 3 miles from city centre in suburbs.

NOTTINGHAM MOAT HOUSE
Mansfield Road, Nottingham NG5 2BT
Tel: (0115) 9359988   Fax: (0115) 9691506
No. of Accessible Rooms: 1. Bath
Accessible Facilities: Lift (to accommodation on 1st floor), Lounge, Restaurant, Bars. Modern hotel north of city centre.

NOTTINGHAM ROYAL MOAT
HOUSE
Wollaton Street, Nottingham NG1 5RH
Tel: (0115) 9369988   Fax: (0115) 9475888
No. of Accessible Rooms: 2.

Accessible Facilities: Restaurants 2, Bars 2
Newly refurbished city centre hotel.

ATTRACTIONS

MUSEUM OF NOTTINGHAM LIFE
Brewhouse Yard, Castle Boulevard,
Nottingham NG7 1FB
Tel: (0115) 9153600   Fax: (0115) 9153601
Nestled in the rock beneath Nottingham
Castle, the museum is housed in a group
of 5 restored cottages built in 1675. It
presents a realistic glimpse of everyday
domestic and working life in the city during
the last 700 years. A number of interactive exhibits and wide variety of displays
are both enchanting and educational.
Behind the museum is a series of caves set
into the castle rock depicting WWII and
other displays. These are accessible with
fairly even brick floors.

SD �&   CP 👟&   E 👟&   RF 👟&
S �&   WC 🚶   RFE 👟&

NOTTINGHAM CASTLE MUSEUM
& ART GALLERY
Nottingham NG1 6EL
Tel: (0115) 9153700   Fax: (0115) 9153653
Interactive "Story of Nottingham" exhibition
on city's history in C17th building.

SD n/a   CP 👟&   E 👟&   RF 👟&

L 🚶   C &   S 🚶   WC 🚶

THEATRES

NOTTINGHAM PLAYHOUSE
Wellington Circus, Nottingham NG1 5AF
Admin: (0115) 9474361
Booking: Box Office: (0115) 9419419
Minicom: (0015) 9476100
Fax: (0115) 9241484
CP 🚶 (North Circus St., East Circus St., Wellington Circus)
RE &   ED &   INT &   L &
WC 👟&   AUD & From entrance foyer lift to level 1 -
enter stairs by side entrance on Row M where wheelchair
seating located.   B/R &

THEATRE ROYAL
Theatre Square, Nottingham NG1 5ND
Part of Royal Centre, which includes Royal
Concert Hall, also accessible.
Admin: (0115) 9895500
Booking: Box Office: (0115) 9895555
Minicom: (0115) 9470025
Fax: (0115) 9503476
CP 🚶 (Disabled bays on Burton Street).
RE &   ED & (except Manual Door)   INT &
WC 🚶 (good, except WC seat 51cm above floor).
AUD & (Stalls only - whole back row removed at
8.00pm).   Ends of all stalls rows A - V accessible for
wheelchair transfer.   B/R &

The views from Nottingham Castle are spectacular.

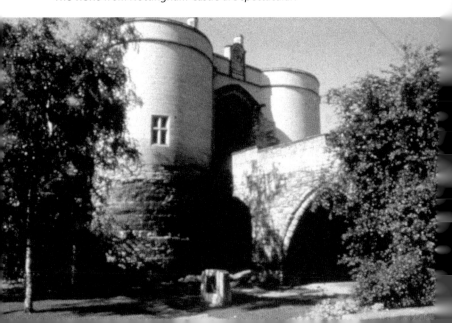

OLLERTON

17 miles north of Nottingham, a small mining town at the junction of the Rivers Rainworth-Water and Maun.

TOURIST INFORMATION CENTRE
Sherwood Heath, Ollerton Roundabout,
Ollerton NG22 9DR
Tel: (01623) 824545

ATTRACTION
RUFFORD COUNTRY PARK – ABBEY END
Ollerton NG22 9DF
Tel: (01623) 822944
NOTE: There are 2 entrances – take Abbey End, not Mill End. Rufford Abbey was founded as a Cistercian Monastery in C12th. After Dissolution of Monasteries in 1536, Rufford passed to private hands and picturesque remains are still standing. There are large areas of woodland and parkland, a craft centre in the former stable block, a Gallery with changing exhibitions and Britain's first Ceramics Centre.

SD ⬚ CP ⬚ E ⬚ RF ⬚ L ⬚
C ⬚ S ⬚ WC ⬚ RFE ⬚

SUTTON-IN-ASHFIELD

ATTRACTION
TEVERSAL VISITOR CENTRE
Carnarvon Street, Teversal,
Sutton-in-Ashfield NG17 3HJ
Tel: (01623) 442021
Displays on wildlife and industrial heritage of Pleasley Trails network, now designated as local Nature Reserves. The Trails themselves, tranquil, through lovely countryside, include the old village of Teversal, one of most unspoilt in the country and with connections with Lord Carnarvon of Tutankhamun fame and D.S. Lawrence's "Lady Chatterley's Love."
Of 6 trails, Areas 1,2,3 and part of 5 are accessible.
NB: Entrance ramped at 1:10.

SD ⬚ CP ⬚ E n/a RF ⬚ C ⬚
S ⬚ WC ⬚ RFE ⬚

WORKSOP

TOURIST INFORMATION CENTRE
Public Library, Memorial Avenue,
Worksop S80 2BP
Tel: (01909) 501148

ATTRACTION
CRESSWELL CRAGS VISITOR CENTRE
Crags Road, Welbeck, Worksop S80 3LH
Tel: (01909) 720378
Fax: (01909) 724726
e-mail: heritage@cresswell.co.uk
Caves and rock shelters of the crags were used by Stone Age hunters and artefacts now in visitor centre whose exhibition and audio-visual displays explain life in prehistoric times.

SD ⬚ CP ⬚ E ⬚ RF ⬚
S ⬚ WC ⬚ RFE ⬚

OXFORDSHIRE

ABINGDON

Lying near the water meadows of the River Thames where it is joined by the Little Ock, the town originally grew up around its Abbey and has some fine early timbered-framed houses and Georgian properties.

BED & BREAKFAST ACCOMMODATION
KINGFISHER BARN ⬚
Rye Farm, Culham, Abingdon OX14 3NN
Tel/Fax: (01235) 537538
e-mail: liz@kingfisherbarn.demon.co.uk
No. of Accessible rooms: 10. Bath
Accessible Facilities: C17th renovated barn with adjacent stable buildings offering wide selection of activities in rural setting.

BANBURY

Flourishing community with one of the oldest breweries in the country and many fine old houses remain plus twisted medieval streets.

TOURIST INFORMATION CENTRE

Banbury Museum, 8 Horsefair,
Banbury OX16 0AA
Tel: (01295) 259855   Fax: (01295) 270556

ATTRACTIONS

UPTON HOUSE (NT)
Nr. Banbury OX15 6HT
Tel: (01295) 670266
e-mail: vuplan@smtp.ntrust.org.uk
Impressive late C17th house remodelled
1927 for the 2nd Viscount Bearsted. Fine
painting collection includes El Greco,
Bruegel, Bosch, Hogarth and Stubbs. Wide
lawns and terraced herbaceous borders
with the National Collection of Asters,
descend to two lakes.

SD ♿   CP ♿   E ⚹ (Side Door)
C ⚹   S ⚹   WC ⚹

SWALCLIFFE BARN MUSEUM

Swalcliffe, Nr. Banbury OX15 5DR
Tel: (01295) 788278
Swalcliffe Barn was built for the Rectorial
Manor of Swalcliffe by New College,
Oxford, who owned the manor.
Constructed between 1400 and 1409 it
retains much of its medieval timber half-
cruck roof intact and is one of the finest
medieval barns in the country. Collection
of agricultural and trade vehicles.

SD ♿   CP ⚹   E ♿   RF ♿   WC ♿

BURFORD

Lovely Cotswolds' town, with a wide
High Street sloping down to the River
Windrush, crossed by a narrow 3-
arched bridge. Golden Cotswold stone
houses everywhere.

TOURIST INFORMATION CENTRE

The Brewery, Sheep Street, Burford OX18 4LP
Tel: (01993) 823558   Fax: (01993) 823590

ATTRACTION

COTSWOLD WILDLIFE PARK
Burford OX18 4JW
Tel: (01993) 823006   Fax: (01993) 823807
Set in 160 acres of gardens and parklands
around listed Victorian manor house.
Several endangered species including Giant

Tortoise and Red Panda with tropical
birds, penguins and mammals in the
walled garden, plus tropical and reptile
houses, aquarium, insect house and fruit
bats.

SD ♿   CP ♿   E ♿   RF ♿
C ♿   S ♿   WC ⚹   RFE ♿

FARINGDON

On the edge of the Cotswolds
between Oxford and Swindon.
Historically famous for its Civil War
stand against the Roundheads, the
town is still a vibrant market centre.

HOTEL

BEST WESTERN SUDBURY HOUSE
HOTEL   ♿
56 London Street, Faringdon SN7 8AA
Tel: (01367) 241272 Fax: (01367) 242346
stay@sudburyhouse.co.uk
www.sudburyhouse.co.uk
No. of Accessible Rooms: 1. Bath
Accessible Facilities: Lounge, Restaurant,
Lift. Originally a fine Regency house, now
extended to a fully equipped hotel. Set in
9 acres of secluded private grounds.

HENLEY-ON-THAMES.

Picturesque Thameside town, with
Victorian houses, separated from the
neighbouring county of
Buckinghamshire by elegant C18th
bridge spanning a wide stretch of the
River.

TOURIST INFORMATION CENTRE

Town Hall, Market Place, Henley RG9 2AQ
Tel: (01491) 578034 Fax: (01491) 411766

HOTEL

HOLMWOOD   ⚹
Shiplake Row, Binfield Heath, Henley-on-
Thames RG9 4DP
Tel: (0118) 9478747   Fax: (0118) 9478637
No. of Accessible Rooms: 2, via vertical
(not stair) lift). Accessible Facilities:
Lounge, Dining Room. Large secluded
Georgian country house with impressive

reception rooms and galleried hall. Set in 4 acres of lovely gardens with additional grounds of 26 acres of paddocks and woods. Extensive views of Thames Valley. Emily Tennyson spent the night here before her wedding to Alfred, Lord Tennyson and Algernon Charles Swinburne composed much poetry here.

ATTRACTION
RIVER AND ROWING MUSEUM
Mill Meadows, Henley-on-Thames RE9 1BF
Tel: (01491) 415600   Fax: (01491) 415601
e-mail: museum@rrm.co.uk
www.rrm.co.uk

Walk the length of River Thames from source to sea, exploring River's role through history from major trading route to boating paradise. Experience highs and low of international rowing with fascinating artefacts and memorabilia brought to life with archive film.

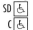   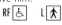
SD CP E RF L
C S WC

OXFORD
Oxford University is the second oldest in Europe, whose fine buildings combine with many other outstanding architectural features. Little back streets and scenes of Christ Church meadows, where the River Isis becomes the Thames, produce a magical atmosphere.

TOURIST INFORMATION CENTRE
The Old School, Gloucester Green, Oxford OX1 2DA
Tel: (01865) 726871   Fax: (01865) 240261

BUSES
Oxford Bus Company: Tel: (01865) 785410
Operate some low floor buses, including Park & Ride, which are all low floor.
Stagecoach Oxford: Tel: (01865) 772250
Operate some low floor kneeling buses, also the "Oxford Tube" to London
Thames Travel: Tel: (01491) 874216

TAXIS
ABC Taxis: Tel: (01865) 770077

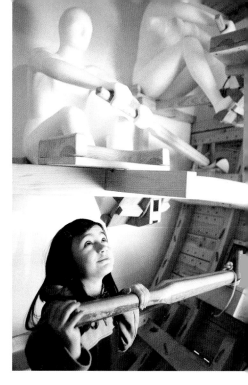

Another budding match-winning cox at the River and Rowing Museum.

20 adapted vehicles
City Taxis: Tel: (01865) 794000
20 adapted vehicles but can't take large electric chairs
AA Taxis: Tel: (01865) 430430
20 adapted vehicles
Radio Taxis: Tel: (01865) 242424
20 adapted vehicles

TRAINS
Thames Trains: Special Needs:
Tel: (0118) 9083607
www.thamestrains.co.uk
Virgin Trains: Special Needs:
Tel: (0845) 7443366
Minicom: (0845) 7443367

Oxford Station has level access to both platforms from car parks, lifts to both platforms, disabled WC on concourse, helpline telephone on both platforms.

CAR PARKS
Disabled badge spaces in all 4 Park & Ride car parks, also plenty of free on-street spaces.
Tel: (01865) 726871

SHOPMOBILITY
Level 1a, Westgate Car Park, Oxford
Tel: (01865) 248737   Fax: (01865) 249536
e-mail: robin@shopmo.oxford.demon.co.uk

HOTELS
WESTWOOD COUNTRY HOTEL   [♿]
Hinksey Hill Top, Nr. Boars Hill,
Oxford OX1 5BH
Tel: (01865) 735408
Fax: (01865) 736536
e-mail: reservations@westwoodhotel.co.uk
www.westwoodhotel.co.uk
No. of accessible Rooms: 2. Roll-in Shower
Accessible Facilities: Lounge, Restaurant.
Charming property, privately owned, set in
3.5 acres of landscaped gardens, backing
onto 160 acres of woodland, 2.5 m. from
city centre.

BOWOOD HOUSE HOTEL   [♿]
238 Oxford Road, Kidlington,
Oxford OX5 1EB
Tel: (01865) 842288   Fax: (01865) 841858
No. of Accessible Rooms: 1
Accessible Facilities: Lounge, Restaurant.
Comfortable, small hotel situated on the
A4260 in village of Kidlington, 3.5 m. from
city centre.

BED & BREAKFAST
BURLINGTON HOUSE   [🚶]
374 Banbury Road, Summerton,
Oxford OX2 7PP
Tel: (01865) 513513   Fax: (01865) 311785
e-mail: stay@burlington-house.co.uk
www.burlington-house.co.uk
No. of Accessible Rooms: 1. Roll-in Shower
Accessible Facilities: Lounge, Dining Room
Large, detached Victorian merchant's
house, dating from 1889, situated in
premier residential area, 5 minutes from
centre of Oxford.

ATTRACTIONS
ASHMOLEAN MUSEUM
Beaumont Street, Oxford OX1 2PH
Tel: (01865) 278000   Fax: (01865) 278018
e-mail: name/dept@ashmus.ox.ac.uk
Oldest museum open to the public in
Britain and a fine example of neo-classical
architecture, containing the University's
collections of European and Near Eastern

Antiquities, Western and Eastern paintings
and sculptures, with ever changing
temporary exhibitions

SD [♿]	CP n/a	E [♿]	RF [♿]	L [🚶]
C [🚶] (access via lift)	S [♿]	WC [🚶]		

THEATRE
OXFORD PLAYHOUSE
Beaumont Street, Oxford OX1 2LW
Admin: (01865) 247134
Fax: (01865) 793748
Booking-Box Office: (01865) 798600
Minicom: (01865) 792196
Complies with Part M, Building Regulations

CP [🚶]	RE [♿]	ED [♿] (except Manual Door)
INT [♿]	WC [♿]	AUD [♿]	B/R [♿]

WALLINGFORD

HOTEL
THE GEORGE   [🚶]
High Street, Wallingford OX10 0BS
Tel: (01491) 836665   Fax: (01491) 825359
No. of Accessible Rooms: 3. Bath
Accessible Facilities: Lounge, Restaurant.
Lovely hotel in centre of town, originally a
16thC coaching inn.

WITNEY
Situated on the River Windrush, on the
edge of the sheep-rearing area, the
town's fame for blanket-making is
worldwide. Mellowed stone-built town
with wide street, gradually narrowing
and continuing for almost 1 mile.

TOURIST INFORMATION CENTRE
26 Market Square, Witney OX28 6BB
Tel: (01993) 775802   Fax: (01993) 709261

HOTEL
FOUR PILLARS HOTEL   [🚶]
Ducklington Lane, Witney OX8 7TJ
Tel: (01993) 779777
Fax: (01993) 703467
e-mail: enquiries@four-pillars.co.uk
www.four-pillars.co.uk
No. of Accessible Rooms: 1. Bath
Accessible Facilities: Lounge, Restaurant,
Bar. Located 2 miles from centre of town,

this is a modern, very comfortable and spacious hotel, built in traditional style immediately off the A40 on A415.

BED & BREAKFAST
CROFTERS GUEST HOUSE
29 Oxford Hill, Witney OX28 3JU
Tel/Fax: (01993) 778165
No. of Accessible Rooms: 2. Shower Accessible Facilities: Lounge, Conservatory Breakfast Room. Family home bursting with knick knacks, run by charming hosts who hope their clients will arrive as "guests and depart as friends". 1.5 miles from town centre.
2nd double with shower and separate access. Separate garden access.

WOODSTOCK
Lovely old country town bisected by a handsome bridge over the River Glyme, with many old stone houses and pleasant streets which lead to the great Palace of Blenheim.

TOURIST INFORMATION CENTRE
Oxfordshire Museum, Park Street, Woodstock OX20 1SN
Tel: (01993) 813276   Fax: (01993) 813632
e-mail: woodstock.vic@westoxon.gov.uk

ATTRACTION
THE OXFORDSHIRE MUSEUM
(Tourist Information Centre) see above, History of the people of Oxfordshire located in charming townhouse.

SD   CP   E   RF
C   S   WC

SHROPSHIRE

SHROPSHIRE TOURISM
Harlescott Barns, Harlscott, Shrewsbury SY1 3SZ
Tel: (01743) 462462   Fax (01743) 462035
e-mail: enquiries@shropshiretourism.info
www.shropshiretourism.info.

SPECIALIST OUTDOOR ACTIVITES
THE LYNEAL TRUST
The Shirehall, Shrewsbury SY2 6ND
Tel: (01743) 251000
The Llangollen Canal weaves across the Cheshire/Shropshire borders through wonderful canal-side country.
The Trust arranges canal based holidays on two canal boats on a do-it-yourself basis, so each party should include some able-bodied adults. For day trips the Trust provides a helmsman. Both boats carry hydraulic lift, steering and ramps and the larger has adapted WCs.

BRIDGNORTH
Both high and low town connected by flights of steps and a railway with steepest gradient in Britain. This setting, part spread across the red sandstone ridge, part at its foot, is unique in England with some fine buildings in the town.

TOURIST INFORMATION CENTRE
The Library, Lidstley Street, Bridgnorth WV16 4AW
Tel: (01746) 763257   Fax: (01746) 766625

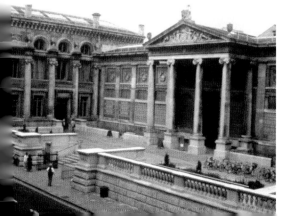

Ashmolean Museum. Neo-classical at its best.

HOTEL
THE OLD VICARAGE HOTEL
Worfield, Nr. Bridgnorth WV15 5JZ
Tel: (01746) 716497
Fax: (01746) 716552
e-mail: admin@the-old-vicarage.demon.co.uk
www.oldvicarageworfield.com
No. of Accessible Rooms: 2. Roll-in Shower
Accessible Facilities: Lounge, Restaurant,
Gardens via Croquet lawn.
Privately owned 14 bedroomed property
full of antique furniture in lovely grounds.

ATTRACTION
DUDMASTON HALL (NT)
Quatt, Bridgnorth WV15 6QN
Tel: (01746) 780866
Fax: (01746) 780744
e-mail: mduefe@smtp.ntrust.org.uk
C17th. house with fine furniture,
contemporary paintings and sculpture and
lovely gardens.
NB: Entrance ramped at 1:10

| SD ♿ | CP n/a | E ♿ | RF ♿ |
| C ♿ | S ♿ | WC ⚹ | |

CHURCH STRETTON
Mary Webb country: she spent her
honeymoon here and the
"Shepwardine" of her novels is Church
Stretton. The surrounding hills and
bleak, heathery Long Mynd offer
magnificent views.

TOURIST INFORMATION CENTRE
County Branch Library,
Church Streeton SY6 6DQ
Tel: (01694) 723133

BED & BREAKFAST
JINLYE
Castle Hill, All Stretton,
Church Stretton   SY6 6JP
Tel/Fax: (01694) 723243
e-mail: kate@jinlye.freeserve.co.uk
No. of Accessible Rooms: 1. Roll-in Shower.
Accessible Facilities: Lounge, Dining Room,
Garden. Excellently situated guest house
standing in 15 acres of grounds adjoining
the Long Mynd - an area of great beauty.
Period furnishings and cottage gardens.

LUDLOW
Historic market town, capital of the
Marches, with Broad Street described
by Nicholas Pevsner as 'the most
beautiful street in England'. To the
south of its Castle lies a medieval grid
of streets mostly rebuilt in C18th.
There are 500 listed buildings in
Ludlow, many half-timbered Tudor and
red-brick Georgian houses.

TOURIST INFORMATION CENTRE
Castle Street, Ludlow SY8 2AS
Tel: (01584) 875053 Fax: (01584) 877931

HOTELS
THE FEATHERS AT LUDLOW ⚹
The Bull Ring, Ludlow SY8 1AA
Tel: (01584) 875261   Fax: (01584) 876030
No. of Accessible Rooms: 9. Bath
Accessible Facilities: Lounge, Restaurant.
Historic hotel in town centre, this Grade I
listed building is the oldest timbered
facade in England. The New York Times
has described this inn as 'the most
handsome in the world'.

THE GABLES ⚹
Broome, Craven Arms SY7 0NX
Tel: (01588) 660667   Fax: (01588) 660799
No. of Accessible Rooms: 3
Accessible Facilities: Dining Room
Lovely house and gardens in glorious
countryside

SELF-CATERING
HOLLY COTTAGE
Sutton Court Farm, Little Sutton,
Ludlow SY8 2AJ
Tel: (01584) 861305 Fax: (01584) 861441
No. of Accessible Units: 1
No. of Beds per Unit: 2. Bath with shower
Accessible Facilities: Lounge, Dining Room,
Kitchen, Garden. 1 of 6 holiday cottages
set in Corve Dale Valley. Located 5.5 miles
from Ludlow.

SPORTING VENUE
LUDLOW RACECOURSE
Bromfield, Ludlow
Tel: (01981) 250052 Fax: (01981) 250192

Booking: No advance booking required.
Tel. above for information

CP ♿   RE ♿   ED ♿   WC 🚹
SS n/a (CCTV in all bars)   B/R ♿

MARKET DRAYTON

Home to gingerbread and Clive of
India, with black and white half-
timbered inns and bustling street
markets, held here for over 750 years.

TOURIST INFORMATION CENTRE
49 Cheshire Street, Market Drayton TF9 1PH
Tel/Fax: (01630) 652139

BED & BREAKFAST
MICKLEY HOUSE   🚹
Faulsgreen, Tern Hill,
Market Drayton TF9 3QW
Tel: (01630) 638505
No. of Accessible Rooms: 2.
Accessible Facilities: Lounge, Dining Room
Victorian farmhouse, within 125 acre cattle
farm, with oak beams and leaded windows
situated between Market Drayton and
Shrewsbury.

ATTRACTION
HODNET HALL GARDENS
Hodnet, Market Drayton TF9 3NN
Tel: (01630) 685202   Fax: (01630) 685853
60 acres of quite superb landscaped
gardens with pools, lush plants and trees.
Set down outside Victorian Tearoom.

SD ♿   CP 🚹   RF ♿
C ♿   S ♿   WC 🚹

SHIFNAL

In 1591 this small town was largely
destroyed by fire, and its architecture is
therefore very varied with some fine
examples of both Norman and
Georgian design.

ATTRACTIONS
WESTON PARK
Weston-under-Lizard, Nr. Shifnal TF11 8LF
Tel: (01952) 850207   Fax: (01952) 850430
Mansion built in 1671, surrounded by
wonderful gardens and park designed by

221

*The superb landscape gardens of
Hodnet Hall, Market Drayton.*

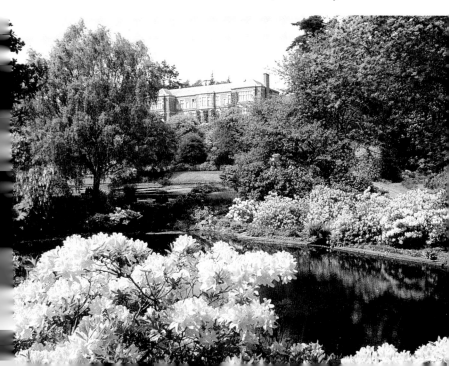

'Capability Brown' with lakes, miniature railway and adventure playground.

SD ♿ CP 🚶 E ♿ RF ♿ C ♿
S ♿ WC 🚶 RFE ♿

ROYAL AIR FORCE MUSEUM COSFORD
Shifnal TF11 8UP
Tel: (01902) 376200
Fax: (01902) 376211
e-mail: rafmuseumcosford@compuserve.com
Large aviation collection including Spitfires and Hurricanes from WW11, Victor and Vulcan Bombers and British Airways exhibition hall

SD ♿ CP 🚶 E ♿ RF ♿ C ♿
S ♿ WC ♿ RFE ♿

SHREWSBURY
One of the best preserved medieval towns in England, the spires of its 2 churches piercing the skyline and its town centre houses of beautiful timber-framing.

222

TOURIST INFORMATION CENTRE
The Music Hall, The Square,
Shrewsbury SY1 1LH
Tel: (01743) 350761
Fax: (01743) 355323

SHREWSBURY & ATCHAM BOROUGH COUNCIL
Director of Health, Tourism & Leisure
Oakley Manor, Belle Vue Road,
Shrewsbury SY3 7NW
Tel: (01743) 231456   Fax: (01743) 271593

BUSES
First PMT: Tel: (01782) 207999
Buses throughout Shropshire & the Potteries.

TAXIS
Clare's Cab: Tel: (01743) 236900
1 adapted vehicle

TRAINS
Virgin Trains: Special Needs:
Tel: (0845) 7443366
Minicom: (0845) 7443367
Wales & West: Special Needs:
Tel: (0845) 3003005
Shrewsbury Station is suitable for wheelchairs using ramp access.

CAR PARKS
Designated parking bays for disabled drivers all over the city-map available from Shopmobility as below.

SHOPMOBILITY
Level 1, Ground Floor, Ravens Meadows Car Park, Shrewsbury SY1 1PL
Tel: (01743) 236900

HOTEL
ALBRIGHT HUSSEY HOTEL   🚶
Ellesmere Road, Shrewsbury SY4 3AF
Tel: (01939) 290571   Fax: (01939) 291143
e-mail: abhotel@aol.com
www.albrighthussey.co.uk
No. of Accessible Rooms: 1
Accessible Facilities: Restaurant, Bar.
Lovely hotel, half timbered, recorded in Domesday Book. Current building dates from 1524, with original wall beams, an architectural treasure. A garrison for Royalist troops in the Civil War. Situated in 4 acres of landscaped gardens in lovely open countryside.

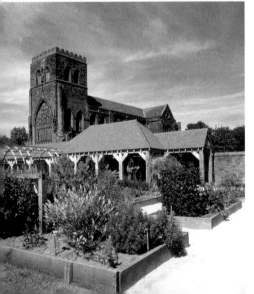

The monk's herb garden,
Shrewsbury Quest.

SELF-CATERING
NEWTON MEADOWS HOLIDAY COTTAGES
Wem Road, Harmer Hill,
Nr. Shrewsbury SY4 3DZ
Tel/Fax: (01939) 290346
e-mail:e.simcox@btopenworld.com
www.virtual-shropshire.co.uk/newton
No. of Accessible Units: 3. Roll-in Showers.
No. of Beds per Unit: 4/7
Accessible Facilities: All have ground floor
bedrooms. Open plan
Lounge/Diner/Kitchen, Patio. 3 newly
renovated spacious adjoining cottages,
converted from old cow shed in rural
hamlet. 6 miles north of Shrewsbury with
country views.

ATTRACTIONS
ATTINGHAM PARK (NT)
Atcham, Shrewsbury
Tel: (01743) 709203
Elegant neo-classical mansions with 250
acres of superb parkland. Deer park,
woodlands and River.

SD   CP   E   RF   L
C   S   WC

THE SHREWSBURY QUEST
193 Abbey Foregate, Shrewsbury SY2 6AH
Tel: (01743) 366355
Fax: (01743) 244342
Staff Training: Yes. The Benedictine Abbey
of St. Peter and St. Paul stood on this site
for 500 years. This is a re-creation of
mediaeval monastic life – the bustle of
tradespeople, delicate sounds of dulcimer,
harp and lute, barrels rolling into the great
store, bells proclaiming Vespers.

SD   CP   E   RF   L
C   S   WC

TELFORD
Britain's first major new city, begun in
1963, comprised of Madely,
Ironbridge, Coalbrookdale, Wellington
and Oakengates. The name was
chosen to commemorate Thomas
Telford whose bridges, viaducts, canals
and churches are endemic to
Shropshire.

TOURIST INFORMATION CENTRE
The Telford Centre, Telford TF3 4BX
Tel: (01952) 230032   Fax: (01952) 291723

HOTELS
HOLIDAY INN TELFORD/IRONBRIDGE
Telford International Centre, St. Quentin Gate,
Telford TF3 4EH
Tel: (01952) 527000
e-mail: holidayinn.telford@virgin.net
www.holiday-inn.com/telforduk
No. of Accessible Rooms: 2. Bath
Accessible Facilities: Lounge, Dining Room.
Modern low-rise property located adjacent
to Telford International Centre with good
access to M54 and town centre

TELFORD MOAT HOUSE
Foregate, Telford Centre, Telford TF3 4NA
Tel: (01952) 429988 Fax: (01952) 292012
No. of Accessible Rooms: 2
Accessible Facilities: Lounge, Restaurant,
Leisure Club. Large modern hotel just off
M54.

223

SOMERSET

SOMERSET TOURISM
www.somerset.gov.uk/tourism/

BATH & NORTHEAST SOMERSET COUNCIL
Tel: (01225) 477000   Fax: (01225) 477637

BASONBRIDGE
Small inland village close to Burnham -
on-Sea, equidistant between Weston -
super-Mare and Bridgewater with
many places of interest within a short
drive.

BED & BREAKFAST
MERRY FARM
Basonbridge TA9 3PS
Tel: (01278) 783655
No. of Accessible Rooms: 1 ground floor
single room. Bath

Accessible Facilities: Lounge, Dining Room 300 year old farmhouse full of character and old beams, with private fishing on 600m of the River Brue.

BATH

Somerset's largest town and the most celebrated of England's spa towns. The main pool today is below the modern street level and open to the sky with original lead flooring and surrounding paving. Major association with the Romans who enjoyed the baths over 4 centuries. Majority of Bath now dates from Georgian times, when fashionable people came to "take the waters". The city still retains fine Georgian terraces and other buildings of mellow Bath stone and virtually all the streets are very attractive with stylish shops. The city has a rich cultural life with an arts festival every May.

TOURIST INFORMATION CENTRE
Abbey Chambers, Abbey Church Yard, Bath BA1 1LY
Tel: (01225) 477101
e-mail: tourism@bathnes.gov.uk
www.visitbath.co.uk

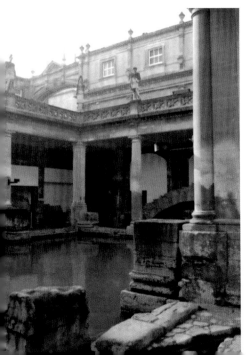

BUSES
Bath Bus Company
1 Pierrepont Street, Bath BA1 1LB
Tel: (01225) 330444 Fax: (01225) 330727
Some low floor routes
First Badgerline: Tel: (01225) 466889
Some low floor/kneeling routes
Abus: Tel: (0117) 9776126
Based in Bristol, some low floor routes.

TAXIS
Taxi rank at station
Rainbow Taxis: Tel: (01225) 460606
2 adapted vehicles

TRAINS
First Great Western:
Special Needs: Tel: (0845) 7413775
Wales & West
Special Needs: (0845) 3003005
Minicom: (0845) 7585469
Bath Spa Station has level access to concourse with ticket counter, level tunnel to westbound platform via long ramp (1:12) and 1:11 to eastbound platform.
Disabled WCs.

CAR PARKING
Free disabled parking permits for parking in Council controlled car parks. Also considerable amount of on-street parking, free to disabled badge holders.
Tel: (01225) 394147

SHOPMOBILITY
4 Railway Street, Bath BA1 1PG
Tel/Fax: (01225) 481744
Minicom: (01225) 481773

HOTELS
HILTON BATH CITY
Walcot Street, Bath BA1 5BJ
Tel: (01225) 463411   Fax: (01225) 464393
No. of Accessible Rooms: 1
Accessible Facilities: Restaurant, Bar. Modern hotel situated in city centre.

The magnificent Roman Baths – still producing hot water after 2000 years.

CENTURION HOTEL ♿
Charlton Lane, Midsomer Norton,
Nr. Bath BA3 4BD
Tel: (01761) 417711 Fax: (01761) 418357
No. of Accessible Rooms: 2. Bath.
Accessible Facilities: Lounge, Restaurant
(rear entrance).
Family run complex, including the
Fosseway Country Club to which it is
linked by the Restaurant with longish
walk to club facilities.
Located 19 miles from Bath in fine setting
midway between Bath and Wells.

ATTRACTIONS
BATH ABBEY
Bath BA1 1LT
Tel: (01225) 422462 Fax: (01225) 429990
C15th Perpendicular style Abbey church
built on site of Saxon Abbey where
coronation took place of England's first
king, Edgar, in 973 AD.

SD ♿   CP 🚶   E ♿   RF ♿
S 🚶   WC 🚶   RFE ♿

MUSEUM OF COSTUME (NT)
Assembly Rooms, Bennett Street, Bath
Tel: (01225) 477789 Fax: (01225) 444793
e-mail: costume_enquiries@bthnes.gov.uk
Large and fine collection of fashionable
dress from late C16th to present day,
house in C18th Assembly Rooms which
are in the basement and lower ground
floor, accessible by lift. Assistance
available if required.

SD ♿   CP n/a   E ♿   RF 🚶
L ♿   S ♿   WC 🚶

PRIOR PARK LANDSCAPE GARDEN (NT)
Ralph Allen Drive, Bath BA2 5AH
Tel: (01225) 833422
Fine example of C18th English landscape,
a haven of peace and a work of art with
panoramic views of the city. There is a
Wilderness area of woodland, Serpentine
Lake and natural springs, a Palladian
Bridge created in 1755, lakes and dams
and a Rock Gate.

SD ♿   CP ♿   E ♿   RF ♿
WC ♿   RFE ♿

THE ROMAN BATHS MUSEUM
Stall Street, Bath BA1 1LZ
Tel: (01225) 477785 Fax: (01225) 477743
e-mail: christine_mclean@bathnes.gov.uk
The baths, built by the Romans nearly 2000
years ago, served those who were ill and
pilgrims who were visiting the adjacent
Temple of Sulis Minerva.
Access for wheelchairs to inner and outer
Terraces overlooking the Great Bath only.
There are special access evenings when it is
possible to take visitors down to the
Museum - tel. above number.

SD ♿   CP n/a   E ♿   RF ♿   C ♿
S ♿   WC 🚶   RFE ♿

BRIDGWATER
Enterprising industrial town with both
old and modern buildings. Castle
Street, running down to the West
Quay is a superb example of the
C17th, whilst St. Mary's Church is
C13th to C15th has some magnificent
features.

BED & BREAKFAST ACCOMMODATION
BLACKMORE FARM ♿
Cannington, Bridgwater TA5 2NE
Tel: (01278) 653442 Fax: (01278) 653427
e-mail: Dyerfarm@aol.com
No. of Accessible Rooms: 3. Roll-in Shower
Accessible Facilities: Lounge, Dining Room.
Built in C14th and retains many of its
period features including stone archways,
garderobes and oak beams. The Stable is
an annexe to the main house in a barn
conversion with disabled facilities.
The farm consists of 2 holdings extending
to 750 acres, with both livestock and arable
crops. Family owned and managed by the
Dyers who have a fascinating history of
the farm.

BRUTON
Picturesque small town on River Bruce,
founded in Saxon times and retaining
many intriguing glimpses of its past
including Jacobean almshouses, Abbey
remains, C15th packhorse bridge,
twin-towers church and famous
dovecote.

SELF-CATERING
DISCOVE FARM
Bruton BA10 0NQ
Tel: (01749) 812284
www.bruton.freeuk.com/discovefarm
The Dovecote:
Owl Barn:
No. of Accessible Units: 2. Roll-in Showers.
No. of Beds per Unit: Dovecote-2,
Owl-4/5
Accessible Facilities: Lounge Dining Room,
Kitchen, Garden with barbecue and picnic
table, elevated level Sundeck.
Purpose-built units for wheelchair users in
peaceful countryside setting.

CASTLE CARY
Vibrant market town with winding
main street of thatch and golden stone
below Lodge Hill. On Bailey Hill stands
the C18th 'pepper pot' lock up, one of
only 4 in the country.

ATTRACTION
HADSPEN GARDEN & NURSERY
Castle Cary BA7 7NG
Tel/Fax: (01749) 813707
e-mail: hadspen@compuserve.com
Five-acre garden noted for herbaceous
borders and roses.

SD | CP | E | RF
C | S | WC | RFE

CHEDDAR
Pale-grey limestone cliffs rise vertically
to 150m. on either side of the town,
with spectacular views from the cliff
top. Cheddar cheese has been made
here in local farmhouses since the
C12th, although its main industries are
now market gardening (particularly
strawberries), limestone quarrying and
cheese straw making.

SELF-CATERING
THE HEATHERS
Westfield Lane, Draycott, Cheddar
Tel: (01934) 744187
No. of Accessible Units: 1. Roll-in Shower.

No. of Beds per Unit: 2
Accessible Facilities: Lounge, Dining Room,
Kitchen, Garden.
A very private unit with wonderful views
across the Cheddar Valley.

DULVERTON
Lies in the beautiful valley of the River
Barle, in an area of densely wooded
steep hillsides. There are narrow
streets, live theatre, craft markets and
special events, attracting artists and
anglers particularly.

SELF-CATERING
NORTHMOOR HOUSE
Dulverton TA22 9QG
Tel: (01398) 323720
No. of Accessible Units: 1. Roll-in Shower.
No. of Beds Per Unit: 2
Accessible Facilities: Lounge, Dining Room.
The House is arranged to accommodate up
to 22 adults plus 3 cots and best suited for
large parties where 1 or 2 people require
wheelchair access.
NB: The kitchen is not suitable for Cat. 2.

ATTRACTION
EXMOOR NATIONAL PARK
Exmoor House, Dulverton TA22 9HL
Tel: (01398) 323665
Fax: (01398) 323150
The rugged nature of Exmoor's 267 square
miles of protected landscape, can seem
challenging but the area's unique
atmosphere is most enjoyable. Cool
wooded valleys, flowing streams and
wildlife, together with spectacular
coastline of rugged cliffs, wild seas, high
moorland and heather.

VISITOR CENTRES AT:
Combe Martin, Devon – Cross Street,
Tel (01271) 883319
Lynmouth, Devon – The Esplanade,
Tel: (01598) 752509
Dunster, Somerset – Dunster Steep,
Tel: (01643) 821835
Dulverton, Somerset – Fore Street,
Tel: (01398) 323841
Well worth visiting:

North West Exmoor: Barbrook, Blackmoor Gate, Brendon Common, Combe Martin, Heddon Valley, Holdstone & Trentishoe Downs, Lee Abbey Estate, Malmsmead, Oare & Doone Country, Martinhoe & Woody Bay, Parracombe, Valley of Rocks, Lynton, Lynmouth, Watersmeet, Countisbury Barna Barrow.

Central & Southern Exmoor: Exford, Heasley Mill Nr. North Molton, Landacre Bridge, Molland, Shoulsbarrow Common, Simonsbath, Tarr Steps, Wimbleball Lake, Winsford, Withypool.

North East Exmoor: Horner Water, Porlock Hill, Selworthy Beacon, Webber's Post, Yenworthy Common.

FROME

Long history from 685AD as market and agricultural town with many historic buildings, particularly around Cheap Street and the Catherine Hill areas. Notable C17th bridge, largely untouched over the past 200 years.

TOURIST INFORMATION CENTRE
The Round Tower, Black Swan, 2 Bridge Street, Frome BA11 1BB
Tel: (01373) 467271

GLASTONBURY

Famous for its connections with history of Christianity, the majestic ruins of its Abbey and its association with the legends of King Arthur, who with his wife, Guinevere, is reputed to be buried in the Abbey grounds. Many of the town centre shops are dedicated to the history, myth and legend which surround Glastonbury, producing a singular ambience.

TOURIST INFORMATION CENTRE
The Tribunal, 9 High Street, Glastonbury BA6 9DP
Tel: (01458) 832954
No. of Accessible Units: 1. Roll-in Shower.
No. of Beds per Unit: 2 + child
Accessible Facilities: Open plan studio with bedroom/Lounge/kitchen, plus additional large hall with bed if needed. Double patio doors lead to lovely private wooden deck. Open at the same times as the house and garden. The garden only is suitable for wheelchairs.

SD 🦽 CP 🚶 S 🦽
E 🚶 (Garden) WC 🚶

STREET

Named after ancient causeway running north across River Brue to Glastonbury. In C19th tanning sheepskin was main trade, prosperity much increasing when, in 1825, C & J Clark founded their shoe factory here.

TOURIST INFORMATION CENTRE
Clark's Village, Farm Road, Street BA16 0BB
Tel: (01458) 447384
www.glastonbury.tic@ukonline.co.uk

227

SHOPMOBILITY
Clark's Village as above.
Tel: (01458) 440155
Free loan of scooters, powerchairs and manual wheelchairs.

ATTRACTION
CLARK'S VILLAGE
As above
Tel: (01458) 840064 Fax: (01458) 841132
www.clarksvillage.co.uk
Factory outlet shopping, with many retail units offering discounts on well-known products in charming surroundings.

SD 🦽 CP 🦽 E 🦽 RF 🦽
C 🦽 S 🦽 (all outlets)
WC 🚶 RFE 🦽

TAUNTON

Prosperous town situated in the centre of one of the country's most fertile plains. A fine Georgian street of deep-red brick and white porticoed houses combine with the late C15th church of St. Mary Magdalene.

TOURIST INFORMATION CENTRE
The Library, Paul Street, Taunton TA1 2XZ
Tel: (01823) 336344
Fax: (01823) 340308
e-mail:Tautic@somerset.gov.uk
www.heartofsomerset.com
Extremely helpful!

BUSES
First Southern National: Tel: (01823) 272033
Some low floor buses

TAXIS
A1 Taxis: Tel: (01823) 323323
1 adapted vehicle

TRAINS
First Great Western: Special Needs:
Tel: (0845) 7413775
Virgin Trains: Special Needs:
Tel: (0845) 7443366
Minicom: (0845) 7443367
Wales & West: Special Needs:
Tel: (0845) 3003005
Minicom: (0845) 7585469
Taunton Station accessible by lift.

CAR PARKS
Disabled badge scheme. Tel: (01823) 338781

SHOPMOBILITY
1st Floor, Pool Street Car Park,
Old Market Centre, Taunton
Tel: (01823) 327900

HOTEL
HOLIDAY INN TAUNTON
Deane Gate Avenue, Taunton TA1 2UA
Tel: (01823) 332222   Fax: (01823) 332266
No. of Accessible Rooms: 2. Bath
Accessible Facilities: Lounge, Restaurant.
Modern property, close to numerous
attractions and with good access to
Exmoor National Park and Cheddar Gorge.

BED & BREAKFAST
REDLANDS
Treble's Holford, Combe Florey, Taunton,
Somerset TA4 3HA
Tel: 01823 433159
e-mail: redlandshouse@hotmail.com
www.escapetothecountry.co.uk
No. of Accessible Rooms: 1. Roll-in Shower

Accessible Facilities: Lounge, Dining Room
and areas of the Garden. The owner is
herself a wheelchair user. Set in quiet
country location by stream, adjacent to
the Quantock Hills. 8 miles from Taunton
and close to the preserved West Somerset
Railway. Both self-catering and b & b, the
latter in the Courtyard Room which is
accessible.

PROCTORS FARM
West Monkton, Taunton TA2 8QN
Tel: (01823) 412269
No. of Accessible Rooms: 2. Roll-in Shower
Accessible Facilities: Lounge, Dining Room.
C17th farmhouse with exposed oak beams
and log fires standing in own grounds and
surrounded by family-run farm. Located 2
miles from Taunton

SELF-CATERING
HOLLY COTTAGE
Stoke St. Gregory, Taunton TA3 6HS
Tel: (01823) 490828
Fax: (01823) 490590
e-mail: robhembrow@btinternet.com
No. of Accessible Units: 1. Roll-in Shower.
No. of Beds per Unit: 4
Accessible Facilities: Lounge, Kitchen/Diner.
The Linny is 1 of 5 cottages converted
from stone barns built by present owner's
great grandfather. Holly Farm is a
traditional working farm in peaceful rural
countryside of Sedgemoor.

TEMPLECOMBE

HOTEL
FOUNTAIN INN MOTEL
High Street, Henstridge,
Templecombe BA8 0RA
Tel: (01963) 362722
No. of Accessible Rooms: 1. Shower.
Accessible Facilities: Lounge, Restaurant.
Henstridge is on the Somerset/Dorset
border and overlooks the Blackmore Vale.

WATCHET
Busy small commercial port with
attractive harbour.

TOURIST INFORMATION CENTRE
The Esplanade, Watchet
Tel: as Minehead.

SELF-CATERING
ROSEVILLE
48A Brendon Road, Watchet TA23 0HT
Tel: (01984) 634199
Fax: (01984) 631572
No. of Accessible Units: 1. Bath(2)
No. of Beds per Unit: 3 bedrooms - 1dbl/1 twin/1 triple.
Accessible Facilities: Lounge/Dining Room, Kitchen. Large bungalow with level parking.

WELLS
Somerset's only city, with fine Cathedral. The wells from which city derives its name rise in the grounds of the Bishop's Palace, producing an average 100 litres of water per second.

TOURIST INFORMATION CENTRE
Town Hall, Market Place, Wells BA5 2RB
Tel: (01749) 672552

ATTRACTION
THE BISHOP'S PALACE
The Henderson Rooms, The Bishop's Palace, Wells BA5 2PD
Tel/Fax: (01749) 678691
Medieval residence built by Bishop Jocelin in early C13th with undercroft still virtually intact. Fortified in the C14th there are several state rooms and a superb long gallery housing portraits of former Bishops. Access through C14th gatehouse only. Located next to Cathedral off Market Square. Ground floor of palace and garden are both accessible by wheelchair. There are 2 mobility electric wheelchairs available for free hire. These can be booked in advance. A stairlift is planned for 2003 which will make the whole building accessible.

SD | E | RF | C | WC

WOOKEY HOLE CAVES & PAPERMILL
Wookey Hole, Wells BA5 1BB
Tel: (01749) 672243   Fax: (01749) 677749

e-mail: witch@wookey.co.uk
www.wookey.co.uk
Although no access to actual caves, worth visiting the Victorian Papermill-watch exquisite paper being made. In the Mill there is a Magical Mirror Maze and a typical Old Penny Arcade.

SD | CP | E | RF
C | S | WC | RFE

WESTON-SUPER-MARE
Somerset's largest seaside resort with fine wide sea-front roads, pavements and gardens.

HOTELS
MOORLANDS
Hutton, Weston-Super-Mare BS24 9QH
Tel/Fax: (01934) 812283
No. of Accessible Rooms: 1. Shower
Accessible Facilities: Lounge, Lovely Georgian house near centre delightful village of Hutton, standing in 2 acres of mature landscaped gardens and paddock. The village lies under steep, wooded slopes of western Mendips. 10 minutes drive from Weston.

LAURISTON HOTEL
6-12 Knightstone Road,
Weston-Super-Mare BS23 2AN
Tel: (01934) 620758   Fax: (01934) 621154
No. of Accessible Rooms: 2
Accessible Facilities: Lounge, Restaurant, Garden. Located opposite the beach, close to the sea front promenade and shopping precinct, this hotel caters specifically for visually impaired guests and most facilities accessible by wheelchair lift.

SELF-CATERING
HOPE FARM COTTAGE
Brean Road, Lympsham,
Weston-Super-Mare BS24 0HA
Tel/Fax: (01934) 750506
No. of Accessible Units: 4. Bath.
No. of Beds per Unit: 4 + cot
Accessible Facilities: Open plan Lounge/Kitchen/Diner, Central Heating. Cottages are set within a courtyard and backing onto open farmland. There is level

paved access to all cottages from carpark. There is also a telephone, games room and laundry. Located on outskirts of small village, 5 miles from Weston-super-Mare and close to Bath and Wells. Being within the Somerset Levels, much of the surrounding area is flat.

ATTRACTIONS
HELICOPTER MUSEUM
The Heliport, Lockine Hook Road, Weston-Super-Mare BS22 8PL
Tel: (01934) 635227 Fax: (01934) 822400
Unique collection of over 60 helicopters with new large undercover displays including restoration hangar and how helicopters work.
Wheelchair available for loan.

SD ♿	CP ♿	E ♿	RF ♿
C ♿	S ♿	WC 🚹	

NORTH SOMERSET MUSEUM
Burlington Street, Weston-Super-Mare BS23 1PR
Tel: (01934) 621028 Fax: (01934) 612526
e-mail: museum.service@n-somerset.gov.uk
Displays on the seaside holiday, apothecary shop, dairy and fountain with Victorian mosaics. Mendip mining and local archaeology also on display. Wheelchair access ground floor only.

SD ♿	CP n/a	E ♿	RF ♿
C ♿	S ♿	WC 🚹	RFE- ♿

YEOVIL
Major town in south Somerset situated in rolling fertile land beside the River Yeo.

TOURIST INFORMATION CENTRE
Petter's House, Petter's Way, Yeovil BA20 1SH
Tel: (01935) 471279

ATTRACTIONS
FLEET AIR ARM MUSEUM
RNAS Yeovilton, Ilchester, Nr. Yeovil BA22 8HT
Tel: (01935) 840565 Fax: (01935) 842630
e-mail: info@fleetairarm.com
www.fleetairarm.com

Leading naval aviation museum with impressive displays on both World Wars and recent conflicts such as Falklands and the Gulf and a Harrier Exhibition. The "Ultimate Carrier Experience", a flight deck built on land, offers special effects with sounds, smell and excitement of a big carrier on a mercy mission. Other attractions include model aircraft and ships, weapons, uniforms and airfield viewing galleries where visitors can watch modern Navy aircrews train.

SD n/a	CP ♿	E ♿	RF ♿
L ♿	C 🚹	S 🚹	WC ♿	RFE ♿

MONTACUTE HOUSE (NT)
Montacute, Yeovil
Tel/Fax: (01935) 823289
Late C16th, this Elizabethan house was the location for the film 'Sense & Sensibility'. Features include Renaissance plasterwork, a long Gallery hung with Tudor and Jacobean court portraits, C17th and C18th furniture and a fine formal garden

SD ♿	CP 🚹	E ♿	C 🚹	S ♿	WC 🚹

HAYNES MOTOR MUSEUM
Sparkford, Nr. Yeovil BA22 7LH
Tel: (01963) 440804 Fax: (01963) 441004
e-mail: mike@haynesmotormuseum.co.uk
www.haynesmotormuseum.co.uk
Spectacular collection of over 350 cars from American monsters to marvellous Minis. A Hall of red sports cars including Ferarris and Cobras combines with Model T Ford of 1903 and the famous Duesenberg of 1931. Not a personal enthusiast, I was nevertheless captivated!

SD ♿	CP ♿	E ♿	RF ♿
C ♿	S ♿	WC ♿	

STAFFORDSHIRE

TOURIST INFORMATION CENTRE
Quadrant Road, Hanley
Stoke-on-Trent ST1 1RZ
Tel: (01782) 236000   Fax: (01782) 236005

ALTON
Stone-built village lying east of
Cheadle on the rocky, wooded slopes
of the Churnet Valley, all towers,
turrets and spires. Alton is one half of
the Rhineland of Staffordshire: every
road and lane is a hill, every bend or
gap in the trees or houses offers a
central European view.

ATTRACTION
ALTON TOWERS
Alton ST10 4DB
Tel: (01538) 703344   Fax: (01538) 702831
www.alton-towers.com
Theme park with a variety of rides, shows
and attractions. Built into the landscape,
the estate provides a delightful green,
wooded backdrop. The park provides a
guide to the rides for those with disabilities
giving entrance details and any restrictions,
but in the majority of cases, a companion
must also come aboard. Nemesis and the
Skyride are not accessible.
SD ♿   CP ♿   E ♿   RF ♿
C ♿ (Towers Family Restaurant particularly)
S ♿   WC ♿ Wheelchairs available just inside
entrance on right hand side.

LEEK
Situated at the southern end of some
of the most impressive scenery in the
county.

BED AND BREAKFAST
CROFT MEADOWS FARM ♿
Horton, Leek ST13 8QE
Tel: (01782) 513039
No. of Accessible Rooms: 1. Roll-in Shower

Accessible Facilities: Lounge, Dining Room.
Self-contained country cottage.

LICHFIELD
From whichever direction one enters
the city, the three magnificent spires of
the cathedral can be seen. There is a
cobbled market square, narrow streets
and many links with Dr. Johnson, a
statue of him is set in the square.
Lichfield has long military associations,
the Staffordshire Regiment being a
famous aspect.

ATTRACTION
STAFFORDSHIRE REGIMENT MUSEUM
Whittington Barracks, Lichfield WS14 9PY
Tel: (0121) 311 3229   Fax: (0121) 311 3205
Regimental militaria including battle
honours, trophies and uniforms.
SD n/a   CP ♿   E ♿   RF ♿
C ♿   WC ♿   RFE ♿

STAFFORD
Birthplace of the world's most
renowned angler, Izaak Walton and
connections with the famous English
playwright, Richard Brinsley Sheridan.
The church of St. Mary, the High
House, a four-storied timbered house
where Charles I and Prince Rupert
stayed in 1642, Royal Brine Baths,
Church of St. Chad and Noel
Almshouses in Mill Street, are all worth
a view.

ATTRACTION
SHUGBOROUGH ESTATE (NT)
Shugborough, Milford, Nr. Stafford ST17 0XB
Tel: (01889) 881388   Fax: (01889) 881323
Truly superb estate built in the late C17th,
enlarged c1750 and again at the turn of
the C19th. Seat of the Earls of Lichfield
and currently home to Patrick Lichfield, the
well-known photographer. Now being
restored as a C19th working estate. The
house has a variety of collections plus
original kitchens and laundry and working

farm museum with educational programmes and demonstrations. The farmhouse has its original working mill, used for grinding flour and providing the many estate animals' food.

A great day out.

Access to ground floor only of the house, but much to see and well worth while. Additional disabled parking at farmhouse. Accessible picnic tables.

SD ⟨♿⟩ CP ⟨♿⟩ E ⟨♿⟩ (Stairclimber)
C ⟨♿⟩ S ⟨♿⟩ WC ⟨♿⟩

RFE ⟨♿⟩ 3 self-drive Batri-cars available for park and garden, with instruction. (kept near museum) 5 wheelchairs available.

STOKE-ON-TRENT

Came into being in 1910 when Stoke-on-Trent was combined with five adjoining towns – Tunstall, Burslem, Hanley, Fenton and Longton. Today it is a large town renowned for its many potteries and ancient buildings.

TOURIST INFORMATION CENTRE
Quadrant Road, Hanley,
Stoke-on-Trent ST1 1RZ
Tel: (01782) 236000
Fax: (01782) 236005
Minicom: (01782) 236004

SOCIAL SERVICES DEPARTMENT
Disability Resource Team
Regent Centre
Regent Road, Hanley
Stoke on Trent ST1 3TD
Tel: (01782) 235200   Fax: (01782) 235206
Minicom (01782) 235285

BUSES
First PMT: Tel: (01782) 207999
Some low-floor buses.
Passenger Transport Team:
Tel: (01782) 234500
Regional Travel Line: Tel: (0870) 6082608

TAXIS
Roseville (Newcastle): Tel: (01872) 613456
Six adapted vehicles
Scraggs Taxis: Tel: (01782) 265109
One adapted vehicle.

TRAINS
First North Western: Special Needs:
Tel: (0845) 6040231
Virgin Trains – Special Needs:
Tel: (0845) 7443366
Minicom: (0845) 7443367

CAR PARKS
Disabled badge spaces in all council owned car parks. Some on-street parking in city centre.
Tel: (01782) 232091

SHOPMOBILITY
Level 1C, Potteries Shopping Centre Car Park, Off Bryan Street, Stoke-on-Trent.
Tel: (01782) 233333   Fax: (01782) 233496
Minicom: (01782) 233334

HOTEL
STOKE-ON-TRENT MOAT HOUSE   ⟨♿⟩
Etruria Hall, Festival Way, Etruria,
Stoke on Trent ST1 5BQ
Tel: (01782) 609988   Fax: (01782) 284500
No. of Accessible Rooms: 3. Bath Accessible Facilities: Lounge, Restaurant, Pool, Sauna, Whirlpool. The former home of Josiah Wedgwood, Etruria Hall is now a quality hotel and conference centre.

ATTRACTIONS
ETRURIA INDUSTRIAL MUSEUM
Lower Bedford Street, Etruria,
Stoke-on-Trent ST4 7AF
Tel: (01782) 233144   Fax: (01782) 233145
Working forge and demonstrations of steam machinery, plus Britain's sole surviving steam powered potter's mill. Visitor Centre (i.e. entrance) is fully accessible: no wheelchair access to Etruscan Bone Mill.

SD ⟨♿⟩   CP ⟨♿⟩   E ⟨♿⟩   RF ⟨♿⟩
L ⟨♿⟩   C ⟨♿⟩   S ⟨♿⟩   WC ⟨♿⟩

GLADSTONE POTTERY MUSEUM
Uttoxeter Road, Longton,
Stoke-on-Trent ST3 1PQ
Tel: (01782) 311378
Fax: (01782) 598640
Cobbled yard within museum possibly problematical – bringing a companion will make it easier. The only remaining complete Victorian pottery. This unique

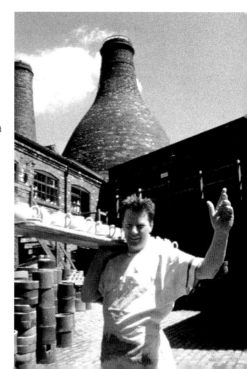

working museum allows visitors to see how potters worked. Traditional skills, original workshops, cobbled yard and huge bottle kilns create a real time-warp. Make your own pot or bone china flower.
There is a large display 'Flush with Pride' which is dedicated to the history of toilets. The tile gallery has been relocated and enlarged. Both are completely accessible.

SD ♿ CP ♿ E ♿ RF 🚶 L ♿
C 🚶 S 🚶 WC ♿ RFE ♿

ROYAL DOULTON VISITOR CENTRE
Nile Street, Burslem, Stoke-on-Trent ST6 2AJ
Tel: (01782) 292434
Fax: (01782) 292424
e-mail: visitor@royal-doulton.com
Combination of magic of Royal Doulton figures with treasures from the company's collection. Includes the biggest range of figurines in the world. There are displays of ceramic skills in the Royal Minton fine art studio where personal orders are all hand painted. The centre is sited on the ground floor of the original factory purchased in 1877. Visitor Centre accessible restaurant/museum. Factory tours NOT ACCESSIBLE.

SD ♿ CP ♿ E ♿ RF 🚶
C ♿ S 🚶 WC ♿ RFE ♿

WEDGWOOD VISITOR CENTRE
Barlaston, Stoke-on-Trent ST12 9ES
Tel: (01782) 282986
Fax: (01782) 374083
Self-guided tour with the aid of audio guide. Comprises of museum items from Josiah's very early days through to present day. There is a factory tour where you can see Jasperware being made. There is also a demonstration area. These are all fully accessible for wheelchairs.

SD ♿ CP ♿ E ♿ RF ♿
C ♿ S ♿ WC 🚶 RFE ♿

The happy potter of Gladstone Pottery museum.

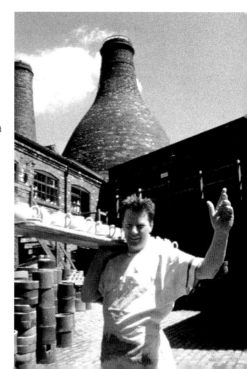

UTTOXETER
Known mainly for its racecourse, reckoned to be the finest National Hunt Steeplechase course in the Midlands. The strangest thing about this small market town is its name, believed to derive from a form of Witta, a man's name and an old word for health.

SPORTING VENUE
UTTOXETER RACECOURSE
Wood Lane, Uttoxeter ST14 8BD
Admin & Booking-Box Office:
(01889) 562561   Fax: (01889) 562786
e-mail: info@uttoxeter-racecourse.co.uk
www. uttoxeter-racecourse.co.uk

CP ♿   RE ♿   ED ♿   INT ♿
L 🚶   WC ♿ (except inward door opening).
3 units in main grandstand 7 in betting hall.
SS ♿   B/R ♿ Woodrows – all level, bistro style
♿ Platinum Suite – lift access, silver service.

233

WOLVERHAMPTON
(Staffs area)
See West Midlands for remainder.

ATTRACTION
MOSELEY OLD HALL (NT)
Moseley Old Hall Lane,
Fordhouses,
Wolverhampton WV10 7HY
Tel: (01902) 782808

This is where Charles II hid after the Battle of Worcester. An exhibition retells the story of this dramatic escape from Cromwell's troops. The garden, recreated in C17th. style with formal knot garden, has varieties of herbs and plants of the period. Three rooms on the ground floor in the house, the exhibition and garden are accessible.

SD [&]   CP [&]   E [太]   RF [&]
C [&]   S [&]   WC [太]

SUFFOLK

SUFFOLK TOURISM
www.suffolkcc.gov.uk

TRAVELINE
Public Transport Group, Environment & Transport Dept. Suffolk County Council, St. Edmund House, County Hall,
Ipswich IP4 1LZ
Tel: (08459) 583358
www.traveline.suffolkcc.gov.uk

For all information on bus, coach and rail services within the county.
Very helpful web site.

SPECIALIST OUTDOOR ACTIVITIES
WALDRINGFIELD BOATYARD LTD.
The Quay, Woodbridge IP12 4QZ
Tel/Fax: (01473) 736260.

Cruising on the River Deben through lovely wooded country, from Felixstowe Ferry to Woodbridge and Wilford Bridge.
Organised parties and individuals between May/September. The M.V. Jahan is especially designed to provide access for up to 4 disabled persons with wide hatches and 2 hydraulic lifts. Accessible WC on quay, but not on board.

ALDEBURGH
Quiet seaside resort of unspoilt charm with an internationally famous Music Festival (see BAFA in Intro.)

TOURIST INFORMATION CENTRE
Tel/Fax: (01728) 453637 (Seasonal)

HOTEL
UPLANDS HOTEL   [太]
Victoria Road, Aldeburgh IP15 5DX
Tel: (01728) 452420   Fax: (01728) 454872

No. of Accessible Rooms: 1
Accessible Facilities: Lounge, TV Lounge (3 steps). Privately owned Regency country house hotel in landscaped gardens a short distance from the sea.

BUNGAY
Market town and yachting centre on the River Waveney. Surrounded by sandy beaches and unspoilt countryside.

ATTRACTION
NORFOLK AND SUFFOLK AVIATION MUSEUM
Flixton, Nr. Bungay NR35 1NZ
Tel: (01986) 896644

Living museum bursting with WW1 and WW2 British, American and German civil and military exhibits and personal memorabilia amongst machinery and over 25 historic aircraft outside. This area of Britain swarmed with aviation sites during WW11 though many exhibits come from farther afield. A must for both aviation fans and laymen alike. N.B. Although there are ramps and paths they do advise a helper to cope with the grassy areas.

CP [&]   E [&] (to hangars)
RF [太]   C [太]   S [太]   WC [太]

BURY ST. EDMUNDS
Began as Benedictine Abbey, founded in 945AD, becoming one of the richest in the country prior to its dissolution in 1539. It is known for its elegant Georgian streets and flower gardens.

TOURIST INFORMATION CENTRE

6 Angel Hill, Bury St. Edmunds IP33 1UZ
Tel: (01284) 764667 Fax: (01284) 757084
Minicom: (01284) 757023
e-mail: appleby@burybo.stedsbc.gov.uk
www.stedmundsbury.gov.uk

BUSES

Suffolk Traveline: Tel: (08459) 583358
www.traveline.suffolkcc.gov.uk
Simonds of Botesdale: Tel: (01379) 898202
R W Chenery: Tel: (01379) 741221
Operates London Service.
Whippet Coaches: Tel: (01480) 463792

TAXIS

No black cabs in Bury.
A1 Cars: Tel: (01284) 766777
2 adapted vehicles.

TRAINS

See Suffolk Traveline above.
Anglia Railways: Tel: (01473) 693333

CAR PARKS

Free disabled badge spaces in all borough
council-owned car parks.
Tel: (01284) 763233

SHOPMOBILITY

The Old Bus Shelter, Angel Hill, Bury St.
Edmunds IP33 1XB
Tel/Fax: (01284) 757175
Minicom: (01284) 757023

ATTRACTIONS

ABBEY VISITOR CENTRE
Abbey Precinct, Abbey Gardens,
Bury St. Edmunds IP33 1RS
Tel: (01284) 763110
Fax: (01284) 757079
e-mail: blake@burybo.stedsbc.gov.uk
Local history museum housed in C11th.
Norman building with permanent
collections and temporary exhibitions and
Visitor Centre with hands-on activities and
interpretation of medieval life in the town.
Nearest car park at Manor House Museum
300m away.
SD CP n/a E RF S WC

MOYSES HALL MUSEUM
Cornhill, Bury St. Edmunds IP33 1DX

Tel: (01284) 757489 Fax: (01284) 707079
e-mail: blake@burybo.stedsbc.gov.uk
Rare C12th. Norman house retaining
many original features. Houses an
important archaeology collection and
many displays on local history. Ground
floor accessible.
SD 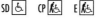 CP E RF S

FELIXSTOWE

Seaside resort with an important port.
Its pier, once 0.5 miles long, was
shortened after WWII, but there is an
amusement park and two miles of
concrete promenade plus a shingle
beach with safe bathing.

TOURIST INFORMATION CENTRE

Tel: (01394) 276770
Fax: (01394) 277456

BED AND BREAKFAST

DORINCOURT GUEST HOUSE
41 Undercliffe Road West,
Felixstowe IP11 8AH
Tel/Fax: (01394) 270447
No. of Accessible Rooms: 2. Bath
Accessible Facilities: Lounge, Dining
Room. Located on the seafront.

FRAMLINGHAM

Pleasant market town with attractive
architecture. 2 sets of Almshouses are
worth noting as are a number of shop
fronts on Market Hill and Castle
Street.

ATTRACTION

FRAMLINGHAM CASTLE
Castle Street,
Framlingham IP13 9BP
Tel/Fax: (01728) 724189
Built between 1177 and 1215, the castle
has fine curtain walls, 13 towers and
many Tudor chimneys. 2 wheelchairs
available. Only ground floor of house
accessible.
SD  CP E RF 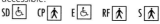 S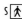

IPSWICH

Probably the first English town founded by the Angles on the River Orwell. Spectacular with a cluster of narrow streets, open parks and dockland area.

TOURIST INFORMATION CENTRE
St. Stephen's Church, St. Stephen's Lane, Ipswich 1P1 1DP
Tel: (01473) 258070
Fax: (01473) 432017

IPSWICH BOROUGH COUNCIL
Tel: (01473) 432000
Access officer.
Produces Ipswich Access Guide.

BUSES
Ipswich Buses: Tel: (01473) 232600
Most low-floor buses with raised kerbs.

TAXIS
Anglia Taxis: Tel: (01473) 252222
Three adapted vehicles.
Avenue Taxis: Tel: (01473) 407777
One adapted vehicles.

TRAINS
Anglia Railways: Assistance:
Tel: (01473) 693333
Minicom: (01603) 630748 or (0845) 6050600
Central Trains: Assistance:
Tel: (0845) 7056027
www.centraltrains.co.uk
First Great Eastern: Special Needs:
Tel: (0845) 9505050
Ipswich Station is NOT accessible to any platform without assistance.

CAR PARKS
Ipswich main shopping streets now pedestrianised, but free 3-hour parking available on-street close by. Normal fee payable in most car parks for disabled badge holders.
Tel: (01473) 738109.

SHOPMOBILITY
Buttermarket Centre, Buttermarket, St. Stephen's Lane, Ipswich.
Tel: (01473) 222225.

HOTELS
COURTYARD BY MARRIOTT
The Havens, Ransomes Europark, Ipswich IP3 9SJ
Tel: (01473) 272244   Fax: (01473) 272484

Experience the Industrial Revolution at Long Shop Steam museum.

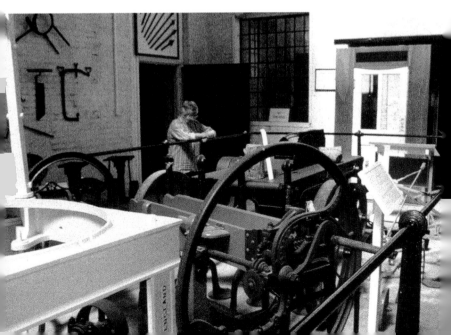

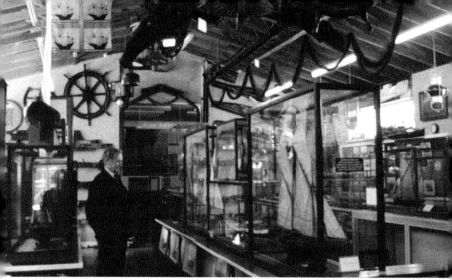

Something for everyone at the excellent Lowestoft Maritime museum.

No. of Accessible Rooms: 2. Bath
Accessible Facilities: Lounge, Restaurant
Modern hotel on the east side of town
centre. East on A14, first slip road after
Orwell Bridge, signposted Nacton and
Ransomes Europark. Good base for
exploring Constable country and Suffolk
Heritage Coast.

IPSWICH COUNTY HOTEL
London Road, Copdock, Ipswich IP8 3JD
Tel: (01473) 209988   Fax: (01473) 730801
No. of Accessible Rooms:1 . Bath.
Accessible Facilities: Lounge, Restaurant.
Comfortable hotel on old A12.

NOVOTEL IPSWICH
Greyfriars Road, Ipswich IP1 1UP
Tel: (01473) 232400   Fax: (01473) 232414
No. of Accessible Rooms: 3. Bath
Accessible Facilities: Lounge, Restaurant,
Bar. Located 0.5 mile from city centre.

SELF-CATERING
STABLE COTTAGES
Chattisham Place, Nr. Ipswich IP8 3QD
Tel/Fax: (01473) 652210
e-mail: Margaret.Langton@talk21.com
No. of Accessible Units: 2
No. of Beds per Unit: 2 - 8
Accessible Facilities: Lounge/diner, Kitchen.
Both have showers.
Converted individual farm buildings
situated around south-east facing

courtyard. Tennis and heated pool. Stable
and Coachmans Cottages are accessible.
Arable farm in small, quiet village near
Constable country and Suffolk River
valleys. Nearby towns of Kersey and
Lavenham worth exploring.

BLACKSMITHS COTTAGE
Hall Farm, Hall Lane, Otley,
Nr. Ipswich IP6 9PA
Tel/Fax: (01473) 890766
www.holidayholmes.com
No. of Accessible Units: 1. Roll-in
Shower.
No. of Bed per Unit:2
Accessible Facilities: Open plan
Kitchen/Lounge. Located in the heart of
rural Suffolk on a 200-acre working farm
on the outskirts of Otley village. Pubs
serving food close by.

LEISTON
Home of Leiston Abbey, probably the
most romantic ruin in the country.

ATTRACTION
LONG SHOP STEAM MUSEUM
Main Street, Leiston,
Nr. Saxmundham   IP16 4ES
Tel: (01728) 832189
www.longshop@care4free.net
The Long Shop was built in 1852 and

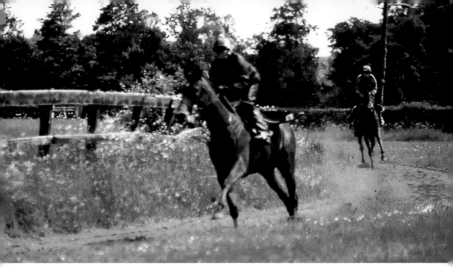

At the gallops, Newmarket is horse training.

was one of Britain's first production lines for steam engines. This award-winning museum has a unique and fascinating collection of exhibits. Travel back in time and explore the industrial heritage of the Victorians.

SD ♿   P ♿   E ♿   RF ♿
S ♿   WC ♿   RFE ♿

LOWESTOFT

Seaside town of some character which pivots around the swing bridge.

TOURIST INFORMATION CENTRE
Tel: (01502) 523000   Fax: (01502) 539023

ATTRACTIONS
LOWESTOFT MARITIME MUSEUM
Sparrows Nest Park, Whapload Road,
Lowestoft NR32 1XG
Tel: (01502) 511260
Lively exhibition on the history of the local fishing fleet from early sail to steam and through to modern diesel vessels. Displays on trawling and herring driftnet fishing, plus the town's wartime association with the Royal Navy.

SD ♿   CP ♿   RF ♿   S ♿

PLEASUREWOOD HILLS
Leisure Way, Corton, Lowestoft NR32 5DZ
Tel: (01502) 586000 Fax: (01502) 567393

e-mail: info@pleasurewoodhills.co.uk
www.pleasurewoodhills.co.uk
Family theme park with over 50 rides, shows and attractions. The rides are mostly ramped, but park staff not allowed (for Health and Safety regulations) to assist disabled guests, a companion is needed. Some rides are inaccessible, and the majority require guests to be able to sit straight and hold onto any restraint on the ride. Situated between Lowestoft and Great Yarmouth just off the A12.

SD ♿   CP ♿   E ♿   RF ♿
C ♿   S ♿   WC 🚶   RFE ♿

SUFFOLK WILDLIFE PARK
Kessingland, Lowestoft NR33 7SL
Tel: (01502) 740291
Fax: (01502) 741105
Within 100 acres of parkland, wild cats, primates and other animals including the only aardvarks in the country living under natural conditions.

SD ♿   CP ♿   E ♿   RF ♿
C 🚶   S ♿   WC 🚶   RFE ♿

NAYLAND

A village set in beautiful country by the River Stour, at one time a busy cloth town. There is an obelisk milestone and a number of attractive cottages and inns.

SELF-CATERING
GLADWINS FARM
Harper's Hill, Nayland CO6 4NU
Tel: (01206) 262261 Fax: (01206) 263001
e-mail: gladwinsfarm@aol.com
No. of Accessible Units: 3. One with roll-in Shower
No. of Beds per Unit: Variable.
Accessible Facilities: Converted Tudor barn and stables. Gainsborough cottage has walk-in shower. Dedham and Hadleigh cottages also accessible. Located on the edge of Dedham Vale, famous for Constable and Gainsborough, in 22 acres of southern countryside overlooking the lovely Stour Valley.

NEWMARKET
On the border of Cambridgeshire and Suffolk. Newmarket has been the headquarters of British horseracing for nearly 400 years. With 3,000 acres of cultivated grassland, more than 2,700 racehorses are in training in 60 yards as well as 40 breeding studs.

TOURIST INFORMATION CENTRE
Tel: (01638) 667200 Fax: (01638) 660394

HOTEL
HEATH COURT HOTEL
Moulton Road, Newmarket CB8 8DY
Tel: (01638) 667171 Fax: (01638) 666533
e-mail: quality@heathcourthotel.com
No. of Accessible Rooms: 42. Bath.
Accessible Facilities: Lounge, Restaurant. Delightful property standing in its own grounds, 400m from the town centre, at the bottom of the famous Newmarket Heath where James I discovered that the heathlands were ideal for racing horses in 1605.

ATTRACTION
NATIONAL HORSERACING MUSEUM
99 High Street, Newmarket CB8 8JH
Tel: (01638) 560622 Fax: (01638) 665600
Museum is completely accessible but a degree of mobility is required to watch horses on the gallops and in their swimming pool and this is a mini-bus tour.

Learn about racing and ask retired jockeys your questions.

SD CP E RF L
C S WC RFE

SAXMUNDHAM
The town straddles the main Ipswich/Lowestoft road, the main street beginning at the southern end with cottages and Georgian houses.

HOTEL
THE CROWN AT WESTLETON
Westleton, Saxmundham IP17 3AD
Tel: (01728) 648777 Fax: (01728) 648239
No. of Accessible Rooms: 1. Bath
Accessible Facilities: Restaurant
A fine Inn, managed by owners with log fires and gardens. Located in delightful village midway between Southwold and Aldeburgh, with thatched C12th church, village green and duck pond.

SELF-CATERING
ROSE FARM
Mill Street, Middleton,
Nr. Saxmundham IP17 3NG
Tel: (01728) 648456
No. of Accessible Units: 2. Roll-in Shower
No. of Beds per Unit: 1 - 3
Accessible Facilities: Lounge, Dining Room, Kitchen, Gardens, Barbecue. Stable Cottage and Thatched Barn can sleep up to 6 and 2 respectively. Located on the edge of rural Middleton, set on eight acres of land with open views across farm land. Approximately halfway between Aldeburgh and Southwold, ideal for exploring Suffolk's Heritage coast.

ATTRACTIONS
BRUISYARD VINEYARD & HERB CENTRE
Church Road, Bruisyard, Saxmundham IP17 2EF
Tel: (01728) 638281 Fax: (08701) 363708
e-mail: ian@bruisyardwines.fsnet.co.uk
Tour 10-acre vineyard and adjoining winery with audio/visual accompaniment followed by wine tasting and visit to tranquil herb and water gardens.

239

SD ♿ CP 🚶 E ♿ RF ♿
S ♿ WC 🚶
RFE- (Building) ♿ (garden) 🚶

MINSMERE RSPB NATURE RESERVE
Westleton, Saxmundham IP17 3BY
Tel: (01728) 648281   Fax: (01728) 648770
e-mail: minsmere@interramp.co.uk
Reasonably firm paths lead to 4 hides
overlooking famous Scrape with avocets
and other waders- all accessible, some
with special viewing places. Cars may be
driven to hides by application to reception.
Disabled badge holders may drive within
400m of island Mere hide with ramped
access. Batricar available free.

SD ♿ CP ♿ E ♿ RF ♿
C ♿ S ♿ WC ♿ RFE ♿

WOODBRIDGE
Originally a busy seaport now mainly a
sailing centre with a winding channel
emerging on the coast between
Bawdsey and Felixstowe.

TOURIST INFORMATION CENTRE
Tel/Fax: (01394) 382240

HOTELS
GROVE HOUSE HOTEL ♿
39 Grove Road, Woodbridge IP12 4LG
Tel: (01394) 382202
No. of Accessible Rooms: 1 roll-in shower.
Accessible Facilities: Dining Room
Newly renovated hotel with garden.

UFFORD PARK HOTEL 🚶
Yarmouth Road, Ufford,
Woodbridge IP12 1QW
Tel: (01394) 383555 Fax: (01394) 383582
e-mail: uffordparkltd@btinternet.com
www.uffordpark.co.uk
No. of Accessible Rooms: 2
Accessible Facilities: Lounge, Restaurants
(2), Leisure Centre.
Set in 120 acres of parkland, this is a
modern hotel and leisure complex.

SELF-CATERING
ST. PETER'S VIEW ♿
The Lodge, Monk Soham,

Woodbridge IP12 7EN
Tel/Fax: (01728) 685358
e-mail: geoffreyclarke@suffolkonline.net
No. of Accessible Units: 4. Shower
No. of Beds per Unit: 2 - 4
Accessible Facilities: Lounge, Dining Room,
Kitchen.
4 cottages in grounds of the Hall.

SURREY

SURREY TOURISM
Room 404, County Hall,Penrhyn
Road,Kingston upon Thames KT1 2DY
Tel: (020) 8541 8092
Fax: (020) 8541 9172
e-mail: surreytourism@surreycc.gov.uk
www.visitsurrey.com

DISS
Harrowlands, Harrowlands Park,
Dorking RH4 2RA
Tel: (01306) 875156
Operates a vast library of information
on all aspects of disability.

WHEELCHAIR TRAVEL
1 Johnston Green, Guildford GU2 6XS
Tel: (020) 8233640
Fax: (020) 8237772
Provides independent transport for
disabled people on self-drive basis, plus
taxi service.

SCILL DISABILITY INFORMATION
3 Robin Hood Lane, Sutton, SM1 2SW
Tel: (020) 8770 4065 Fax: (020) 8770 4067
e-mail: information@scill.org.uk
www.scill.org.uk
Free, impartial and confidential
information on all aspects of life, including
employment, benefits, education, support
groups, equipment, access, holidays,
transport and recreation.

CAMBERLEY
Known for the Royal Staff College and
nearby Royal Military Academy,
Sandhurst.

ATTRACTIONS
ROYAL LOGISTIC CORPS MUSEUM
Deepcut, Camberley GU16 6RW
Tel: (01252) 340871 Fax: (01252) 833484
e-mail: query@rlcmuseum.freeserve.co.uk
The story of support to the Army in transport, ordinance, pioneers, catering and post in hands-on artefacts, hardware, words and pictures. There is a large display area and seating areas.

SD [♿] CP [♿] E [♿] RF [♿]
S [♿] WC [♿] RFE [♿]

BASINGSTOKE CANAL VISITOR CENTRE
Mytchett Place Road, Mytchett,
Nr. Frimley GU16 6DD
Tel: (01252) 370073 Fax: (01252) 371758
e-mail: info@basingstoke-canal.co.uk
Completed in 1794, 37 miles long with 29 locks, the canal survived through a series of local developments, was privately owned at one time and is now much restored. From North Warnborough, through Crookham Village, Fleet, Aldershot, Pirbright, St. John's and West Byfleet, it ends at Woodham. Displays on the sights and sounds of Greywell Tunnel and the lives of barge skippers over 100 years ago. History, restoration and wildlife habitats of the canal also on display.

SD [♿] CP [♿] E [♿] RF [🚶] C [🚶]
S [🚶] WC [🚶] RFE- (Exhibition) [♿]

FRIMLEY LODGE PARK
Sturt Road, Frimley Green,
Nr. Camberley GU16 6NG
Tel: (01252) 836970 Fax: (01252) 836970
Woodland and canalside walks, miniature railway and play area.

SD [♿] CP [♿] E [♿] RF [♿]
C [♿] WC [🚶] RFE [♿]

CHERTSEY

FAMILY ATTRACTION
THORPE PARK
Staines Road, Chertsey KT16 8PN
Tel: (01932) 569393 Fax: (01932) 566367
e-mail:thorpepark@mail.bogo.co.uk
www.thorpepark.co.uk
Rides/attractions at large amusement park.

SD [♿] CP [♿] E [♿] RF [♿]

C [🚶] S [♿] WC [♿] RFE [♿]

DORKING
Ancient market town delightfully set between Box Hill and the Downs rising to the north.

SELF-CATERING
BADGERHOLT [🚶]
Bulmer Farm, Holmbury St. Mary,
Nr. Dorking RH5 6LG
Tel: (01306) 730210
No. of Accessible Units: 1. Shower
No. of Beds per Unit: 2
Accessible Facilities: Open plan Lounge/Kitchenette, Garden. This is a working farm with the s/c units converted from original farm buildings. Holmbury is a lovely village with pubs, Victorian cottages and a famous church. Surrounded by the Surrey Hills.

ATTRACTION
POLESDEN LACEY (NT)
Great Bookham, Nr. Dorking RH5 6BD
Tel: (01372) 452048
Fax: (01372) 452023
Regency villa remodelled in 1906-9. Fine collection of paintings, furniture, porcelain and silver. Extensive grounds include walled rose garden and landscape walks through open countryside and woodland.

SD [♿] CP [♿] E [♿] RF [♿] C [🚶]
S [♿]
WC [🚶] RFE- [🚶] (Landscaped walk of 1.5 miles)

BOX HILL (NT)
National Trust Information Centre, The Old Fort, Box Hill Road, Tadworth,
Nr. Dorking KT20 7LB
Tel: (01306) 885502
Fax: (01306) 875030
Outstanding area of woodland and chalk downland with wonderful views toward South Downs. Access to summit area and slopes via wheelchair path to viewpoint.

SD [♿] CP [🚶] E [♿] RF [♿]
C [♿] S [🚶] WC [♿] RFE [♿]

241

EGHAM

Historic town skirted by the River Thames and the fields of Runnymede, scene of the signing of the Magna Carta in 1215.

HOTEL

RUNNYMEDE HOTEL AND SPA
Windsor Road, Egham TW20 0AG
Tel: (01784) 436171
Fax: (01784) 436340
e-mail: info@runnymedehotel.com
www.runnymedehotel.com
No. of Accessible Rooms: 47. Bath
Accessible Facilities: Lift, Lounge, Restaurants (2), Spa (3 steps). Quality hotel on the banks of the River Thames, beside Bell Weir. Riverside gardens and lawns.

SAVILL COURT HOTEL
Wick Lane, Englefield Green, Egham TW20 0XN
Tel: (01784) 472000
Fax: (01784) 472200
No. of Accessible Rooms: 1. Bath
Accessible Facilities: Lounge, Restaurant.
Jacobean style mansion set in 22 acres of secluded parkland. Located 5 minutes from M25 (J.13) and Heathrow airport.

ATTRACTION

THE SAVILL GARDEN
Windsor Great Park, Wick Lane, Englefield Green, Egham SL4 2HT
Tel: (01753) 847518   Fax: (01753) 847536
www.savillgarden.co.uk
Within Windsor Great Park, 35 acres created to be the best and finest woodland garden for all seasons. Flower gardens blend with open vistas, secret glades and alpine meadows. Wheelchairs on site.

EPSOM

15 miles south-west of London and home to the famous race course, Epsom Downs, and the English Derby.

ATTRACTION

HORTON PARK CHILDREN'S FARM
Horton Lane, Epsom KT19 8PT
Tel: (01372) 743984
Animals chosen for friendliness. Children can stroke and cuddle some of them, otherwise watch and talk to them. Farm walks, adventure play grounds.

ESHER

Residential town on River Mole.

ATTRACTION

CLAREMONT LANDSCAPE GARDEN (NT)
Portsmouth Road, Esher KT10 9JG
Tel: (01372) 467806   Fax: (01932) 464394
e-mail: claremount@ntrust.org.uk
Claremont was laid out before 1720, and is the earliest known surviving English landscaped garden with 50 acres including

On stage at Birdworld's Heron Theatre.

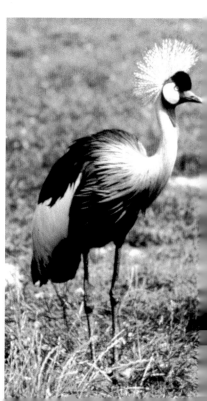

a lake, grotto and turf amphitheatre.

SD ♿   CP ♿   E ♿   RF ♿
C ♿   S ♿   WC 🚹   RFE ♿

SPORTING VENUE
SANDOWN PARK RACECOURSE
Esher KT10 9AJ
Tel: (01372) 464348/463072
Fax: (01372) 465205
Booking: as above.
CP ♿   RE ♿   ED ♿ (except Manual Door)
INT ♿   L ♿   WC ♿ (2 units in main foyer
& near end of Surrey hall)
SS ♿ (follow signs to bottom of Grandstand)
B/R ♿ (lift access)

EWELL

ATTRACTION
BOURNE HALL MUSEUM
Spring Street, Ewell KT17 1UF
Tel: (020) 8394 1734
Low-lying circular modern building of
1960s, with open-plan galleries accessed
by lift. Displays draws on a collection of
over 5,000 items promoting area history,
including collection of toys, old costume
and medical items, a primitive fire engine
and a hansom cab.
SD ♿   CP ♿   E ♿   RF ♿
L ♿   C ♿   S ♿   WC 🚹

FARNHAM
Noted for its Georgian architecture,
particularly in Castle and West Streets.

TOURIST INFORMATION CENTRE
Vernon House, 28 West Street,
Farnham GU9 7DR
Tel: (01252) 715109   Fax: (01252) 717377

BED AND BREAKFAST AND SELF-CATERING
AUDUBON HOUSE   ♿
High Wray, 73 Lodge Hill Road,
Farnham GU10 3RB
Tel/Fax: (01252) 715589
e-mail: sdqq@dial.pipex.com
B & B: No. of Accessible Rooms: 1. Bath
Accessible Facilities: Lounge, Dining Room.
S/C: No. of Accessible Units: 2. Roll-in

shower   No. of Beds per Unit: 2/5
Purpose-built flats for wheelchair users, a
mile from town centre.

ATTRACTION
BIRDWORLD
Holt Pont, Farnham GU10 4LD
Tel: (01420) 22140   Fax: (01420) 23715
Wide variety of waterfowl and land birds in
18 acres of gardens and parkland. Meet
the keepers in the Heron Theatre and
enjoy a picnic in a covered area of the
gardens.
SD ♿   CP 🚹   E ♿   RF ♿
C ♿   S ♿   WC 🚹   RFE ♿

GODALMING
An old town suffering from congested
streets which contain several old
buildings some dating back to the
C16th. The first town in UK to have
electric street lighting. Home of
Charterhouse School, founded in
1611, now located on outskirts.
Surrounded by open countryside and
lovely villages.

ATTRACTION
WINKWORTH ARBORETUM (NT)
Hascombe Road, Nr. Godalming GU8 4AD
Tel: (01483) 208477
Hillside woodland, created in C20th. with
over 1,000 different shrubs and trees,
many of them rare. Impressive displays in
spring for azaleas and in autumn for
amazing colours. 2 lakes and an
abundance of wildlife. Located 2 miles SE
of Godalming on E. side.
SD ♿   CP 🚹   E- ♿   RF ♿
C 🚹 /S 🚹 (combined)   WC 🚹   RFE 🚹

GUILDFORD
Historic old town rich in parks, gardens
and open spaces. Natural amphitheatre
close to town centre, used for open-air
theatre. There is an attractive riverside
along the River Wey, one of the first
rivers to be converted to a navigable
waterway.

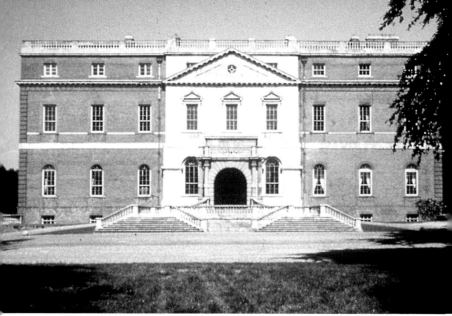

Clandon Park House has some wonderful exhibts.

TOURIST INFORMATION CENTRE
14 Tunsgate, Guildford GU1 3QT
Tel: (01483) 444333   Fax: (01483) 302046

GUILDFORD BOROUGH COUNCIL
Millmead House, Millmead,
Guildford GU2 5BB
Tel: (01483) 505050
Fax: (01483) 302221
www.guildfordborough.co.uk
Produce Access in Guildford.

BUSES
Arriva: Tel: (01483) 505693
Some low-floor buses.

TAXIS
Wheelchair Travel: Tel: (01483) 233640
36 adapted vehicles.

TRAINS
South West Trains: Special Needs:
Tel: (0845) 6050440
Minicom: (0845) 6050441
www.setrains.co.uk
Virgin Trains: Special Needs:
(0845) 7443366
Minicom: (0845) 7443367
Helpline: Tel: (01703) 213600
Guildford Station has level access from the
street though not from Farnham Road:
platforms are accessible via the subway,
standard-height (149cm) telephones, and a
ramp for wheelchairs.

CAR PARKS
Free unlimited disabled badge spaces in all
borough council car parks, also some on-
street parking.
Tel: (01483) 505050

SHOPMOBILITY
Level 3, Bedford Road Car Park,
Guildford GU1 4SA
Tel: (01483) 453993

HOTEL
FORTE POSTHOUSE GUILDFORD
Egerton Road, Guildford GU2 5XH
Tel: (01483) 574444   Fax: (01483) 302960
No. of Accessible Rooms: 1. Bath
Accessible Facilities: Open plan public
rooms. Modern property located 2 miles
from town centre. Good location for
Chessington and Thorpe Park.

ATTRACTIONS
CLANDON PARK (NT)
West Clandon, Nr. Guildford GU4 7RQ
Tel: (01483) 222482   Fax: (01483) 223479
The house contains spectacular ceilings,
porcelain, furniture and tapestries, and the

gardens include a parterre on the south side and a Maori house and sunken Dutch garden on the east side. The Queen's Royal Surrey Regiment Museum is in the basement.

SD ♿   CP 🚶 Entrance ♿🚶 – an electric stair-climber is available to negotiate the few steps at the main entrance. Access generally easy apart from the first floor. RF ♿   C ♿   S ♿   WC ♿🚶 Wheelchairs and wheeled walkers/seats are available.

DAPDUNE WHARF (NT)
River Wey and Godalming Navigations, Dapdune Wharf, Wharf Road, Guildford GU1 4RR
Tel: (01483) 561389 Fax: (01483) 531667
e.mail: riverwey@ntrust.org.uk
A barge-building site on the river Wey. Navigations and parts of the wharf have been restored with stable, smithy, barge-building shed and original Wey barge. There are a series of exhibitions, models and displays which tell the story of the people who lived and worked on the river. The Wey barge accessible with care. Some parts of the towpath and some fishing sites accessible. Contact the Navigations Office on telephone number above for inform-ation and advice on parking and access.

SD ♿   CP 🚶   E ♿   RF ♿
C 🚶   S 🚶   WC 🚶   RFE ♿

HORLEY
(GATWICK AIRPORT)
Small town close to West Sussex border with C14th church. Good access to M25 and A23.

HOTELS
CHEQUERS THISTLE HOTEL   🚶
Brighton Road, Horley RH6 8PH
Tel: (01293) 786992 Fax: (01293) 820625
No. of Accessible Rooms: 39. Bath
Accessible Facilities: Lounge.
Located close to Gatwick Airport

GATWICK MOAT HOUSE   🚶
Longbridge Roundabout, Horley RH6 0AB
Tel: (01293) 899988 Fax: (01293) 899904
No. of Accessible Rooms: 2 (2nd floor via accessible lift).

Accessible Facilities: Lounge, Restaurant (1st floor via lift)
Located close to Gatwick Airport

LEATHERHEAD
An old town home to the Royal School for the Blind established here in 1799.

ATTRACTION
BOCKETTS FARM PARK
Young Street, Fetcham,
Nr. Leatherhead KT22 9BS
Tel: (01372) 363764 Fax: (01372) 361764
Working family farm with old and modern animal breeds. Displays of agricultural bygones, outdoor paddocks and large covered areas. Farm Park area is flat earth.

SD ♿   CP ♿🚶   E ♿   RF ♿
C ♿🚶   S ♿🚶   WC 🚶   RFE ♿

OXTED

BED AND BREAKFAST
ARAWA   🚶
58 Granville Road, Oxted RH8 0BZ
Tel/fax: (01883) 714107
e-mail: gibbsdj@compuserve.com
No. of Accessible Rooms: 1. Bath
Accessible Facilities: Lounge, Dining Room.
Family home taking guests.

REDHILL
Part of the Borough of Reigate and almost a railway creation. Quickly grew in importance, outstripping its parent to become virtually the commercial centre of the borough, a role further increased by the creation of London Gatwick Airport three miles south.

HOTEL
CRABHILL HOUSE (Winged Fellowship)
Kings Cross Lane, South Nutfield,
Redhill RH1 5PA
Tel: (01737) 822221
In the heart of rural Surrey countryside, within easy distance of Brighton and London. All rooms have en-suite facilities and hoist tracking and variable bed

heights. Indoor heated pool. Shop. Bar. Library. Lounger. Conservatory. Lawns and gardens. Adaptive transport.

ATTRACTION
THE OLD MILL
Outwood Common, Nr. Redhill RH1 5PW
Tel: (01342) 843644   Fax: (01342) 843458
e-mail: sheila@jimnutt.cix.co.uk
Oldest working windmill in England, dating from 1665, and the best preserved. Ground floor only is accessible.

SD 🚶	CP 🚶	E ♿
RF ♿	S 🚶	WC 🚶

WEYBRIDGE
An old town on the site where, according to tradition, Julius Caesar crossed the Thames in 55BC. Home to Brooklands Motor Course.

ATTRACTION
BROOKLANDS MUSEUM
Brooklands Road, Weybridge KT13 7QN
Tel: (01932) 857381   Fax: (01932) 855465

Brooklands racing circuit was the home of British motorsport and aviation. This museum, on 30 acres of the original 1907 racing circuit, has many of the original buildings, now restored, in which vehicles and aircraft are displayed.

SD ♿	CP ♿	E ♿	RF ♿
C ♿	S ♿	WC ♿	

WOKING
Comparatively new town, developed with the railway line in the late 1830s.

ATTRACTION
RHS GARDEN WISLEY
Wisley, Woking GU23 6QB
Tel: (01483) 224234 Fax: (01483) 211750
e-mail: rhs@rhs.org.uk
Major experimental gardens of the Royal Horticultural Society. 240 acres of both gardens and vegetable gardens with greenhouses and specialist areas with many unusual plants and shrubs.

SD ♿	CP ♿	E ♿	RF ♿
C ♿	S ♿	WC 🚶	

The house at Wisley in the gardens of the Royal Horticultural Society.

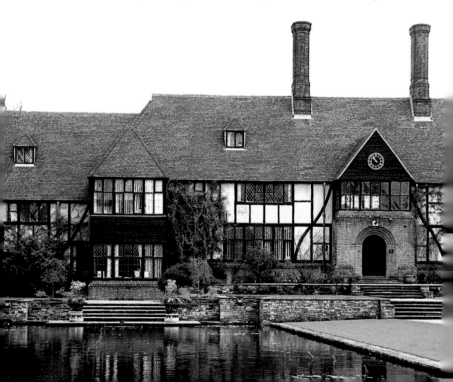

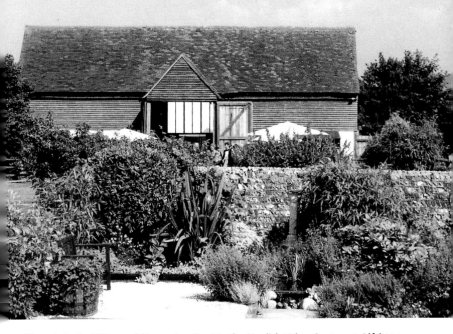

The original off-licence? No, not quite, it's the English Wine Centre at Alfriston.

SUSSEX

EAST SUSSEX

ALFRISTON

Ancient town with first building to be
acquired by the National Trust: the
C14th Clergy House, and example of a
pre-Reformation vicarage, purchased
in 1896 for £10. The C15th Star Inn is
one of the oldest in England.

ATTRACTION
DRUSILLAS PARK
Alfriston BN26 5QS
Tel: (01323) 870656   Fax: (01323) 870846
e-mail: drusilla@drusilla.demon.co.uk
Fine small zoo with wide variety of animals
in naturalistic environments including a
walk-through Bat Enclosure and Pet
World. Children's activities include
Playland, Train, Panning for Gold, Wacky
Workshop, Maasai Exhibition and Animal
Encounter sessions.

SD ♿	CP ♿	E ♿	RF ♿
C ♿	S ♿	WC ♿	RFE ♿

ENGLISH WINE CENTRE
Alfriston Roundabout, Alfriston BN26 5QS
Tel: (01323) 870164   Fax: (01323) 870005
e-mail: bottles@englishwine.co.uk
www.englishwine.co.uk
Wine tastings and tour of museum.

SD ♿	CP ♿	E ♿	RF ♿
C ♿	S ♿	WC ♿	RFE ♿

BATTLE

Built on the site of the Battle of
Hastings, the town contains many old
buildings, some of C13th & C14th,
but interest centres mainly around the
abbey and the historic events of 1066.

TOURIST INFORMATION CENTRE
88 High Street, Battle, TN33 0AQ
Tel: (01424) 773721   Fax: (01424) 773436

ATTRACTION
BATTLEFIELD OF HASTINGS AND ABBEY
RUINS (EH)
Battle Abbey, Battle TN33 0AD
Tel: (01424) 773792   Fax: (01424) 775059
Tour the battlefield and step back in time
to October 1066. See interactive displays
and exhibitions and audio-visual

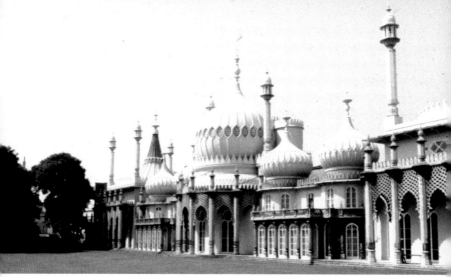

Now returned to its original palatial splendour, Brighton's Royal Pavilion.

interpretation of the Battle. Of the abbey, the Great Gatehouse is the best preserved. Separate entrance up a slight incline with York paving stones, through gate into abbey grounds.

SD ⬤ CP   E ⬤ S ⬤ F ⬤

BRIGHTON

Largest resort in the SE, combining gracious C18th architecture with modern amusements. Its wonderful Royal Pavilion, Palace Pier and an amble along the promenade sit rather oddly with an exploration of the famous Lanes, with restaurants and antique shops.

TOURIST INFORMATION CENTRES

10 Bartholomew Square,
Brighton BN1 1JS
Tel: (01273) 292599
www.brighton.co.uk

Hove Town Hall, Church Road, Hove BN3 3BQ. Telephone number as above

BRIGHTON AND HOVE FEDERATION OF DISABLED PEOPLE

Snowdon House, 3 Rutland Gardens,
Hove BN3 5PD
Tel: (01273) 208934
Produces Access to Brighton & Hove.

BRIGHTON AND HOVE DISABILITY ADVICE CENTRE

Tel: (01273) 203016
Hire out wheelchairs.

BUSES

Brighton and Hove Bus Company:
Tel: (01273) 886200
Some low-floor buses.
Community Transport: Tel: (01273) 292599
Usually for residents, but do take visitors if space available.

TAXIS

Brighton Streamline Taxis:
Tel: (01273) 747474
10 adapted vehicles.
Brighton & Hove Radio Cabs:
Tel: (01273) 324245
1 adapted vehicle.
Hove Streamline Taxis: Tel: (01273) 202020
Southern Taxis: (01273) 205205
2 adapted vehicles.

TRAINS

Connex Southcentral: Disabled Traveline:
Tel: (0870) 6030405
Fax: (0870) 6030505
Minicom: (01273) 617621
Thameslink: Special Needs:
Tel: (0207) 6206333
Minicom: (0207) 6205561
Stationlink bus: Tel: (0207) 9183312
Virgin Trains: Special Needs: (0845) 7443366

Minicom: (0845) 7443367
Wales & West: Special Needs:
Tel: (0845) 3003005
Minicom: (0845) 7585469
Brighton Railbus: Tel: (01273) 886200
Valid on all Brighton and Hove bus services
within a given area.
Brighton Station is suitable for wheelchairs
using ramp access.

CAR PARKS
Free unlimited disabled badge spaces in
Pay & Display and in council car parks.
Tel: (01273) 203016

WHEELCHAIR HIRE
Red Cross Medical Loans,
29-31 Prestonville Road, Brighton.

HOTELS
BRIGHTON THISTLE 🚶
Kings Road, Brighton BN1 2GS
Tel: (01273) 206700   Fax: (01273) 820692
No. of Accessible Rooms: 3.
Accessible Facilities: Public areas accessible
by Lift. Quality hotel on the seafront.

DE VERE GRAND HOTEL 🚶
Kings Road, Brighton BN1 2PW
Tel: (01273) 321188   Fax: (01273) 202694
e-mail: general@grandbrighton.co.uk
No. of Accessible Rooms: unknown
Accessible Facilities: Ramped entrance,
Lounge, Restaurant. Majestic property
designed in elaborate Italian Renaissance
style, in commanding position on the
seafront.

QUALITY HOTEL BRIGHTON 🚶
West Street, Brighton BN1 2RQ
Tel: (01273) 220033   Fax: (01273) 778000
e-mail: admin@gb057.u-net.com
www.choice hotelseurope.com
No. of Accessible Rooms: 2 (via
accessible lift)
Accessible Facilities: all public areas (level or
lift access).
Large modern hotel adjacent to the
Conference Centre and close to seafront.

ACCESSIBLE ATTRACTION
BOOTH MUSEUM OF NATURAL HISTORY
194 Dyke Road, Brighton BN1 5AA

Tel: (01273) 292777 Fax: (01273) 292778
e-mail: boothmus@pavilion.co.uk
Creation of Victorian ornithologist Edward
Booth, and built in 1874 to house his
collection of stuffed British birds. The
birds now share display with over half a
million other specimens from the natural
world - butterflies, beetles, skeletons,
fossils, minerals and rocks, plants and
microscope slides. Displays on taxidermy,
flint knapping, fossil collecting and
butterfly mounting etc. All galleries on
one level.
SD ♿   CP ♿   E ♿ (via rear entrance)
S ♿

THE ROYAL PAVILION
Brighton BN1 1EE
Tel:(01273) 290900   Fax:(01273) 2902821
Former seaside residence of George IV
with domes and minarets and sumptuous
interior. Recently undergone a massive
structural restoration and a must to visit.
SD ♿   CP 🚶 (Book in advance in both cases)
E ♿   C n/a   S ♿   WC 🚶

BURWASH
Half way between Hastings and
Tunbridge Wells, famous particularly
as the home of Rudyard Kipling
(Bateman's) but also worth a visit for
its redbrick and weatherboard
cottages.

ATTRACTION
BATEMAN'S (NT)
Burwash, Etchingham TN19 7DS
Tel: (01435) 882302   Fax: (01435) 882811
The home of Rudyard Kipling from
1902/1936, this is a delightful C17th
ironmaster's house. Kipling's study is as it
was, as is his 1928 Rolls-Royce. Lovely
gardens with restored watermill. After
reporting to the ticket office, those with
mobility problems can drive down an
alternative entrance, entering property by
a path that, although of uneven stones,
has no slope. House: Wheelchair access
possible on ground floor of house and
tea-room, but ambulant access only
available to shop and mill. Gardens:

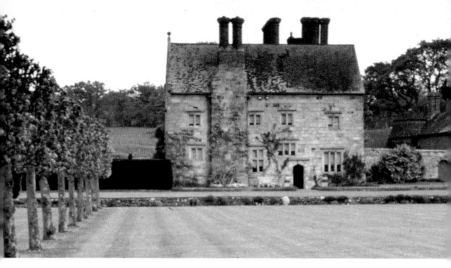

Batemans, Rudyard Kipling's home.

Garden paths have varying surfaces, and so a wheelchair access map is provided. Generally accessible.

SD 🦽   CP ♿   E 🦽   C 🚶
S 🚶   WC 🚶   RFE ♿

EASTBOURNE

Much favoured by those in retirement, Eastbourne has a fine three-mile seafront, the coastline is dominated by miles of chalk cliffs and Beachy Head.

TOURIST INFORMATION CENTRE
3 Cornfield Road, Eastbourne BN21 4QL
Tel: (01323) 411400   Fax: (01323) 649574

TOURISM AND COMMUNITY SERVICES
College Road, Eastbourne, BN21 4JJ
Tel: (01323) 415437   Fax: (01323) 430093

ACCESS OFFICER
Department of Environmental Services, 68 grove Road, Eastbourne BN21 1DF
Tel: (01323) 415281   Fax: (01323) 415995
Minicom: (01323) 415111
Produces Access, information on all aspects of Eastbourne.

WHEELCHAIR/SCOOTER HIRE
Mobility Hire.
149 Tideswell Road, Eastbourne BN21 3RT
Tel: (01323) 721223/638046
Rental of Scooters and Electric and Manual Wheelchairs.

BRITISH RED CROSS CENTRE
The Redoubt, Royal Parade, Eastbourne
Tel: (01323) 732471
Hires out wheelchairs as above.

BEACH LIFEGUARD STATION
Wish Tower, Eastbourne
Tel: (01323) 412290
Summer Season – a wheelchair available for daily hire and a Beach Wheelchair to help across shingle.

BUSES
Bus Stop Shops: Tel: (01323) 416416
Arndale Centre (Bankers Corner Entrance)
Railway Station for all bus information.

TAXIS
Town & Country Cabs: Tel: (01323) 727766
Nine adapted vehicles.
Ranks outside the station, the Pier, Bolton Road.

TRAINS
Connex Southcentral.
Disabled Traveline: Tel: (0870) 6030405
Fax: (0870) 6030505
Minicom: (01233) 617621
Eastbourne Station has a wheelchair ramp.

CAR PARKS

Some free disabled badge spaces in council-owned car parks, others are charged. On-street parking on yellow lines for 3 hours.
Tel: (01323) 415218

HOTELS

CONGRESS HOTEL
31-41 Carlisle Road, Eastbourne BN21 4LS
Tel: (01323) 732118   Fax: (01323) 720016
e-mail: Congresshotels@msn.co.uk
www.Congresshotels@msn.co.uk
No. of Accessible Rooms: 4. Bath
Accessible Facilities: Lounge/Bar (ramped),
Restaurant. Family owned and managed
hotel near town centre and seafront.

HEATHERDENE HOTEL
26-28 Elms Avenue, Eastbourne BN21 3DN
Tel/Fax: (01323) 725811
No. of Accessible Rooms: 2
Accessible Facilities: Dining Room, Bar.
Privately owned attractive property in
pleasant avenue close to Grand Parade.

ATTRACTIONS

BEACHY HEAD COUNTRYSIDE CENTRE
Beachy Head, Eastbourne BN20 7YA
Tel: (01323) 737273
Innovative exhibition on local wildlife and
history with rock pool, mock cliff face,
micrarium, talking shepherd, Bronze Age
man and 3-D colour slide show.
SD [&] CP n/a E [&]   RF [&]   C [&]
S [&]   WC [人] RFE [&]

LIFEBOAT MUSEUM
King Edwards Parade, Eastbourne
Tel: (01323) 730717
Memorabilia and lifeboats models trace the
history of these sturdy vessels.
This is a very small museum and shop with
room for no more than 2 wheelchairs at a
time. Lovely views onto the beach and sea
from the flat outside area.
SD [&]   CP [人]   E [&]

HAILSHAM

An important market town as far back
as Norman times and still has one of
the largest markets in East Sussex,
covering more than 3 acres.

ATTRACTION

CUCKOO TRAIL
Accessible route for wheelchairs through
attractive countryside following route
between Polegate and Heathfield. Stretch
between Polegate and Hailsham (3 miles)
particularly suitable for wheelchair users.

MICHELHAM PRIORY (EH)
Upper Dicker, Hailsham BN27 3QD
Tel: (01323) 844224
Fax: (01323) 844030
A moat and range of gardens surround
the medieval priory with Tudor additions.
Home to fascinating collection tracing
Michelham's religious origins, through its
life as a working farm to country house. A
watermill, Elizabethan barn and imposing
C14th gatehouse give further evidence of
the priory's importance. A wonderful
setting. Wheelchairs available for hire.
SD [&]   CP [人&]   E [&]   RF [&]
C [&]   S [&]   WC [人]   RF [人]

HASTINGS

Famous as the base from which
William the Conqueror set out to fight
the Battle of Hastings, there is an
extensive shingle beach and long pier
supplying the usual seaside
amusements.

TOURIST INFORMATION CENTRE

Town Hall, Queens Road, Hastings
TN34 1QR
Tel: (01424) 781111
Fax: (01424) 781186

HOTEL

GRAND HOTEL
Grand Parade, St. Leonards,
Hastings TN8 0DD
Tel/Fax: (01424) 428510
No. of Accessible Rooms: 2. Bath
Accessible Facilities: Lounge, Restaurant.
Located within town, 200m from beach.

HERTSMONCEAUX

The castle, a fine example of a fortified manor house, is home to the C15th Royal Greenwich Observatory. The village is noted for its woodcrafts, traditional in this area.

BED & BREAKFAST
CONQUERORS
Cowbeech Hill, Hertsmonceaux BN27 4PR
Tel/Fax: (01323) 832446
No. of Accessible Rooms: 1. Roll-in Shower
Accessible Facilities: Lounge, Restaurant, Gardens with horses, peacocks and sheep.
This is a working farm.

LEWES

Narrow and steep streets here, the High Street has many Georgian buildings and interesting little corners to delight the eye.

TOURIST INFORMATION CENTRE
187 High Street, Lewes BN7 2DE
Tel: (01273) 483448   Fax (01273) 484003
Car Parking – disability parking at precinct, Cliffe High Street and Main High Street.

COMMUNITY TRANSPORT
Tel: (01273) 517 332
Car with ramped rear access available to hire, accommodating 3 passengers, including 1 in wheelchair. Minibus with ramped rear access available for hire carrying 16 passengers or 14 and 2 seated in wheelchairs.

BUSES
CountyRider/Lewes Area Dial-a-Ride wheelchair accessible transport, routes vary on different days.
Contact: (01273) 478 007

TAXIS
Farmer/Saltdean Taxis
Tel: (01273) 307 827

7/8 seater minibus accommodating 2 wheelchairs.

VERSACAB, HURSTPIERPOINT
Tel: (01273) 832 832
6-seater taxi capable of being adjusted to carry up to 2 wheelchairs.

ATTRACTION
TREKKERS DISABLED CYCLE CENTRE
Granary Barn
Seven Sisters County Park, Lewes
Tel: (01323) 870 310
Range of wheelchair and side by side tandem bikes specially designed. These can be used on paths and forest trails within the park. There is disabled parking close to Hiring Centre and an accessible WC and shower.

NEWHAVEN

Car Parking – disability parking in Meeching Road and multi-storey car park.

PARADISE FAMILY LEISURE PARK
Avis Road, Newhaven BN9 0DH
Tel: (01273) 512123   Fax: (01273) 616005
e-mail: enquiries@paradisepark.co.uk
web: www.paradisepark.co.uk
Leisure and Botanic gardens, Planet Earth Exhibition, including Dinosaur Museum, Natural Science and History displays, Maritime Museum and a play zone with rides, railway, boats and pirate ship. A great day out for all.

| SD ♿ | CP ♿ | E ♿ | C ♿ |
| S ♿ | WC ♿ | RFE ♿ | |

NUTLEY

Small village in Ashdown Forest a short drive from the south coast.

SELF-CATERING
WHITE HOUSE FARM HOLIDAY HOMES
Hornley Common, Nutley TN22 3EE
Tel/Fax: (01825) 712377
No. of Accessible Units: 1. Shower.
No. of Beds per Unit: 4

Accessible Facilities: Lounge/Diner, Kitchen, Patio. 5 self contained single storey cottages with views across Ashdown Forest and undulating countryside.

PLUMPTON

SPORTING VENUE
PLUMPTON RACECOURSE
Plumpton BN7 3AL
Tel: (01273) 890383   Fax: (01273) 891557
Booking: as above.

CP   RE   ED   (except manual door)
INT   WC   (2 units on ground level)
SS   B/R

RYE

Truly one of the most attractive towns in England which has managed to retain its ancient character despite the influx of visitors. Standing near the mouth of the River Rother, its hilly streets (many are cobbled, which can be tricky), there is a wealth of medieval, Tudor, Stuart and Georgian houses.

TOURIST INFORMATION CENTRE
The Heritage Centre, Strand Quay, Rye TN31 7AY
Tel: (01797) 226696   Fax: (01797) 223460

ACCESSIBLE ATTRACTIONS
GREAT KNELLE FARM
Beckley, Rye TN31 6UB
Tel: (01797) 260250   Fax: (01797) 260347
Working farm, encouraging visitors to hands-on-experience. Disabled fishing platforms for seasonal coarse fishing on River Rother. Woodland trail is the only area which is not hard surfaced and open to the vagaries of climate.
CP   E   C   S   WC   RFE

SEAFORD
Located on Sussex Downs on the coast between Newhaven and Eastbourne.

TOURIST INFORMATION CENTRE
Station Approach, Seaford BN25 2AR

Central location but small entrance step means access is difficult. Level promenade approximately 1.5 miles long, stretching from the Buckle to Splash Point. Disabled parking at Splash point in Esplanade car park. Viewing point allowing wheelchairs to get close to the sea at Splash Point.

ATTRACTION
SEVEN SISTERS COUNTRY PARK
Exceat, Seaford BN25 4AD
Tel: (01323) 870280   Fax: (01323) 871070
The park is 700 acres of open Downland, meadows, salt marsh, shingle beach and wetland, one of the few undeveloped valleys in the south east of the country. Within a site of Special Scientific Interest and an area of Outstanding Natural Beauty. At the valley bottom there is a 2km concrete track suitable for wheelchair users with resting places along main route.

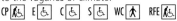

SD   CP   E   RF   C
S   WC

 RFE   Wheelchairs and two self-drive cars available.

UCKFIELD

ATTRACTIONS
BLUEBELL RAILWAY
Sheffield Park Station,
Nr. Uckfield TN22 3QL
Tel: (01825) 723777   Fax: (01825) 724139
A leisurely journey through both the Sussex Weald and time, from the Victorian age at Sheffield Park, to the 1950s at Kingscote. Both stations accessible, although no parking at Kingscote and so it's more practical to begin and end at Sheffield Park. Intermediate station at Horsted Keynes not accessible. Sheffield Park is the HQ with a locomotive collection and a small museum.
SD   CP   E   RF   C   S
WC   (located at Sheffield Park and Kingscote.)

HEAVEN FARM
Furners Green, Uckfield TN22 3RG
Tel: (01825) 790226   Fax: (01825) 790881
Buildings erected in early 1820s comprise the Farm Museum with cowshed, dairy, wood corners, oasthouse and cooling floor,
These illustrate farming in that period.

Sadly the wood parkland and waterside walks are undulating and hard work and therefore inaccessible.

SD ♿   CP 🚶   E 🚶   RF 🚶
C 🚶   S 🚶   WC 🚶

SHEFFIELD PARK GARDEN (NT)
Sheffield Park, Uckfield TN22 3QX
Tel: (01825) 790231
Fax: (01825) 791264

Four large lakes linked by cascades and waterfalls with rare shrubs and colourful flowers in this garden laid out by famous landscape gardener Capability Brown.
WARNING: Unmade car park unsuitable, but disabled passengers can be set down directly at concrete ramps leading into the admissions area, before parking. If travelling alone, this option isn't feasible.

SD ♿   CP ♿   E ♿   RF ♿
C ♿ (not NT but ramp & level access)
S ♿   WC 🚶   RFE ♿

WEST SUSSEX

WEST SUSSEX TOURISM INITIATIVE
12 Steyne, Worthing BN11 3DU
e-mail: wsti@enta.net
www.westsussex.gov.uk

WEST SUSSEX ASSOCIATION FOR THE DISABLED
10 South Pallant, Chichester PO19 1SU
Tel: (01243) 774088

WEST SUSSEX TRAVELINE:
Tel: (0345) 959099

WEST SUSSX COUNTY COUNCIL.
Tel: (01243) 777100

ARUNDEL
Peaceful town nestles below the battlements of one of the most impressive castles in the country. Quaint narrow streets are brim-full of tearooms and antique shops. The warm stone of the castle stands over the red tiled roofs of the town rambling down to the river Arun.

TOURIST INFORMATION CENTRE
61 High Street, Arundel BN18 9AJ
Tel: (01903) 882258   Fax: (01903) 882419

BED AND BREAKFAST
MILL LANE HOUSE   🚶
Slindon, Arundel BN18 0RP
Tel: (01243) 814440
Fax: (01243) 814436

No. of Accessible Rooms: 2. Roll-in Shower
Accessible Facilities: Dining Room.
C17th house in National Trust downland village with superb views. Accommodation is in Coach House across drive from main house with own entrance. Breakfast can be taken in room or in main house (one step).

WOODYBANKS   🚶
Crossgate, Amberley, Nr. Arundel BN18 9NR
Tel: (01798) 831295

No. of Accessible Rooms: 2. Shower.
Accessible Facilities: Lounge, Dining Room,
Low lying windows affording elevated views across the Wildbrooks of Amberely ranging for 10 miles.
Amberley is a tranquil village nestling in the South Downs. The owners have a disabled daughter and sound extremely understanding and pleasant.

Arundel - home to an amazing castle and church, high above narrow streets packed with antique shops.

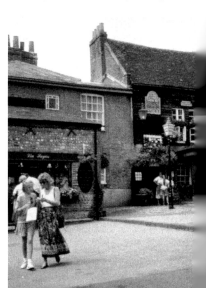

ATTRACTIONS
AMBERLEY MUSEUM
Amberley, Nr. Arundel BN18 9LT
Tel: (01798) 831370
Fax: (01798) 831831
e-mail: office@amberleymuseum.co.uk
www.amberleymuseum.co.uk
Established to preserve and record the working heritage of the South East, its collections include timber-working, brick-making, road-building, blacksmithing, pottery and recent histories of printing, mechanised transport and radio.

SD | CP | E | RF | C
S | WC | | RFE (AV Room)

DENMANS GARDENS
Denmans Lane, Fontwell,
Nr. Arundel BN18 0SU
Tel: (01243) 542808
Fax: (01243) 544064
3.5 acre site, gradually developed over the past 50 years to include a wonderful walled garden, bursting with perennials and old-fashioned roses: a gravel stream with a pond and grasses and a south garden with maple and cherry trees, plus rare species. There is a school of garden design in the clockhouse.

SD n/a | CP | E | RF
C | S | WC | RFE

THE WILDFOWL AND WETLANDS TRUST
Mill Road, Arundel BN18 9PB
Tel: (01903) 883355
Fax: (01903) 884834
60 acres of ponds, lakes and reedbeds with thousands of tame and wild and migratory birds. Four activity stations spark interest and many birds can be hand fed.

SD | CP | E | RF | C
S | WC | RFE | G

SPORTING VENUE
FONTWELL PARK RACECOURSE
Fontwell, Nr. Arundel BN18 0SX
Admin & Booking - Box Office:
(01243) 543335   Fax: (01243) 543904
CP (Disabled badge parking on request)
RE   ED (except Manual Door)
INT   L
WC (2 units, one in each enclosure)
SS n/a (No designated seating as such)

BOGNOR REGIS
Popular seaside resort with soft sands and calm seas. It lies in the lee of Selsey Bill and sheltered by the Isle of Wight and the South Downs.

TOURIST INFORMATION CENTRE
Belmont Street, Bognor Regis PO21 1BJ
Tel: (01243) 823140   Fax: (01243) 820435

HOTEL
THE ALDWICK HOTEL
Aldwick Road, Aldwick, Bognor Regis PO21 2QU
Tel: (01243) 821945   Fax: (01243) 821316
No. of Accessible Rooms: 1. Bath with Hydraulic Transfer Chair.
Accessible Facilities: Lounge, Restaurant. Located 5 miles from Chichester close to the seafront and town centre.

SELF-CATERING
27 NELSON ROAD
Bognor Regis
Book through Grooms Holidays
No. of Accessible Units: 1
No. of Beds per Unit: 8
Accessible Facilities: Lounge, Kitchen, Diner. Specially designed, spacious house located in quiet residential area of town, 8 minutes' walk from seafront and shops.

BEACH LODGE
Flepham, Nr. Bognor Regis
Book through Grooms Holidays
No. of Accessible Units: 1
No. of Beds per Unit: 9
Accessible Facilities: Garden
Spacious, split level modern house on private seaside estate in small village. Located at entry to level promenade stretching for miles along sandy seafront.

CHICHESTER
Founded by the Romans c.AD70 who laid out the main street plan and built the original city walls, rebuilt in flint in medieval times. Notable now for its Georgian architecture, especially in the street Little London.

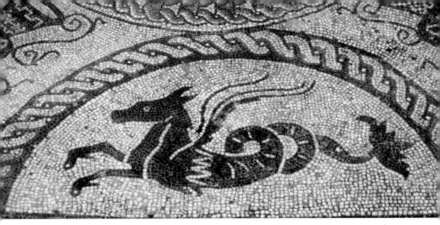

A floor mosiac.at Fishbourne Roman Palace, Chichester.

TOURIST INFORMATION CENTRE
29A South Street, Chichester PO19 1AH
Tel: (01243) 775888   Fax: (01243) 539449

BUSES
Stagecoach Coastline: Tel: (01243) 539953
No low-floor buses as yet.

TAXIS
Central Taxis: Tel: (0800) 789432
1 adapted vehicle.
Blueline Taxis: Tel: (01243) 774077
1 adapted vehicle.
Direct Line Taxis: Tel: (01243) 533335
3 adapted vehicles.
Many more available from ICIS:
Tel: (0800) 859929

TRAINS
Connex Southcentral. Disabled Traveline:
Tel: (0870) 6030405
Fax: (0870) 6030505
Minicom: (012333) 617621
Wales & West: Special Needs:
Tel: (0845) 30030005
Minicom: (0845) 585469
Chichester Station is suitable for
wheelchairs using ramp access.

CAR PARKS
Disabled badge spaces. Tel: (01243) 777100

HOTELS
CROUCHERS BOTTOM COUNTRY HOTEL ♿
Birdham Road, Chichester PO20 7EH
Tel: (01243) 784995   Fax: (01243) 539797
e-mail: Crouchers_bottom@hantslife.co.uk
Crouchers_bottom@hantslife.co.uk

No. of Accessible Rooms: 2. Bath
Accessible Facilities: Lounge, Restaurant.
Early 1900s farmhouse converted to small
hotel with bedrooms in outside barn and
coach house and bar and restaurant in
main house. Situated between Chichester
Marina and Del Quay.

ST. ANDREWS LODGE ♿
Chichester Road, Selsey
Nr. Chichester PO20 0LX
Tel: (01243) 606899   Fax: (01243) 607826
No. of Accessible Rooms: 1. Roll-in Shower
Accessible Facilities: Lounge, Restaurant.
Family run hotel situated on the Manhood
Peninsula, 7 miles south of Chichester and
close to unspoilt beaches and countryside.

SELF-CATERING
SEAGULLS
Bill Point, Grafton Road, Selsey, Nr.
Chichester
Book through Grooms Holidays
No. of Accessible Units: 1
No. of Beds per Unit: 6. Shower
Accessible Facilities: Garden. Ramp down
to the beach. Located on southernmost tip
of Selsey Bill, this lovely bungalow enjoys
panoramic view across English Channel.

TAMARISK
Farm Road, Bracklesham Bay,
Nr. Chichester
Book through Grooms Holidays.
No. of Accessible Units: 1. Shower
No. of Beds per Unit: 6
Accessible Facilities: Garden
New purpose-built bungalow a few

minutes from the sea. Bracklesham Bay has many isolated havens.

SELSEY COTTAGE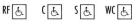
Selsey, Nr. Chichester.
Bookings: Mrs. Sue Graves, 28 Wise Lane, London NW7 2RE
e-mail: sue@suegraves.demon.co.uk
No. of Accessible Units: 1. Roll-in Shower
No. of Beds per Unit: 2
Accessible Facilities: Lounge, Dining Room, Kitchen. Spacious seafront house with fine views. Pets welcome. 20 minutes from Chichester.

10 CULIMORE CLOSE
West Wittering, Chichester PO20 8HD
Tel: (01243) 672723
No. of Accessible Units: 1
No. of Beds per Unit: 2 + sofa-bed
Accessible Facilities: Lounge, Kitchen/Diner, Private Garden.
Fully self-contained annexe of family home in quiet cul-de-sac. 2 minutes from the sea and village, 6 miles from Chichester.

ATTRACTIONS
EARNLEY GARDENS
133 Almodington Lane, Earnley, Nr. Chichester PO20 7SR
Tel: (01243) 512637   Fax: (01243) 673658
Tropical butterflies, exotic birds. Theme gardens, small animals, pottery, shipwreck museum and Rejectamenta the Nostalgia Museum, all under cover. Follow the Butterflies & Gardens signs off the A286 Chichester/Witterings Road.

SD   CP   E   RF   C   S   WC   RFE

GOODWOOD HOUSE
Goodwood, Chichester PO18 0PX
Tel: (01243) 755048   Fax: (01243) 755005
e-mail: debora@goodoowd.co.uk
Ancestral home of the Dukes of Richmond for 300 years and now lived in by the Earl of March and his family. Soon after Napoleon's 1798 Campaign on the Nile, the 3rd Duke created his Egyptian State Dining Room which has now been recreated and open to the public together with the other newly restored state apartments.

SD   CP   E (Ballroom E.)

RF   C   S   WC   RFE

FISHBOURNE ROMAN PALACE
Salthill Road, Fishbourne, Chichester PO19 3QR
Tel: (01243) 785859   Fax: (01243) 539266
Largest known Roman residence in Britain with many original mosaic floors restored. The museum relates the history of the palace with full-size reconstruction of one room and a museum of Roman gardening and a reconstructed Roman garden.

SD   CP   E   RF   C
S   WC   RFE (Gardens)

MECHANICAL MUSIC AND DOLL COLLECTION
Church Road, Portfield, Chichester PO19 4HN
Tel: (01243) 372646   Fax: (01243) 370299
Rare barrel organs and musical boxes combine with fine examples of Victorian china and wax dolls housed in well-preserved Victorian church.

SD   CP   E   RF   S   RFE

WEST DEAN GARDENS
West Dean, Chichester PO10 04Z.
Tel: (01243) 818201/811301
Fax: (01243) 811342
25 acres noted for a 100m long pergola. Newly restored walled garden contains Victorian glasshouses, large working kitchen garden and tool/mower collection. Glasshouses and pergola not suitable for wheelchairs.

SD   CP   E   C
S   WC   RFE

SPORTING VENUE
GOODWOOD RACECOURSE
Goodwood, Chichester PO18 9OS
Admin & Booking-Box Office: (01243) 755022 Fax: (01243) 755025
Credit Card bookings: (0800) 0818191
Wheelchair loan available.

CP   (Park in CP 8 - need disabled sticker)
RE   ED   INT   L
WC   (5 units, in March Stand Floor, East & West. Sussex Stand Floor and Public Enclosure)
SS   (Viewing ramps for access on Richmond Enclosure Lawn, Sussex Stand Lawn and Parade Ring (in Gordon Enclosure)
B/R   (Access to all areas except Bentinck Bar in Richmond Enclosure)

EAST GRINSTEAD

Notable for Sackville college in the
High Street, Jacobean Almshouses
founded in 1609 by Robert Sackville
2nd Earl of Dorset and still a home for
the elderly.

ATTRACTION
STANDEN (NT)
West Hoathley Road,
East Grinstead RH19 4NE
Tel: (01342) 323029 Fax: (01342) 316424
e-mail: sstpro@smtp.ntrust.org.uk
Built in 1890s, a showpiece of the arts
and crafts of the William Morris period.
Hillside garden and wooded walks.

SD ♿	CP ♿	E 🚹	RF ♿
C ♿	S ♿	WC 🚹	

GATWICK AIRPORT

TRAINS
Connex: Customer Services:
Tel: (0870) 6030405
Fax: (0870) 6030505
Minicom: (01233) 617621
Gatwick Express: Assistance:
Tel/Minicom: (099) 301530
Thameslink: Special Needs:
Tel: (0207) 6206333
Minicom: (0207) 6205561
Stationlink bus: Tel: (0207) 9183312
Virgin Trains: Special Needs:
Tel: (0845) 7443366
Minicom: (0845) 7443367

HOTELS
COPTHORNE EFFINGHAM PARK   🚹
West Park Road,
Copthorne RH10 3EU
Tel: (01342) 714994 Fax: 901342) 716039
No. of Accessible Rooms: 1. Bath
Accessible Facilities: Lounge, Restaurant,
Outdoor seating area. Fine modern hotel
built around an historic country house in
40 acres of parkland and delightfully
landscaped gardens.

COPTHORNE LONDON GATWICK   🚹
Copthorne Way, Copthorne RH10 3PG

Tel: (01342) 348800 Fax: (01342) 348833
No. of Accessible Rooms: 13. Bath
Accessible Facilities: Lounge,
Restaurants (2).
Built around a C16th farmhouse, set in
100 acres of wooded, landscape gardens
in village of Copthorne. Very close to M23
(J10), close to Gatwick Airport.

HILTON LONDON GATWICK   🚹
South Terminal, Gatwick Airport RH6 0LL
Tel: (01293) 518080 Fax: (01293) 528980
No. of Accessible Rooms: 2. Roll-in Shower
Accessible Facilities: Lift (Cat.1), Lounge,
Garden Restaurant, Pool, Sauna, Spa.

LE MERIDIEN LONDON GATWICK   🚹
North Terminal, Gatwick Airport RH6 0PH
Tel: (01293) 567070 Fax: (01293) 567739
No. of Accessible Rooms: 2. Bath
Accessible facilities: Lounge, Restaurant,
Pool, Sauna, Spa.

HAYWARDS HEATH

Large market town with both urban
and rural aspects as an important
agricultural centre.

ATTRACTIONS
BORDE HILL GARDENS
Balcombe Road, Haywards Heath RH16 1XP
Tel: (01444) 450326
Fax: (01444) 440427
www.bordehill.co.uk
Botanical and tranquil gardens with rich
variety of seasonal colour set in 200 acres of
parkland and woodland. Extensive planting
with rose and herbaceous gardens.

SD ♿	CP ♿	E ♿	RF ♿
C 🚹	S 🚹	WC 🚹	RFE ♿

NYMANS GARDEN (NT)
Handcross, Nr. Haywards Heath RH17 6EB
Tel: (01444) 400321 Fax: (01444) 400253
Flowering shrubs, roses, rare trees, a secret
sunken garden and old walled orchard.

SD ♿	CP 🚹	E ♿	C 🚹	S 🚹	WC 🚹

WAKEHURST PLACE GARDEN
Royal Botanic Gardens, Ardingly, Haywards
Heath EH17 6TN

Tel: (01444) 894049   Fax: (01444) 894069
www.rbgkew.org.uk
170 acres of gardens and woodlands
contain many species not found at Kew
Gardens. 4 national collections of birch,
hypericum, southern beech and skimmia.
Woodlands with temperate trees from 4
continents, Loder Valley Nature Reserve for
conservation of plants and animals of the
Sussex Weald. Winter Garden, Walled
Gardens, Pinetum and Asian Heath Garden.

SD ♿   CP ♿   E ♿   RF ♿
C ♿   S 🚶   WC ♿   RFE ♿

PETWORTH

The town has a number of very old
houses, some timber-framed and many
in narrow streets around the little
market square, dating from Tudor to
Georgian times.

TOURIST INFORMATION CENTRE
(Weekends only during winter)
Market Square, Petworth GU28 0AF
Tel: (01798) 343523   Fax: (01798) 343942

BED AND BREAKFAST
THE OLD RAILWAY STATION   🚶
Petworth GU28 0JF
Tel/Fax: (01798) 342346
e-mail: query@old-station.co.uk
www.old-station.co.uk
No. of Accessible Rooms: 1. Bath
Accessible Facilities: Lounge, Dining Room
Colonial style splendour at Victorian station,
a Grade 11 listed building. Pullman railway
carriages are your home here. In summer
take breakfast on the old platform.

ATTRACTIONS
THE DOLL HOUSE MUSEUM
Station Road, Petworth GU28 0BF
Tel: (01798) 344044   Fax: (01798) 343858

259

*England's largest herd of deer are just
out of this shot of this view of
Petworth House.*

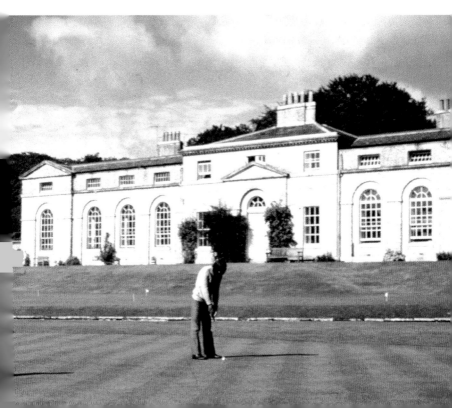

Amazing collection, mainly modern 1/12th scale showing present day life in all types of buildings, e.g. ballet boarding school, prison, log cabin, Shaker, Mozart Bicentenary. Also room and collection boxes and fully furnished house in 1/24th scale.

SD ♿ CP 🚶 E 🚶 RF ♿
L ♿ S ♿ WC 🚶 RFE ♿

PETWORTH HOUSE (NT)
Petworth GU28 0AE
Tel: (01798) 342207
Fax: (01798) 342963

Rebuilt in 1688 around the ancient manor house of the Percy family, Petworth houses the finest collection of paintings and sculpture in the care of the National Trust. Highlights include Turner oil paintings in Red Room and North Gallery, Van Dycks in Square and little Dining Rooms and Grinling Gibbon's limewood carvings in the Carved Room. Also a 30-acre woodland garden and 700-acre Petworth Park designed by Capability Brown and home to England's largest herd of fallow deer. All main showrooms, except chapel and some bedrooms are accessible.

SD ♿ CP ♿ E ♿ RF ♿
C ♿ (wheelchair lift to C) S ♿
WC 🚶 RFE ♿

PULLBOROUGH

ATTRACTION
PARHAM HOUSE AND GARDENS
Parham Park, Nr. Pullborough
Tel: (01903) 742021   Fax: (01903) 746557
e-mail: Parham @dial.pipex.com

Major Elizabethan house, family-owned for many hundreds of years and containing a fine collection of paintings, furniture and carpets. Surrounded by 7 acres of gardens and C18th pleasure grounds with lake, and brick and turf maze. In turn surrounded by 875 acres of working agricultural and forestry land. Please give prior notice if entrance ramp is required.

SD ♿ CP 🚶 E ♿ RF ♿
C ♿ S ♿ WC 🚶

PULLBOROUGH BROOKS
RSPB NATURE RESERVE

Wiggonholt, Pullborough RH20 2EL
Tel: (01798) 875851
Fax: (01798) 873816

Excellent for viewing wintering and wading birds, with water meadows, ditches and pools, higher meadows, hedgerow and woodland. Nature trail on all-weather hardcore of 2 miles leading to 3 hides. Demanding journey for manual chair and requires pusher. Batricar available on loan, but cannot be taken into the hides.

SD ♿ CP ♿ E ♿ RF ♿
C n/a S ♿ WC 🚶 RFE ♿ & 🚶

SHOREHAM
Popular seaside resort and an ancient town. Old Shoreham lies north of the main centre, established by south Saxons in C5th. It is now separated from the sea by the Ader, the harbour and shingle of Shoreham Beach.

ATTRACTION
MUSEUM OF D-DAY AVIATION
Shoreham Airport, Shoreham BN43 5FJ
Tel: (01374) 971971

Aircraft engines for Hurricanes, Spitfires and Hawker Typhoons, plus Typhoon cockpit being restored. Unique collection of artefacts, uniforms, medals and photos.

SD ♿ CP ♿ E ♿ RF ♿ WC 🚶
RFE ♿

STEYNING

ATTRACTION
STEYNING MUSEUM
Church Street, Steyning BN44 3YB
Tel: (01903) 813333

Celebration of Steyning's history, the Normans and their successors established the town. Exhibits on crafts and industries.

SD ♿ CP ♿ E ♿ S ♿
WC 🚶

WORTHING

Popular seaside resort with extensive sands and shingle beaches. The C19th pier is one of the oldest. Several parks and gardens.

TOURIST INFORMATION CENTRES
Town Hall, Chapel Road,
Worthing BN11 1HL
Tel: (01903) 210022
Fax: (01903) 236277
e-mail: wbctourism@pavilion.co.uk
www.worthing.gov.uk/wbc

Marine Parade, Worthing BN11 3PX
Tel: (01903) 210022
(Summer months only)
Produces a guide for disabled visitors.

WORTHING BOROUGH COUNCIL
Address as TIC. Tel: (01903) 239999

BUSES
Compass Travel: Tel: (01903) 233767
Stagecoach Coastline: Tel: (01903) 237661
Some low-floor buses.

TAXIS
Worthing Taxi Association:
Tel: (01903) 232523
One adapted vehicle, but has contact with other firms.
Baz Cabs:Tel: (mobile) (07710) 992131
One adapted vehicle.

TRAINS
Connex South Central: Customer Services:
Tel: (0870) 6030405
Fax: (0870) 6030505
Minicom: (01233) 617621
Wales & West: Tel: Special Needs:
Tel: (0845) 3003005
Minicom: (0845) 7585469
Worthing Station is suitable for wheelchairs using ramp access.

CAR PARKS
Free, unlimited parking in Pay & Display car parks, Council-run car parks, also many disabled parking bays around town.
Tel: (01903) 204436

SHOPMOBILITY
United Reform Church, Shelley Road,
Worthing BN11 1TT
Tel: (01903) 820980
Also has range of single and 2-seater electric vehicles for hire: Towns to Downs.

HOTELS
BEACH HOTEL
Marine Parade, Worthing BN11 3QJ
Tel: (01903) 234001   Fax: (01903) 234567
e-mail: Thebeachhotel@Btinternet.com
No. of Accessible Rooms: 2. Shower
Accessible Facilities: Lounge, Restaurant, all ground floor public rooms. Family owned and managed for 40 years with restaurant and rooms overlooking the sea.

BEST WESTERN BERKELEY HOTEL
86 - 95 Marine Parade, Worthing
BN11 3GD
Tel: (01903) 820000   Fax: (01903) 821333
No. of Accessible Rooms: 1. Bath
Accessible Facilities: Lounge, Restaurant.
Seafront hotel overlooking promenade.

LANTERN HOTEL
54 Shelley Road, Worthing BN11 4BX
Tel: (01903) 238476   Fax: (01903) 602429
No. of Accessible Rooms: 13. Roll-in
Shower
Accessible Facilities: All.
Hotel is owned by British Polio Fellowship.

KINGSWAY HOTEL
117 Marine Parade, Worthing BN11 3QQ
Tel: (01903) 237542   Fax: (01903) 204173
No. of Accessible Rooms: 2.
Accessible Facilities: Lounges (2), Bar, Restaurant, Buttery. Family-owned, seafront hotel .

WINDSOR HOUSE HOTEL
16 Windsor Road, Worthing
Tel: (01903) 239655
Fax: (01903) 210763
e-mail: thewindsorhotel@compuserve.com
No. of Accessible Rooms: 1. Shower
Accessible Facilities: Lounge, Restaurant
Refurbished in 1998.

TYNE AND WEAR

DISABILITY DIRECTORY
Tel: (01772) 631690
Covers the whole of the North East.

GATESHEAD
A fire in 1854 destroyed most of the historical buildings, and much is now modern. There are fine views of the famous five Tyne bridges linking Gateshead to Newcastle-upon-Tyne. Known for the superb MetroCentre shopping centre.

TOURIST INFORMATION CENTRE
Central Library, Prince Consort Road, Gateshead NE8 4LN
Tel: (0191) 4773478
Gateshead Metrocentre, Portcullis, 7 The Arcade, MetroCentre NE11 9YL
Tel: (0191) 460 6345

HOTELS
NEWCASTLE/GATESHEAD MARRIOTT
Metro Centre, Gateshead NE11 9XF
Tel: (0191) 4932233
No. of Accessible Rooms: 2. Bath
Accessible Facilities: Lounge, Dining Room, most of Bar.
Quality hotel by Metro Centre.

SWALLOW HOTEL
High West Street, Gateshead NE8 1PE
Tel: (0191) 4771105   Fax: (0191) 4787214
No. of Accessible Rooms: 1. Bath
Accessible Facilities: (Via accessible lift) Lounge, Restaurant. Busy modern hotel located a mile from Newcastle city centre.

JARROW
Part of the industrial Tyneside, lying at the Durham end of the Tyne tunnel. Intense poverty marked the closing of shipyards in 1933 followed by the famous hunger march that warned of dependence on one industry. Now new houses and flats replace slums and small factories and workshops have been introduced to prevent another civic crisis.

Bede's World, a worthy reminder of Britain's first historian.

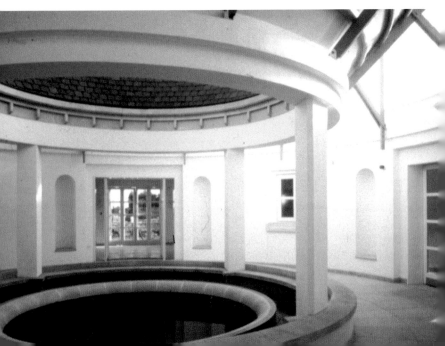

ATTRACTION
BEDE'S WORLD
Church Bank, Jarrow NE32 3DY
Tel: (0191) 4282106   Fax: (0191) 4282361
e-mail: visitor.info@bedesworld.co.uk
The Venerable Bede (AD673-735), early
medieval Europe's greatest scholar, was
the first to record the history of England,
He lived and worked as a monk at Jarrow.
Explore the golden age of saints and kings
in Northumbria via an Anglo-Saxon Farm,
Jarrow Hall Exhibition and St. Paul's
Church and Monastic site where Bede
spent much of his life. Great museum.

| SD 🚾 | CP 🚾 | E 🚾 | RF 🚾 |
| L 🚾 | C 🚾 | S 🚾 | WC 🚹 |

NEWCASTLE-UPON-TYNE
A complex scene of blackened masses
of old buildings, tall new blocks, the
ornamental crown of St. Nicholas
Cathedral, the pretty spire of All Saints,
the square-shouldered castle keep, the
quays, warehouses and industry. Main
area for visitors is the square mile
between the Riverside and the Town
Moor. The Moor gives this highly
industrialised city a unique breathing
space of 927 windswept acres on which
freemen can – and do – pasture cows.

TOURIST INFORMATION CENTRES
City First Stop and Information Centre,
City Library, Princess Square,
Newcastle upon Tyne NE99 1DX
Tel: (0191) 2610610

Main Concourse, Central Station, Newcastle
upon Tyne NE1 5DL
Tel: (0191) 2300300

Unit 1, Royal Quays Outlet Shopping Centre,
Coble Dene, North Shields NE29 6DW
Tel: (0191) 2005895

Museum and Art Gallery, Ocean Road,
South Shields NE33 1HZ
Tel: (0191) 4546612

BUSES
Arriva Northumbria: Tel: (0191) 2121313
Fax: (0191) 2818999
www.arriva.co.uk
Some low-floor buses.
Stagecoach: Tel: (0191) 2761411
Some low-floor buses.

TAXIS
Metro Taxis: Tel: (0191) 2611891
50 adapted vehicles
Noda: Tel: (0191) 2221888
40 adapted vehicles outside Central
Station.
Transcab (South Shields):
Tel: (0378) 783614
3 adapted vehicles.

TRAINS
Great North Eastern Railway: Special Needs:
Tel: (0345) 225444
Minicom: (0191) 2330173
Virgin Trains: Special Needs:
Tel: (0845) 7443366
Minicom: (0845) 7443367

METRO
Tel: (0191) 2325325
ASSISTANCE required

CAR PARKS
Free unlimited disabled badge parking in
council-owned car parks.

SHOPMOBILITY
Eldon Square Shopping Centre, Eldon Court,
Percy Street, Newcastle upon Tyne NE1 7JB
Tel: (0191) 2611891
Fax: (0191) 2616340

HOTELS
QUALITY FRIENDLY HOTEL   🚾
Witney Way, Boldon, Newcastle NE35 9PE
Tel: (0191) 5191999
No. of Accessible Rooms: 3
Accessible Facilities: Lounge, Restaurant.
Modern hotel located on junction of A19
and A184 east of Newcastle.

COPTHORNE NEWCASTLE   🚹
The Close, Quayside, Newcastle NE1 3RT
Tel: (0191) 2220333   Fax: (0191) 2301111
No. of Accessible Rooms: 1. Bath
Accessible Facilities: Lounge, Restaurant,
Bar. Quality hotel in city centre.

HOLIDAY INN 🚶
Great North Road, Seaton Burn,
Newcastle NE13 6BF
Tel: (0191) 2019988
Fax: (0191) 2368091
No. of Accessible Rooms:
Accessible Facilities:
Purpose-built hotel located 3m west of
Tyne Tunnel toward Morpeth

NEWCASTLE AIRPORT MOAT HOUSE 🚶
Woolsington, Newcastle NE13 8DJ
Tel: (0191) 4019988   Fax: (01661) 860157
No. of Accessible Rooms:
Accessible Facilities: Restaurant, Bar (lift)
Modern hotel within airport complex.

NOVOTEL NEWCASTLE 🚶
Ponteland Road, Kenton,
Newcastle 0633
Tel: (0191) 2140303
Fax: (0191) 2140633
No. of Accessible Rooms: 4. Bath
Accessible Facilities: Lounge, Restaurant,
Lift. Bright, modern hotel located off the
A1 western by-pass 4 miles from
Newcastle town centre.

ATTRACTIONS
TYNE AND WEAR
INTERNATIONAL CENTRE FOR LIFE
Market Keepers House, Times Square,
Scotswood Road,
Newcastle upon Tyne NE1 4EP
Tel: (0191) 243 8223
Fax: (0191) 261 4150
www.centreforlifeco.uk
Interactive-science centre which takes
visitors on an exciting inter-active jouney
through the life sciences.

MUSEUM OF ANTIQUITIES
University and Society of Antiquities,
Newcastle upon Tyne NE1 7RU
Tel: (0191) 2227849   Fax: (0191) 2228561
e-mail: m.o.antiquities@ncl.ac.uk
Main museum for Hadrian's Wall with
historical displays from prehistoric times.
SD ♿   CP 🚶   E ♿   S ♿

SPORTING VENUE
NEWCASTLE UNITED FOOTBALL CLUB
St. James' Park, Newcastle NE1 4ST

Admin: (0191) 2018634
Booking: Box Office: (0191) 2018457 or
2611571
Fax: (0191) 2018609
web: www.nufc.co.uk
Complies with Building Regulations Part M.
CP ♿   RE ♿   ED ♿   INT ♿
L ♿   WC ♿   SS ♿   B/R ♿

THEATRE
THEATRE ROYAL
100 Grey Street, Newcastle NE1 6BR
Admin: (0191) 2320997
Booking: Box Office: (0191) 2322061
Fax: (0191) 2611906
CP 🚶   RE 🚶
ED ♿   (Except for non-automatic door)
INT ♿   L ♿   WC ♿
AUD - Alternative rear entrance leads past adapted WC to
back of stalls with wheelchair user positions.
B/R ♿

STOCKTON-ON-TEES
Famous for the open air market started
in 1310 and still held twice weekly in
the broadest high street in England.
History was made here when the
world's first passenger railway steamed
in on 27th September 1825.

TOURIST INFORMATION CENTRE
Theatre Yard, off High Street,
Stockton on Tees TS18 1AT
Tel: (01642) 393936

SPORTING VENUE
SEDGEFIELD RACECOURSE
The Bungalow,
Sedgefield,
Stockton-on-Tees TS21 2HW
Booking/Admin :Tel: (01740) 621925
Fax: (01740) 620663
CP ♿ (pre-book)   RE ♿
ED ♿ (except manual door)
INT ♿   L ♿
WC ♿ (4 units situated on each level of pavilion and
first level of Fosters stand)
SS ♿ (viewing area). Tarmac from turnstiles to viewing
area.
B/R ♿   Main bar ramped, lift to restaurant level

TYNEMOUTH

A walk along the 0.75mile North Tyne Pier has been called a trip to sea without leaving land. It is an excellent vantage point for ship-watching and viewing the priory ruins and coastline. Tynemouth occupies the cliffs on the north side of the river mouth and has been a seaside resort for at least 200 years. There are fine sands, overlooked by amusement centre and park.

ATTRACTION
TYNEMOUTH PRIORY AND CASTLE (EH)
East Street, Tynemouth,
North Shields NE30 4BZ
Tel: (0191) 2571090
Castle walls and gatehouse enclose substantial remains of Benedictine priory founded c1090 on a Saxon monastic site.

SD [ ]   CP [ ]   E [ ]   RF [ ]   S [ ]

TYNEMOUTH SEA LIFE CENTRE
Grand Parade, Tynemouth,
North Shields NE30 4JF
Tel: (0191) 2581031   Fax: (0191) 2572116
www.sealife.co.uk
Close encounters with marine life from starfish to sharks, octopus to eels: feeding demonstrations and touchpools in unique aquariums.

SD [ ]   CP [ ]   E [ ]   RF [ ]
C [ ]   S [ ]   WC [ ]   RFE [ ]

WASHINGTON

A new town has risen on this former colliery village, and streets of miners' houses have been demolished. Pit-head buildings are converted to a museum and the pit heap moved away.

ATTRACTION
THE WILDFOWL AND WETLANDS TRUST
District 15,
Washington NE38 8LE
Tel: (0191) 4165454   Fax: (0191) 416801
e-mail: wetlands@globalnet.co.uk

Situated on north bank of the River Wear, a 100 acre site, home to many exotic wildfowl. Discovery centre, waterfowl nursery and viewing gallery. Wheelchairs available.

SD [ ]   CP [ ]   S [ ]

WHITLEY BAY

Most popular of Northumbria's resorts, the beach has grassy banks and runs the length of the town. Fine lighthouse on St. Mary's island lying off the north end of the bay.

TOURIST INFORMATION CENTRE
Park Road, Whitley Bay NE26 1EJ
Tel: (0191) 2008535

HOTEL
YORK HOUSE HOTEL   [ ]
28-32 Park Parade, The Promenade,
Whitley Bay NE26 1AP
Tel: (0191) 2528313 Fax: (0191) 2513953
No. of Accessible Rooms: 3. Shower.
Accessible Facilities: Lounge, Restaurant
Located in town centre.

Above us the waves, the amazing view at Tynemouth sea life centre.

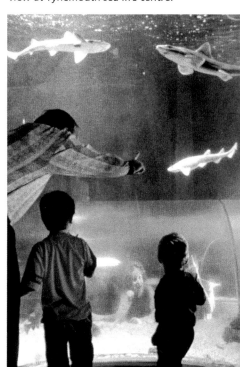

BED AND BREAKFAST
MARLBOROUGH HOTEL
20- 21 East Parade,
Whitley Bay NE26 1AP
Tel: (0191) 2513628   Fax: (0191) 2525033
No. of Accessible Rooms: 2. Shower
Accessible Facilities: Lounge, Restaurant.
Entrance has ramped access.
Privately owned hotel overlooking beach.
Evening meals available but not at
weekends. Restaurant next door with two-
step access to the main door.

WARWICKSHIRE

SHAKESPEARE COUNTRY TOURISM
Conoco Centre, Warwick Technology Park,
Gallows Hill CV34 6DB
Tell: (01926) 404891   Fax: (01926) 404893
e-mail: info@shakespeare-country.co.uk
www.shakespeare-country.co.uk

ALCESTER
Small town 8 miles from Stratford at
the confluence of rivers Arrow and
Alne. Particularly attractive is the
narrow Butter Street, off the High
Street, with its jumble of ancient roofs.

ATTRACTION
RAGLEY HALL
Alcester B49 5NJ
Tel: (01789) 762090   Fax: (01789) 764791
Family home of the Marquis of Hertford
since it was built in 1680 and surrounded
by 27 acres of gardens, within vast
parkland. The house contains a fine
collection of treasures, particularly notable
for James Gibb's elegant baroque
plasterwork. All rooms are one floor,
accessed by a lift close to parking in right
hand courtyard side of main entrance.
The Stables and Woodland Walk reached
along fairly steep gravel and grass paths:
slope uphill on the return. The Rose
Garden has steps and is not accessible.

SD 🚻 CP 🚻 E 🚻 RF 🚻 L 🚻

C 🚻 S 🚻 WC 🚹 G 🚻

ATHERSTONE

SELF-CATERING
HIPSLEY FARM COTTAGES 🚻
Hipsley Lane, Hurley, Atherstone CV9 2LR
Tel/Fax: (01827) 872437
No. of Accessible Units: 1
No. of Beds per Unit: 2
Accessible Facilities: Kitchen/Living
Room. Farm barns and a cowshed
converted to individual cottages with
garden and BBQ and garden furniture.
Wainwright Cottage is single-storey
stone cottage. Situated in rolling
countryside, well placed for Birmingham,
National Exhibition Centre and Stratford
and Warwick.

ATTRACTION
TWYCROSS ZOO
Atherstone CV9 3PX
Tel: (01827) 880250
Fax: (01827) 880700
Run by a devoted crew specialising in
primates, there is an enormous variety of
species together with other animals
including lions and tigers, sealion and
penguin pools.

SD 🚻 CP 🚻 E 🚻

C 🚻 S 🚻 WC 🚹

HATTON
Located between Warwick and
Solihull on A41/A4177 or M40
(Jct.15).

ATTRACTION
HATTON COUNTRY WORLD
Dark Lane, Hatton CV35 8XA
Tel: (01926) 843411
Fax: (01926) 842023
Rural crafts, farm park and shopping
village under one roof. A great deal to
do, see and to buy in 35 shops. Housed
in redundant farm buildings, access has
been made wherever possible. Farm park
has hard core pathways.

SD n/a CP 🚻 & 🚹 E 🚻 RF 🚻

C 🚻 S 🚹 WC 🚹

HUNTS GREEN

Tiny village between Birmingham and Tamworth.

ATTRACTION
MIDDLETON HALL TRUST, WARWICKSHIRE.
(postal address is Staffordshire)
Middleton, Tamworth, Staffs B78 2AE
Tel: (01827) 283095 Fax: (01827) 285717
Originally built c1300, with an 11-bay
Georgian west wing and C16th Great hall,
restored in 1994. A display of 24 framed
embroideries depicting history of Sutton
Coldfield decorates the first-floor corridor.
Craft Centre in the former stable block.
Walled gardens plus nature reserve,
orchard and woodland.

SD   CP   E   RF
C   S   WC

LEAMINGTON SPA

Owes its being to the passion for taking
the waters, following in the wake of
Bath. Lovely Georgian, Regency and early
Victorian terraced houses to be seen on
the north side of the River Leam.

SELF-CATERING
HOME COTTAGE
Knightcote Farm, Knightcote,
Southam CV47 2EF
Tel: (01295) 770637 Fax: (01295) 770135
e-mail: fionawalker@farmcottages.com
www.farmcottages.com
No. of Accessible Units: 1. 2 Roll-in
Showers.
How many Beds per Unit: 5
Accessible Facilities: Open plan
Lounge/Diner, Kitchen, Patio garden with
barbecue. Taxi service with wheelchair
access. Local pubs with wheelchair access.
Award winning self-catering cottage with
views of far stretching farmland. Located
between Leamington Spa and Banbury,

STRATFORD-UPON-AVON

The least spoilt cult town. England's
prime tourist centre outside London, its
famous resident William Shakespeare is
celebrated all over the town. Apart
from the Shakespeare connections
there is much to see. The canal wharf
is lovely and the southern section of
the Stratford-upon-Avon Canal has
been completely restored by the
National Trust.

STRATFORD-UPON-AVON TOURIST INFORMATION CENTRE
Bridgefoot, Stratford-upon-Avon CV37 6GW
Tel: (01789) 293127
Fax: (01789) 295262

CENTRO (Coventry): Tel: (024) 76 559559
www.centro.org.uk
All information on public transport in West
Midlands.

TRAVELINE
(0870) 6082608

BUSES
See Centro, some low-floor buses.

TAXIS
A & M Cars: Tel: (01926) 612487
Six adapted vehicles.
Mervs Taxis: Tel: (01789) 764981

TRAINS
Railtrack Property Major Stations:
Tel: (0121) 6544288
Minicom: (0121) 6544292
Information on all stations on UK mainland.

Central Trains: Assistance:
Tel: (0845) 7056027
www.centraltrains.co.uk
Thames Trains: Special Needs:
Tel: (0118) 9083607
www.thamestrains.co.uk

CAR PARKS
Free unlimited disabled badge parking in
council car parks, 3 hours' parking in
Sheep Street.
Tel: (01789) 260691

SHOPMOBILITY
Sheep Street, Stratford upon Avon CV37 6HX
Tel: (01789) 414534

HOTELS
FALCON HOTEL 🚶
2 Chapel Street,
Stratford-upon-Avon CV37 6HA
Tel: (01789) 279953
No. of Accessible Rooms: 1
Accessible Facilities: Lounge, Restaurant
Delightful C16th inn right in centre of
town. There has been an alehouse on the
site since then.

GROVENOR HOUSE HOTEL 🚶
Warwick Road, Stratford-upon-Avon
CV37 6YT
Tel: (01789) 269213   Fax: (01789) 266087
www.groshotel/stratford.co.uk
No. of Accessible Rooms: 3. Bath
Accessible Facilities: Lounge, Restaurant
(ramped). Built between 1832/43 as
private homes in both Regency and
Elizabethan style, this 3 star listed hotel is
within two minutes of Stratford's high
street.

MARSTON/STRATFORD MANOR 🚶
Warwick Road, Stratford-upon-Avon
CV37 0PY
Tel: (01789) 731173
Fax: (01789) 731131
No. of Accessible Rooms: 5
Accessible Facilities: Lounge, Restaurant,
Pool, Sauna. Charming, modern hotel, set
in 21 acres of lovely countryside, 3 miles
from Stratford.

STRATFORD MOAT HOUSE 🚶
Bridgefoot, Stratford-upon-Avon CV37 6YR
Tel: (01789) 279988 Fax: (01789) 298589
No. of Accessible Rooms: 2
Accessible Facilities: Lounge, Restaurant,
Bar. Large modern hotel with attractive
setting on banks of River Avon.

WELCOME HOTEL 🚶
Warwick Road,
Stratford-upon-Avon CV37 0NR
Tel: (01789) 295252
No. of Accessible Rooms: 7
Accessible Facilities: Lounge, Restaurant.

Country house hotel; a spectacular C19th.
Jacobean-style mansion with many original
antiques. Set within 157 acres of parkland
and an 18-hole golf course.

BED AND BREAKFAST
CHURCH FARM ♿
Dorsington, Stratford-upon-Avon CV37 8AX
Tel: (01789) 720471   Fax: (01789) 720830
www.churchfarmstratford.co.uk
No. of Accessible Rooms: 1
Accessible Facilities: Lounge, Dining Room
Georgian farmhouse set in pretty and quiet
village, close to Stratford.

PENSHURST GUEST HOUSE ♿
34 Evesham Place,
Stratford-upon-Avon CV37 6HT
Tel: (01789) 205259 Fax: (01789) 295322
www.penhurst.net
No. of Accessible Rooms: 1. Roll-in
Shower.
Accessible Facilities: Dining room.
Holiday Care Service winner 1996.
Pretty Victorian townhouse 10 minutes
from town centre.

ATTRACTIONS
SHAKESPEARE BIRTHPLACE TRUST
The Shakespeare Centre, Henley Street,
Stratford-upon-Avon CV37 6QW
Tel: (01789) 204016 Fax: (01789) 296083
e-mail: info@shakespeare.org.uk
www.shakespeare.org.uk
The Trust manages the 5 Shakespeare
houses in and around Stratford-upon-
Avon. 3 in the town, The Birthplace,
Nash's House and New Place and Halls'
Croft: Anne Hathaway's cottage and Mary
Arden's House a few miles outside. The
houses do present some difficulties for
disabled visitors, although in some cases
ground floor rooms and gardens are
accessible. Anne Hathaway's Cottage is
not accessible. In all the 4 sites visited, we
found the staff to be extremely helpful and
attentive.The Birthplace Trust is in the
process of improving the physical access to
all the historic houses, with the help of
consultation by South Warwickshire Access
Group. These include detailed access
guides, new exterior pathway surfaces,
external entrances and exits, adaptive

WC's where not yet in place, firm hand rails on ramps, wheelchair availability and more.

SHAKESPEARE'S BIRTHPLACE:
Born here in 1564, the tour begins in the very accessible Visitor's Centre exhibition, telling the story of Shakespeare's life and background with many original items and specially constructed scenes. The Birthplace is approached from the garden's wide paving stones, has one large step and one narrow doorway accessible by the site's own manual chair, but not by an electric wheelchair. Uneven flooring throughout, but ground floor rooms accessible. Plans to have CD on upper rooms for disabled only.

SD   CP   E 🔽 H 🔽 WC 🔽
S -Exhibition 🔽   House 🔽

NASH'S HOUSE & NEW PLACE
Chapel Street, Stratford-upon-Avon
Tel: (01789) 292325
Adjoins the site of New Place, Shakespeare's home for the last 18 years of his life. It belonged to Thomas Nash, who married Shakespeare's granddaughter in 1626, 10 years after the dramatist's death. The house, accessed by external and internal ramps, gradients 1:10, has notable oak furniture and paintings. Ground floor accessible. A passageway beyond the entrance hall leads to a small step onto the site and gardens of New Place, sadly no longer there. Paths in the first garden are too narrow for access, but the beautiful Great Garden beyond is accessible along Chapel Lane to the right of the entrance.

E 🔽   RF 🔽   WC 🔽

HALL'S CROFT
Old Town, Stratford-upon-Avon
Tel: (01789) 292107
Fine half-timbered, gabled house, owned by John Hall who married Shakespeare's daughter, Susanna, in 1607. Fine paintings inside and lovely walled garden. Entrance via stone step, ground floor mainly flat and level. Shop and restaurant via shallow ramp. Garden and seating area reached via flat access from house, lawn area ramped.

E 🔽 RF 🔽 C 🔽 S 🔽 WC 🔽 G 🔽

MARY ARDEN'S HOUSE
Wilmcote
Tel: (01789) 293455
Located 3 miles from Stratford-upon-Avon, this was probably the home of Shakespeare's mother before she married. It is a fine Tudor farmhouse with many old outbuildings, a delightful homestead and a must to visit. Accessed in and out by shallow ramp, with flat and level access throughout most of the site although the house has some thresholds of 8cm. Flooring is stone flagging and there is room to manoeuvre between exhibits. 1 step into Glebe Farm and 1 step into the farming exhibit. Garden has flat picnic area. Wheelchair available for loan.

CP 🔽 E 🔽 RF 🔽 C 🔽 S 🔽 WC 🔽

STRATFORD BUTTERFLY FARM
Swan's Nest Lane,
Stratford-upon-Avon CV37 7LS
Tel: (01789) 299288 Fax: (01789) 415878
Largest butterfly and insect exhibition in Europe with many of the world's most spectacular varieties of butterflies in tropical setting. Also Insect City and deadly spiders in Arachnoland.

SD 🔽 CP 🔽 E 🔽 RF 🔽 S 🔽
WC n/a (Accessible WC 30m away-owned by council)
RFE 🔽

No mock-Tudor at Mary Arden's house.

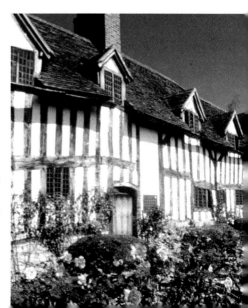

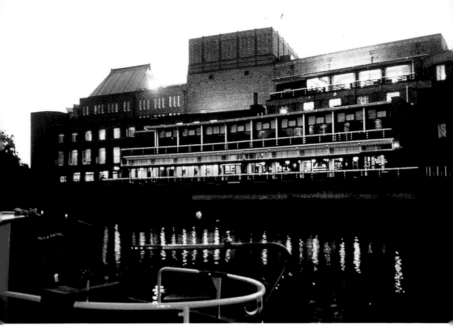

Royal Shakespeare Theatre.

THEATRE
ROYAL SHAKESPEARE COMPANY
Waterside, Stratford-upon-Avon
Admin-Minicom: (01789) 412658
Fax: (01789) 412639
Booking-Box Office: (01789) 295623,
Minicom/Fax: (01789) 261974
Complies with Part M, Building
Regulations.
CP ♿ Public   CP-Market Place
Taxi Rank—200m or by phone in front of theatre.
RE ♿   ED ♿   INT ♿
WC ♿ (ground floor)   AUD ♿   B ♿

WARWICK
One of most unspoilt of all county
towns, standing on a north rise from
the river Avon, which is crossed by two
bridges. Delightful pre-1694 houses in
Castle Street. The castle itself is truly
magnificent, but inaccurate.

WARWICK TOURIST INFORMATION CENTRE
Jury Street, Warwick CV34 4EW
Tel: (01926) 492212   Fax: (01926) 494?

HOTEL
CHARLECOTE PHEASANT COUNTRY HOTEL   🚶
Charlecote CV35 9EW
Tel: (01789) 279954 Fax: (01789) 470222
No. of Accessible Rooms: 6
Accessible Facilities: Lounge, Restaurant.
Charming rural retreat converted from
farm buildings, sitting alongside Charlecote
Manor. Located in old village a short
distance from both Warwick and Stratford-
upon-Avon.

HILTON NATIONAL WARWICK/STRATFORD   🚶
Stratford Road, Warwick CV34 6RE
Tel: (01926) 499555 Fax: (01926) 410020
No. of Accessible Rooms: 1
Accessible Facilities: Lounge, Restaurant
Located on M40 (J15).

ATTRACTION
CHARLECOTE PARK (NT)
Warwick CV35 9ER
Tel: (01789) 470277   Fax: (01789) 470544
e-mail: vclgrismpt.ntrust. org
Strong associations with Elizabeth 1 and
Shakespeare in this essentially Tudor
house. Early Victorian interior and deer
park designed by Capability Brown.
SD ♿   CP 🚶   E ♿   RF ♿
C ♿   S ♿   WC 🚶   RFE – H & G 🚶

HERITAGE MOTOR CENTRE
Banbury Road, Gaydon, Warwick CV35 0BJ
Tel: (01926) 641188   Fax: (01926) 641555
Largest purpose-built road transport museum in the UK, with the largest collection of historic British cars in the world. Directed at the whole family, displays include the Corgi collections and activities, and the quad bike circuit.

SD ♿ CP ♿ E ♿ RF ♿ L ♿
C ♿ S ♿ WC ♿ RFE ♿

WEST MIDLANDS

BIRMINGHAM
Second largest city in Britain with a population of one million with a great concentration of industries, and their legacy of excellent heritage museums. Now a post-manufacturing centre, the city is dominated by wide roads, banked by large buildings with a shopping centre terraced beneath the flyovers. This area is traffic free and linked by subways.

TOURIST INFORMATION CENTRES
130 Colmore Row, Victoria Square, Birmingham B3 3AP
Tel: (0121) 6936300   Fax: (0121) 6939600

2 City Arcade, Birmingham B2 4TX
Tel: (0121) 6432514   Fax: (0121) 6161038

CENTRO Hotline: Tel: (0121) 2002700
Minicom: (0121) 2147777
All information on buses in West Midlands.

TRAVELINE
(0870) 6082608

BUSES
Easyrider: Tel: (0121) 3333108 (Birmingham North) : Tel: (0121) 4862663 (South).
Low steps, lifts, trained staff.

TAXIS
BB Cabs. Tel: (0121) 3032624
10 adapted vehicles

TOA: Tel: (0121) 4278888
300 adapted vehicles.

TRAINS
Central Trains: Assistance:
Tel: (0845) 7056027
www.centraltrains.co.uk
Chiltern Railways: Mobility Impaired:
Tel: (01296) 332113/4
www.chilternrailways.co.uk
Silverlink: Special Needs:
Tel: (01923) 207818
Fax: (01923) 207023
Minicom: (01923) 256430
Virgin Trains: Special Needs:
Tel: (0845) 7443366
Minicom: (0845) 7443367
Wales & West: Special Needs:
Tel: (0845) 30030005
Minicom:(0845) 7585469
Centro Hotline: Tel: (0121) 2002700

Birmingham New Street Station:
Tel: (0121) 6544288
Minicom: (0121) 6544292
Information covers whole of UK mainland.

CAR PARKS
3-hour free parking in council-owned car parks, some on-street parking.
Tel: (0121) 3033634

METRO
Tel: (0121) 2002700
Minicom: (0121) 2147777
All trams are easy access with ramps/lifts to platforms.

SHOPMOBILITY
The Central Library, Chamberlain Square, Birmingham B3 3HQ
Tel: (0121) 6936613   Fax: (0121) 7850104

Birmingham Markets, Markets Customer Centre, Edgbaston Road, Birmingham B5 4RB
Tel: (0121) 6434130

HOTELS
COPTHORNE BIRMINGHAM 🚶
Paradise Circus, Birmingham B3 3HJ
Tel: (0121) 2002727 Fax: (0121) 2001197
www.millenium-hotels.com
No. of Accessible Rooms: 1

Accessible Facilities: Lounge, Restaurants 2.
Quality large city-centre hotel overlooking
Centenary Square.

NOVOTEL BIRMINGHAM AIRPORT
Birmingham International Airport,
Birmingham B26 3QL
Tel: (0121) 7827000 Fax: (0121) 7820445
No. of Accessible Rooms: 6. Bath
Accessible Facilities: Lounge, Restaurant, Lift.
Modern hotel with walkway connection to
airport.

ATTRACTIONS
BIRMINGHAM BOTANICAL GARDENS
Westbourne Road, Edgbaston,
Birmingham B15 3TR
Tel: (0121) 4541860 Fax: (0121) 4547835
www.birminghambotanicalgardens.org.uk
15 acres of ornamental gardens including
Rock, Historic, Herb & Cottage and
Themed Gardens, plus exotic birds in
indoor and outdoor aviaries on the Loudon
Terrace, cactus and succulent house and
Japanese gardens.

SD   CP   E   RF ⟨⟩   C ⟨⟩
S ⟨⟩   WC ⟨⟩   RFE ⟨⟩

SOHO HOUSE MUSEUM
Soho Avenue, Handsworth, Birmingham
Tel: (0121) 5549122 Fax: (0121) 5545929
Elegant home of industrial pioneer,
Matthew Bolton from 1766 to 1809.
Possibly the first centrally heated house
since Roman times, it has been restored to
its C18th appearance and contains original
furniture. Also an opportunity to see
products of his nearby factory where
ormolu clocks and vases and Sheffield plate
silverware were made, and where he
developed the steam engine in partnership
with James Watt. The VC is a community
exhibition centre with changing
programmes.
The main entrance to the house has 2
steps of 5cm and 7cm, avoidable by
portable ramp, or via ramped access at the
side of the house. WC, shop and catering
are in adjacent Visitor Centre (Cat. 3. as
ramp is 1:11.2).

SD ⟨⟩   CP   E   RF
L   C ⟨⟩   S ⟨⟩   WC ⟨⟩

COVENTRY
A thriving city in which the legend of
Godiva, who, it is said, rode naked
through the city in order to obtain
relief for the town from the taxes
levied by her husband Leofric, is still
part of its heritage. Much of the old
city was devastated by the German
air raid in November 1940, but the
city centre is dominated by its new
cathedral. Early wealth derived from
textiles, but now is associated with
car manufacture.

TOURIST INFORMATION CENTRE
Bayley Lane, Coventry CV1 5RN
Tel: (024) 76 832303

**COVENTRY COUNCIL OF DISABLED
PEOPLE**
101 Broad Park Road, Henley Green,
Coventry CV2 1DB
Tel: (024) 76 61400

TRAVELINE
(0870) 6082608

BUSES
Easyrider: Tel: (024) 76 602293
Low steps, lifts, trained staff.

TAXIS
Alan's Taxis: Tel: (024) 76 555555
25 adapted vehicles.
Central Taxis: Tel: (024) 76 333333
80 adapted vehicles.
Lewis Taxis: Tel: (024) 76 666666
2 adapted vehicles.

TRAINS
Silverlink: Special Needs: (024) 76 207818
Fax: (024) 76 207023
Minicom: (024) 76 256430
Virgin Trains: Special Needs:
Tel: (0845) 7443366
Minicom: (0845) 7443367
Coventry Station accessible via level route.

CAR PARKS
Free unlimited disabled badge parking in
Pay & Display car parks.

SHOPMOBILITY
Barracks Car Park, Upper Precinct,
Coventry CV1 1DD
Tel: (024) 76 832020   Fax: (024) 76 832017

HOTELS
HILTON NATIONAL COVENTRY
Paradise Way, Walsgrave Triangle,
Coventry CV2 2ST
Tel: (024) 76 603000   Fax: (024) 76 841001
No. of Accessible Rooms: 2
Accessible Facilities: Open plan Public
Areas. Bright modern property situated just
outside Coventry.

NOVOTEL COVENTRY
Wilsons Lane, Longford, Coventry CV6 6HL
Tel: (024) 76 365000 Fax: (024) 76 362422
No. of Accessible Rooms: 2
Accessible Facilities: Lounge, Restaurant
(ramped access)
Modern bright hotel 11 miles from NEC
Birmingham. Located on M6 (J.3)

ATTRACTIONS
COVENTRY CATHEDRAL
Priory Street, Coventry
Tel: (024) 76 227597   Fax: (024) 76 631448
e-mail: information@coventrycathedral.org
The remains of the old cathedral, bombed
in 1940, have been preserved. The new
pink-sandstone cathedral, designed by Sir
Basil Spence and consecrated in 1962,
houses superb contemporary works
including John Piper's baptistery window,
tapestry by Graham Sutherland and
bronzes by Epstein.

SD | CP | E | RF | L | C | S | WC

HERBERT ART GALLERY AND MUSEUM
Jordan Well, Coventry CV1 5QP
Tel: (024) 76 832381   Fax: (024) 76 832410
e-mail: artsandheritage.gov.uk
History of Lady Godiva's city told through
interactive displays and paintings.

SD | CP | E | RF | L | C | S | WC | RFE

MUSEUM OF BRITISH ROAD TRANSPORT
Hales Street, Coventry CU1 1PN
Tel: (024) 76 832425
Fax: (024) 76 832465
www.mbrt.co.uk
Largest display of British-made road
transport in the world, under one
enormous roof. Explore Memory Lanes
display of Edwardian and vintage vehicles
set in period street scenes: trace the
progress of the cycle from Hobby Horse
to Mountain Bike: see old and new buses
and public vehicles: experience the
Coventry Blitz in an emotionally
interpreted display. A charming, easily
accessible museum.

SD | CP | E | RF | L | C | S | WC

273

Cathedrals old and new at Coventry.

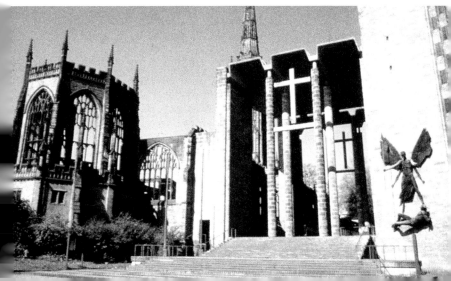

SPORTING VENUE
COVENTRY CITY FOOTBALL CLUB
Highfield Road Stadium, King Richard Street, Coventry CV2 4FW
Admin: (024) 76 234000
Fax: (024) 76 234099
www.ccfc.co.uk
Booking: Wheelchair spaces for car park and viewing: (01203) 234020 for credit card or by post.

CP ♿   RE ♿   ED ♿ (except manual door)
L ♿   WC ♿ (2 units)

SOLIHULL
A suburb of Birmingham with some Tudor houses in the High Street.

HOTEL
SOLIHULL MOAT HOUSE　　🚶
Homer Road, Solihull B91 3QD
Tel: (0121) 6239988 Fax: (0121) 7112696
No. of Accessible Rooms:
Accessible Facilities: Lounge, Bar, Restaurant
Modern hotel well located for NEC or shopping centre very close by.

ATTRACTIONS
BADDESLEY CLINTON HALL (NT)
Knowle, Solihull
Tel: (01564) 783294 Fax: (01564) 782706
The written history of Baddesley began long before the C13th when the Clintons settled here, dug the moat and gave the place their name. The house has grey stone walls, tiled roofs and tall red-brick chimneys emblazoned in trees in the hollow of a park which has never been formally planted or landscaped.

SD ♿   CP 🚶   E 🚶   RF ♿
C 🚶   S ♿   WC 🚶   RFE 🚶

PACKWOOD HOUSE
Lapworth, Solihull B94 6AT
Infoline: (01684) 855362
Tel: (01564) 783294 Fax: (01564) 782706
e-mail: packwood@ntrust.org.uk
Cromwell's general, Henry Ireton, stayed here before the Battle of Edgehill in 1642, but many of the interiors were designed in the 1920s and 30s as an idealised

Elizabethan or Jacobean manor and offer great insight into the taste, rich decoration and way of life of a wealthy amateur connoisseur between the wars. The house is surrounded by tranquil gardens.
NB: Access to ground floor only.

SD ♿   E 🚶   RF 🚶   C n/a   S 🚶
WC 🚶   RFE 🚶 Wheelchairs available for hire.

STOURBRIDGE
Early importance as glass-making centre, introduced by religious refugees from Hungary in C16th. Situated on south bank of river Stour on edge of the Black Country.

ATTRACTION
BROADFIELD HOUSE GLASS MUSEUM
Compton Drive, Kingswinford,
Nr. Stourbridge DY6 9NS
Tel: (01384) 812745
Fax: (01384) 812746
Fine collection of C19th and C20th glass cut in nearby Stourbridge. Ground floor only is accessible.

SD ♿   CP 🚶   E ♿   RF ♿
C 🚶   S ♿   WC 🚶

WOLVERHAMPTON
Capital of the Black Country with many striking buildings of Victorian civic architecture, but little else.

HOTEL
NOVOTEL WOLVERHAMPTON　　Q
Union Street, Wolverhampton WV1 3JN
Tel: (01902) 871199
Fax: (01902) 870054
No. of Accessible Rooms: 3. Bath
Accessible Facilities: Lounge, Restaurant.
Located within easy reach of city centre.

ATTRACTION
WOLVERHAMPTON ART GALLERY
Lichfield Street, Wolverhampton WV1 1DU
Tel: (01902) 552055
Fax: (01902) 552053
www.artgall.scit.wlv.ac.uk
Changing art, sculpture and photographic

exhibitions throughout the year, plus hands-on Ways of Seeing Room, an exploration of art through eyes, ears and hands. Very accessible gallery.

SD ♿ CP ♿ E ♿ RF ♿
L ♿ C ♿ S ♿ WC 🚹

WILTSHIRE

CHIPPENHAM

King Alfred spent much time here, hunting in the nearby forests. There is a C15th Town Hall and some attractive half-timbered houses, and others in stone dating from the C18th.

TOURIST INFORMATION CENTRE
The Citadel, Bath Road, Chippenham SN15 2AA
Tel: (01249) 706333   Fax: (01249) 460776

ATTRACTION
LACOCK ABBEY (NT)
Lacock, Chippenham SN15 2LG
Tel: (01249) 730227
Founded in 1232, Lacock became secular after the Dissolution of the Monasteries by Henry VIII. The church was destroyed but fine medieval cloisters remain. In the mid C19th William Henry Fox Talbot remodelled south elevation and added 3 oriel windows. The abbey and most of the village was donated to the NT in 1944/46, and the village retains its unique mixture of architecture spanning 700 years. The museum commemorates the life and work of W H F Talbot who invented the positive/negative process in 1840, and was known as the Father of Modern Photography. Abbey is not accessible, but cloisters and museum are. Museum has stair lift to upper floor. The present cloisteral walkway is of C14th and C15th.

SD ♿ CP ♿ E ♿ RF ♿
C ♿ S 🚹
WC ♿ (Radar key obtained from Stable Cafe)
RFE ♿

DEVIZES

An old market town with some C16th buildings, the town is particularly rich in C18th structures.

TOURIST INFORMATION CENTRE
Cromwell House, The Market Place,
Devizes SN10 1JG
Tel: (01380) 729408

Lacock Abbey spans 700 years from monks to photography.

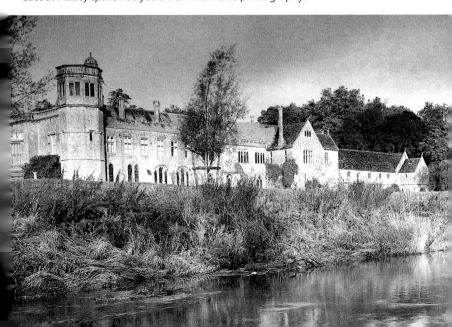

SELF-CATERING
ABBOTTS BALL FARM 🧍
Pound Hill, Worton Road, Potterne,
Devizes SN10 5PW
Tel: (01380) 721661
No. of Accessible Units: 1. Roll-in Shower
No. of Beds per Unit: 2D +1S.
Accessible Facilities: Lounge/diner,
Kitchen, Garden. The cottage is an
annexe onto the farmhouse on edge of
village of Potterne with far reaching
views. 30 minutes from Salisbury, Bath
and Stonehenge.

MARLBOROUGH
Situated in the Kennet Valley and on a
main road, Marlborough was popular
in coaching times. Most of the older
half-timbered houses are hidden in
small back lanes off the High Street,
itself an impressive wide road
sweeping down the centre of the
town. Overall effect is Georgian, but
there are a number of periods
manifest here.

TOURIST INFORMATION CENTRE
George Lane Car Park, Marlborough
SN18 1EE
Tel: (01672) 513989

ATTRACTION
ALEXANDER KEILLER MUSEUM (NT)
Avebury, Nr. Marlborough SN8 1RF
Tel: (01672) 539250   Fax: (01672) 539388
Museum is a site museum for Avebury
Monuments, situated 250m from the
stone circle on the western side of
Avebury Manor farmyard. New museum
gallery in C17th thatched barn in
farmyard designed with access. Avebury
Manor, just behind the Museum is not
accessible to wheelchairs.
SD ♿ CP 🧍 E ♿ RF 🧍 S 🧍
WC 🧍

SALISBURY
Built on the junction of the rivers Avon
and Nadder, the city's history

dates back to C13th when the bishop's
see was moved from old Sarum and
the famous cathedral's foundations
were laid here in 1220. It has been a
market town since its inception. There
is much of interest in the streets,
flanked by gabled houses and in
buildings of all periods set in
comfortable juxtaposition. See C16th
facade of Joiner's Hall in St. Ann Street;
C17th Shoemaker's Guildhall: C15th
Poultry Cross in Silver Street, etc.

TOURIST INFORMATION CENTRES
Fish Row, Salisbury SP1 1EJ
Tel: (01722) 334956   Fax: (01722) 422059
Also at Salisbury Station (summer months).

ENABLE
3 Priory Square, The Maltings, Salisbury
SP1 1BD
Tel: (01722) 416189
General information on all aspects of
disability, very helpful.

TRAVELINE
(0870) 6082608

BUSES
Wilts and Dorset: Tel: (01722) 336855
Some low-floor buses

TAXIS
Value Cars: Tel: (01722) 505050
Seven adapted vehicles.

TRAINS
South West Trains: Special Needs:
Tel: (0845) 6050440
Minicom: (0845) 6050441
www.swtrains.co.uk
Wales & West: Special Needs:
Tel: (0845) 3003005
Minicom: (0845) 585469

CAR PARKS
2 hours free parking in city council-owned
car parks, free unlimited disabled badge
spaces. If staying with a resident, a free
parking permit may be obtained.
Tel: (01722) 713000

SHOPMOBILITY
The Maltings Car Park, Malthouse Lane,
Salisbury S02 7TL
Tel/Fax: (01722) 328068

HOTEL
GRASMERE HOUSE HOTEL   [♿]
70 Harnham Road, Salisbury SP2 8JN
Tel: (01722) 338388   Fax: (01722) 333710
No. of Accessible Rooms: 4. Bath
Accessible Facilities: Lounge, Restaurant,
Garden. Victorian family residence, set in
1.5 acres of mature gardens laid largely to
lawn, with towering beech trees and small
woodland fir copse. Built in 1896 of red
brick with attractive pointed filials on the
roof gables. Converted and extended with
ambience of comfortable Victorian home.

BED AND BREAKFAST
WEBSTERS   [♿]
11 Hartington Road, Salisbury SP2 7LG
Tel: (01722) 339779   Fax: (01722) 421103
e-mail: websters.salis@eclipse.co.uk
No. of Accessible Rooms: 1. Roll-in Shower
Accessible Facilities: Lounge, Dining Room
1996 Holiday Care Service Award winner.
Situated in cul-de-sac on end of colourful
Victorian terrace.

ATTRACTION
SALISBURY CATHEDRAL
33 The Close, Salisbury SP1 2EJ
Tel: (01722) 555120   Fax: (01722) 555116
www.visitors@salcath.co.uk
Built between 1220 and 1258, a medieval
masterpiece of Early English Gothic
architecture with an elegant spire, the
tallest in England at 123m. Artefacts
include one of the original Magna Carta
documents and probably the oldest
working clock in the world, c.1386.
Accessibility leaflet available.
WARNING: ENTRANCE RAMPED AT 1:8.
THE BUILDING HAS BEEN INCLUDED
BECAUSE OF ITS IMPORTANCE.
SD [&]   CP [♿]   E n/a   C [♿]   S [♿]   WC [♿]

SALISBURY AND SOUTH WILTSHIRE MUSEUM
The King's House, 65 the Close,
Salisbury SP1 2EN
Tel: (01722) 332151   Fax: (01722) 325611

e-mail: museum
@salisburymuseum.freeserve.co.uk
www.salisburymuseum.org.uk
One of several beautiful buildings in
Cathedral Close, with fascinating displays
including galleries on Stonehenge, Early
Man, History of Salisbury, Pitt Rivers
collection, ceramics and Wedgwood room.
Good exhibitions all year round.
SD [&]   CP [♿]   E [&]   RF [&]   C [&]
S [&]   WC [♿]   RFE [&]

WILTON HOUSE
The Estate Office, Wilton, Salisbury SP2 0BJ
Tel: (01722) 746728   Fax: (01722) 744447
e-mail: Tourism@Wiltonhouse.com
www.wiltonhouse.com
Set in 21 acres of landscaped parkland,
Wilton House is the famous family home
of the 17th Earl of Pembroke and
considered one of the premier houses of
England. The Palladian-style house
contains a fine art collection, Victorian
laundry and Tudor kitchen. Setting for
scenes from Sense and Sensibility and Mrs.
Brown. Video provides introduction to
house and family. Grounds include
Palladian bridge, Woodland Walk and Old
English Rose Garden.
SD [&]   CP [♿]   E [&]   RF [♿]   C [&]
S [&]   WC [♿]   RFE [♿]

WARMINSTER
Situated 130m. above sea-level, above
the valley of the Wylye, the town grew
rich from the manufacture of cloth and
the sale of wheat. There are Georgian
houses and cottages and some lovely
inns in this rather graceful town.

TOURIST INFORMATION CENTRE
Central Car Park, Warminster BA12 9BT
Tel: (01985) 218548 Fax: (01985) 846154
www.visitwarminster@westwiltshire.gov.uk

ATTRATION
STOURTON HOUSE FLOWER GARDEN
Stourton, Zeals, Warminster BA12 6QF
Tel: (01747) 840417
4-acre plant lovers' garden lies hidden just
before the car park of Stourhead House

(NT). Grassy paths lead through the 12 Apostles walk, through hedged borders, ponds, and varied vistas of colourful shrubs, trees and unusual plants. Delicious cream teas.

SD 🚶 CP 🚶 E ♿ RF 🚶
C 🚶
S 🚶 WC 🚶 RFE 🚶

LONGLEAT HOUSE AND SAFARI PARK
Warminster BA12 7NW
Tel: (01985) 844400 Fax: (01985) 844885
e-mail: enquiries@longleat.co.uk
www.longleat.co.uk
Superb stately home of high Elizabethan architecture with enormous grounds. Information sheet for visitors with disablties. Only three wheelchair users allowed in the house at any one time, and each must be accompanied by two able bodied companions. Wheelchair access is via the Victorian Kitchen at the back of the house, via Lady Bath's Shop, where the guide will call for lift, up to Great Hall. Lift access to both floors, with wide, level wooden surfaces. Tour follows normal route exceept no access to State Drawing Room. Wheelchair progress logged in lift against fire and accident. Access to Cellar Cafe is via the Victorian Kitchen. Accessible WC in main square. Accessible attractions: Butterfly Garden/King Arthur's Mirror Maze, Lord Bath's Bygones, Railway - 1 adapted carriage.
Not accessible: Safari Boats, Virtualscope, Maze, Life and Time, Dolls Houses. The Safari Park is accessed by car with the usual warnings of accessing the monkey section at your own risk to your car.

SD ♿ CP 🚶 E ♿ L ♿
C ♿ S ♿ WC ♿

YORKSHIRE

YORKSHIRE – NORTH AND EAST

YORKSHIRE TOURIST BOARD
312 Tadcaster Road, York YO24 1GS
Tel: (01904) 707961 Fax: (01904) 701414
e-mail: info@ytb.org.uk
www.yorkshirevisitor.com

NORTH YORK MOORS NATIONAL PARK
North York Moors National Park,
The Old Vicarage, Bondgate,
Helmsley YO62 5BP
Tel: (01439) 770657 Fax: (01439) 770691
Bleak, but glorious wide open spaces and panoramic views across the heather moorland and out to sea.
Wheelchair hire.

PICKERING TOURIST INFORMATION CENTRE
Eastgate Car Park. Tel: (01751) 473791
Park and View
Cowhouse Bank. 3 miles north of Helmsley on Bransdale Road. No restroom.
Newgate Bank. 6 miles north-west of Helmsley on B1257. No adaptive restroom.
Clay Bank. 3 miles north of Chop Gate on B1257. Refreshments, no restroom.
Sheepwash. 2 miles north of Osmotherley on Swainby Road.
Hazel Heads. 3 miles north-west of Helmsley on Osmotherly Road. No restroom.
Peak Scar. 3 miles north of Sutton Bank. No restroom.
Helmsley Bank. 4.5 miles north of Helmsley on road to Baxtons. No restroom.
Thimbley Moor and Chequers. Both are on the road to Osmotherly from Hawnby.
Carlton Bank. 1 mile south-east of Carlton-in-Cleveland on the road to Chop Gate. Café.
Rudland Rigg. 6 miles north-north-west of Kirkbymoorside. On road to Bransdale from Kirkby there are several viewing places.
Gillamoor, Surprise View. In Gillamoor village, 3 miles north of Kirkbymoorside, by the side of the church.
Saltergate Bank. 7/5 miles north-east of Pickering on A169. No restroom.
Blue Bank. 1 mile south of Sleights on A169. No restrooms.
Bell Heads. Nr. Hackness at top of steep hill on road to Silpho. No restroom.
Highwood Brow. Forest Enterprise car

park. No restroom.

Scaling Dam. 7 miles west of Sandsend on A1717 at Scaling Reservoir. Facilities for angling for the disabled. Enquiries, call 01287 640214. Restroom.

Ravenscar. Roadside lay-by. Restroom.

Sandsend. Car park at foot of Lythe Bank, fronting onto sea. Ramp access to sandy beach.

Runswick Bay. Car park in village with sea views.

Whitby. Abbey Plains car park. Follow signs from Whitby to the abbey.

Public restrooms with disabled facilities:

Farndale, Hutton-le-Hole, Goathland, Grosmont Station, Kildale, Thornton-le-Dale, Low Dalby, Staindale Lake (Dalby Forest), Kirkbymoorside, Pickering (Ropery and Eastgate Car Parks), Coxwold, Newton-under-Roseberry, Ravenscar, Danby Moors Centre, Sutton Bank, Swainby, Scaling Dam, Helmsley (Cleveland Way Car Park and Borogate).

Accessible Trails and Paths

Farndale. Daffodil path suitable from Low Mill car park. Able-bodied companion recommended.

Mulgrave Woods, Sandsend. Parking at East Row Car Park, walk borders two steep ravines reaching almost to the sea. Mixed woodland, meadow and beckside glade.

Cawthorn Roman Camps, Nr. Cropton. Only short part of archaeological trail is accessible, but possible to see earth ramparts of the most westerly of the camps.

CLEVELAND WAY NATIONAL TRAIL

110 miles long, running from Helmsley around the North York Moors to Saltburn and along the coast to Filey. The accessible routes below spread throughout the length of the walk. These routes have compact hard surface or are fairly smooth with compact earth/short even grass and a gradient of not more than 1/20. Remember to take your RADAR key with you.

Sutton Bank, Nr. Thirsk. From Thirsk take A170 towards Scarborough. Visitor Centre is at the top of Sutton Bank on the left, about 7 miles beyond Thirsk. Go south for

1.5 miles towards the Kilburn White Horse, or north for 0.5 mile to overlook Lake Gormire. Both walks start from Visitor Centre (accessible restroom) car park. For walk south, follow stone path towards Bank and cross road. Walk follows escarpment edge along smooth stone surface to finish at White Horse. Going north, head for escarpment and turn right. Path remains flat and smooth as far as views over Lake.

Hambleton Drove Road, Nr. Kepwick. Kepwick is north-east of Thirsk. Turn off A19 at Knayton, 3 miles north of Thirsk. Follow signs to Kepwick, and carry straight on up steep and climbing hill, ignoring sign saying no motor vehicles. There are 2 gates along this road that must be opened before reaching start of walk. Park beyond top gate on reaching the moor and head downhill on gentle grass slope. This is a linear moor land walk of 0.65 mile, there and back. You will reach the ruins of Limekiln House after 0.33 mile.

279

BEDALE

An important meeting point since Saxon times, Bedale flourished as a thriving country town, particularly at the height of the coaching era. With its long, curving High Street, flanked by Georgian buildings and a market cross at its centre, Bedale forms the gateway to the Yorkshire Dales.

TOURIST INFORMATION CENTRE

(Open Easter-end September)
Bedale Hall, North End, Bedale DL8 1AA
Tel: (01677) 424604   Fax: (01677) 427146

SELF-CATERING

ELMFIELD HOUSE COTTAGES
Arrathorne, Bedale DL8 1NE
Tel: (01677) 450558   Fax: (01677) 450557
stay@elmfieldhouse.freeserve.co.uk
No. of Accessible Units: 2. Roll-in Shower
No. of Beds per Unit: 3
Accessible Facilities: Open plan Kitchen, Dining Room, Lounge.
Cottages adjacent to country guest house.

ATTRACTION
BEDALE MUSEUM
Beadale Hall, Bedale DL8 1AA
Tel: (01677) 423797
Fax: (01677) 425393
Building of C17th with famous exhibit of 1742 fire engine. Artefacts give interesting account of the lives of ordinary people.
SD [♿]   CP [♿]   E [♿]   RF [♿]

BROUGH
A coaching town in the last century. Brough is at the foot of the long ascent over Stainmore, with a castle dating from C11th. The National Trust has a protected area to the north, Musgrave Fell, which is a limestone pavement.

BED AND BREAKFAST
RUDSTONE WALK   [♿]
South Cave, Brough, East Yorkshire
Nr. Beverley HU15 2AH
Tel: (01430) 422230   Fax: (01430) 424552
e-mail: office@rudstone-walk.co.uk
www.rudstone-walk.co.uk
No. of Accessible Rooms: 3. Roll-in Shower/Bath. Accessible Facilities: 400-year-old farmhouse forms the heart of this property, with cottages, including adapted Woodland Cottage, converted from the farm buildings adjacent to the house, where meals are served. Set in its own grounds and wooded hills, overlooking the Vale of York. Located a few miles from historic Beverley, and 1.5 miles from the village of South Cave.

DARLINGTON
Busy town, renowned for locomotives and known as the cradle of railways although locomotive engineering shops were closed in 1966.

TOURIST INFORMATION CENTRE
13 Horsemarket, Darlington DL1 5PW
Tel: (01325) 388666

TRAINS
Great North Eastern Railway: Special Needs:
Tel: (0845) 7225444
Mincom: (0191) 2330173
Virgin Trains: Special Needs:
Tel: (0845) 7443366
Minicom: (0845) 7443367

HOTEL
ST. GEORGE AIRPORT HOTEL   [♿]
Teesside Airport, Darlington DL2 1RH
Tel: (01325) 332631
Fax: (01325) 333851
No. of Accessible Rooms: 1
Accessible Facilities: Restaurant, Lounge/Bar. Originally the officer's mess on site of WWII bomber airfield of Middleton St. George, now converted into a modern hotel.

BED AND BREAKFAST
CLOWBECK HOUSE   [♿]
Monkend Farm, Crofton-on-tees, Darlington DL2 2SW
Tel: (01325) 721075   Fax: (01325) 720419
e-mail: reservations@clowbeckhouse.co.uk
www.clowbeckhouse.co.uk
No. of Accessible Rooms: 1
Accessible Facilities: Lounge (1 step), Dining Room. Charming country residence, set in rolling countryside and deriving its name from the Beck, winding its way through the farm to the River Tees. Dinner also available.

GRASSINGTON
This Wharfedale village is very appealing: its buildings crowd around a small market place paved with cobblestones and along irregular passages. The river is crossed by a stone bridge of 1603. There are numerous prehistoric sites here.

SELF-CATERING
THE BARN   [♿]
24 Broughton Fold, Grassington BD23 5AL
Tel: (01756) 753037
To book: Call Mrs. Evans on
(01274) 561546
No. of Accessible Units: 1. Bath,
No. of Beds per Unit: 1D/2S
Accessible Facilities: Lounge/Dining Room,

Kitchen, Garden, secluded, south facing with patio.
Ground floor cottage forming part of converted Dales barn, situated in quiet private part of the village square.

HARROGATE
A stately and genteel town in a high and airy location with spacious parks, an abundance of trees and lavish flower beds. Famous for fine shopping and rich teas, Edwardian and Victorian buildings in its centre and its annual flower show that is a social must.

TOURIST INFORMATION CENTRE
Royal Baths Assembley Rooms, Crescent Road, Harrogate HG1 2RR
Tel: (01423) 537300   Fax: (01423) 537305

BUSES
Local bus and rail information:
Tel: (01423) 566061
Harrogate District Travel:
Tel: (01423) 507227

TAXIS
Blueline Cars: Tel: (01423) 530830
Eight adapted vehicles.
Central Radio Cabs: Tel: (01423) 505050
Five adapted vehicles, two minibuses.

TRAINS
Northern Spirit: Special Needs:
Tel: (0845) 6008008

CAR PARKS
Free unlimited disabled badge parking, either in car parks or off-street.

SHOPMOBILITY
Victoria Car Park, East Parade, Harrogate
Tel: (01423) 500666

HOTEL
HARROGATE MOAT HOUSE   [🏃]
Kings Road, Harrogate HG1 1XX
Tel: (01423) 849988   Fax: (01423) 524435
No. of accessible Rooms: 1. Bath
Accessible Facilities: Lounge, Restaurant.
Quality town-centre hotel.

SELF-CATERING
OLD SPRING WOOD LODGES   [🏃]
Hartwith Bank, Summerbridge, Harrogate HG3 4DR
Tel: (01423) 780279
Fax: (01423) 780994
No. of Accessible Units: 4. Bath
No. of Beds per Unit: 2 - 10
Accessible Facilities: Open plan Lounge/Dining Room/Kitchen
Scandinavian lodges in woodland overlooking the Nidd Valley.

ATTRACTIONS
RHS HARLOW CARR
Crag Lane, Harrogate HG3 1QB
Tel: (01423) 565418   Fax: (01423) 530663
58 fine acres of ornamental and woodland gardens with courses and activites throughout the year.

SD [♿]   CP [♿]   E [♿]   RF [♿]   C [♿]
S n/a   WC [🏃]   RFE [♿]

RIPLEY CASTLE
Ripley, Harrogate HG3 3AY
Tel: (01423) 770152
Fax: (01423) 771745
e-mail:khodgson@ripleycastle.co.uk
www.ripleycastle.co.uk
Home of the Ingilby family, dating from 1320s in extensive Capability Brown designed estate. Fine paintings, furnishings and Civil War memorabilia. Home to the National Hyacinth collection.

SD [♿]   CP [♿]   E [♿]   RF [♿]
C [♿]   S [🏃]   WC [♿]   RFE - Gardens [🏃]

HELMSLEY
Helmsley lies in a hollow of the River Rye, an excellent gateway to Ryedale and the North Yorkshire Moors. The view dropping into it from the south takes in the red-roofed house, spacious market square, pinnacled church tower and the gaunt shell of Helmsley Castle.

TOURIST INFORMATION CENTRE
Town Hall, Market Place, Helmsley YO6 5DL
Tel: (01439) 770173
www.ryedale.gov.uk

SELF-CATERING
ANGEL COTTAGE
Wheatfield, Newton Grange,
Oswaldkirk YO62 5YE
Tel/Fax: (01439) 788493
No. of Accessible Units: 1. Roll-in Shower
No. of Beds per Unit: 4
Accessible Facilities: Lounge, Kitchen/Diner
Holiday cottage 3 miles from Helmsley.

ATTRACTIONS
NUNNINGTON HALL (NT)
Nunnington, Nr. Helmsley YO62 5UY
Tel: (01439) 748283   Fax: (01439) 748284
C16th. country manor house with
panelled rooms and a superb staircase,
plus display of the Carlisle collection of
miniature rooms.

SD 🦽   CP 🚶   E 🦽   RF 🚶   C 🚶
S 🚶   WC 🚶   RFE 🚶

RIEVAULX TERRACE AND TEMPLES (NT)
Rievaulx, Helmsley YO61 5LJ
Tel: (01439) 798340 Fax: (01439) 748284
Firm gravel path through woodland or
wheelchair route straight onto Terrace.
Picnic along elegant half-mile created over
300 years ago. Superb views of Rievaulx
Abbey and landscape of Hambleton Hills.
Two C18th. classical temples, neither
accessible inside, but well worth a look.
Pre- book Batteriicar or wheelchair.

SD 🦽   CP ♿   E ♿   S ♿

INGLETON
At the north-west extreme of
Yorkshire, with hills and moors above
the village showing weathered
limestone outcrops so typical of the
area. There are 5 pubs and 3 cafes
with reasonable access.

TOURIST INFORMATION CENTRE
Community Centre Car Park,
Ingleton LA6 3HG
Tel: (015242) 41049

BED AND BREAKFAST
RIVERSIDE LODGE
24 Main Street,
Ingleton, via Carnforth LA6 3HJ

Tel: (015242) 41359
No. of Accessible Rooms: 2. Shower
Accessible Facilities: Lounge, Restaurant,
Country guesthouse with conservatory
with beautiful views, level access to top
garden, sauna, games room (the latter two
on lower ground floor, accessible from
outside with 1 step, then 3 steps).

KINGSTON-UPON-HULL
Severely damaged during WWII, with
modern, rather unexciting buildings
combining with the lawns, flower-beds
and pools of Queens Gardens. Third
largest port in UK, its docks run for
seven miles along the north bank of
the Humber, and the country's largest
fishing operation

.

HULL TOURISM
1 Paragon Street,
Kingston-upon-Hull HU1 3NA
Tel: (01482) 223559
www.hull700.co.uk

HOTEL
QUALITY ROYAL HOTEL
170 Ferensway, Hull HU1 3UF
Tel: (01482) 325087   Fax: (01482) 323172
email: admin@gb611.u-net.com
No. of Accessible Rooms: 2. Bath
Accessible Facilities: Lounge, Restaurant
Located in city centre.

ATTRACTIONS
THE DEEP, KINGSTON-UPON-HULL
HU1 4DP
Tel: (01482) 381000   Fax: (01482) 381010
e-mail: info@thedeep.co.uk
www.thedeep.co.uk
World Ocean Discovery Centre based
around an aquarium with supplementary
buildings creating marine complex. Located
at confluence of Rivers Hull and Humber.
Built on four levels, it includes exhibits
using IT and interactive displays to examine
the sea life of the world's oceans from prehistoric times to present day. The
attraction takes 2 - 3 hours to get round.
Wheelchair access to all public areas
although it is worth bearing in mind that

there will be a queuing system in operation on busy days.

SD ♿ CP ♿ E ♿ RF ♿ L ♿
C 🚶 S ♿ WC ♿

BURTON CONSTABLE HALL
Burton Constable, Sproatley, Nr. Hull HU11 4LN
Tel: (01964) 562400 Fax: (01964) 563229
Lovely Elizabethan house built in 1570 with fine reception rooms and Tudor long gallery and much Chippendale furniture. 200-acre park designed by Capability Brown. Located a few miles NW of Hull.

SD ♿ CP ♿ E ♿ RF ♿ L ♿
C ♿ S ♿ WC ♿ RFE ♿

KIRBYMOORSIDE
Just off the Pickering-Helmsley road, its main street climbs steeply toward the hills. On the Vivers hill behind the church are the sketchy remains of a Norman castle.
Fine Georgian houses in its broad main street and a cobbled market square.

BED AND BREAKFAST
THE CORNMILL 🚶
Kirby Mills, Kirbymoorside, York YO62 6NP
Tel: (01751) 432000 Fax: (01751) 432300
e-mail: cornmill@kirbymills.demon.co.uk
www.kirbymills.demon.co.uk
No. of Accessible Rooms: 1. Roll-in Shower
Accessible Facilities: Lounge/Bar, Dining Room. Renovated C18th watermill and farmhouse with glass-floored dining room over millrace. Accommodation in annexed Victorian farmhouse.

LEYBURN
A broad mile-long terrace shaded with evergreens, oaks and sycamores allows fine views over Wensleydale. Among other landmarks are Bolton and Middleham castles.

TOURIST INFORMATION CENTRE
4 Central Chambers, Railway Street, Leyburn DL8 5BB

Tel: (01969) 623069 Fax: (01969) 622833

HOTEL ACCOMMODATION
EASTFIELD LODGE
1 St. Matthews Terrace, Leyburn DL8 5EL
Tel: (01969) 623196
No. of Accessible Rooms: 1. Bath
Accessible Facilities: Lounge, Restaurant. Private hotel, built in mid-1800s, in lovely Wensleydale with attractive south-facing public rooms and garden.

GOLDEN LION HOTEL
Market Place, Leyburn DL8 5AS
Tel: (01969) 622161 Fax: (01969) 623836
No. of Accessible Rooms: Several (via accessible lift)
Accessible Facilities: Dining Room (1 step), Bar. Dating from 1765, a traditional family hotel of 15 rooms. Ideal base for exploring Yorkshire Dales.

MALTON
Historic centre of Ryedale since Roman times. North of Roman fort site at Orchard Fields is the original town of Old Malton, in the centre of which stands a fragment of St. Mary's the only Gilbertine Priory in use in England. Traditional agricultural town, holding thrice-weekly cattle market.

MALTON TOURIST INFORMATION CENTRE
58 Market Place, Malton YO17 7LW
Tel: (0800) 137233

RYEDALE TOURISM NORTH YORKSHIRE
Rydedale District Council, Rydedale House, Malton YO17 0HH
Tel: (01653) 600666 Fax: (01653) 696801
www.ryedale.gov.uk

ATTRACTIONS
EDEN CAMP MODERN HISTORY THEME MUSEUM
Malton YO17 6RT
Tel: (01653) 697777 Fax: (01653) 698243
e-mail: admin@edencamp.co.uk
The People's War, a fascinating range of WWII exhibits on the Home Guard, Street

283

at War, U-Boat Menace, Prisoners of War, Civil Defence, The Blitz etc. Also six new exhibitions on military and political events complementing the civilian story.

| SD ♿ | CP ♿ | E ♿ | RF ♿ |
| C ♿ | S ♿ | WC ♿ | RFE ♿ |

MALTON MUSEUM
Town Hall, Market Place, Malton YO17 0LT
Tel: (01653) 695136
Well known for its rich archaeological collection, there are depictions of the famous Roman settlements in the area, particularly of the Roman fort at Derventio.

| SD ♿ | CP 🚶♿ | E ♿ | RF 🚶 | S 🚶 |

MIDDLESBROUGH
Large town, administrative centre of Tees-side with several museums and galleries.

TOURIST INFORMATION CENTRE
(Open April-end October)
High Green Car Park, Great Ayton, Middlesbrough TS9 68J
Tel: (01642) 722835

ATTRACTIONS
CAPTAIN COOK BIRTHPLACE MUSEUM
Stewart Park, Marton, Middlesbrough TS7 8AT
Tel: (01642) 311211   Fax: (01642) 515655
Unique perspective on the life and times of Captain James Cook through this superb museum with films, special effects, inter-active hands-on exhibits about Cook's three great voyages. Discover the creaking timbers, the perils of the ocean and the recordings of artists and scientists among the strange plants and animals of the South Seas and the Americas. Superb in content and access. Not to be missed. NB. Entrance is through The Grove, not the main car park.

| SD n/a | CP 🚶♿ | E 🚶♿ | RF 🚶♿ | C ♿ |
| S ♿ | WC ♿ | L ♿ |

ORMESBY HALL (NT)
Church Lane, Ormesby, Middlesbrough TS7 9AS
Tel: (01642) 324188

Fax: (01642) 300937
e-mail: yorkor@smtp.ntrust.org.uk
C18th. Palladian mansion, noted for plasterwork and carved wood decoration.

| SD ♿ | CP 🚶 | E 🚶♿ | RF 🚶 |
| C 🚶♿ | S 🚶♿ | WC 🚶 | RFE 🚶♿ |

NORTHALLERTON
Set in the rich farmland of the Vale of Mowbray, Northallerton is the county town with elegant redbrick buildings. It has a long history and a town trail points out sites and buildings with historical connections. The Church of All Saints at the north end of the High Street dates from 1120 and just outside the town a memorial stone marks the site of the Battle of the Standard.

TOURIST INFORMATION CENTRE
Applegarth, Northallerton DL7 8LZ
Tel/Fax: (01609) 776864

BED AND BREAKFAST
LOVESOME HILL FARM   🚶
Lovesome Hill, Northallerton DL6 2PB
Tel: (01609) 772311
No. of Accessible Rooms: 1. Shower
Accessible Facilities: Dining Room.
Dinner is available. 165-acre working farm four miles north of Northallerton with accommodation in granary conversion, Granary Mill is accessible. Fine touring base being between Yorkshire Dales and North Yorkshire Moors.

PICKERING
Reputed to be one of the oldest towns in the area dating back to 270BC. Skyline dominated by fine spire of the Church of St. Peter and St. Paul. Hidden high above the town are the ruins of Pickering Castle. Narrow streets lead off in all directions, the market place straggling along the hilly main street.

TOURIST INFORMATION CENTRE
The Ropery, Pickering YO18 8DY
Tel: (01751) 473791

SELF-CATERING
MOONPENNY COTTAGE
Levisham, Pickering YO18 7NL
Tel: (01751) 460311
e-mail.mici@supranet.com
No. of Accessible Units: 1. Shower
No. of Beds per Unit: 2
Accessible Facilities: Lounge, Dining Room, Kitchen, Patio, Garden. Tourist board award-winning renovation of a Grade II listed C18th farm, preserving its historic character. The village is full of stone-built houses and wide grass verges along a main street, surrounded by moorland and forest.

CLOTH FAIR COTTAGE
Rawcliffe House Farm, Stape,
Nr. Pickering YO18 8JA
Tel: (01751) 473292   Fax: (01751) 473766
e-mail: office@yorkshireaccommodation.com
No. of Accessible Units: 1. Roll-in Shower
No. of Beds per Unit: 2
Accessible Facilities: Kitchen, Lounge, Dining Room. The farm is set in 42 acres of rolling pasture and wild flower meadows in heart of North York Moors National Park. Three cottages converted from old stone barns are arranged around stone courtyard.

DAIRY HOUSE
Manor Farm, Newton upon Rawcliffe,
Pickering YO18 8QA
Tel: (01751) 472601
e-mail: emkirkmanorfarm@aol.com
No. of Accessible Units:1
No. of beds: 4
Accessible Facilities: Kitchen/Diner, Lounge. Stone-built cottage in small, unspoilt village cluster of stone farms around village green and duckpond. Much of interest within easy reach.

ATTRACTION
RYEDALE FOLK MUSEUM
Hutton-le-Hole, Nr. Pickering YO6 6UA
Tel/Fax: (01751) 417367
Open air museum with 13 historic buildings showing the lives of ordinary people from earliest times to know. Roman artefacts. Saxon stone crosses, medieval crofter's cottage and an Elizabethan manor house combine with C18th Stangend, a

Victorian Cottage and a C20th Edwardian studio.

SD 🦽	CP n/a	E 🦽	RF 🦽
S 🦽	WC 🦽	RFE 🦽	

REDCAR
Holiday resort for Teesside with 3 beaches and long rocky reefs running out to sea that are left bare, but for seaweed at low tides.

TOURIST INFORMATION CENTRE
West Terrace, Esplanade, Redcar TS10 3AE
Tel: (01642) 471921

SPORTING VENUE
REDCAR RACECOURSE
Redcar TS10 2BG
Admin & Booking-Box Office: (01642) 484068 Fax: (01642) 488272
Open venue with large open concourse served by tarmac walkways and areas providing free movement to facilities.

CP 🦽   RE 🦽   ED 🦽 (No door entrance, through gates adjoining Main entrance)
INT 🦽   L 🦽
WC 🦽 (3 sites at centre of course, behind Tattersalls and in Members' Paddock Rooms)
SS 🦽 (1 space in viewing area)
B/R - Ground floor facilities have level access: first floor accessed by manned lift.

RICHMOND
Set dramatically at the entrance to steep-sided Swaledale. Striking ruined Norman fortress on its sheer rock. Large, cobbled market place surrounded by an easy blend of Georgian and Victorian stone buildings.

TOURIST INFORMATION CENTRE
Friary Gardens, Victoria Road,
Richmond DL104AJ
Tel: (01748) 850252

BED AND BREAKFAST
MOUNT PLEASANT FARM
Whashton, Richmond DL11 7JP

Tel: (01748) 822784
No. of Accessible Rooms: 1. Shower
Accessible Facilities: Lounge, Dining
Room. The accessible Piggery Room is
one of several cottage style rooms in a
converted stable on a working farm of
sheep and beef cattle. The stone
farmhouse of 1850 is situated in rolling
countryside 3 miles from Richmond and
just outside peaceful Whashton, with fine
views of Vale of York.

SPORTING VENUE
CATTERICK RACECOURSE
Catterick Bridge, Richmond
Admin & Booking-Box Office: (01748)
811478 Fax: (01748) 811082
Complies with Part M, Building
Regulations
Open venue with open concourses served
by tarmac walkways providing free
movement to enclosures and facilities.

CO 🦽   RE 🦽   ED 🦽 (except manual door)
INT 🦽   L 🦽
WC 🦽 (1 site in Gods Solution Bar)
SS 🦽 (1 space only in viewing area, no seating in stands)
B/R 🦽

RIPON
Small market town with great cathedral
and rectangular market place.

SELF-CATERING
SWALLOW COTTAGE   🚹
Moor End Farm, Knaresborough Road,
Accessible Facilities: Lounge/Diner,
Kitchen. Detached cottage recently
converted from an old byre, retaining old
trusses and beams, located on small
working sheep farm. Set in its own
courtyard adjacent to main farmhouse.
Three miles from Ripon.

ATTRACTION
BLACK SHEEP BREWERY VISITOR CENTRE
Wellgarth, Mashon, Ripon HG4 4EN
Tel: (01765) 689227   Fax: (01765) 689746
e-mail: visitor.centre@blacksheep.co.uk
The brewhouse and fermenting rooms
included in the Brewery Tour, make the
whole tour inaccessible, but wheelchair

users can see a video of the brewing process
and the history explained by a tour guide.
Ingredients are shown and tasted by visitors,
smell the hops and taste the malts. Good
photographic display of the whole process.

SD 🦽   CP 🦽   E 🦽   RF 🦽
C 🦽   S 🦽   WC 🚹

THE NIDDERDALE MUSEUM
King Street, Pateley Bridge, Nr. Ripon
HG3 5LE
Tel: (01423) 711225
10 rooms illustrating past local life
including Victorian sitting room and
kitchen, schoolroom and cobblers' shop.

SD 🦽   CP 🚹   E 🦽   RF 🦽
L-Stair lift from ground floor entrance to first floor.
WC 🦽   RFE-See lift
Wheelchair available on first floor to tour museum all on
one level

SCARBOROUGH
Big, breezy North Sea resort that
combines castle ruins, a fishing village,
working port, luxury hotels, boarding
houses, sands, terraced gardens, long
wave-swept promenades, views and
carnival-style amusements.
Scarborough is built below and on top
of a cliff with steep steps, footpaths
and lifts connecting the parts.

SCARBOROUGH AND DISTRICT
DISABLEMENT ACTION GROUP
Allatt House, West Parade,
Scarborough YO12 5ED
Tel/Fax and Minicom: (01723) 379397
e-mail: scardag@onyxnet.co.uk
scardag@onyxnet.co.uk
Produces a guide for accdessible holidays,
accommodation and attractions in the
Scarborough and Filey area.

TOURIST INFORMATION CENTRE
Unit 3, Pavilion House, Valley Bridge Road,
Scarborough YO11 2UZ
Tel: (01723) 373333   Fax: (01723) 363785

SCARBOROUGH, WHITBY & FILEY
TOURISM
Londesborough Lodge, The Crescent

Scarborough, YO11 2PW
Tel: (01723) 232323   Fax: (01723) 376941

SCARBOROUGH MOBILITY CENTRE
8/9 Hanover Road, Scarborough
Tel: (01723) 500045
Manual wheelchairs available for hire.

WHEELCHAIR HIRE
Spring Hill House, Springhill Close,
Scarborough, Yorkshire YO12 4AD
Tel: (01723) 353177
Manual wheelchairs available for hire.

TRAVELINE
(0870) 6082608

BUSES
East Yorkshire Motor Services:
Tel: (01482) 327142
Some low-floor buses.

TAXIS
Station Taxis: Tel: (01723) 366366
Eight adapted vehicles.

TRAINS
ArrivaTrains North: Special Needs:
Tel: (0845) 6008008

CAR PARKS
Three-hour free parking in the city centre,
free unlimited further hour. Council-
owned car parks charge.

HOTEL
THE GRAINARY HOTEL   [♿]
Keasbeck Hill Farm, Harwood Dale,
Scarborough YO13 0DT
Tel/Fax (01723) 870026
e-mail:thesimpsons@grainary.co.uk
www.grainary.co.uk
No. of Accessible Rooms: 4. Roll-in
Shower
Accessible Facilities: Lounge, Restaurant
Family run hotel on 300-acre mixed farm
in the heart of the National Park. Located
midway between Scarborough and
Whitby.

THEATRE
STEPHEN JOSEPH THEATRE
Westborough, Scarborough YO11 1JW

Admin: (01723) 370540
Booking-Box Office: (01723) 370541
Minicom: (01723) 370555
Fax: (01723) 360506
Complies with Part M, Building
Regulations.

CP [♿]   RE [♿]   ED [♿] (except Manual Door)
INT [♿]   L [♿]
WC [♿] (2 sites on 1st floor, 1 on 2nd floor)

SETTLE
Narrow streets, tiny courtyards and
fine Georgian houses contribute to
an interesting townscape in this
picturesque centre for touring in an
area of great limestone hills and
crags, across the Ribble from
Giggleswick.

TOURIST INFORMATION CENTRE
Town Hall, Cheapside, Settle BD24 9EJ
Tel: (01729) 825192
e-mail: settle@ytbtic.co.uk
www.settle.org.uk

ATTRACTION
YORKSHIRE DALES FALCONRY AND
CONSERVATION CENTRE
Crows Nest, Nr. Giggleswick, Settle LA2 8AS
Tel: (01729) 822832 Fax: (01729) 823160
Privately owned falconry centre with
many species of birds of prey from
around the world: eagles, vultures,
hawks, falcons and owls in natural
habitats. Regular free-flying
demonstrations, the star attraction being
an Andean Condor, the largest bird in
the world. Children's Area, Hawk Walk,
bird feeding and educational talks.

SD [♿]   CP [♿]   E [♿]   RF [♿]
C [♿]   S [♿]   WC [♿]   RFE [♿]

SKIPTON
A good gateway to Wharfedale, the
town has charming old houses and
courtyards, an old toll-booth and
stocks in Sheep Street. Very lively
market four times a week, a medieval
church and a beautiful castle.

TOURIST INFORMATION CENTRE
35 Coach Street, Skipton BD23 1QL
Tel: (01756) 792809

HOTEL
CRAVEN HEIFER INN 🚶
Grassington Road, Skipton BD23 3LA
Tel: (01756) 792521 Fax: (01756) 794442
e-mail: philandlynn@cravenheifer.co.uk
www.cravenheifer.co.uk
No. of Accessible Rooms: 1. Shower
Accessible Facilities: Lounge, Restaurant.
Traditional dales country inn serving ales
and home cooked food with adjoining
barn converted to a selection of rooms.

SELF-CATERING
THE GHYLL COTTAGES ♿
Dalegarth, Buckden, Skipton BD23 5JU
Tel/Fax: (01756) 760877
e-mail: dalegarth@aol.com
www.dalegarth.co.uk
No. of Accessible Units: 3. Roll-in Shower
No. of Beds per Unit: 4 - 6
Accessible Facilities: Lounge, Dining Room,
Kitchen, Spa Bath, Indoor Pool with
ramped entrance, assistance required with
steps. National award-winning cottages
offering tranquillity with wonderful views
of Dales National Park.

CAWDER HALL COTTAGES 🚶
Cawder Lane, Skipton BD23 2TD
Tel: (01756) 791579 Fax: (01756) 797036
e-mail: info@cawdorhallcottages.co.uk
www.cawdorhallcottages.co.uk
No. of Accessible Units: 1. Shower or Bath
No. of Beds per Unit: 4-5
Accessible Facilities: Living Room, Kitchen.
The Smithy is 1 of 5 traditional farm
buildings now converted. Peaceful rural
setting, surrounded by fields and
moorland. A mile from Skipton.

ATTRACTIONS
BOLTON ABBEY GARDENS
Bolton Abbey, Skipton BD23 6EX
Tel: (01756) 718009 Fax: (01756) 710535
e-mail: boltonabbey@dalesweb.co.uk
Bolton Abbey Estate has been in the family
of the Dukes of Devonshire since 1754,
providing 75 miles of footpaths through
wonderful scenery of moorland, woodland

and riverside with walks for all ages and
abilities. There are three car parks, we have
selected the most accessible:

BOLTON ABBEY VILLAGE CAR PARK:
From the village green head north along
the main road (no pavement), Turn down
drive marked No Cars. On reaching the
priory door proceed around the north side
to avoid obstacles. Firm path. No steps into
church.
SD ♿   CP 🚶   E ♿   RF ♿
S ♿   WC 🚶   RF ♿

STRID WOOD CAR PARK:
The Cumberland Trail is accessible, it winds
through the wood with resting places and
viewing platform overlooking Barden Beck.
Fully accessible bird hide.
SD ♿   CP 🚶   S ♿   WC ♿   TRAIL ♿

EMBSAY & BOLTON ABBEY STEAM RAILWAY
Bolton Abbey Station, Bolton Abbey,
Skipton BD23 6AF
Tel: (01756) 710614
Fax: (01756) 710720
e-mail: embsay.steam@btinternet.com
www.embsayboltonabbeyrailway.org.uk
Journey through delightful Yorkshire Dales
scenery. N.B. No ramp access to Victoria
Coaches
SD ♿   CP ♿   E ♿   RF ♿
S 🚶   WC ♿   RF ♿

MALHAM NATIONAL PARK CENTRE
Malham, Skipton BD23 4DA
Tel: (01729) 830363 Tel: (01729) 830673
e-mail: malham@ytbtic.co.uk
www.destinationdales.org
Set high in glorious country, the Centre
offers displays and information on the
Yorkshire Dales. They offer a list of
detailed "Easy Access Trails" which include
access to the foot of the Malham cove and
to the exhibition in Townhead Barn,
Malham.
SD ♿   CP ♿   RF ♿   E ♿   WC ♿

THIRSK
Small market town, prosperous in
medieval times as evidenced by a large,

cobbled market place, and also in Georgian times, with many houses still standing on Kirkgate. Known to many as James Herriot's town, Thirsk is closely associated with this famous author vet, and the surgery where the real Mr. Herriot worked can be seen in Kirgate. Horse racing has been popular here since C18th. Sutton Bank, housing the National Park Visitor Centre, is reached via the A170 with a 1:4 incline as it climbs 170m, to offer incredible views across the Vale of York to the Pennines.

TOURIST INFORMATION CENTRE
14 Kirkgate, Thirsk YO7 1PQ
Tel: (01845) 522755
Fax: (01845) 526230
(Seasonal)

SUTTON BANK VISITOR CENTRE
Sutton Bank, Thirsk YO7 2EK
Tel: (01845) 597426

BED AND BREAKFAST
DOXFORD HOUSE
73 Front Street, Sowerby, Thirsk YO7 1JP
Tel/Fax: (01845) 523238
No. of Accessible Rooms: 1. Bath
Accessible Facilities: Lounge, Dining Room.
Comfortable Georgian guest house overlooking village greens.

ATTRACTION
FALCONRY UK
Sion Hill Hall, Kirby Wiske,
Nr. Thirsk YO7 4EU
Tel: (01845) 587522
Fax: (01845) 523735
www.falconrycentre.co.uk
Birds of prey centre where eagles, hawks and owls swoop and dive around you in a lovely English garden. Skilled handlers explain all there is to know. The flying displays and information on breeding and training programmes is fascinating.

SD    CP   E 🖐   RF 🖐

C 🖐   S 🖐   WC   RFE 🖐

WHITBY
Charming town on the coast, with the Esk emptying into the sea. It divides the town, connected by a swing bridge. Associated with seagulls, the smell of fish, the sight of red roofs up the steep banks from the quay, and above the ruin of the C7th. Abbey on the cliff. Captain Cook served an apprenticeship here in 1746.

WHITBY AND DISTRICT DISABLEMENT ACTION GROUP
Church House, Flowergate, Whitby YO21 3BA
Tel: (01947) 821991

TOURIST INFORMATION CENTRE
Langbourne Road, Whitby TO21 1YN
Tel: (01947) 602674

SELF-CATERING
THE BYRE 🖐
Millinder House, Westerdale,
Whitby YO21 2DE
Tel: (01287) 660053
No. of Accessible Units: 1. Roll-in Shower
No. of Beds per Unit: 5
Accessible Facilities: Lounge/Diner, Kitchen.
Cottage in courtyard

CAPTAIN COOK'S HAVEN 🖐
Larpool Lane, Whitby UO22 4JE
Tel: (01947) 601396   Fax: (01947) 893573
No. of Accessible Units: 1. Roll-in Shower
No. of Beds per Unit: 4
Accessible Facilities: Open plan Lounge/Kitchen
Resolution Bungalow is in a modern cottage complex located on the Esk, a mile from Whitby.

YORK
Normans, Saxons and Danes preceded our own Plantagenets for whom York became the commercial capital of the north. Although much restored, the city's fine walls are mainly C14th, though fragments of Norman work still survive. Medieval York is everywhere,

289

not least in the web of narrow streets. The city contains England's greatest concentration of medieval stained glass, mainly in York Minster, Britain's largest Gothic building. Start a city tour here, visit the Shambles or walk around the walls to Exhibition Square and Museum Street and then the Jorvik Centre.

TOURIST INFORMATION CENTRES
The de Grey Rooms, Exhibition Square, York YO1 2HB
Tel: (01904) 621756
e-mail: tic@york-tourism.co.uk
www.visityork.org

Railway Station, Outer Concourse, York YO2 2AY
Tel: (01904) 621756

DISABILITY INFORMATION AND ADVICE CENTRE
Room 2, Nursery Block, Priory Street Centre, 12 Priory Street, York YO1 6ET
Tel: (01904) 638467

TRAVELINE
(0870) 6082608

BUSES
General Enquiries: Tel: (01904) 551400
Also includes train information.

TAXIS
Station Taxis: Tel: (01904) 554455
Five adapted vehicles.
K Jibb: Tel: (01904) 654500
Two adapted vehicles.
A & P Transport: Tel: (01904) 471300
Seven adapted minibuses.

TRAINS
Great North Eastern Railway: Special Needs: Tel: (0845) 7225444
Minicom: (0191) 2330173
Arriva : Special Needs:
Tel: (0845) 6008008
Virgin Trains: Special Needs:
Tel: (0845) 7443366
Minicom: (0845) 7443367

York and Selby Line (York-Leeds):
Tel: (0345) 484950

York Station has disabled parking bays, disabled WCs, underpass tunnel to far platform. Also accessible via lifts, Minicom telephones available, automatic doors into ticket office/travel information.

CAR PARKING
Limited disabled badge parking for 3 hours. Much of York is pedestrianised.
Tel: (01904) 613161

SHOPMOBILITY
2nd Floor, Piccadilly Car Park, the Coppergate Centre, Piccadilly, York
Tel/Fax: (01904) 679222

WHEELCHAIR HIRE
Easyway Healthcare, Unit 3, Enterprise Complex, Walmgate, York
Tel: (01904) 611516

HOTELS
YORK MARRIOTT
Tadcaster Road, Dringhouses, York YO24 1QQ
Tel: (01904) 701000   Fax: (01904) 702308
No. of Accessible Rooms: 2. Bath
Accessible Facilities: Lounge, Restaurant, Lift, Beauty Salon. Quality hotel near the racecourse.

NOVOTEL YORK
Fishergate, York YO10 4FD
Tel: (01904) 611660   Fax: (01904) 610925
No. of Accessible Rooms: 4
Accessible Facilities: Lounge, Restaurant, Pool. Modern hotel a mile from city centre.

CLIFTON BRIDGE HOTEL
Water End, Clifton, York YO30 6LL
Tel: (01904) 610510   Fax: (01904) 640208
No. of Accessible Rooms: 3. Bath
Accessible Facilities: Lounge, Restaurant Private hotel opposite Homestead Park and beside the river. 0.5 mile from city centre.

RAMADA JARVIS HOTEL
Shipton Road, Skelton, York YO3 6XW
Tel: (01904) 670222   Fax: (01904) 670311
www.jarvis.co.uk

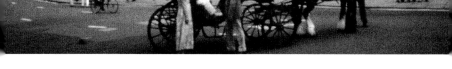

Masterful York Minster seems almost bigger inside.

No. of Accessible Rooms: 2. Bath
Accessible Facilities: Lounge, Restaurant
Very spacious Georgian country house,
modernised, but retaining many original
features, in six acres of grounds. All public
areas easily accessed. Located close to A19
York ring road and A1. 4 miles from York
city centre.

HEWORTH COURT HOTEL
76 - 78 Heworth Green, York YO31 7TQ
Tel: (01904) 425156   Fax: (01904) 415290
e-mail: hotel@heworth.co.uk
www.heworth.co.uk
No. of Accessible Rooms: 2, in courtyard,
ground floor.
Accessible Facilities: Restaurant, Bar
Charming family run hotel within 1 mile of
city centre. Located off A1036 Malton
Road

SAVAGES HOTEL
St. Peter's Grove, Clifton, York YO3 6AQ
Tel: (01904) 610818
No. of Accessible Rooms: 3. Bath
Accessible Facilities: Lounge, Restaurant
Victorian hotel in peaceful tree-lined street
close to city centre and attractions.

HILTON YORK
1 Tower Street, York YO1 9WD
Tel: (01904) 648111
No. of Accessible Rooms: 3. Bath
Accessible Facilities: Lounge, Restaurant.
Well situated within city walls, close to the
Minster, the Shambles and main
attractions.

SELF-CATERING
YORK LAKESIDE LODGES
Moor Lane, York YO24 2QU
Tel: (01904) 702346   Fax: (01904) 701631
No. of Accessible Units: Several
No. of Beds per Unit: Beech - 4/6, Rowan
Lodge 6-8, Roll-in Shower Cat2.
Accessible Facilities: Beech Lodges. Some
are Cat.3 with Lounge/Diner, Kitchenette.
Family owned and run, these attractive
lodges are situated along one side of a 10-
acre lake, facing south with fine views over
the water. Reached via south outer ring
road (A64), close to Tesco and Park & Ride.

ATTRACTIONS
JORVIK VIKING CENTRE
Coppergate, York YO1 9WT
Tel: (01904) 643211   Fax: (01904) 627097

e-mail: jorvik@jvcyork.demon.co.uk
www.jorvik-viking-centre
Jorvik was the Viking name for York and
the centre takes you on a journey from
audio-visual introduction, on time-cars
(one is accessible for wheelchairs) from
WWII back to Norman times and then a
full-scale reconstruction of the C10th.
Coppergate where remarkable discoveries
were made, and the dig of the 1970s.
Voices speak in old Norse language and
the smells and sounds give an authentic
air. NOT TO BE MISSED.
NB. Although the centre does not have
parking facilities, there are disabled spaces
at Piccadilly car park within easy reach of
the centre and with its own Shop Mobility
department. Piccadilly is at a right angle to
Coppergate. Free disabled badge parking.

SD n/a   CP n/a   E 🚻   RF 🚻   L 🚻
C 🚻   S 🚻   WC 🚹   RFE 🚻

MERCHANT ADVENTURERS' HALL
Fossgate, York YO1 9RD
Tel/Fax: (01904) 654818
Medieval, mid C14th guild hall where
merchants carried out business with early

furniture, paintings and other artefacts.
Also an Undercroft (ramped) where the
poor were cared for.

SD 🚻   CP n/a   E 🚹   RF 🚹
WC 🚹   RFE 🚹

NATIONAL RAILWAY MUSEUM
Leeman Road, York YO26 4XJ
Tel: (01904) 621261   Fax: (01904) 631319
e-mail: nrm@nmsi.ac.uk
www.nrm.org.uk
The story of the train. From Stephenson's
rocket and giant steam trains to Eurostar
and miniature railways, rail is brought to
life with interactive displays and
exhibitions. FREE ADMISSION.

SD 🚻   CP 🚻   E 🚻   RF 🚻   L 🚻
C 🚻   S 🚻   WC 🚹

THE ORIGINAL GHOST WALK OF YORK
C/o King's Arms Pub, Ouse Bridge, York
Tel/Fax: (01759) 373090
e-mail: york@talk21.com
This is a guided tour around the city, i.e.
outdoors, leaving the pub at 22.00 every
night. The walk aims to be accurate and
authentic, exploring a world of folklore,
legend and dreams. Guides will amend the
route to avoid steps.

SD 🚻   CP n/a (street parking adjacent to pub)

YORK CITY ART GALLERY
Exhibition Square, York YO1 2EW
Tel: (01904) 551861   Fax: (01904) 551866
e-mail: art.gallery@york.gov.uk
600 years of superb paintings represented
here by Bellotto, Lowry and Nash, plus a
fine pottery collection. Stairlift to upper
collections of Victorian and modern
paintings and modern stoneware pottery.

SD 🚻   CP n/a Nearest CP in Marygate   E 🚻
RF 🚻   L 🚻   S 🚻   WC 🚹

YORK MINSTER
Deangate, York YO1 7HH
Tel: (01904) 557216   Fax: (01904) 557218
e-mail: visitors@yorkminster.org
www.yorkminster.org
The minster was built between 1220 and

Early shopping mall –the Shambles.

1472, although parts of a previous Norman church survive in the building. It is the largest medieval cathedral north of the Alps, and renowned for its original stained glass. The main area of the minster is on one level. There is a ramped facility into the choir area, but crypt is not accessible to wheelchairs that are available on loan. NB. Call in advance for hire and to book parking spaces.

SD [♿] CP [🚶] (NE side of the Minster)
E [♿] (Chapter House Yard)
RF [🚶] S [🚶] WC [🚶]

BURNBY HALL GARDENS
The Balk, Pocklington, York YO42 2QF
Tel: (01759) 302068

Age Concern award winner. 7 wonderful acres of park and garden with fine varieties of trees and shrubs, a picnic area and lakes.
National collection of water lilies is here. 14 miles east of York.

SD [♿] CP [♿] E [♿] RF [♿]
C [♿] S [♿] WC [♿]

CASTLE HOWARD
Castle Howard Estate Office, York YO60 7DA
Tel: (01653) 648444 Fax: (01653) 648501
e-mail: house@castlehoward.demon.co.uk

C18 palace designed by Vanbrugh, with 2 original Vanburgh rooms. He later created Blenheim Palace. Built for the 3rd Earl of Carlisle, Charles Howard, his descendants still call it home. An immense painted and gilded dome tops the facade and the interior contains richly furnished rooms and a superb family chapel that is not accessible. 1,000 acres of gardens.
Near Malton, 15 miles from York off A 64. Stable courtyard entrance adjacent to car park with 4 shops, cafeteria and WC. Land train, ramped with 2 wheelchair places, transports visitors to the house that is 300m from the courtyard. Main area also has cafeteria, a shop and WC.
Main floor of house accessed through the shop, round to main staircase and up by wheelchair lift, staff member always on duty to assist. Once on main floor, surfaces flat, wooden or tiled.

SD [♿] CP [♿] E [♿] RF [♿] C [♿]
S [♿] WC [🚶] G [♿]

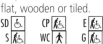

SPORTING VENUE
YORK RACECOURSE
The Knavesmire, York YO23 1EX
Admin & Booking-Box Office: (01904) 620911 Fax: (01904) 611071
CP [♿] (D2 Car park outside Stands Enclosure near Paddock Gates) RE [♿]
WC [🚶] (4 sites at Course Enclosure, Silver Ring, County and Melrose Stands)
SS - Silver Ring [♿]. Raised race viewing platform
Tattersalls - Access to Stand and Parade Ring. Raised viewing platform
County Stand - Raised viewing platform
Parade Ring - raised viewing platform

THEATRE
YORK THEATRE ROYAL
St. Leonard's Place, York YO1 7HD
Admin: (01904) 658162
Fax: (01904) 611534
Booking-Box Office: (01904) 623568
SD [♿]
CP [🚶] Public car park. Taxi Rank-around corner.
RE [♿] ED [♿] INT [♿]
WC [♿] (ground floor). AUD [♿]
B/R [♿] accessed via disabled lift..
Add. Notes: access straight through front doors to Stall doors, 1.5m from doors to spaces.

YORKSHIRE – SOUTH AND WEST

KIRKLEES FEDERATION
Oldgate House, 2 Oldgate Huddersfield HD1 6QF
Tel: (01484) 225078 Fax: (01484) 225360
www.kirkleesmc.gov.uk

TRAVELINE
(0870) 6082608

BARNSLEY
Positioned in the exact centre of the Yorkshire coalfield. A huge market that started in 1249 is still held weekly on the original town centre site.

SPORTING VENUE
BARNSLEY FOOTBALL CLUB
Oakwell Stadium, Barnsley S71 1ET
Admin & Booking-Box Office: (01226)

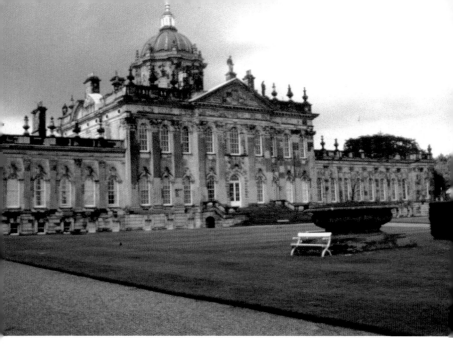

TV classic 'Brideshead Revisited' was filmed at Castle Howard.

211211 Fax: (01226) 211444
e-mail: thereds@barnsleyfc.co.uk
www.barnsleyfc.co.uk
Complies with Part M, Building
Regulations.

CP 🦽   RE 🦽   ED 🦽   INT 🚶
WC 🦽 (4 units, close to disabled seating areas)
SS 🦽 Route via Entrance 1 to Van Damme Stands
B/R 🚶 (Access via lift)

BATLEY
ATTRACTION
BAGSHAW MUSEUM
Wilton Park, Batley WF17 0AS
Tel: (01924) 326155 Fax: (01924) 326164
Victorian Gothic mansion in wooded park.
Collections include Life and death in Egypt
in the Kingdom of Osiris.

SD 🦽   CP 🚶   E 🚶   RF 🦽
WC 🦽   RFE 🚶

OAKWELL HALL GARDEN
Nutter Lane, Birstall, Batley WF17 9LG
Tel: (01924) 326240 Fax: (01924) 326249
Grade 1 Elizabethan Manor House, set in 100
acres of Yorkshire country park, displayed as
a later C17th home. Associations with
English Civil War and Charlotte Bronte. The
hall is not accessible, but the country park

with a wildlife garden is.

SD n/a   CP 🚶   RF 🦽   S 🦽
WC 🚶   RF 🦽

BRADFORD
In its prime, the town was the world's
largest producer of worsted cloth and
much of the town looks confidently
Victorian, but there is considerable
new building. Bradford was the first
town to have a variety of educational
services, such as school meals and a
nursery school, plus a municipal
hospital.

TOURIST INFORMATION CENTRE
City Hall, Bradford, BD1 1HY
Tel: (01274) 753678

HOTEL
NOVOTEL BRADFORD   🚶
Merrydale Road, Bradford BD4 6SA
Tel: (01274) 683683   Fax: (01274) 651342
No. of Accessible Rooms: 2. Bath
Accessible Facilities: Open plan Lounge/Bar,
Restaurant.

One of first Novotels to be built in Britain. Three miles from the city centre.

ATTRACTION
THE COLOUR MUSEUM
Perkin House, 1 Providence Street,
Bradford BD1 2PW
Tel: (01274) 390955
Fax: (01274) 392888
e-mail: museum@sdc.org.uk
Britain's only Museum of Colour with 2 galleries full of exhibits on the effects of light and colour-optical illusions and the story of dyeing and textile printing. There is no setting down point nor car park, all else is varyingly accessible.

SD n/a	CP n/a	E 	RF ♿
L ♿	S ♿	WC ♿	RFE ♿

DONCASTER

Modern town, transformed from an agricultural to an industrial centre by the arrival of the railway in 1848. Ringed by mining villages, it now manufactures agricultural equipment and the famous butterscotch.

TOURIST INFORMATION CENTRE
Central Library, Waterdale,
Doncaster DN1 3JE
Tel: (01302) 734309

HOTELS
DONCASTER MOAT HOUSE
Warmsworth, Doncaster DN4 9UX
Tel: (01302) 799988   Fax: (01302) 310197
No. of Accessible Rooms: 3. Roll-in Shower.
Accessible Facilities: Lounge, Restaurant
Near A1M (J36), close to Earth Centre and several cultural/art/industrial sites.

MOUNT PLEASANT HOTEL
Great North Road, Rossington,
Doncaster DN11 0HW
Tel: (01302) 868696   Fax: (01302) 875130
No. of Accessible Rooms: 14. Bath.
Accessible Facilities: Lounge, Restaurant
Former estate house for Rossington Hall. This family-owned, Georgian house stands in 100 acres of private wooded parkland.

ATTRACTION
THE EARTH CENTRE
Doncaster Road, Denaby Main, Doncaster,
South Yorks DN12 4EA
Tel: (01709) 512000
Fax: (01709) 512010
e-mail: info@earthcentre.org.uk
www.earthcentre.org.uk
Earth Centre's 26 acres of indoor and outdoor attractions, gardens, play areas, events, theatre, a restaurant and shop, all focus on sustainable living in an entertaining and thought-provoking way. The centre is a working example of sustainable living, built using environmentally sound materials and methods, on the regenerated sites of two former coal mines.The exhibitions and gardens are enthralling in their own right, but also are part of messages the centre wants to convey. Through the sound and light exhibition of Planet Earth Experience the message is that we are destroying the planet on which we live. Action for the Future exhibition delivers the message that we need not despair because people worldwide are taking action for a sustainable future. The centre brings hope for the future in a practical way showing we can take action at home, at work, and at school.

DONCASTER MUSEUM AND ART GALLERY
Chequer Road, Doncaster DN1 2AE
Tel: (01302) 734293
Fax: (01302) 735409
Home to collections of the Kings Own Yorkshire Infantry and a wide variety of decorative art and sculpture.

SD ♿	CP ♿	E ♿	L ♿
S ♿	WC ♿		

SPORTING VENUE
DONCASTER RACECOURSE
The Grandstand, Leger Way,
Doncaster DN2 6BB
Admin & Booking-Box Office:
(01303) 320066   Fax: (01302) 323271

CP ♿	RE ♿	ED ♿	L 🚶

WC 🚶 (10 units)
SS ♿ (Disabled stand position by winning post)
B/R ♿

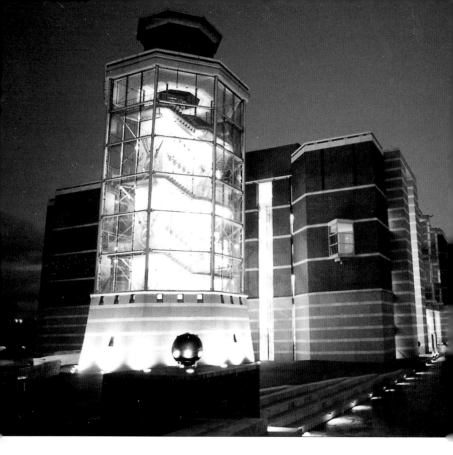

The Royal Armouries, Leeds

HALIFAX

Built on the cloth trade from C13th. The town is set in the Pennine foothills, rising on steep hills from Hebble Brook, and is largely C19th in appearance.

TOURIST INFORMATION CENTRE
Piece Hall, Halifax HX1 1RE
Tel: (01422) 368725

ACCESS FOR ALL IN CALDERDALE
Calderdale Borough Council,
Tourist Information Centre,
1 Bridge Gate, Hebden Bridge HX7 8EX
Tel: (01422) 843831
www.calderdale.gov.uk
Information on access to public buildings in Halifax, Brighouse, Elland, Hebden Bridge, Sowerbybridge and Todmorden.

ATTRACTION
EUREKA! THE MUSEUM FOR CHILDREN
Discovery Road, Halifax HX1 2NE
Tel: (01422) 330069
24hr Information Line: (07626) 983191
e-mail: info@eureka.org.uk
www.eureka.org.uk
First hands-on museum in Britain designed for children up to 12 with over 400 different exhibitions to explore. Touch, listen, smell and look at four main areas - Me and My Body, Living and Working Together, Invent, Create, Communicate and Things. Programme of workshops.

SD   CP   E   RF
L   C   S
WC   (hinged support rail 30cm from seat centre)
RFE

HAWORTH

Home to the Bronte family, the village is all grey-stone houses, slate roofs and smoking chimney pots. The main street, paved with stones, and requiring a strong pusher, struggles up a very steep bank. Near the top the street widens into a little square with the Black Bull Hotel, where Branwell Bronte drank. At the top is the parsonage, the Bronte's home, behind lies moorland and a hint of the windswept isolation recalled from the Bronte sisters' writings. The parsonage is not accessible, and the village a tourist spot, but it is very evocative and not to be missed.

TOURIST INFORMATION CENTRE
2-4 West Lane, Haworth BD22 8EF
Tel: (01535) 642329

BRONTE COUNTRY TOURISM
See Keighley.

SELF-CATERING
STABLE COTTAGE 🖰
West Field Farm, Tim Lane, Haworth
BD22 7SA
Tel: (01535) 644568
Fax: (01535) 646686
e-mail:cottages@brontecountycottages.co.uk
www.brontecountycottages.co.uk
No. of Accessible Units: 1. Roll-in Shower
No. of Beds per Unit 2. One of 5 cottages converted from old farm buildings in an elevated south position near the village. Stunning views. NB: Steep hill to village centre, requires powered wheelchair or car.

HUDDERSFIELD

Extremely hilly town covering a spectacular site in the Colne Valley on the edge of the Pennines. Huddersfield has been the centre of textile production for centuries, and the town is still famous for worsted, and more recently, music.

TOURIST INFORMATION CENTRE
3-5 Albion Street, Huddersfield HD1 2NW
Tel: (01484) 223200

ATTRACTIONS
KIRKLEES LIGHT RAILWAY
Park Mill Way, Clayton West, Nr.
Huddersfield HD8 8SX
Tel: (01484) 865727
www.kirkleeslightrailway.com
3 steam locomotives operating on narrow 37cm gauge railway running through gently rolling farmland for 4 miles. Picnic facilities provided at both ends. CARRIAGES CANNOT TAKE WHEELCHAIRS From platform to carriages there is one step, approx. 200m high.

| SD 🖰 | CP 🚶 | E 🖰 | RF 🖰 |
| C 🚶 | S 🚶 | WC 🚶 | RFE 🚶 |

TOLSON MEMORIAL MUSEUM
Ravensknowle Park, Wakefield Road,
Huddersfield HD5 8DJ
Tel: (01484) 223830
Fax: (01484) 223843
Discover Huddersfield's past from the tools of earliest settlers to modern collections from local people. Ground floor galleries on one level or shallow ramp. First floor has 2 short flights of steps (3 steps) and a Stannah stairlift.

| SD 🖰 | CP 🖰 | E-(REAR) 🚶 | RF 🚶 |
| C 🚶 | S 🚶 | WC 🚶 | |

KEIGHLEY

BRONTE COUNTRY TOURISM
Cedar House, Aire Valley Business Centre,
Lawkholme Lane, Keighley BD21 3DD
Tel: (01535) 670700   Fax: (01535) 671373
e-mail: espencer@brontecountry.co.uk
www.brontecountry.co.uk

ATTRACTIONS
CLIFFE CASTLE MUSEUM AND PARK
Spring Gardens Lane, Keighley BD20 6LH
Tel: (01535) 618231   Fax: (01535) 610536
Completed in 1833 in Elizabethan style, the owner re-constructed the castle and grounds from a wide range of medieval architectural styles in 1875. Permanent displays on the local area including its natural history, minerals and domestic,

297

social, agricultural and industrial bygones.

SD [♿] CP [♿] E [♿] RF [♿]
C [🚶] S [🚶] WC [🚶] RFE [🚶]

VINTAGE RAILWAY CARRIAGE MUSEUM
Ingrow Railway Centre, Keighley BD22 8NJ
Tel: (01535) 680425 Fax: (01535) 610796
e-mail: admin@vintagecarraigestrust.org
www.vintagecarraigestrust.org
Unique display of historic railway
carriages with sound presentations
bringing the story to life. Railway
memorabilia available in large shop.

SD [♿] CP [🚶] E [♿] RF [♿]
S [♿] WC [🚶] RFE [♿]

LEEDS

Spread over a large, hilly area, the
town centres on Victoria Square.The
Town Hall is a successful example of
classic revival architecture. Briggate
Street offers examples of the typical
Leeds arcades, with delightful glass-
roofed passages lined with shops.

**GATEWAY YORKSHIRE REGIONAL
TOURIST INFORMATION CENTRE**
The Arcade, Leeds City Station, Leeds
LS1 1PL
Tel: (0800) 808050
www.leeds.gov.uk

TRAVELINE
(0870) 6082608

BUSES
Black Prince Coaches: Tel: (0113) 2532305
Some low-floor buses.

TAXIS
Streamline: Tel: (0113) 2443322
40 adapted vehicles.
Telecabs: Tel: (0113) 2792222
20 adapted vehicles.
City Cabs: Tel: (0113) 2469999
5 adapted vehicles.

TRAINS
Midland Mainline: Special Needs:
Tel: (0114) 2537654
Minicom: (0845) 7078051

Arriva: Special Needs:
Tel: (0845) 6008008
Great North Eastern Railway: Special Needs:
Tel: (0845) 7225444
Minicom: (0191) 2330173
Virgin Trains: Special Needs:
Tel: (0845) 7443366
Minicom: (0845) 7443367

CAR PARKS
Free unlimited disabled badge parking in
all council car parks, 4 free hours in
marked bays, some on-street parking
Tel: (0113) 2477500

SHOPMOBILITY
White Rose Shopping Centre, Dewsbury
Road, Leeds LS11 8LU
Tel: (0113) 2773636 Fax: (0113) 27778772
Unit 92, Merrion Centre, Merrion Way,
Leeds LS2 8LY
Tel/Minicom: (0113) 2460125

HOTELS
HILTON NATIONAL LEEDS CITY   [🚶]
Neville Street, Leeds LS1 4BX
Tel: (0113) 2442000   Fax: (0113) 2433577
No. of Accessible Rooms: 1
Accessible Facilities: Restaurant, Lounge
(3rd Floor), Lift. Bright, modern hotel
adjacent to railway station.

CROWNE PLAZA HOTEL   [🚶]
Wellington Street, Leeds LS1 4DL
Tel: (0113) 244 2200 Fax: (0113) 2440460
www.crowneplaza.com
No. of Accessible Rooms: 2
Accessible Facilities: Restaurant,
Lounge/Bar (first floor via accessible lift).
Quality hotel located in city centre.

ATTRACTIONS
LOTHERTON HALL
Rangers Office, Stable Courtyard,
Lotherton Hall Estate, Towton Road,
Nr. Aberford, Leeds LS25 3EB.
Tel/Fax: (0113) 2813068
Rebuilt in present form during Victorian
and Edwardian times, Lotherton was
owned by the Gasgoigne family until given
to Leeds City Council in 1968. The hall,
despite its rich collection, retains a family
ambience – the type of home we would al

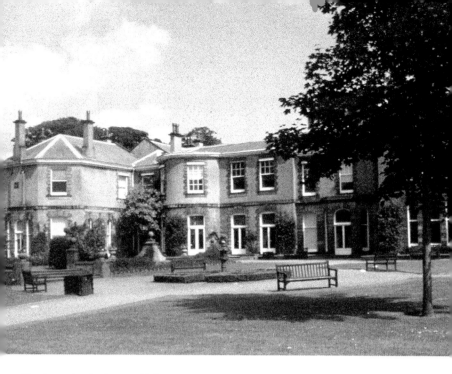

The imposing Lotherton Hall.

love to live in. Beyond delightful bird and formal gardens, the estate offers lovely countryside walks. The hall is accessed by 3 steps. The ground-floor flat and wide corridors, formal gardens, paths and countryside walks and bird garden.

SD ♿ CP ♿ RF ♿ C ♿
S ♿ WC ♿ Hall 🚶 G ♿

MIDDLETON RAILWAY

The Station, Moor Road, Hunslet,
Leeds LS10 2JQ
Tel: (0113) 2710230
e-mail: howill@globalnet.co.uk

World's oldest working railway, established by the first British Railway Act of Parliament in 1758. Built to carry coal from the mines of Middleton to Leeds Bridge. Steam trains run each weekend in the season.

SD ♿ CP 🚶 E ♿ RF ♿
C ♿ S ♿ WC 🚶 RFE 🚶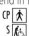

ROYAL ARMOURIES

Armouries Drive, Leeds LS10 1LT
Tel: (0113) 2201899 Fax: (0113) 2201954
e-mail: enquiries@armouries.org.uk
www.armouries.org.uk

Experience 3,000 years of history through this famous collection of arms and armour. Live interpretations, fine displays and exhibits.

SD ♿ CP 🚶 E ♿ RF ♿
L 🚶 C ♿ S ♿ WC ♿

THACKRAY MUSEUM

Beckett Street, Leeds LS9 7LN
Tel: (0113) 244 4343 Fax: (0133) 247 0219
e-mail: info@thackereymuseum.org

The story of health care and medicine told through audio-visual displays, reconstructions, and hands-on exhibits showing how developments and improvements have transformed our lives.

SD ♿ CP ♿ E ♿ RF ♿
L ♿ C 🚶 S ♿ WC ♿

THWAITE MILLS MUSEUM

Thwaite Lane, Stourton, Leeds LS10 1RP
Tel: (0113) 249 6453 Fax: (0133) 2776737

Water-powered mill whose enormous cogs crushed stone for putty and paint during C19th. The Georgian mill-owner's house has been restored, displays tell the mill's history.

SD ♿ CP 🚶 E ♿ RF ♿
S 🚶 WC 🚶

THEATRE
WEST YORKSHIRE PLAYHOUSE
Playhouse Square, Quarry Hill, Leeds LS2 7UP
Tel: (0113) 2137800 Fax: (0113) 2137250
www.wyp.com
Box Office: Tel: (0113) 2137700. Minicom:
(0113) 2137299 Fax: (0113) 2137210
Complies Part M, Building Regulations.

CP [♦]   RE [♦]   ED [♿] (except Manual Door)
INT [♿]   L [♿]   WC [♦]
AUD [♦] Quarry – lift (in foyer) to level 1, access to Row
H via disabled entrance. Courtyard - as above but
accessed through main theatre doors.
B/R [♿] all accessed by lift, low level counters in
restaurant and low-level tables.

SPORTING VENUE
LEEDS UNITED FOOTBALL CLUB
Elland Road. Leeds LS11 0ES
Admin & Booking-Box Office:
(0845) 1211992

CP [♿] RE [♿] ED [♿] (except Manual Door)
INT [♿] L [♿] WC [♿] SS [♿] (West Stand Paddock
40 spaces & helper seating and 80 ambulant spaces: North
Stand 25 spaces & helper seating and 58 ambulant spaces:
South West Corner 26 spaces & helper seating and 40
ambulant spaces: Family Stand 10 spaces & helper seating.
Route through either NW tunnel or up low gradient ramp in
SW corner) B/R [♿] DISABLED LOUNGE open 1.5 hours
prior to kick off, tea/coffee at subsidised rate.

PONTEFRACT
There are some fine C18th and C19th
buildings and the town is famous for
the liquorice in its Pontefract Cakes.

SPORTING VENUE
PONTEFRACT RACECOURSE
Administration: 33 Ropergate,
Pontefract WF8 1LE
Admin & Booking-Box Office: (01977)
703224 Fax: (01977) 600577
Booking: As above
Complies with Part M, Building
Regulations

CP [♿]   RE [♿] Gate adjacent Paddock Ent.
Second Enclosure not accessible, Third Enclosure open to cars
at a charge.   ED [♿]
INT [♿] Access along back of both Main Stands which
connect all Enclosures.
WC [♦] (2 sites, in Club and in Paddock by Main Stairs).

SS [♿] No. special viewing area. Enclosures pronounced
slope provides good all-round visibility but some obstacles
for those with mobility problems.
B/R [♿]

ROTHERHAM
Coal mines, iron, steel, brass and glass
works dominate its situation in the Don
Valley. There has been much rebuilding
in recent years, but some of the
medieval street plan remains.

TOURIST INFORMATION CENTRE
Central Library, Walker Place,
Rotherham S65 1JH
Tel: (01709) 823611

HOTEL
HELLABY HALL HOTEL   [♿]
Old Hellaby Lane, Hellaby, Rotherham
S66 8SN
Tel: (01709) 702701   Fax: (01709) 700979
No. of Accessible Rooms: 2. Bath
Accessible Facilities: Lounge, Restaurant,
Pool, Sauna, Whirlpool
Unique C17th building, Flemish in style
with baronial reception rooms.

ATTRACTIONS
MAGNA
Sheffield Road, Templeborough,
Rotherham S60 1DX
Tel: (01709) 720002   Fax: (01709) 820092
e-mail: info@magnatrust.co.uk
www.magnatrust.org.uk
Magna is an exciting exploration of Earth,
Air, fire and Water, a chance for visitors to
create their own adventure through hands-
on interactive challenges. visit the four
Adventure Pavilions, two shows and the
outdoor adventure park and have fun
unearthing the mysteries of our world.

SD [♿]   CP [♿]   E [♿]   RF [♿]   L [♿]
C [♦]   S [♿]   WC [♿]   RFE [♿]

ROTHERHAM ART GALLERY/YORKS AND
LANCASTER REGIMENTAL MUSEUM
Rotherham Arts Centre, Walker Place,
Rotherham S65 1JH
Tel: (01709) 823635   Fax: (01709) 823631
www.rma.org.uk

Regularly changing exhibitions of contemporary and fine art.

SD ♿   CP ♿   E ♿   RF ♿
L ♿   C ♿   WC 🚹

SHEFFIELD

England's fourth largest city, still famous for its steel, cutlery, engineering and toolmaking industries, but the city centre is being transformed as work begins on the Heart of the City Millennium project.

TOURIST INFORMATION CENTRE
Peace Gardens, Sheffield S1 2HH
Tel: (0114) 2734571

TRAVELINE
Tel: (0870) 6082608
Information on buses, trams and trains

BUSES
First Mainline: Tel: (01709) 566000
TAXIS
Central Cabs: Tel: (0114) 2769869
30 adapted vehicles.
Shefftax: Tel: (0114) 2720000
30 adapted vehicles

TRAMS
Accessible to wheelchairs.

TRAINS
First North Western: Special Needs:
Tel: (0845) 6040231
Midland Mainline: Special Needs:
(0114) 2537654
Minicom: (0845) 7078051
Virgin Trains: Special Needs: (0845) 7443366
Minicom: (0845) 7443367
Sheffield Station has some lifts, but lots of stairs and no subways.

CAR PARKING
Free unlimited disabled badge parking in council-owned car parks, some on-street parking also.

SHOPMOBILITY
Bank Street, Sheffield
Tel: (0114) 2812278   Fax: (0114) 2787173

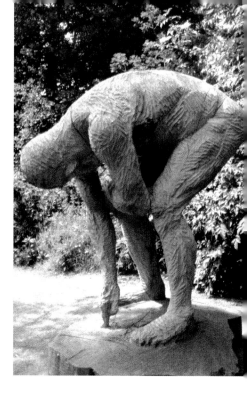

Famous artists and their works have brought monumental acclaim to Wakefield.

HOTEL
SHEFFIELD MOAT HOUSE   🚹
Chesterfield Road South,
Sheffield S8 8BW
Tel: (0114) 2829988
Fax: (0114) 2378140
No. of Accessible Rooms: 4. Bath
Accessible Facilities: Lounge, Restaurant, Bar, Pool. Located near M1 motorway south of the city.

SPORTING VENUE
SHEFFIELD WEDNESDAY FOOTBALL CLUB
Hillsborough, Sheffield S6 1SW
Admin: (0114) 2212121
Fax: (0114) 2212122
Booking: Tel: (0114) 2212400
Fax: (0114) 2212401
Complies with part M, Building Regulations.

CP ♿ (request in advance)   RE ♿
ED ♿ (except Manual Door)
WC ♿ (Located on North Stand)

SS 🏠 (Westfield Enclosure with ramp access in north Stand – 56 spaces and helper seating: West Lower Disabled Enclosure – 32 spaces and helper seating)
B/R 🏠 (Ramped/Lift access to some)

WAKEFIELD

City centre is the Bull Ring, redeveloped with modern shops, but some good Georgian houses remain on the South and West parades.

TOURIST INFORMATION CENTRE

Town Hall, Wood Street,
Wakefield WF1 2HQ
Tel: (01924) 305000

ATTRACTIONS

NATIONAL COAL MINING MUSEUM FOR ENGLAND
New Road, Overton, Wakefield WF4 4RH
Tel: (01924) 848806
Award-winning museum offering visitors the working world of mining. See the conditions in a 75cm. seam and meet genuine pit ponies, now in retirement. New visitor centre with access. Underground tour available for wheelchair users. Contact in advance for details.

SD 🏠   CP 🏠   E 🏠   RF 🏠
C 🏠   S 🏠   WC 🏠

YORKSHIRE SCULPTURE PARK
Bretton Hall, West Bretton,
Wakefield WF4 4LG
Tel: (01924) 830579
Fax: (01924) 832600
www.ysp.co.uk
Over 500 acres of C18th parkland are used to display some of the best sculpture in the country produced by artists worldwide. Alongside changing exhibitions permanent features include C19th bronzes by Rodin, contemporary sculptures and Henry Moore bronzes in the adjacent 100-acre Bretton country park. The blend of landscape and sculpture is extraordinary: the soothing peace of the countryside arrested and stimulated by the sight of a single piece of work alongside sheep, the park's natural inhabitants. But it works. Not to be

missed! Four scooters and one powerchair for use in the park free of charge from the Information Centre.

SD 🏠   CP 🏠   C 🏠
  E 🏠 (Information Centre at Car Park)
  S 🏠 (Information Centre)
  🏠 (Pavilion Gallery Bookshop)
  🏃 (Bothy Shop)   WC - Several 🏃
RFE 🏠 (Access Sculpture Trail)
  🏠 Lakeside, Hillside, Driveside, Bothy Garden, Bretton Country Park.
Formal Garden (can be viewed from terrace)

WETHERBY

TOURIST INFORMATION CENTRE

24 Westergate, Wetherby LS22 6NL
Tel: (0113) 247 7251

SPORTING VENUE

WETHERBY RACECOURSE
York Road, Wetherby LS22 5ET
Admin & Booking-Box Office:
(01937) 582035
Fax: (01937) 588021
Complies with Part M, Building Regulations. Open venue with large viewing concourses served by tarmac paths/walkways providing freedom of movement to all enclosures and facilities.

CP 🏠   RE 🏠
ED 🏠 through main gate onto centre of course
INT 🏠   L 🏠
WC 🏠
SS 🏠   B/R 🏠

SCOTLAND

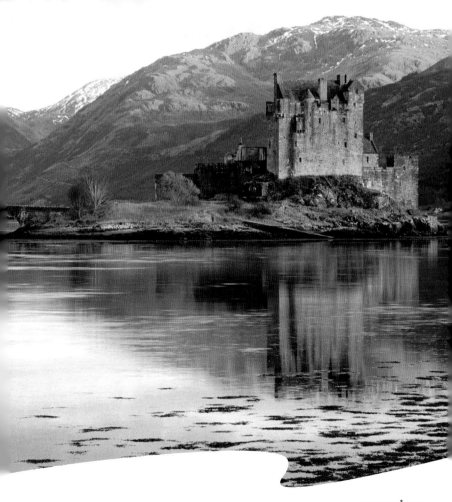

Eilean Donan Castle.

gowrings
mobility

Apart from the Central Information Department, Scotland is now divided into eight areas, some with several tourist boards within each of these regions.

VISIT SCOTLAND
Tel: (08457) 2255122
www.visitscotland.com

REGION 1
SOUTH OF SCOTLAND

DUMFRIES and GALLOWAY TOURIST BOARD
64 Whitesands, Dumfries DG1 2RS
Tel: (01387) 253862   Fax: (01387) 245551
e-mail: info@dgtb.visitscotland.com
www.dumfriesandgalloway.co.uk

AYRSHIRE and ARRAN TOURIST BOARD
Burns House, Burns Statue Square,
Ayr KA7 1UP
Tel/Fax: (01292) 262555
Fax: (01292) 288686
e-mail: ayr@ayrshire-arran.com
www.ayrshire-arran.com

SCOTTISH BORDERS TOURIST BOARD
Tourist Information Centre, Murray's Green,
Jedburgh TD8 6BE
Tel: (0870) 6080404
Fax: (01835) 864099
e-mail: info@scot-borders.co.uk
www.visitscottishborders.com

REGION 2
EDINBURGH AND LOTHIANS

EDINBURGH and LOTHIANS TOURIST BOARD
4 Rothesay Terrace, Edinburgh EH3 7RY
Tel: (0131) 4733600   Fax: (0131) 4733626
e-mail: info@visitscotland.com
www.edinburgh.org

REGION 3
GREATER GLASGOW AND CLYDE VALLEY

GREATER GLASGOW and CLYDE VALLEY TOURIST BOARD
11 George Square, Glasgow G2 1DY

Tel: (0141) 2044400
Fax: (0141) 2213524
e-mail: enquiries@seeglasgow.com
www.seeglasgow.com

REGION 4
ARGYLL, THE ISLES, LOCH LOMOND, STIRLING AND TROSSACHS TOURIST BOARD

Dept. SOS, 7 Alexandra Parade, Dunoon, Argyll PA23 8AB
Tel: (01369) 703755
Fax: (01369) 706085
e-mail: info@scottish.heartlands.org.uk
www.visitscotland.com

REGION 5
PERTHSHIRE, ANGUS & DUNDEE & THE KINGDOM OF FIFE

ANGUS and DUNDEE TOURIST BOARD
21 Castle Street, Dundee DD1 3AA
Tel: (01382) 527527
Fax: (01382) 527551
e-mail: enquires@angusanddundee.co.uk
www.angusanddundee.co.uk

KINGDOM OF FIFE TOURIST BOARD
70 Market Street, St. Andrews KY16 9NU
Tel: (01334) 472021   Fax: (01334) 478422
www.standrews.com/fife

PERTHSHIRE TOURIST BOARD
Lower City Mills, West Mill Street,
Perth PH1 5QP
Tel: (01738) 627958   Fax: (01738) 630416
e-mail: perthtouristb@perthshire.co.uk
www.perthshire.co.uk

REGION 6
GRAMPIAN HIGHLANDS, ABERDEEN AND THE NORTH EAST COAST

ABERDEEN and GRAMPIAN TOURIST BOARD
27 Albyn Place, Aberdeen AB10 1YL
Tel: (01224) 288828   Fax: (01224) 581367
e-mail: info@castlesandwhisky.com
www.agtb.org

REGION 7
THE HIGHLANDS AND SKYE

HIGHLANDS OF SCOTLAND TOURIST BOARD
Peffery House, Strathpeffer, Ross-shire IV14 9HA
Tel: (01997) 423019   Fax: (01997) 421168
e-mail: info@host.co.uk
www.host.co.uk

PORTREE TOURIST INFORMATION CENTRE
Bayfield House, Bayfield Road, Portree IV51 9EL
Tel: (01478) 612137   Fax: (01478) 612141
e-mail: portree@host.co.uk
www.highlandfreedom.com

REGION 8
OUTER ISLANDS

WESTERN ISLES TOURIST BOARD
26 Cromwell Street, Stornoway,
Isle of Lewis HS1 2DD
Tel: (01851) 703088   Fax: (01851) 705244
e-mail: witb@visitthehebrides.co.uk
www.witb.co.uk

ORKNEY TOURIST BOARD
6 Broad Street, Kirkwall, Orkney KW15 1NX
Tel: (01856) 872856   Fax: (01856) 875056
e-mail: info@otb.ossian.net
www.visitorkney.com

SHETLAND ISLANDS TOURISM
Market Cross, Lerwick, Shetland ZE1 0LU
Tel: (01595) 693434   Fax: (01595) 695807
e-mail: shetland.tourism@zetnet.co.uk
www.visitshetland.com

USEFUL ORGANISATIONS
HISTORIC SCOTLAND
Longmore House, Salisbury Place,
Edinburgh EH9 1SH
Tel: (0131) 6688800   Fax: (0131) 6688888
www.historic-scotland.gov.uk

NATIONAL MUSEUMS OF SCOTLAND
Chambers Street, Edinburgh EH1 1JF
Tel:(0131) 2257534   Fax: (0131) 2204819
www.nms.ac.uk

SCOTTISH AIRPORTS LTD
St. Andrew's Drive, GLASGOW Airport,

Paisley, Renfrewshire PA3 2SW
Tel: (0141) 8484441
Fax: (0141) 8421412
www.baa.co.uk

THE NATIONAL TRUST FOR SCOTLAND
28 Charlotte Square, Edinburgh EH2 4ET
Tel: (0131) 2439300   Fax: (0131) 2439301
e-mail: information@nts.org.uk
www.nts.org.uk

DISABILITY ORGANISATIONS
DIAL SCOTLAND
Braid House, Labrador Avenue, Mowden,
West Lothian EH54 6DU
Tel: (01506) 433468   Fax: (01506) 431201
Information service for disabled people.

DISABILITY RESOURCE CENTRE
130 Langton Road, Pollock, Glasgow G53
Tel: (0141) 8832997

DISABILITY SCOTLAND
Princes House, 5 Shandwick Place,
Edinburgh EH2 4RG
Tel: (0131) 2298632   Fax: (0131) 2295168
Information on all aspects of disability.

MULTIPLE SCLEROSIS IN SCOTLAND
National Office, Ratho Park, 88 Glasgow
Road, Ratho Station, Edinburgh EH28 8PP
Tel: (0131) 2253600   Fax: (0131) 2205188

PHAB SCOTLAND
Princes House, 5A Warriston Road,
Edinburgh EH3 5LQ
Tel: (0131) 5589912

SCOTTISH SPORTS ASSOCIATION FOR THE
DISABLED
Fife Institute PRE, Viewfield Road,
Glenrothes KY6 2RA
Tel: (01592) 771700   Fax: (01592) 415710

SCOTRAIL RAILWAYS
Caledonian Chambers, 87 Union Street,
Glasgow G1 3TA

SPINAL INJURIES SCOTLAND (SIS)
The Festival Business Centre, 150 Brand
Street, Glasgow G51 1DH
Tel: (0141) 3140056
Equivalent of SIA in Scotland.

REGION 1
SOUTH OF SCOTLAND

DUMFRIES & GALLOWAY

CASTLE DOUGLAS
Laid out in the C18th by local lad, William Douglas, this is a planned village, which Douglas hoped would become a major commercial and industrial centre - but it didn't happen.

SELF-CATERING
BARNCROSH LEISURE CO.   🦽
Barncrosh, Castle Douglas DG7 1TX
Tel: (01556) 680216   Fax: (01556) 680442
No. of Accessible Units: 4
No. of Beds per Unit: 2 - 9
Accessible Facilities: Lounge, Kitchen. Comfortable cottages on working farm with access to seashore, hills, forests and botanical gardens.

ATTRACTION
THREAVE GARDEN (NT for S)
Castle Douglas DG7 1RX
Tel: (01556) 502575   Fax: (01556) 502683
64 acres with fine springtime displays of daffodils, colourful summer herbaceous borders and trees and heathers in autumn.

SD 🦽   CP 🦽   E 🦽   RF 🦽
C 🦽   S 🦽   WC 🦽   RFE 🦽

DALBEATTIE
Forms the meeting point of A710 and A711 around north coast of Solway Firth. Good day's tour from Dumfries, driving through Dalbeattie Forest and hamlets of Kippord and Colvend.

HOTELS
CLONYARD HOUSE   🦽
Colvend, Dalbeattie, DG5 4QW
Tel: (01556) 630372   Fax: (01556) 630422
No. of Accessible Rooms: 1. Shower

Accessible Facilities: Lounge Bar, Restaurant. The Garden Wing houses the room for disabled guests, modern, ground floor with own small patio overlooking quiet area of the gardens. Small, family run hotel situated in 7 acres of woodland in secluded position on Solway Coast between Rockliffe and Kipord. This is Scotland's waiting-to-be-discovered south west corner with high cliffs, sheltered creeks, lochs and forest clad hills.

DUMFRIES
Known as Queen of the South, Dumfries was a seaport in the Middle Ages. Regularly invaded by the English, this red sandstone town beside River Nith is still important as a focus for the area's agricultural prosperity.

TOURIST INFORMATION CENTRE
64 Whitesands, Dumfries DG1 2RS
Tel: (01387) 245550

SOCIAL WORKS DEPARTMENT
5-8 Gordon Street, Dumfries DG1 1EG
Tel: (01387) 261234

BUSES
Stagecoach/Western Buses:
Tel: (01387) 253496
4 low-floor buses each taking 1 wheelchair.

TAXIS
Red Rose Taxis: Tel: (01387) 263103
Only firm with wheelchair facilities.

TRAINS
GNER – Special Needs Tel: (08457) 225444
Minicom: (0191) 2330173
Wheelchair space in both first and standard class. Dumfries Station offers assistance when booked in advance.

SHOPMOBILITY
Holywood Trust Building, Old Assembly Close, Dumfries.
Tel: (08457) 090904
Fax: (08457) 269026

HOTEL
BEST WESTERN HETLAND HALL HOTEL
Carrutherstown, Dumfries DG1 4JX
Tel: (01387) 840201   Fax: (01387) 840211
No. of Accessible Rooms: 1
Accessible Facilities: Lounge, Restaurant,
Pool, Sauna. Charming hotel in countryside
location, situated by main A75, 8 miles
from Dumfries.

SELF-CATERING
CAIRNYARD HOLIDAY LODGES
Nether Cairnyard House, Beeswing,
Dumfries DG2 8JE
Tel: (01387) 730218
No. of Accessible Units: 4
No. of Beds per Unit: 2 sleeping 2,
2 sleeping 4.
Accessible Facilities: Unit for 2. Open plan
Kitchen/Dining/Lounge, Verandah. Unit for
4 – Kitchen/Diner, Lounge, Verandah.
Located 5 miles from Dumfries, in the
former orchard of a large Victorian house
set in mature grounds and surrounded by
countryside.
www.cairnyard.fsnet.co.uk
e-mail: lodges@cairnyard.fsnet.co.uk

ATTRACTION
DUMFRIES MUSEUM
The Observatory, Dumfries DG2 7SW
Tel: (01387) 253374   Fax: (01387) 265081
e-mail: info@dumfriesmuseum.demon.co.uk
Largest museum in southwest Scotland,
with 150 years' worth of collections and
exhibits on the history and landscape of
the region.

SD | CP | E | RF
L | S | WC

ROBERT BURNS CENTRE
Mill Road, Dumfries DG2 7BE
Tel: (01387) 264808
Situated in the town's C18th watermill on
west bank of River Nith. Tells the story of
Burns' last years in Dumfries in the 1790s.
Exhibition illuminated by original
documents and personal relics, plus scale
model of Dumfries at the time and AV
presentation.

SD | CP | E | RF
C (Stannah Stairlift) | S | WC

NEWTON STEWART
Typical Galloway town on banks of river
Cree, where gamefishing is popular.

BED AND BREAKFAST
ROWANTREE GUEST HOUSE
38 Main Street, Glenluce,
Newton Stewart DG8 0PS
Tel: (01581) 300244
No. of Accessible Rooms: 1
Accessible Facilities: Lounge, Dining Room.
C19th guest house, formerly the shoe
shop, in peaceful village midway between
Stranraer and Newton Stewart.

ATTRACTION
CREETOWN GEM ROCK MUSEUM
Chain Road, Creetown DG8 7HJ
Tel: (01671) 820357   Fax: (01671) 820554
e-mail: gen.rock@btinternet.com
Fine privately owned collection of
gemstones, crystals, minerals, gemstone,
objects d'art and fossils. Almost every
known gemstone and mineral is
represented plus recent additions of a
fossilised dinosaur egg and dung along
with meteorites from outer space. Located
19km from Newton Stewart.

SD | CP | E | RF
C | S | WC | RFE

PORTPATRICK
Harbour town and holiday resort with
charming streets and cottages and a
calm harbour backed by low cliffs.

HOTEL
FERNHILL HOTEL
Heugh Road, Portpatrick DG9 8TD
Tel: (01776) 810220   Fax: (01776) 810596
No. of Accessible Rooms: 3
Accessible Facilities: Lounge, Restaurant
High above the village, fine harbour views.

WANLOCKHEAD
Scotland's highest village at 421m, and
the centre of the metal mining industry.

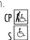

ATTRACTION
THE MUSEUM OF LEAD MINING
Wanlockhead, by Biggar ML12 6UT
Tel: (01659) 74387   Fax: (01659) 74481
Guided tour of Lochnell Lead Mine plus
Visitor Centre, housing a collection of rare
minerals. There are hands-on displays,
mineral collecting areas and a 1.5 mile
walkway to C18th lead mine and miners
cottages. Gold panning tuition available at
Gold Panning Centre. Fascinating museum.

SD ⬚ CP ⬚ E ⬚ RF ⬚
C ⬚ S ⬚ WC ⬚ RFE ⬚

AYRSHIRE & ISLE OF ARRAN

ALLOWAY
Robert Burns was born here in 1759,
his cottage standing on Monument
Road, and much of the village is
associated with his poetry, particularly
the Burns National Heritage Park.

ATTRACTION
BURNS COTTAGE
Alloway KA7 4PY
Tel: (01292) 441215
Home for his first 7 years of the most
famous Scottish poet, born in Alloway in
January 1759. Interpretative presentation,
including audio/visual, offers an interesting
experience of how cottage looked when
the Burns family lived here.

SD ⬚ CP ⬚ E ⬚ RF ⬚
C ⬚ S ⬚ WC ⬚ RFE ⬚

ISLE OF ARRAN
Two ferry services to the island.
Caledonian McBrayne all year round
from Ardrossan (rail link to Glasgow) –
55-minute crossing by modern roll-on
roll-off ferry with facilities for the
disabled. Smaller ferry between
Lochranza and Kintyre during the
summer. Passengers may remain in
their cars. 20 miles long and about 57
miles around, Arran has mountainous
peaks, dense forests and ever-

changing shoreline. Lying across the
path of the gulf stream, Arran enjoys
sub-tropical conditions, palm trees
grow well and basking sharks and
dolphins can be seen from the shore.

BRODICK
The main village on Arran, busy but
unspoilt, with a wide beach stretching
around Brodick Bay.

HOTEL
AUCHRANNIE COUNTRY HOUSE HOTEL ⬚
Brodick, Arran KA27 8BZ
Tel: (01770) 302234   Fax: (01770) 302812
No. of Accessible Rooms: 1
Accessible Facilities: Lounge, Restaurant,
Pool, Sauna, Spa, Fitness Suite, Snooker
Room, Hairdressing Salon,
Aromatherapy Room.

BED AND BREAKFAST
STRATHWHILLAN HOUSE ⬚
Brodick, Aran KA27 8BQ
Tel: (01770) 302331
e-mail: strathwillan@talk21.com
www. strathwillan.co.uk
No. of Accessible Rooms: 8
Accessible Facilities: Lounge Dining Room,
Gardens. Privately owned, the original
house is over 150 years old, carefully
renovated with a new wing. It lies in lovely
grounds of courtyards, lawns and flower
beds with views over Brodick Bay to the
castle and mountains beyond. Situated 0.5
mile from Brodick, with shore and ferry
terminal within 200m.

LAMLASH
3 miles south of Brodick, a secluded
village with some jolly pubs. Coming
down into Lamlash there are fine
views across the golf course and bay
to Holy Island.

LILYBANK HOTEL ⬚
Shire Road, Lamlash, Arran KA27 8LS
Tel: (01770) 600230
No. of Accessible Rooms: 1. Shower

Accessible Facilities: Lounge.
Guest House on the seafront.

MAYBOLE
Robert Burns' parents were said to
have met close to a clock tower in the
high street.

SELF-CATERING
ROYAL ARTILLERY COTTAGE
Culzean Castle, Maybole KA19 8LE
Tel: (01655) 884455   Fax: (01655) 760615
No. of Accessible Units: 1
No. of Beds per Unit: 4
Accessible Facilities: Lounge, Kitchen.
Owned by the National Trust for Scotland.

ATTRACTION
CULZEAN CASTLE & COUNTRY PARK (NT for S)
Maybole KA19 8LE
Tel: (01655) 884400   Fax: (01655) 884522
Built on clifftop 50m above the sea, this is
one of Scotland's finest castles. Built in
C18th, designed by Robert Adam for 10th
Earl of Cassillis. Noted for oval staircase,
circular drawing room and plasterwork.
Country park of 560 acres with walled and
terraced gardens. All castle rooms on
display accessible (lift to first floor). Firm
gravel and grass paths with ramps in
Walled Garden. Access to Fountain Court
Garden via graded path down side of
Viaduct. Dropping off point below Viaduct
for easier access. Woodland area not very
accessible, but hide at Swan Pond
accessible by ramp. Wheelchairs and
batricars available at Castle, Visitor Centre
and kiosk. Batricars should be booked in
advance.

SD   CP   E   RF
L   C   S   WC

AYR
Important seaport and commercial
centre. A popular resort in Victorian
times, the beach still is so. Ayr
racecourse is the most prestigious in
Scotland.

HOTEL
MONKTON LODGE TRAVEL INN
Kilmarnock Road, Monkton,
Nr. Ayr KA29 2RJ
Tel: (01292) 678262
Fax: (01292) 678248
No. of Accessible Rooms: 2
Accessible Facilities: Restaurant
Situated on A77/A78 roundabout by
Prestwick Airport, north of Ayr.

DISABILITY RESOURCE CENTRE
Ground Floor, Burns House, Burns Statue
Square, Ayr KA7 1UP
Tel: (01292) 616261

BUSES
Stagecoach/Western Buses: Tel: (01292)
613700/613500
12 low-floor buses, limited wheelchair
space.

TAXIS
All Black Cabs fully equipped
Tel: (01292) 284545

TRAINS
Scotrail: Special Needs Tel: (0845) 6057021
Ayr Station offers wheelchair unassisted
access and ramps.

SHOPMOBILITY
33 Carrick Street, Ayr KA7 1NS
Tel: (01292) 618086

GIRVAN
Traditional family resort with a lovely
harbour, once a major landing site
for herring catch.

ATTRACTION
BARGANY GARDEN
Bargany Estate, by Girvan KA26 9PQL
Tel: (01465) 871249   Fax: (01465) 871282
Woodland gardens with a main area
with rhododendrons and azaleas and a
pond. Flat walled garden with slightly
inclined approach.
N.B. Gardens are now only open
weekends and Mondays in May.

SD   CP   E   RF

GALSTON
East of Kilmarnock, off the A71.

ATTRACTION
LOUDOUN CASTLE THEME PARK
Galston KA4 8PE
Tel: (01563) 822296 Fax: (01563) 822408
e-mail: loudouncastle@btinternet.com
Scotland's biggest theme park
surrounding Loudoun Castle, the whole
park is steeped in history. The Museum
and Visitor Centre tells the story of the
Earl of Loudon who inhabited the castle
c1714. 500 acres of entertainment
including rides, gentle countryside walks
and children's farm.

SD	🚹	CP	🚹	E	🚹	RF	🚹
C	🚹	S	🚹	WC	🚹	RFE	🚹

IRVINE
Originally a maritime settlement, some
remains visible around the harbour.
Centre of town is cobbled.

HOTEL
THE THISTLE IRVINE 🚹
46 Annick Road, Irvine KA11 4LD
Tel: (01294) 274272 Fax: (01294) 277287
No. of Accessible Rooms: 1
Accessible Facilities: Lounge, Restaurant,
Pool, Jacuzzi. Quality hotel designed in
Moroccan style.

TURNBERRY
Along the south-west Ayrshire coast,
40 minutes from Glasgow. Renowned
as home of one of the great hotels.

HOTEL ACCOMMODATION
THE WESTIN TURNBERRY RESORT
SCOTLAND 🚹
Ayrshire KA26 9LT
Tel: (01655) 331000 Fax: (01655) 331706
No. of Accessible Rooms: 1
Accessible Facilities: Lounge, Restaurant.
Luxury hotel, created at the turn of the
century by the Marquess of Ailsa who

built a private golf course on his estate in
1902. Turnberry is about golf, but also
about the Edwardian love of ease and
luxury which is reflected in the antiques,
paintings and oriental art.

WEST KILBRIDE
HUNTERSTON VISITOR CENTRE
West Kilbride KA23 9QJ
Tel: (0800) 838557 Fax: (01294) 826008
Advanced gas-cooled reactor type of
nuclear power station. Purpose-built
centre with exhibits, inter-active models
and videos.

SD	🚹	CP	🚹	E	🚹	RF	🚹
S	🚹	WC	🚹	RFE	🚹		

SCOTTISH BORDERS

COLDSTREAM
Known as the birthplace of the
Coldstream Guards, the regiment's
history is featured in the local
museum. August sees the ride to
Flodden Field to honour the dead in
battle in 1513.

TOURIST INFORMATION CENTRE
Tel: (0870) 6080404

ATTRACTIONS
COLDSTREAM MUSEUM
12 Market Square, Coldstream TD12 4BD
Tel: (01890) 882630 Fax: 01890 882631
Displays explore the history of
Coldstream and its people with a special
section on the Coldstream Guards.

SD n/a	CP 🚹	E 🚹	RF 🚹	C n/a
S 🚹	WC 🚹	RFE 🚹	Outside Courtyard	

HIRSEL COUNTRY PARK
Hirsel Estate Office, Coldstream TD12 4LP
Tel/Fax: (01890) 882834
Museum of Estates, past and present,
arts and crafts centre, picnic area and
playground.

SD	🚹	CP	🚹	E	🚹	RF	🚹
C	🚹	S	🚹	WC	🚹		

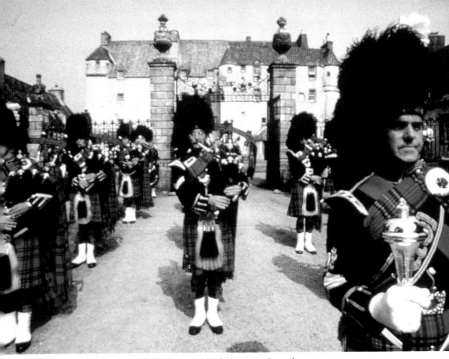

Coldstream, birthplace of the famous Coldstream Guards.

EYEMOUTH

Historic town lying 5m. north of the border where the mouth of the River Eye provides a natural harbour and sandy beaches. People have fished here since C13th and the harbour is still busy.

TOURIST INFORMATION CENTRE
Auld Kirk, Market Place, Eyemouth TD14 5JE
Tel: (01890) 750678

BED AND BREAKFAST
WESTWOOD GUEST HOUSE
Houndwood, Eyemouth TD14 5TP
Tel: (01361) 850232   Fax: (01361) 850333
e-mail: info@westwoodweb.co.uk
www.westwoodweb.co.uk
No. of Accessible Rooms: 1
Accessible Facilities: Lounge, Dining Room, Tea Room, Garden. Mary Queen of Scots hunted with her hounds in the woods here, hence the name. Originally an C18th coaching inn, the property retains much character and is set in over an acre of landscaped gardens with ducks and rare chickens roaming around.

HAWICK

Famous for wool production, located on the banks of the River Teviot.

TOURIST INFORMATION CENTRE
Drumlanrig's Tower, Tower Knowe, Hawick TD9 9EN
Tel: (08706) 080404

SELF-CATERING
CHERRY COTTAGE
Blacklee Square, Bonchester Bridge, Hawick TD9 9TD
Tel/Fax: (01450) 860678
e-mail: kate@blacklee.demon.co.uk
www.aboutscotland.co.uk/quince/cherry.html
No. of Accessible Units: 1
No. of Beds per Unit: 6
Accessible Facilities: Sun Lounge, Dining Room, Kitchen, ramped access to Garden. Originally tradesmen's workshops for local estate, Blacklee Square comprises 4 stone built cottages in traditional courtyard setting with unspoilt countryside of hills, forests, woods and rivers.

INNERLEITHEN

Tweedsdale village, famous in C19th for its spa. A pump room was built by the owners in Traquair House.

ATTRACTIONS
TRAQUAIR HOUSE
Innerleithen EH44 6PW.
Tel: (01896) 830 323   Fax: (01896) 830 639
www.traquair.co.uk
e-mail: enquiries@traquair.co.uk
The oldest inhabited house in Scotland. N.B. wheelchair access to ground floor only. Once a pleasure ground for Scottish kings, a refuge for catholic priests in times of terror, the Stuarts of Traquair supported Mary Queen of Scots and the Jacobite cause. Imprisoned, fined and isolated for their beliefs, their home, untouched by time, reflects the tranquillity of their family life. Secret stairs, spooky cellars, books, embroideries, modern Scottish art in the gallery. Search for the centre of the maze.

SD 🦽 CP 🦽 E 🦽 RF 🦽 C 🚶 S 🦽 WC 🚶

ROBERT SMAIL'S PRINTING WORKS
7-9 High Street, Innerleithen EH44 6HA
Tel: (01896) 830206
This museum contains a Victorian office, paper store, composing and press rooms. Machinery is in full working order and visitors can see the printer at work and try their hands at typesetting. All bottom levels can be reached by various routes, top area is not accessible but staff will bring items downstairs for visitors.

SD 🦽 CP n/a E 🦽 S 🚶

MELROSE
Quiet small hamlet set around a square. Ruins of Melrose Abbey has very limited disabled access.

TOURIST INFORMATION CENTRE
Abbey House, Abbey Street, Melrose TD5 7HE
Tel: (08706) 080404

SELF-CATERING
EILDON HOLIDAY COTTAGES 🦽
Dingleton Mains, Melrose TD6 9HS
Tel/Fax: (01896) 823258
www.aboutscotland.co.uk/eildon/cottages.html
No. of Accessible Units: 5
No. of Beds per Unit: 2 - 6 (Showers in Hamiltons, Langrig and The Croft.)
Accessible Facilities: various room combinations. Converted C18th farm steading with fine views of the Tweed Valley to the Lammermuir and Moorfoot Hills. 4 miles from Abbotsford (see below). Able-bodied and disabled visitors can holiday here without differentiation. Alternatively disabled people can holiday with their carers. Electric hoists are fitted with continuous ceiling track to transport from bed to bath (Single Tree) and bed to shower (Langrig). Portable hoist available for use in other cottages.

ATTRACTION
DRYBURGH ABBEY
Dryburgh, St. Boswells, Melrose TD6 0RG
Tel/Fax: (01835) 822381
Remarkably complete ruins, much of which are of C12th and C13th origin. Sir Walter Scott and Field Marshall Earl Haig are both buried here. Flat approach to the Abbey, mostly accessible, apart from cloisters.

CP 🦽 E 🦽 WC 🚶

PRIORWOOD DRIED FLOWER GARDEN (NT FOR SC)
Abbey Street, Melrose TA6 9PX
Tel/Fax: (01896) 822493
Walled garden and orchard specialising in flowers for drying and historic apple varieties. Picnic area.

SD 🚶 CP 🚶 E 🦽 RF 🚶 S 🚶

PEEBLES
Large town with country shops lining the high street. Famous for the annual display of local horse power in Common Riding of the Marches.

TOURIST INFORMATION CENTRE
High Street, Peebles EH45 8AG
Tel: (08706) 080404

HOTEL
HORSESHOE INN
Eddleston, Peebles EH45 8QP
Tel: (01721) 730225   Fax: (01721) 730268
e-mail: horseshoe.inn@virgin.net
www.ladon.co.uk/horseshoe
No. of Accessible Rooms: 1
Accessible Facilities: Lounge, Restaurant (2
steps). The inn was originally a forge on the
stagecoach route Edinburgh/London, now
an oak-beamed traditional inn, with
bedrooms in separate building, once the old
village school. 30 minutes from Edinburgh.

SELKIRK
Standing above Ettrick and Yarrow
valleys and known for waterpowered
textile mills in C19th. Cashmere,
tweed and tartan are still produced
here, plus Selkirk Glass. Statue of Sir
Walter Scott at one end of the town
with Battle of Flodden memorial at the
other end. And the main A7 goes
through the town centre,

TOURIST INFORMATION CENTRE
Halliwell's House, Selkirk TD7 4BL
Tel: (01750) 20054

ACCESSIBLE ATTRACTIONS
BOWHILL HOUSE and COUNTRY PARK
Bowhill, Selkirk TD7 5ET
Tel/Fax: (01750) 22204
Home of the Duke of Buccleuch and
Queensberry, with superb collection of
paintings by Van Dyck, Gainsborough and
Canaletto and others. Also porcelain and
furniture. Lovely wooded grounds. All
accessible by wheelchair.
SD [♿]   CP [♿]   E [↟]   R [↟]
C [↟]   S [↟]   WC [↟]

SELKIRK GLASS VISITORS CENTRE
Selkirk TD7 5EF
Tel: (01750) 20954   Fax: (01750) 22883
Watch skilled craftsmen at work creating
art glass paperweights, candlesticks and
visit the showroom to take advantage of
reduced factory prices.
SD [♿]   CP [♿]   E [♿]   C [↟]
S [♿]   WC [♿]

REGION 2
EDINBURGH AND LOTHIANS

LOTHIAN COALITION OF DISABLED PEOPLE
Norton Park, 57 Albion Road,
Edinburgh EH7 5QY
Tel/Minicom: (0131) 4752360
Fax: (0131) 4752392
Full information service and publishers of
excellent Guide to Access in Lothian.

ABERLADY
Aberlady Bay was the first area in
Britain to be called a Local Nature
Reserve in 1952 and there is much
wildlife here in this charming pantile-
roofed village.

HOTEL
KILSPINDIE HOUSE HOTEL [↟]
High Street, Aberlady, East Lothian EH32 0RE
Tel: (01875) 870682   Fax: (01875) 870504
No. of Accessible Rooms: 3. Bath
Accessible Facilities: Lounge, Restaurant.
Coastal hotel Northeast of Edinburgh.

313

ATTRACTION
MYRETON MOTOR MUSEUM
Aberlady, East Lothian EH32 0PZ
Tel: (01875) 870288
Dating from 1996, a large collection of
cars, motorcycles, commercials plus
collection of period advertising, posters
and enamel signs.
SD [♿]   CP [↟]   E [↟]   RF [↟]   WC [↟]

EAST FORTUNE
ATTRACTION
MUSEUM OF FLIGHT
East Fortune Airfield, East Fortune,
East Lothian EH39 5LF
Tel: (01620) 880308   Fax: (01620) 880355
www.nms.ac.uk/flight
Housed in former airship base with exhibit
of Airship R34 which flew to New York in
1919. Aircraft on display include Hawker

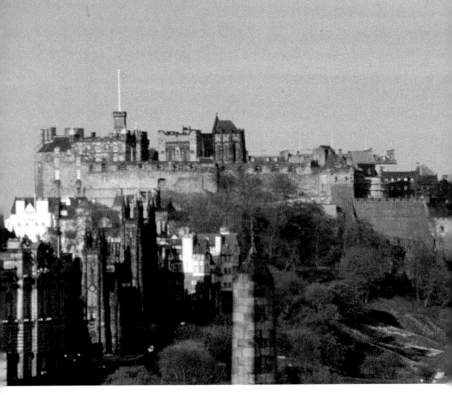

Edinburgh Castle dominates the city skyline.

Sea Hawk and Spitfire MK 16.

| SD ♿ | CP ♿ | E ♿ | RF ♿ |
| C ♿ | S ♿ | WC 🚶 | RFE ♿ |

EDINBURGH

Capital of Scotland whose Castle Rock, overlooking the Firth of Forth, has been a stronghold since 1,000BC. Holyrood Palace, a mile to the east, was built by James IV in 1498. The town growing along this route became known as The Royal Mile which offers a wealth of historic sights, including the house of John Knox and the seat of Scotland's new Parliament. Overcrowding in this part of the city led to a Georgian New Town to the north in the 1700s. The city is divided in half by Princes Street, the principal shopping street with the Royal Mile to its south and New Town to its north. It is a compact city and easy to get around, although the centre is best avoided by car.

TOURIST INFORMATION CENTRE
3 Princes Street, Edinburgh EH2
Tel: (0131) 4733800

BRITISH RED CROSS
Beaverhall House, 27 Beaverhall Road, Edinburgh EH7 4JE
Tel: (0131) 557 9898

TRAVEL LINE
2 Cockburn Street, Edinburgh EH1 1BL
Tel: (0131) 2253858

TAXIS
City Taxis: (0131) 2281211
Computercabs:
Tel: (0131) 2259000/2256736

HANDICABS
58 Canaan Lane, Edinburgh EH10 4SG
Tel: (0131) 4479949

Dial a Bus: Tel: (0131) 4471718
Monday to Friday.

TRAINS
Scotrail: Tel: for disabled assistance:
(0845) 6057021
Tel: for booking in advance for assistance:
(0131) 5502301
Tel: for any other facilities: (0131) 5502263

LOTHIAN SHOPMOBILITY
King's Stables Yard, King's Stables Road,
Edinburgh EH1 2YJ
Tel: (0131) 2259559

Unit 42D, The Gyle Shopping Centre, South
Gyle, Broadway, Edinburgh West EH12 9JY
Tel: (0131) 3171460

HOTELS IN CITY CENTRE & WEST END
SIMPSONS
79 Lauriston Place, Edinburgh EH3 9HZ
Tel: (0131) 622 7979   Fax: (0131) 622 7900
e-mail: reception@simpsons-hotel.demon.co.uk
www: hotel.demon.co.uk
No. of Accessible Rooms: 3
Accessible Facilities: Lounge, Lift.
Continental breakfast is served in guests'
rooms. Opened in 1998, close to Princes
Street and the castle.

SHERATON GRAND & SPA
1 Festival Square, Edinburgh EH3 9SR
Tel: (0131) 2299131   Fax: (0131) 2284510
No. of Accessible Rooms: 2
Accessible Facilities: Lounge, Restaurants (2).
Luxury modern property in the centre of
West End of city with imposing public areas.

THISTLE EDINBURGH
St. James Centre, Edinburgh EH1 3SW
Tel: (0131) 5560111   Fax: (0131) 5575333
No. of Accessible Rooms: 1 with roll-in
shower.
Accessible Facilities: Lounge, Restaurant
Modern hotel in good location just off
Princes Street.

THE CALEDONIAN
Princes Street, Edinburgh EH1 2AB
Tel: (0131) 4599988   Fax: (0131) 2256632
No. of Accessible Rooms: 2
Accessible Facilities: Lounge, Restaurants
(2), Pool, Sauna, Spa. Renowned hotel of
Victorian splendour in heart of the city,
with good views of the castle.

HOLIDAY INN EDINBURGH NORTH
107 Queensferry Road, Edinburgh EH4 3HL
Tel: (0131) 3322442   Fax: (0131) 332 3408
No. of Accessible Rooms: 1
Accessible Facilities: Lounge, Restaurant
Modern hotel on western side of city with
panoramic views.

HOTEL IBIS
Hunter Square, Edinburgh EH11 1QR
Tel: (0131) 2407000   Fax: (0131) 2407007
No. of Accessible Rooms: 2
Accessible Facilities: Open plan Lounge/Bar.
Located in City Centre, close to Royal Mile
with modern accommodation converted
from old warehouses.

HILTON EDINBURGH GROSVENOR
5-21 Grosvenor Street, Edinburgh EH12 5EF
Tel: (0131) 2266001   Fax: (0131) 2202387
No. of Accessible Rooms: 3. Bath
Accessible Facilities: Lounge, restaurant.
city-centre elegant Victorian building, well
refurbished.

BARNTON HOTEL
Queensferry Road, Barnton,
Edinburgh EH4 6AS
Tel: (0131)339 1144   Fax: (0131) 339 5521
No. of Accessible Rooms: 1
Accessible Facilities: Lounge, Restaurant.
Located on A90, 4m. from city centre,
Forth road bridge and airport. Comfortable
public areas.

EDINBURGH CAPITAL MOAT HOUSE
187 Clermiston Road, Edinburgh EH12 6UG
Tel: (0131) 5359988   Fax: (0131) 3349712
No. of Accessible Rooms: 4
Accessible Facilities: Restaurant, Bar.
Modern hotel located close to
Corstorphine Park, 3 miles from airport
and city centre.

KING'S MANOR HOTEL
100 Milton Road East, Edinburgh EH15 2NP
Tel: (0131) 6690444   Fax: (0131) 6696650
No. of Accessible Rooms: 2
Accessible Facilities: Lounge, Dining room,
Bar. Former Laird's home, now family
owned and managed hotel in east end of
the city, close to by-pass.

BED AND BREAKFAST
ARDGARTH GUEST HOUSE ♿
1 St. Mary's Place, Portobello,
Edinburgh EH15 2QF
Tel: (0131) 6693021   Fax: (0131) 4681221
e-mail: enquiries@ardgarth.demon.co.uk
No. of Accessible Rooms: 2
Accessible Facilities: Dining Room.
Lounge has 2 steps. Evening meals can be
provided. Special diets catered for. Owners
hold RADAR WC keys for guests. Adapted
from large Victorian home with well
proportioned rooms in a wide, quiet street
close to the beach and 3.5 miles east of
Princes Street, Edinburgh. Portobello is on
the south shore of the Firth of Forth with a
beach and promenade.

TREFOIL HOUSE ♿
Gogarbank EH12 9DA
Tel: (0131) 339 3148   Fax: (0131) 317 7271
e-mail: info@trefoil.org.uk
No. of Accessible Rooms: 12
Accessible Facilities:
Lounge, Dining Room, Pool, Library,
Games Room, Shop, Bar, Minibus with tail
lift, Woodland Walk, Nature Trail,
Roundabout and Swings. Manor house set
in lovely countryside, a few miles from city
centre and totally adapted holiday centre
for both groups and individuals.

ATTRACTIONS
CITY ART CENTRE
2 Market Street, Edinburgh EH1 1DE
Tel: (0131) 5293993   Fax: (0131) 5293957
e-mail: enquiries@city-art-centre.demon.co.uk
Home to Edinburgh's permanent fine art
collection and temporary world-wide
exhibitions on 6 floors of display galleries
(lift).
SD ♿   E ♿   L ♿   C ♿
S ♿   WC ♿

EDINBURGH CASTLE
Castle Rock, Edinburgh
Tel: (0131) 2259846   Fax: (0131) 2204733
The castle stands of the precipitous crag of
Castle Rock. In 1018 King Malcolm
defeated the English at the Battle of
Carham and a royal castle at Edinburgh
emerges at the end of that century, of

which only the C11th chapel of Queen
Margaret remains. The last siege here was
in 1745. Shortly after the esplanade was
built, it became the site of the Military
Tattoo. Apartments of Mary Queen of
Scots can be seen. The Scottish crown is
displayed in the crown room. Route to
features includes vehicle available from
esplanade to top of the castle - Cat 1: to
Crown Jewels - Cat. 3. The guided tour
includes 26 areas of most interest.
The Lower Ward:
1-Gatehouse,
2-Old Guardhouse
3-Inner Barrier all accessible:
4-Portcullis- Cat. 3
   The Middle Ward:
5-Lang Stairs,
6-Argyle Battery - n/a:
7-Cartshed (restaurant) accessible:
8-Governor's House,
9-New Barracks-n/a:
The Upper Ward:
10-Foog's Gate - vehicle passes through
11-St. Margaret's Chapel
12-Dog Cemetery -not inside, but good
   view of both from platform
13- Argyle Tower - n/a
14-Forwall Battery
15 -Fore Well
16-Half-Moon Battery - all accessible
Buildings in Crown Square:
17-Palace - Crown Room via lift accessible:
18-Great Hall - via ramp:
19-Queen Anne Building - via
   rear entrance:
20-Scottish National War Memorial -
   accessible. Off the beaten track
21-Castle Vaults - majority accessible:
22-Military Prison
23-Dury's Battery-n/a
24-Ordnance Storehouse
25-Hospital
26 -Back Well - all accessible.
S ♿   CP ♿   E ♿   RF ♿
L ♿ Stair Climber.   C ♿   S ♿
WC ♿ ♿ -   RFE ♿ 🚶

PALACE OF HOLYROOD HOUSE
Edinburgh EH8 8DX
Tel: (0131) 5567371   Fax: (0131) 5575256
e-mail: hh@royalcollections.org.uk

The Queen's Scottish residence at the end of the Royal Mile. Founded in 1128, Holyrood evolved from a fortress into a palace. Home to the court of Mary Queen of Scots 1561/67. C17th state rooms and picture galleries are open when the Queen is not in residence.

SD ♿ CP ♿ E ♿ L 🚶
S ♿ WC 🚶 RFE 🚶

NATIONAL GALLERY OF SCOTLAND
The Mound, Edinburgh EH2 2EL
Tel: (0131) 6246200 Fax: (0131) 3433250
Scotland's greatest collection of European paintings and sculpture from renaissance to post-impressionist, including Raphael, Constable, Velasquez, Gaugin and Van Gogh. The collection of Scottish paintings is particularly extensive.

SD ♿ E ♿ L 🚶
S ♿ WC 🚶

MUSEUM OF SCOTLAND
Chambers Street, Edinburgh EH1 1JF
Tel: (0131) 2474422 Fax: (0131) 2204819
e-mail: info@nms.ac.uk
www.nms.ac.uk
Stand adjacent to Royal Museum and together Present the World to Scotland

and Scotland to the World. Chronological history of Scotland from 900AD to C20th. through rich national collections and colour-coded themes. NB: No car park but 2 designated spaces in layby near entrance. Otherwise main street metered parking.

SD ♿ CP n/a E ♿ RF ♿ C ♿
S ♿ WC ♿ L ♿

ROYAL MUSEUM
Chambers Street, Edinburgh EH1 1JF
Tel: (0131) 2474219 Fax: (0131) 2204819
e-mail/web: as above
Victorian building housing fine international collections of decorative arts, science and industry, archaeology and the natural world.
NB. Single yellow line parking adjacent or meters in Chamber Street or at rear in Lothian Street. Level entry through the Museum of Scotland is available.

SD ♿ P n/a E ♿ RF ♿
C ♿ S ♿ WC ♿ L ♿

SCOTCH WHISKY HERITAGE CENTRE
354 Castlehill, the Royal Mile, Edinburgh EH1 2NE
Tel: (0131) 2200441 Fax: (0131) 2206288
e-mail: enquiry@whisky-heritage.co.uk
www.whisky-heritage.co.uk

317

Palace of Holyrood House.

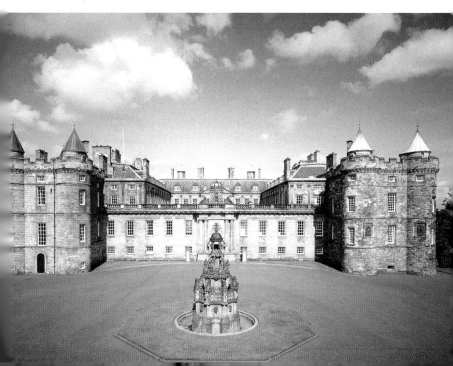

Travel through time exploring the history of this famous export. Meet the Ghostly Blender and enjoy the sights, sounds, smells and the secrets of whisky making.

SD [♿] CP n/a E [🚶] RF [♿] L [♿]
C [🚶] S [♿] WC [🚶] RFE [🚶]

SCOTTISH NATIONAL PORTRAIT GALLERY
1 Queen Street, Edinburgh EH2 1JD
Tel: (0131) 6246200 Fax: (0131) 3433250
Portraits of prominent people who shaped Scotland's history, including Mary Queen of Scots and Sir Walter Scott. All the portraits are of Scots, but not all are by Scots, with works by Van Dyck, Gainsborough, Copley and Rodin.

SD [🚶] E [♿] RF [♿] C [♿]
S [♿] WC [🚶]

SCOTTISH NATIONAL GALLERY OF MODERN ART
73 Bedford Road, Edinburgh EH4 3DR
Tel: (0131) 6246200 Fax: (0131) 3433250
Home to Scotland's finest collection of C20th and C21st paintings including works by Picasso, Matisse, Sickert and Hockney. Also Scottish modern art and important Dada and Surrealist collection with masterpieces by Dali, Magritte and Ernst. Extensive grounds are home to sculptures by Moore, Hepworth, Paolozzi and others.

SD [♿] CP [♿] E [♿] RF [♿]
C [♿] S [♿] WC [🚶]

CRAIGMILLAR CASTLE (HS)
Craigmillar Castle Road, Edinburgh EH16 4SY
Tel/Fax: (0131) 6614445
Fifteenth century stronghold where the plot to murder Darnley, the second husband of Mary Queen of Scots, was hatched. C16th and C17th apartments.

SD [♿] CP [♿] E [♿] RF [♿]
C [🚶] S [🚶] WC [🚶]

EDINBURGH BUTTERFLY & INSECT WORLD
Dobbies Garden World, Lasswade, Midlothian EH18 1AZ
Tel: (0131) 6634932 Fax: (0131) 6542774
e-mail: info@edinburgh-butterfly-world.co.uk
www.edinburgh-butterfly-world.co.uk
Exotic rainforest, splashing waterfalls and pools provide a setting for watching hundreds of the world's spectacular and colourful butterflies flying all around you. Ten minutes from Edinburgh city centre.

SD [♿] CP [♿] E [♿] C [♿]
S [♿] WC [🚶] RFE [♿]

EAST LINTON
East Lothian was one of the foremost grain-growing areas in Scotland when technological changes in the C18th led to a rapid increase in grain production. East Linton's Preston Mill has always been of major importance in this river-side setting with the sea and Lammermuir hills only a short distance away.

ATTRACTION
PRESTON MILL (NT for S)
Preston Road, East Linton, East Lothian EH40 3DS
Tel: (01620) 860426
Oldest water-driven mill in Scotland, last used commercially in 1957. Old mill pond with ducks. No access to upper floor of mill or kiln. Excellent brochure for information and history.

CP [🚶] E [♿] RF [♿] S [♿]
WC [♿] RFE [♿]

LINLITHGOW
Lively town centre surrounded by dismal 1960s concrete blocks. St. Michael's Parish church dedicated in C12th, was rebuilt in C16th. A modern spire was added in 1946.

ATTRACTION
HOUSE OF THE BINNS (NT for S)
Linlithgow EH49 7NA
Tel: (01506) 834255
Historic home of the Dalyell family, General Tam Dalyell raised the Royal Scots Greys here in 1681. Originally a fortified stronghold when built in 1612 it gradually became a large mansion. Notable particularly for fine C17th moulded plaster ceilings.

SD [♿] CP [🚶] E [♿]
RF [♿] C n/a S n/a WC [🚶]
No shop or catering facility on site.

LIVINGSTON
Medium-sized community west of Edinburgh off the M8

HOTEL
RAMADA JARVIS LIVINGSTON
Almondview, Livingston, West Lothian EH54 6QB
Tel: (01506) 431222   Fax: (01506) 434666
No. of Accessible Rooms: 4
Accessible Facilities: Lounge, Restaurant, Pool, Sauna, Spa. Situated between Edinburgh and Glasgow on the M8.

ATTRACTION
ALMOND VALLEY HERITAGE CENTRE
Millfield, Livingston Village, Livingston, West Lothian EH54 7AR
Tel: (01506) 414957   Fax: (01506) 497771
e-mail: info@almondvalley.co.uk
www.almondvalley.co.uk
20-acre site exploring history of the local environment with animals on Mill Farm, vintage farm machinery in Livingstone Mill and a shale oil museum. Lovely family day out.

SD   CP   E   RF
C   S   WC

NEWTOWNGRANGE
Located south of Bonnyrigg, that is SE of Edinburgh off the A72.

ATTRACTION
SCOTTISH MINING MUSEUM
Lady Victoria Colliery, Newtowngrange, Midlothian EH22 4QN
Tel: (0131) 6637519   Fax: (0131) 6541618
At 800 years old, this is the oldest documented coal mining site in Britain. See the Cornish beam engine plus several relevant sites and exhibitions: Cutting the Coal; A Race Apart; Pithead; Smithy; Interactive and audio visual areas; Coal Roadway; At the Coal Face Exhibition; and Old Washer.

SD   CP   E 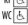   RF
L   C   S   WC

SOUTH QUEENSFERRY
Small village on the bank of the River Forth, 10 miles west of Edinburgh. Famous for its Forth Bridge, below which the old ferry is still used for pleasure craft.

ATTRACTION
DALMENY HOUSE
South Queensferry, West Lothian EH30 9TQ
Tel: (0131) 3311888   Fax: (0131) 3311788
Built in 1815 in Tudor Gothic style, and home to the Earl and Countess of Rosebery, with collections of French and early Scottish furniture, tapestries and china from the Rothschild Mentmore Collection.
Situated on the Firth of Forth.

SD   CP n/a   E   RF
WC   C

WEST CALDER
Located on north side of the Pentland Hills, 18 miles west of Edinburgh city centre. Less than an hour's drive away are palaces, castles, stately homes and many other attractions.

SELF-CATERING
CROSSWOODHILL FARM
By West Calder, West Lothian EH55 8LP
Tel: (01501) 785205   Fax: (01501) 785308
No. of Accessible Units: 1
No. of Beds per Unit: 6
Accessible Facilities: Lounge/Dining Room. NB Kitchen too narrow for a wheelchair. 1,700-acre livestock farm. Steading Cottage is for those happy to be at the heart of the farm. Set back from the road with a small garden, it nestles right beside the farm buildings and a field. Despite thick walls and double glazing you may hear tractors, cattle or perhaps smell the odd farm whiff outside!

REGION 3

GREATER GLASGOW AND CLYDE VALLEY

STRATHCLYDE PASSENGER TRANSPORT
DIAL-A-BUS
Tel: (0141) 3333252
Mon/Sat: easy and flexible door-to-door service. Sunday service in SE Glasgow, Renfrew and Kilmarnock and Thursday evening service in NW Glasgow, Hamilton, East Kilbride, Cumbernauld and Monklands.

GLASGOW

Occupied by the Romans 2,000 years ago, Glasgow's modern city grew wealthy from the British Empire and the Industrial Revolution to become the UK City of Architecture in 1999. In 1991 it was European City of Culture. The streets run on a grid system on the north bank of the River Clyde, which includes rail stations and main shopping facilities. Outside the centre is the West End with bars and restaurants. A vibrant and exciting city to visit.

TOURIST INFORMATION CENTRE
11 George Square, Glasgow G2 1DY
Tel: (0141) 2044400

CENTRE OF INDEPENDENT LIVING
117-127 Brook Street, Bridgeton, Glasgow G40 3AP
Tel: (0141) 5504455   Fax: (0141) 5504858

GLASGOW CITY COUNCIL
Cultural and Leisure Service
20 Trongate, Glasgow G1 1EY
Tel: (0141) 287997 Fax: (0141) 2875151
Contact for general queries pertaining to museums, theatres etc.

TAXIS
Taxis Owner's Association

21 Lawmoor Road, Glasgow G5
Tel: (0141) 429 7070
Wheelchair accessible metro and facility cabs. If you require portable ramps, request the facility car when booking.

TRAINS
Scotrail, Caledonian Chambers, 87 Union Street, Glasgow G1 3TA
Tel: (0141) 3354590
Tel: Disabled Users: (0845) 6057021

National Rail Travel
Passenger Enquiries: (08457) 484950

Glasgow Station offers unassisted wheelchair access and ramps. 24 hours' notice is advisable.

CAR PARK
Charing Cross Car Park, Embankment Crescent, Glasgow.
Tel: (0141) 2219320
Disabled badge parking available.

SHOPMOBILITY
Glasgow Shobmobility, Ground Floor, Buchanan Galleries, Glasgow G3
Tel: (0141) 3540416

HOTELS
HILTON GLASGOW ♿
1 William Street, Glasgow G3 8HT
Tel: (0141) 2045555   Fax: (0141) 2045004
No. of Accessible Rooms: 4
Accessible Facilities: Lift, Lounge, Restaurant, Pool, Sauna, Spa.
Located 0.5 miles from the city centre.

GLASGOW MOAT HOUSE ♿
Congress Road, Glasgow G3 8QT
Tel: (0141) 3069988   Fax: (0141) 2212022
No. of Accessible Rooms: 2
Accessible Facilities: Lounge, Restaurant, Pool, Sauna, Spa. Impressive hotel overlooking the Clyde is located beside the SECC and Armadillo Conference Centre, a mile from the railway station.

THE SHAWLANDS HOTEL & TRAVEL LODGE ♿
Ayr Road, Larkhall, Nr. Hamilton ML9 2TZ
Tel: (01698) 791111   Fax: (01698) 792001

No. of Accessible Rooms: 2
Accessible Facilities: Lounge, Restaurant.
Privately owned with accessible
accommodation in Lodge. Located south of
Glasgow.

HILTON EAST KILBRIDE
Stewartfield Way, East Kilbride G74 5LA
Tel: (01355) 236300   Fax: (01355) 233552
No. of Accessible Rooms: 2
Accessible Facilities: Lounge, 2 Restaurants,
Cafe, Bar, Pool, Sauna, Whirlpool.
Located on the southern outskirts of
Glasgow, this is a modern hotel with a
Living Well healthclub.

BED AND BREAKFAST
GLASGOW GUEST HOUSE
56 Dumbreck Road, Glasgow G41 5NP
Tel/Fax: (0141) 4270129
No. of Accessible Rooms: 2
Accessible Facilities: Lounge, Dining Room.

ATTRACTIONS
THE BURRELL COLLECTION
Pollock Country Park, Glasgow G43 1AT
Tel: (0141) 2872550   Fax: (0141) 2872597
Superb collection of art works ranging
from Chinese ceramics, European medieval
art, stained glass and British silverwork to
paintings and sculptures from C15th to the
early C20th with works by Rembrandt,
Degas and Cezanne. An absolute must,
this really needs two visits!

SD n/a   CP   E   RF
L   C   S   WC

GLASGOW ART GALLERY AND MUSEUM
Kelvingrove, Glasgow G3 8AG
Tel: (0141) 2872699
Fine collection of French Impressionists,
Post-Impressionists and Scottish artists
from C17th onward, plus works by
Rembrandt and Giorgione. The Glasgow
style represented by Charles Rennie
Mackintosh furniture is now as well known
for silver jewellery design.

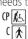
SD   CP   E   L
C   S   WC

GALLERY OF MODERN ART
Queen Street, Glasgow G1 3AZ
Tel: (0141) 2291996   Fax: (0141) 2045316

Opened in 1996 and set in a marvellous
refurbished neo-classical building in the
city centre. Houses contemporary art from
living artists. International and Scottish
artists. All three levels are accessible via
either of the two lifts, and each gallery is
accessible.

SD   CP n/a   E   RF
L   C   S   WC

GLASGOW BOTANIC GARDENS
730 Great Western Road, Glasgow G12 0UE
Tel: (0141) 3342422   Fax: (0141) 339 6964
Dedicated to education, conservation and
research there are 10 main points of
interest, of which the riverwalk and sorbus
and birch areas of arboretum are not
accessible. The main range Glasshouse and
the area around Kibble Palace are
particularly fine. Many of the plants
represent temperate geographical regions:
Mediterranean, Australasian, South
American and temperate Asian. All paths
around the gardens are tarmac, mostly
level or slightly sloping.

SD   CP   E   RF
C   WC   RFE

McLELLAN GALLERIES
270 Sauchiehall Street, Glasgow G2 3EH
Tel: (0141) 3311854   Fax: (0141) 3329957

Glasgow Art Gallery.

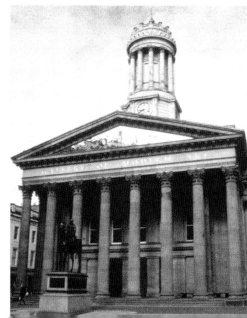

Range of major and changing international exhibitions.

SD ♿ CP n/a E 🚶 L ♿ WC 🚶

PEOPLE'S PALACE
Glasgow Green, Glasgow G40 1AT
Tel: (0141) 554 0223   Fax: (0141) 5500892
Victorian building purpose-built in 1898 as a cultural museum, which houses a wide range of exhibits on the city's social history from the C12th to the C20th. A fine conservatory at the rear of building contains a winter garden and tropical plants and birds.

SD ♿ CP 🚶 E ♿
L ♿ S ♿ WC ♿

UNIVERSITY OF GLASGOW VISITOR CENTRE
University of Glasgow, University Avenue, Glasgow G12 8QQ
Tel: (0141) 3305511   Fax: (0141) 3305225
e-mail: visitorcentre@gla.ac.uk
Starting point for guided tours of the university's many attractions.

SD ♿ CP ♿ E 🚶 RF ♿
C 🚶 S ♿ WC 🚶 RFE 🚶

THEATRE
THE KING'S THEATRE
297 Bath Street, Glasgow
Admin: (0141) 2875006   Fax: (0141) 2483361
Booking-Box Office: (0141) 2875511
Fax: (0141) 2875016

CP 🚶 RE (accessible entrance in Elmbank Street.)
ED ♿ INT ♿
WC ♿ (except inward opening door)
AUD ♿ (5 spaces). B/R ♿

GREENOCK
Developed through industrial growth on the Clyde. Good new leisure development on Inverclyde's waterfront.

HOTEL
JAMES WATT COLLEGE
Halls of Residence, Custom House Way, Greenock PA15 1EN
Tel: (01475) 731360   Fax: (01475) 730877
No. of Accessible Rooms: 16

Accessible Facilities: Lounge, Restaurant. Located 0.25 mile from the town centre.

LANGBANK
30 minutes west of Glasgow, between Glasgow and Greenock,

ATTRACTION
FINLAYSTONE COUNTRY ESTATE
Langbank
Tel: (01475) 540505   Fax: (01475) 540505
e-mail: info@finlaystone.co.uk
www.finlaystone.co.uk
Delightful Victoriana exhibition in the house, but the grounds are particularly splendid with formal and walled gardens, including a scented garden, and woodland walks.

SD ♿ CP ♿ E ♿ RF ♿
C ♿ S ♿ WC ♿ RFE ♿

NEW LANARK
The village, founded in 1785 as a completely new industrial settlement, is now A World Heritage Village and restored as a living and working community. New Lanark is the gateway to the Scottish Wildlife Trust's Falls of the Clyde Wildlife Reserve (limited access for wheelchairs) and there is a Wildlife Centre in the village, together with shops, craft workshops and various exhibitions, all advised as accessible.

TOURIST INFORMATION CENTRE
Horsemarket, Ladyacre Road, Lanark ML11 7LQ
Tel: (01555) 661661   Fax: (01555) 666143

HOTEL
NEW LANARK MILL HOTEL ♿
Mill One, New Lanark ML11 9DB
Tel: (01555) 667200   Fax: (01555) 667222
e-mail: hotel@newlanark.org
www.newlanark.org
No. of Accessible Rooms: 5. Roll-in Shower
Accessible Facilities: Lounge, Restaurant. Set on the upper reaches of the River Clyde in unique surroundings of restored C18th mill village.

REGION 4

WEST HIGHLANDS AND ISLANDS, ARGYLL, LOCH LOMOND, STIRLING AND TROSSACHS

ALLOA

Industrial town of coalmining, textiles and glass-making, close to the north bank of the River Forth.

ATTRACTION
ALLOA TOWER (NT for S)
Alloa FK10 1PP
Tel/Fax: (01259) 211701
A C15th medieval tower house, now restored, is all that remains of the ancestral home of the Earls of Mar. It has rare medieval features, particularly the timber roof. Flat access to ground floor, wide shallow stairs to first floor. Other floors are inaccessible because of a turnpike staircase.

SD	♿	CP	♿	E	♿
RF	♿	S	🚶	WC	🚶

ABERFOYLE

ATTRACTION
QUEEN ELIZABETH FOREST PARK
Visitor Centre, Aberfoyle
Tel: (01877) 382258
30 miles from Glasgow, the park takes in east Loch Lomond and the Trossachs with breath-taking scenery. Wheelchair loan scheme operates from the Visitor Centre. Woodlands walks and trails.

APPIN

Between Ballahulish and Oban

SELF-CATERING
APPIN HOUSE APARTMENTS AND LODGES
Appin House, Appin PA38 4BN
Tel: (01631) 730207   Fax: (01631) 730567
Shuna Apartment
No. of Accessible Units: 1
No. of Beds per Unit: 2
Accessible Facilities: Open plan Lounge/Dining/Kitchen
Pine Lodge
No. of Accessible Units: 1
No. of Beds per Unit: 4
Accessible Facilities: Lounge, Dining room
Both the above are in landscaped gardens of five acres in an elevated position overlooking Loch Linnhe with the hills of Mull in the background and the mountains of Morven to the west.
Oak Tree Cottage
No. of Accessible Units: 1
No. of Beds per Unit: 10
Accessible Facilities: Lounge, Dining room.
Located in Duror, five miles north of Appin House, and under the same ownership. Standing on its own at the head of a peaceful glen, overlooked by Bheinn Beithir, it is five minutes from the local shop and restaurant/pub with Cuil Bay beach and Glencoe very close.

BALLOCH

Visitors to Loch Lomond often by-pass Balloch and head up the road on the west side of the loch. However, it is well worth the minor detour to the Country Park at Balloch at the south end of Loch Lomond and a starting point for loch cruises. Fine view of loch can be had at Duncryne, a small hill three miles NE of Balloch.

ATTRACTION
BALLOCH CASTLE COUNTRY PARK
Balloch G83 8LX
Tel: (01389) 758 216 Fax: (01389) 755 721
At the southern end of Loch Lomond, the castle, built in 1808, has a visitor centre with an introduction to local

history and wildlife. It overlooks the park that offers trails, a walled garden and lawns for picnics.

SD ♿ CP ♿ E ♿ RF ♿
C 🚶 S 🚶 WC 🚶 RFE ♿

CALLANDER
Busy capital of the Trossachs, a good starting point for touring the area with good accommodation and restaurants.

HOTEL
ROMAN CAMP COUNTRY HOUSE HOTEL 🚶
off Main Street, Callander FK17 8BG
Tel: (01877) 330003 Fax: (01877) 331533
e-mail: mail@roman-camp-hotel.co.uk
No. of Accessible Rooms: 1
Accessible Facilities: Lounge (1 step), Restaurant. Built in 1625 in 20 acres of secluded gardens by the River Teith.

BED AND BREAKFAST
AIRLIE HOUSE ♿
Main Street, Strathyre, Callander FK18 8NA
Tel: (01877) 384247 Fax: (01877) 384305
No. of Accessible Rooms: 1
Accessible Facilities: Lounge, Dining Room Victorian house built in late 1800s. Being converted into a guesthouse with 4 bedrooms, one specially adapted. Tourist Board assistance on access compliance requirements. Check when booking.

ATTRACTION
ROB ROY & TROSSACHS VISITOR CENTRE
Ancaster Square, Callander FK17 8ED
Tel: (01877) 331267 Fax: (01877) 330784
The story of Scotland's most famous outlaw shown through multi-media theatre and "Life and Times" exhibition. Well worth a visit. N.B. Ramp entrance on right hand side of main door.

SD ♿ CP ♿ E ♿ RF ♿
S ♿ WC 🚶 RFE ♿ L ♿

DALMALLY
Quiet village with good access to Western Isles, located on A85 from Perth and Crieff heading west toward Oban.

BED AND BREAKFAST
CRUACHAN ♿
Dalmally PA33 1AA
Tel: (01838) 200496 Fax: (01838) 200650
email: mborrett@onetel.net.uk
www.cruachan-dalmally.co.uk
No. of Accessible Rooms: 2. Roll-in Shower
Accessible Facilities: Lounge, Dining room, Garden. Traditional villa with lovely scenery.

ATTRACTION
CRUACHAN THE HOLLOW MOUNTAIN POWER STATION
Dalmally PA33 1AN
Tel: (01866) 822618 Fax: (01866) 922509
e-mail: VISIT.cruachan@scottishpower.plc.uk
Free exhibition contains touch-screen information on the vast cavern hidden inside Ben Cruachan, containing 400,000-kilowatt hydro-electric power station. Access to the surface exhibition only. Buses going inside the mountain cannot take wheelchairs. Visitors with their own diesel transport can be taken in by prior arrangement.

SD ♿ CP ♿ E ♿ RF ♿
C ♿ S ♿ WC ♿

DRYMEN
Located north-west of Glasgow, almost at the south-western tip of Loch Lomond.

ATTRACTION
LOCH LOMOND PARK CENTRE
Balmaha, by Drymen
Tel: (01360) 870470 Fax: (01360) 870471
info@visit-lochlomond.com
www.visit-lochlomond.com
The main exhibition explores the geography of Loch Lomond landscapes. The centre is the focal point for the Millennium Trail with boat yard, pier, car park and shops all set round a lovely bay below Conic Hill.

SD ♿ CP 🚶 E ♿ RF ♿
S ♿ WC 🚶 RFE ♿

324

FALKIRK

This thriving industrial town of the C18th and C19th, maintains a busy shopping centre. Five miles away at Rough Castle are remains of the Antonine Wall, built by the Romans in AD142.

BED AND BREAKFAST

ASHBANK GUEST HOUSE
105 Main Street, Redding, Falkirk FK2 9UQ
Tel: (01324) 716649 Fax: (01324) 712431
e-mail: ashbank@guest-house.co.uk
No. of Accessible Rooms: 1
Accessible Facilities: Dining Room, Garden
Detached stone house situated on the east side of the town with gardens on all sides and views over the Forth Valley. Falkirk is 10 minutes' drive away, Stirling 20 minutes, and Edinburgh 30 minutes.

ATTRACTION

CALLENDAR HOUSE
Callendar Park, Falkirk FK1 1YR
Tel: (01324) 503770 Fax: (01324) 503771
900 years of history demonstrated in the Story of Callendar House exhibition. Costumed interpreters explain local C19th life.

SD ⬚ CP ⬚ E ⬚ RF ⬚ L ⬚
C ⬚ S ⬚ WC ⬚ RFE ⬚

HELENSBURGH

Holiday town, home of John Logie Baird who invented the TV in 1926, and of the designer Charles Rennie Mackintosh.

HOTELS

ARDENCAPLE HOTEL
Shore Road, Rhu, Nr. Helensburgh G84 8LA
Tel: (01436) 820200 Fax: (01436) 821099
No. of Accessible Rooms: 1
Accessible Facilities: Lounge, Restaurant.

ROSSLEA HALL HOTEL
Ferry Road, Rhu, Helensburgh G84 8NF
Tel: (01436) 439955 Fax: (01436) 820897
No. of Accessible Rooms: 2

Accessible Facilities: Lounge, Restaurant
Country house hotel.

ISLE OF ISLAY

Most southerly of Western Isles, home to fine Highland heavily peated malt whiskies with much to see of historical and archaeological interest.

ATTRACTION

LOCH GRUINART NATURE RESERVE (RSPB)
Bushmill Cottages, Gruinart, Bridgend, Islay PA44 7PP
Tel: (01496) 850505 Fax: (01496) 850575
e-mail: yvonnebrown@rspb.org.uk
Super beaches on Islay support a variety of bird life at the reserve. Hide is accessible with wheelchair viewing window. NB: Visitor Centre is ramped at 1:8 and is not accessible.

SD n/a CP   RF-(WC) ⬚
WC ⬚ RFE ⬚

ISLE OF MULL

Largest of the Inner Hebrides with most roads following an irregular coastline backed by mountains. Tobermory, the capital in the north, has colourful houses and a sheltered harbour. Several mountain peaks are over 2,000 feet, Ben More is the highest at 3,169. Some lovely beaches.

HOTEL

THE TOBERMORY HOTEL
53 Main Street, Tobermory, Isle of Mull PA75 6NT
Tel: (01688) 302091 Fax: (01688) 302254
No. of Accessible Rooms: 2. Roll-in Shower
Accessible Facilities: Lounge, Restaurant (both with 1 step). Family hotel situated in the lovely Tobermory Bay.

ATTRACTIONS

MULL AND WEST HIGHLANDS NARROW GAUGE RAILWAY CO.
Craignure, Isle of Mull PA65 6AY
Tel: (01680) 300389
Steam and diesel trains run from Torosay

LOCHGILPHEAD

A market town and hub for smaller communities with bank, supermarket etc. A good base for a tour of the Kintyre Peninsula.

BED AND BREAKFAST

EMPIRE TRAVEL LODGE   🚹
Union Street, Lochgilphead PA31 8JS
Tel: (01546) 602381
No. of Accessible Rooms: 1
Accessible Facilities: Breakfast served in bedrooms. There are five steps to the breakfast room. Built originally as a cinema, now fully refurbished to create mid-Argyll's only purpose-built travel lodge.

ATTRACTION

RSPB LOCHWINNOCH NATURE RESERVE
Larges Road, Lochwinnoch PA12 4JF
Tel: (01505) 842663   Fax: (01505) 813026
e.mail:lochwinnoch@rspb.org.uk
Useful information sheet for people with disabilities visiting the Reserve.
Visitor Centre shop/reception and visitor's area accessible. The observation tower is not accessible. A wheelchair is available free of charge.
Trails and Hides – two trails (Dubbs Water and Aird Meadow) and three bird-watching hides are all accessible to wheelchair users. Open water is a most obvious feature of the reserve with many species – great crested grebes being a summer favourite. Trails follow marsh and meadow and also a small woodland.

SD n/a CP 🚹 E 🚹 RF 🚹
C 🚹 WC 🚹 RFE 🚹

LUSS

Attractive C19th estate village where many cottages were erected to house factory workers. Now restored, Luss is a Conservation Village, famous for the

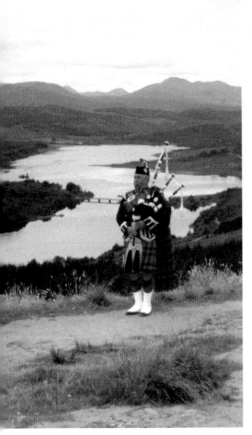

Traditional Piper plays before a dramatic backdrop

Castle to Craignure, 1.5 miles, with woodland and mountain scenery.

SD 🚹 CP 🚹 E 🚹 RF 🚹
S 🚹 WC 🚹

TOROSAY CASTLE

Craignure, Isle of Mull PA65 6AY
Tel: (01680) 812421   Fax: (01680) 812470
Victorian castle of Scottish baronial architecture with a fascinating variety of interior displays. Edwardian library and archive rooms. Italian terraced gardens include statue walk and water gardens. The castle has been built on a slight slope and so access to the gardens with a wheelchair can be difficult.

roses around the doors. Set at the foot of the glen, on the shores of Loch Lomond, where the Luss runs into the loch.

ATTRACTION
LOCH LOMOND PARK CENTRE
Luss Village
Tel: (01436) 860601
The main exhibit provides an insight into landscape, wildlife and the cultural history of Loch Lomond.

SD   CP   E   RF
S   WC

OBAN
Known as the Gateway to the Isles, this is a busy port on the Firth of Lorne with good views of the Argyll coast, and an attractive sea-front shopping area with fresh fish for sale on the pier. The town is dominated by McCraig's Tower (1800). August attracts yachtsmen for West Highland Week.

SELF-CATERING
MELFORT PIER AND HARBOUR
Kimelford, by Oban PA34 4XD
Tel: (01852) 200333   Fax: (01852) 200329
e-mail: melharbour@aol.com
No. of Accessible Units: 4
No. of Beds per Unit: 2 - 6
Accessible Facilities: Lounge/Diner, Kitchen, Balcony. Self-contained harbour houses in superb and unique location right on the shores of Loch Melfort, protected on seaward side by uninhabited islands and sheltered by the hills of Melfort to the North.

ELERAIG HIGHLAND CHALETS
Kilninver, by Oban PA34 4UX
Tel/Fax: (01852) 200225
www.Scotland2000.com/eleraig
No. of Accessible Units: 1. Bath
No. of Beds per Unit: 6
Accessible Facilities: Open plan Lounge/dining/kitchenette.

One of seven Norwegian chalets in a private glen with wonderful scenery and close to Loch Tralaig, 1.5 miles long.

ATTRACTION
ARDUAINE GARDENS (NT for S)
Arduaine, Oban PA34 4XQ
Tel/Fax: (01852) 200366
C19th garden planted on a hillside beside the sea, notable for rhododendrons and azaleas, with variable terrain. Two wheelchair-friendly waymarked routes around the garden. Wheelchair on site.

SD   CP   E
RF   WC

SCOTTISH SEA LIFE SANCTUARY
Barcaldine, Oban PA37 1SE
Tel: (01631) 720386   Fax: (01631) 720529
Set among pine trees on the shore of Loch Creran, this is Scotland's leading marine animal rescue centre. Crystal clear waters allow exploration of over 30 natural marine habitats and dramatic loch-side wildlife trails, seal sanctuary and multi-level viewing enhance this fascinating attraction.

SD   CP   E   RF
C   S   WC

STIRLING
The town grew up around its castle, one of the most important fortresses in Scotland, built in C15th and C16th. Beneath the castle, the Old Town is protected by original C16th walls and is well preserved with a fine medieval church of the Holy Rude, guild hall, tolbooth and wide market place. North of the city is the Bridge of Allan, established as a Victorian spa town and now home to the University of Stirling with landscaped wooded grounds which are worth visiting.

BED AND BREAKFAST
UPPER GARTINSTARRY
Buchlyvie, Nr. Stirling FK8 3PD
Tel/Fax: (01360) 850309
e-mail: goldings@bigfoot.com

No. of Accessible Rooms: 2
Accessible Facilities: Lounge, Dining Room
Country guesthouse a few miles west of
Stirling.

ATTRACTIONS
OLD TOWN JAIL
St. John Street, Stirling FK8 1EA
Tel: (01786) 450050 Fax: (01786) 471301
Built in 1847, this Victorian architectural
gem offers a living history performance
about the daily life of its prisoners. The lift
accesses the rooftop but there is a spiral
staircase to the viewpoint which has
panoramic views of Stirling and beyond.
Guided tour takes place in a level, wide
corridor.

SD n/a CP E RF
L S WC

STIRLING CASTLE
Stirling FK8 1EJ
Tel: (01786) 450000 Fax: (01786) 464678
Strategically built on the Firth of Forth,
much remaining from C15th and C16th.
James II was born here in 1430: Mary
Queen of Scots spent time here. All
apartments are accessible apart from the
museum of Argyll and Sutherland
Highlanders. The lower level of Queen
Anne Gardens is also accessible. Only
medieval kitchens and Elphinstone Tower
are not accessible.

SD CP E RF
C S WC

SMITH ART GALLERY AND MUSEUM
Dumbarton Road, Stirling
Tel: (01786) 471917 Fax: (01786) 449523
e-mail: museum@smithartgallery.demon.co.uk
Located beneath Stirling Castle, with a fine
collection of Scottish painting, and an
important and little-known history
collection, including the Stirling Jug
(1457), the oldest dated curling stone in
the world (1511) and ancient tartans.

SD CP E (not main entrance)
RF L C
S WC RFE

REGION 5
PERTHSHIRE, ANGUS AND DUNDEE, KINGDOM OF FIFE

ANGUS & DUNDEE

ARBROATH
Fishing and holiday town famous for
red stonework, C12th, and Arbroath
Smokies, smoked haddock. Many
fishmongers gather on the seafront
where visitors can watch the smoking
process and enjoy a treat in one of the
wonderful fish and chip shops.

ATTRACTION
ARBROATH ABBEY (HS)
Abbey Street, Arbroath
Tel/Fax: (01241) 878756
Robert the Bruce was declared king in this
C12th abbey in 1320. A rose garden
along the south wall of the abbey church
is accessible. The Abbot's House and
sacristy are not accessible.

SD CP E RF
L WC (50m from Abbey)

CARNOUSTIE
Pleasant seaside town best known for
its championship golf course.

HOTEL
CARLOGIE HOUSE HOTEL
Carlogie Road, Carnoustie DD7 6LD
Tel: (01241) 853185 Fax: (01241) 856528
No. of Accessible Rooms: 4
Accessible Facilities: Lounge, Restaurant.
Set in secluded grounds and close to over
50 golf courses. Situated just off the A92
road from Dundee to Arbroath, the latter
five miles away.

DUNDEE

Major shipbuilding centre in C18th and C19th and the country's fourth largest city. Good views over the River Tay to Fife from its riverfront, where at Victoria Dock lies HM Frigate Unicorn, the oldest British-built warship still afloat (1824). Several historic relics include the Howff, an old burial ground and Old Steeple, C15th tower fragment of the largest medieval church in Scotland.

BUSES
Strathtay Scottish: Tel: (01382) 228345
Thistle Coaches: Tel: (01382) 623456
16-seater vehicles with ramps, straps and private hire if required.

TAXIS
Blackcabs:
505050 Taxis: Tel: (01382) 732111/731222
Findhorn: Tel: (01382) 504040
Four adapted vehicles.
Handytaxis: Tel: (01382) 225825
Two adapted vehicles.

TRAINS
Dundee Scotrail: Tel: (08457) 484950
Disabled passengers: Tel: (0845) 6057021
Ramps and staff assistance available with 24 hours' notice.
GNER – Special Needs: Tel: (0845) 225444
Minicom: (0191) 2330173
Wheelchair space in first and standard class. Assistance available at stations when booked in advance.

HOTEL
HILTON DUNDEE
Earl Grey Place, Dundee DD1 4DE
Tel: (01382) 229271   Fax: (01382) 200072
No. of Accessible Rooms: 3. 1 room has a shower, 2 have baths. Accessible Facilities: Lounge, Restaurant. Quality hotel set on the banks of the River Tay, five minutes' drive from the A90.

SWALLOW HOTEL
Kingsway West, Invergowrie, Dundee DD2 5JT
Tel: (01382) 641122

No. of Accessible Rooms: 3
Accessible Facilities: Lounge, Restaurant, Pool, Sauna, Spa. Victorian mansion in delightful gardens, located off the by-pass, 10 minutes' drive from the city centre.

BED AND BREAKFAST
ALCORN GUEST HOUSE
5 Hyndford Street, Dundee, Angus DD2 1HQ
Tel: (01382) 668433
No. of Accessible Rooms: 1. Bath
Accessible Facilities: Lounge, Dining Room

SELF-CATERING
KINGENNIE LODGES
The Kingennie Fishings, Kingennie, Broughtyferry, Dundee DD5 3RD
Tel: (01382) 350777   Fax: (01382) 350400
e-mail: kingennie@easynet.co.uk
No. of Accessible Units: 1
No. of Beds per Unit: 3
Accessible Facilities: Lounge, Kitchen/Diner, Trout Fishing. Luxury self-catering lodges of which Glenclova is fully accessible. Situated in woodland overlooking trout lakes and old boathouse of 1855. Located five miles north of Dundee. Some areas of the lake are wheelchair accessible.

ATTRACTION
DISCOVERY POINT
Discovery Quay, Dundee DD1 4XA
Tel: (01782) 201245   Fax: (01382) 225891
e-mail: dundeeheritage@sd.co.uk
Home of Captain Scott's Antarctic ship RRS Discovery. There are eight exhibition areas with lighting, special effects and graphics telling the Discovery story. A must.

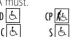

FORFAR
Market town, once a jute and flax milling centre, now producing man-made fabrics and agricultural products.

ATTRACTION
GLAMIS CASTLE GROUNDS
by Forfar DD8 1RJ
Tel: (01307) 840393 Fax: (01307) 840733
e-mail: glamis@great-houses-scotland.co.uk
Unfortunately this wonderful turreted and battlemented castle is not accessible, apart from the ground floor, but worth viewing from outside. Home of the Bowes-Lyon family since C14th, this was the childhood home of the late Queen Mother. The grounds are lovely, details below.

SD   CP   E   RF
C [♿]   S [♿]   WC [↟]

KIRRIEMUIR
Typical Angus town with red sandstone buildings, agricultural and textile works and famous as birthplace of J. M. Barrie, a little cottage at 9 Brechin Road. Statue of Peter Pan in town square.

ATTRACTION
LOCH OF KINNORDY RSPB RESERVE
The Flat, Kinnordy Home Farm, Kirriemuir DD85ER
Tel: (01738) 630783
The lochs, mires and fens of the nature reserve are surrounded by farmland. It is one of the best places in Scotland to see black-necked grebes, which nest in the midst of a colony of black-headed gulls. Ospreys regularly visit in the summer. 3 bird-watching hides, two are accessible. Gullery hide is accessed via a wooden boardwalk. The door opens outwards; there are two adapted places, but help may be needed to move the bench. Swamp hide has an outwards opening door; two adapted places, help may be needed to move the bench. East hide is accessed via six steps.
The reserve is situated 1.6km west of Kirriemuir on the B951. The car park is surfaced with rolled stone and has a slight downward gradient running from the road. N.B. No toilets at the reserve. The nearest adapted toilets are in Kirriemiur 1.6 km away.

SD n/a   CP    E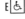

MONTROSE
A wealthy town accumulated through rich agricultural land and more recently oil revenues. Situated at the mouth of river, South Esk is an important area for wintering geese, many thousands roost here. There is a medieval market square and the seafront offers a fine beach.

HOTEL
THE LINKS HOTEL
Mid Links, Montrose, Angus DD10 8RL
Tel: (01674) 671000   Fax: (01674) 672698
No. of Accessible Rooms: 1
Accessible Facilities: Lounge, Restaurant. Small hotel situated in the Links in the centre of Montrose.

KINGDOM OF FIFE
For all information regarding accessible transport throughout Fife, contact Anne Cowan, Transport Department, Fife House, Glenrothes.
Tel: (01592) 414141

ANSTRUTHER
Once the home of Scotland's main fishing fleet, now leisure boats fill the harbour.

ATTRACTION
SCOTTISH FISHERIES MUSEUM
Harbourhead, Anstruther KY10 3AB
Tel: (01333) 310628
Both real and model boats and fisherman's cottages are housed in various C16th and C19th buildings.

SD [♿]   CP [♿]   E [♿]   RF [↟]
C [♿]   S [♿]   WC [↟]

DUNFERMLINE
Capital of Scotland in 1603, dominated by the ruins of the C12th abbey. The abbey church contains the tombs of 22 Scottish kings and queens including Robert the Bruce.

HOTEL
PITBAUCHLIE HOUSE HOTEL
Aberdour Road, Dunfermline KY11 4PB
Tel: (01383) 722282   Fax: (01383) 620738
No. of Accessible Rooms: 1
Accessible Facilities: Lounge, Restaurant.
Family-run hotel on the south side of town
set in wooded, landscaped grounds with
modern public rooms.

SELF-CATERING
BENARTY HOLIDAY COTTAGES
Benarty House, Kelty, Nr. Dunfermline KY4 0HT
Tel/Fax: (01383) 830235
No. of Accessible Units: 1. Bath
No. of Beds per Unit: 6
Accessible Facilities: Living/Dining Room,
Kitchen. The Steading is 1 of 2 cottages
situated on a working farm in woodland
adjacent to Lochore Meadows Country
Park and over the hill from Loch Leven.
Located 4 miles north of Dunfermline.

ATTRACTION
ABBOT HOUSE
Maygate, Dunfermline KY12 7NE
Tel: (01383) 733266 Fax: (01383) 624908
Journey through 1,000 years of history in
this medieval house which has born
witness to the intrigues of church and
state.

SD   CP   E   RF
C   S   WC

GLENROTHES
Planned town of 1950s built to house
Fife's colliery workers, it is full of 60s
architecture. Transport details for
Kirkcaldy, a few miles south, are also
given.

DIAL A RIDE
Rothesay House, Glenrothes DY7 5LT
Tel: (01592) 413434
Useful for information on Taxicard.

SHOPMOBILITY
Multi Storey Car Park, Kingdom Centre,
Glenrothes. Tel: (01592) 414199

HOTEL
BALBIRNIE HOUSE HOTEL
Balbirnie Park, Markinch,
by Glenrothes KY7 6NE
Tel: (01592) 610066 Fax: (01592) 610529
e-mail: balbirnie@btinternet.com
www.balbirnie.co.uk
No. of Accessible Rooms: 4
Accessible Facilities: Lounge, Restaurant.
Listed Grade A Georgian mansion set in
416 acre estate with trees and
rhododendrons. Restored with open fires
and antiques, providing a wonderful
ambience. 30 minutes from Edinburgh
and St. Andrews.

TRAVELINE
Tel: (0870) 6082608

Kirkcaldy Transport
PUBLIC TRANSPORT INFORMATION
HELPLINE   Tel: (01592) 416060

BUSES
First Fife Bus: limited bus service, one
throughout Fife with low-floor access but
no restraints.

TAXIS
Ellis Taxis: Tel: (01592) 654100
One adapted 4-seater vehicle takes one
wheelchair.

Regal Taxis: Tel: (01592) 200300
Various taxis which have been adapted to
take wheelchairs. 3 x 8 seater minibus
and 1x7 seater minibus. One of the 8
seater vehicles can hold 2 normal sized
wheelchairs.

TRAINS
Scotrail, Platform 14, Edinburgh Waverley
Station.
Super-Sprinter and Class 158 trains,
wheelchair spaces.
Train Enquiries for Disabled Users:
Tel: (0845) 6057021
Staff Assistance: Tel: (0845) 6057021

SHOPMOBILITY
Mercat Centre Car Park, Tolbooth Street,
Kirkcaldy KY1 1NJ
Tel: (01592) 412199/414199

KILLIECRANKIE

Killiecrankie is a site of Special Scientific Interest with a magnificent wooded gorge above the River Garry.

ATTRACTION
KILLIECRANKIE VISITOR CENTRE (NTS)
Killiecrankie PH16 5LG
Tel/Fax: (01796) 473233
e-mail: bnotley@nts.org.uk www.nts.org.uk
In 1689 the first shots of the Jacobite uprising were fired at the Pass of Killiecrankie. The centre tells the story of the battle and natural history of the area. The "Soldier's Leap" is a wooded gorge where one soldier evaded capture by jumping across River Garry. Although the paths leading to the "Leap" are steep and rough and not recommended, a viewing balcony at the centre gives good views of the Pass. The Centre offers inter-active war models and fascinating natural history display. Both upper and lower level car parks have one disabled space with clear tarmac. Park on the upper level for level entry into Visitor Centre, and on the lower level for WC and cafe.

CP   E RF
C S WC

NORTH QUEENSFERRY

Important originally as a north terminal for ferry crossing to carry pilgrims to nearby Dunfermline. Ferry lasted 800 years until road bridge opened in 1964.

ATTRACTION
DEEP SEA WORLD
North Queensferry KY11 1JR
Tel: (01383) 411880   Fax: (01383) 410514
e-mail: info@deepseaworld.co.uk
Amazing underwater world viewed from moving walkway travelling along viewing tunnel through the sea bed. Come face to face with sharks, giant rays and conger eels.

SD   CP   E  RF
C S WC   RFE

PITTENWEEM

Home of the Fife fishing fleet with bustling early morning harbour. Overlooking harbour is St. Fillan's Cave, a refuge in the C17th for a Christian missionary. Pittenweem means place of the cave in Pict dialect.

ATTRACTION
KELLIE CASTLE GARDENS (NTS)
Pittenweem KY10 2RF
Tel: (01333) 720271   Fax: (01333) 720326
The castle is not accessible, but smooth paths run round the lovely Victorian walled garden where plants and shrubs are grown organically.

SD   CP E RF
C S WC

ST. ANDREWS

Scotland's oldest university town and one time ecclesiastical capital, now synonymous with golf. Charming crooked housefronts in streets and alleyways, medieval churches and C12th cathedral.

TOURIST INFORMATION CENTRE
70 Market Street, St. Andrews KY16 9NU
Tel: (01334) 472021

HOTEL
RUFFLETS COUNTRY HOUSE
Strathkinness Low Road, St. Andrews KY16 9TX
Tel: (01334) 472594   Fax: (01334) 478703
No. of Accessible Rooms: 1. Roll-in Shower
Accessible Facilities: Unknown
Lovely country house set in 10-acre gardens, 1.5 miles from the famous golf course. Close to several visitor attractions.

SELFCATERING
ST. ANDREW'S COUNTRY COTTAGES
Mountquhanie Estate, Cupar,
Nr. St. Andrews KY15 4QJ
Tel: (01382) 330252   Fax: (01382) 330480
e-mail: enquiries@standrews-cottages.com
www.standrews-cottages.com

No. of Accessible Units: 1
No. of Beds per Unit: 6
Accessible Facilities: Lounge, Kitchen/Diner
One of several charming, secluded cottages and farmhouses on Nydie Mains Farm, three miles west of St. Andrews. Formerly two traditional farm cottages, it has its own enclosed garden. It overlooks the valley of the river Eden with panoramic views towards the Tay and the foothills of the Grampians.

ATTRACTION
ST. ANDREWS CASTLE
The Scores, St. Andrews KY16 9AR
Tel: (01334) 477196   Fax: (01334) 475068
C13th defence with visitor centre showing multi-media exhibition describing castle's history and that of St. Andrews Cathedral.

SD 🚹♿   E ♿   RF ♿
S 🚹   WC 🚹   RFE ♿

PERTHSHIRE

ABERFELDY
Popular, but less touristy than its neighbours though busy in summer with some cafes and shops. Close to the town centre is the 1733 Wades Bridge, and the water mill – powered by Moness Burn that runs through the town centre – has been restored to a working mill again.

TOURIST INFORMATION CENTRE
The Square, Aberfeldy PH15 2DD
Tel: (01887) 820276   Fax: (01887) 829495

SELF-CATERING
LOCH TAY LODGES   ♿
Remony, Aberfeldy PH15 2HR
Tel: (01887) 830209   Fax: (01887) 830802
e-mail: remony@btinternet.com
No. of Accessible Units: 1
No. of Beds per Unit: 6
Accessible Facilities: Lounge, Dining Room, Kitchen. Laggan Lodge is one of six lodges, originally constructed by the Earl of Breadalbane in the mid 1800s as estate workers cottages, now rebuilt. Situated on the eastern side of the small village of

Acharn, close to Loch Tay in tranquil countryside of hill farms and sporting estates. Fine views in all directions.

BLAIRGOWRIE
Main centre for skiing in Glen Shee Ski area, 39km to the north. Famous as major raspberry growing area since 1898. Woollen mill, shops and cafes add to a pleasant ambience.

TOURIST INFORMATION CENTRE
26 Wellmeadow, Blairgowrie PH10 6AS
Tel: (01250) 872960   Fax: (01250) 873701

HOTEL
KINLOCH HOUSE HOTEL   ♿
By Blairgowrie PH10 6SG
Tel: (01250) 884237   Fax: (01250) 884333
No. of Accessible Rooms: 4
Accessible Facilities: Lounge, Restaurant. Country house hotel in 25 acres of woods, parkland and highland cattle.

CRIEFF
Located on the cultural and physical border between the Highlands and Lowlands, Once a famous cattle market town, Crieff sits on the southern slope of the Knock, a large hill with woods.

TOURIST INFORMATION CENTRE
Town Hall, High Street, Crieff PH7 3HU
Tel: (01764) 652578   Fax: (01764) 655422

HOTEL
BEST WESTERN CRIEFF HYDRO HOTEL   🚹
Ferntower Road, Crieff PH7 3LQ
Tel: (01764) 655555   Fax: (01764) 653087
No. of Accessible Rooms: 2
Accessible Facilities: Lift (Cat.1), Lounge, Restaurant, Pool, Sauna, Spa, Cinema, Disabled Riding School, Victorian Garden, Beauty Salon, Boutique, Coffee Shop, Ballroom. Well-known, quality hotel on northern edge of the town combining traditional values and all modern conveniences, plus enormous range of sporting and leisure facilities.

ATTRACTION
FAMOUS GROUSE EXPERIENCE GLENTURRET DISTILLERY
The Hosh, Crieff PH7 4HA
Tel: (01764) 656565   Fax: (01764) 654366
www.famousgrouse.com
Oldest distillery in Scotland, dating back to 1775, uses water from the Turret Burn to make award-winning whiskies.

SD   CP   E   RF
C   S   WC   L

DUNKELD
Situated by river Tay and almost destroyed in the Battle of Dunkeld in 1689. The little houses lining Cathedral Street were the first to be rebuilt. Ruins of a C14th cathedral can be seen.

TOURIST INFORMATION CENTRE
The Cross, Dunkeld PH8 0AN
Tel/Fax: (01350) 727688

ATTRACTIONS
THE HERMITAGE (NT for S)
11 The Cross, Dunkeld PH8 0AN
Tel: (01350) 728641
A designed landscape with a woodland walk leading to St. Ossian's Hall, an C18th folly overlooking the dramatic Falls of Braan.
Disabled badge holders park at Ossian's Hall by going from the car park through an unlocked barrier behind the main notice board and following the track for 0.25 mile.

CP

BI ARTS COMMUNITY & BEATRIX POTTER EXHIBITION
Station Road, Birnam by Dunkeld PH8 0DS
Tel: (01350) 727674 Fax: (01350) 727748
e-mail: admin@birnaminstitute.com
www.birnaminstitute.com
Fascinating permanent Beatrix Potter and monthly changing art exhibition. It was here that Beatrix Potter found the inspiration for the Peter Rabbit stories.

SD CP L RF
C S WC

LOCH OF THE LOWES VISITOR CENTRE
Scottish Wildlife Trust, Dunkeld PH8 0HH
Tel/Fax: (01350) 727337
e-mail: lochlowes@swt.org.uk
www.swt.org.uk
Star attraction from early April until late August is a pair of breeding ospreys. These and other species can be seen from the observation Hide. Otters, deer and wildfowl can also be seen. Fascinating wildlife exhibition at Visitor Centre.
N.B. Upper hide not accessible, but lower is fine with wide door and wheelchair space. The Visitor Centre has two entrance doors of 75 and 79cm, but have four steps Staff will open side entrance to rear of Visitor Centre and to lower hide with small gradient path.

SD   CP   E   RF
S   WC

FORGANDENNY
Located in the River Earn valley, a few miles from Perth, lying within a short distance of an ancient Roman road connecting a string of outposts, forts and camps along the valley.

BED AND BREAKFAST
BATTLEDOWN BED AND BREAKFAST
Battledown, Forgandenny PH2 9EL
Tel/Fax: (01738) 812471
e-mail: ian@battledown34.freesave.co.uk
No. of Accessible Rooms: 1
Accessible Facilities: Lounge, Dining Room.
Late C18th cottage that once belonged to the village baker. Set in a mature garden with trees and shrubs, including rare rowans. Secluded and sheltered in an old part of Forgandenny village that was on the stage route from Perth until early this century.

KILLIN
Charming little village dominated by Ben Lawers. The river Dochart runs through the centre with much photographed scenic falls.

HOTEL
DALL LODGE COUNTRY HOUSE HOTEL
Main Street, Killin FK21 8TN
Tel: (01567) 820217   Fax: (01567) 820726
e-mail: wilson@dalllodgehotel.co.uk
www.dalllodgehotel.co.uk
No. of Accessible Rooms: 1. Bath
Accessible Facilities: Lounge, Restaurant.
Country house hotel at the head of Loch
Tay.

SELF-CATERING
THE SHIELING
Aberfeldy Road, Killin FK21 8TX
Tel/Fax: (01567) 820334
No. of Accessible Units: 3. Bath
No. of Beds per Unit: 1-4
Accessible Facilities: Lounge, Kitchen,
Verandah with patio furniture, barbecue.
Log cabins and chalets (accessible) situated
adjacent to woodland and overlooks rolling
hills at west end of Loch Tay. Located on
the north (A827) side of Loch Tay, close to
Killin Golf Course.

KINROSS
Located at the south entrance to
Tayside, with fine C17th tolbooth.

HEART OF SCOTLAND
TOURIST INFORMATION CENTRE
Service Area, J.6, M90 Kinross
Tel: (01577) 863680   Fax: (01577) 863370

HOTELS
LOMOND COUNTRY INN
Main Street, Kinneswood,
Kinross KY13 9HN
Tel: (01592) 840253   Fax: (01592) 840 693
e-mail: info@lomandcountryinn.com
www.lomandcountryinn.com
No. of Accessible Rooms: 1
Accessible Facilities: Lounge, Restaurant
Charming, small hotel lying in the slopes
of the Lomond Hills, overlooking Loch
Lomond in a small village, with wonderful
Loch views. Good base for touring.

Pitlochry boat station.

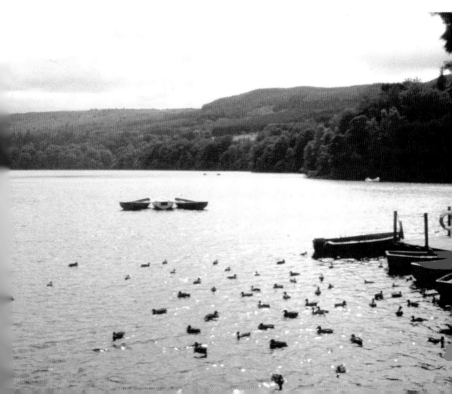

WINDLESTRAE HOTEL
The Muirs, Kinross KY13 8AS
Tel: (01577) 863217   Fax: (01577) 864733
No. of Accessible Rooms: 2. Bath
Accessible Facilities: Lounge, Restaurant (3 steps). Attractive hacienda style frontage leads into this rather cosy 45-roomed property, located close to M90 (J6).

ATTRACTION
KINROSS HOUSE GARDENS
Kinross KY13 8ET
Tel: (01577) 862900
C17th house, not open to the public, but lovely formal gardens with yew, roses and herbaceous borders to view.

SD   CP   E   RFE

PERTH
Once the capital of medieval Scotland with wonderful historic buildings remaining – the Fair Maid's House c1600, on North Park, is the oldest in town. The River Tay runs through the centre. John Knott preached his fiery sermons here in the Church of St. John in 1559.

TOURIST INFORMATION CENTRE
(01738) 450600

NATIONAL TRAVELINE
Tel: (0870) 6082608

PERTH AND KINROSS COUNCIL
Recreation/Outdoor Divisions
3-5 High Street, Perth PH1 5JS
Tel: (01738) 475200   Fax: (01738) 441690

Arts and Heritage Division
George Street, Perth , PH1 5LB
Tel: (01738) 632488   Fax: (01738) 443505

BUSES
Tel: (0870) 602608 (ask for Traffic Manager). Service 1 and 2 are wheelchair accessible and run every 12 minutes.

TAXIS
A & M King Taxis: Tel: (01738) 622255
Fully equipped but advisable to book.

TRAINS
Scotrail: Tel: for special assistance
(0845) 6057021

GNER: Special Needs Tel: (0845) 7225444
Wheelchair spaces in first and standard class trains, advisable to book. One space in each with straps. Perth station has no wheelchair unassisted access but there are ramps and staff assistance when notified 24 hours in advance.

HOTEL
SUNBANK HOUSE HOTEL
50 Dundee Road, Perth PH2 7BA
Tel: (01738) 624882   Fax: (01738) 442515
No. of Accessible Rooms: 3
Accessible Facilities: Lounge, Restaurant. Small hotel close to city centre.

SPORTING VENUE
THE PERTH HUNT
Perth Racecourse, Scone Palace Park, Perth
Tel: (01738) 551597   Fax: (01738) 553021
Complies with Part M, Building Regulations.

CP 🦽   RE 🦽   ED 🦽   INT 🦽

WC 🦽 (2 adapted WC's on ground level of public enclosure)

SS 🦽 Route from main entrance around paddock to racecourse on rails – good viewing. 6 spaces

B 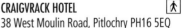 (ground floor)

PITLOCHRY
One of Queen Victoria's favourite European resorts, the town is surrounded by the pine-covered hills of the central Highlands. A busy town with good shops and restaurants along its main street.

TOURIST INFORMATION CENTRE
22 Atholl Road, Pitlochry PH16 5BX
Tel: (01796) 472215   Fax: (01796) 474046

HOTELS
CRAIGVRACK HOTEL
38 West Moulin Road, Pitlochry PH16 5EQ
Tel: (01796) 472399   Fax: (01796) 473990
No. of Accessible Rooms: 2
Accessible Facilities: Lounge, Restaurant
Comfortable holiday hotel, with elevation

located beside Braemar Road and fine views over surrounding wooded hills.

BED AND BREAKFAST
BALLINDUIN BOTHY

Strathtay, by Pitlochry PH9 0LP
Tel: (01887) 840275   Fax: (01887) 840275
No. of Accessible Rooms: 3
Accessible Facilities: Lounge, Dining Room, Garden. Converted farm buildings, quiet, with lovely views of wildlife and birds.

ATTRACTIONS
BLAIR ATHOLL DISTILLERY VISITOR CENTRE
Perth Road, Pitlochry PH16 5LY
Tel: (01796) 482003   Fax: (01796) 482001
By 1579 whisky making took so much barley that food supplies were threatened. Sadly, much of the actual tour of this Bells-owned distillery is inaccessible, but join in beneath the stills room and continue to the bonded warehouse with rolling stock of 15 million litres. Blair Atholl, 12 year old malt is produced here. Home of Bells Whisky. There is a ramp to the whisky tasting room. Special tutored tastings can be arranged. The distillery is part of the Diago Group with a choice of 27 malts available.

SD 🦽   CP 🧍   E 🦽   RF 🦽
C 🦽   S 🦽   WC 🧍

BLAIR CASTLE
Blair Atholl, Pitlochry PH18 5TL
Tel: (01796) 481207   Fax: (01796) 431487
www.blair-castle.co.uk
Scotland's most visited privately owned home of the Dukes of Atholl with 30 fully furnished rooms of beautiful furniture, a fine collection of paintings, armour, china, lace and embroidery displays. Extensive parklands, deer park, highland cattle, picnic area and nature trail in the grounds.

SD 🦽   CP 🦽   E 🦽   RF 🦽
C 🦽   S 🦽   WC 🧍   RFE 🦽

EDRADOUR DISTILLERY
Pitlochry PH16 5JP
Tel: (01796) 472095   Fax: (01796) 472002
Scotland's smallest distillery producing a handmade malt in limited quantity. Enjoy a wee dram in the Malt Barn where the history and whisky maker's art will be revealed, and then tour the distillery.

SD 🦽   CP 🧍   E 🦽   C n/a
RF 🦽   S 🦽   WC 🧍   RFE 🧍

GLENGOULANDIE DEER PARK
Glengoulandie, Foss, by Pitlochry PH15 5NL
Tel/Fax: (01887) 820272
Drive-through park with herds of red deer and cattle and numerous native birds and animals in natural surroundings.

S 🧍   WC 🧍

PITLOCHRY ANGLING CLUB
Sunnknowe, 7 Nursing Home Brae, Pitlochry PH16 5HP
Tel: (01796) 472 484
Fly fishing for trout and grayling on Loch Kindardochy. Information and permits available in local tackle shops. Parking 50m up the slope from the lochside. There is provision on one loch for a boat with an accessible seat for boat fishing. Booking is necessary.

PITLOCHRY BOATING STATION
Loch Faskally, Cluniebridge Road, Pitlochry
Tel: (01796) 472919
Charming spot on lovely loch with coffee shop and picnic facilities, boats and ducks.

CP 🦽   E 🦽   RF 🦽
C 🦽   S 🦽   EC 🦽

STANLEY
River Tay runs close to the village of Stanley that is close to Perth, Dunkeld, Blairgowrie and Pitlochry.

BALLATHIE HOUSE HOTEL

Kinclaven, by Stanley PH1 4QN
Tel: (01250) 883268   Fax: (01250) 883396
No. of Accessible Rooms: 2, 1 being a suite. Twin-shower: Suite-Spa bath. Accessible Facilities: Lounge, Restaurant Lovely country house in a delightful location overlooking River Tay.

REGION 6

GRAMPIAN HIGHLANDS, ABERDEEN & NORTH EAST COAST

ABERDEEN

Maritime city and one-time royal burgh, the sea is the essence of this city, where gas and oil, rather than fish, are now paramount. It has a distinctive townscape formed by the many buildings of locally quarried silver granite used since the C18th to shape the town, hence it is known as the granite city. There are many shopping malls, and continuous floral displays in the gardens of Duthies Park and other city parks. The university was founded here in 1494. 3km of sands between the mouths of the rivers Dee and Donn maintain its seaside town appeal.

TOURIST INFORMATION CENTRE

Aberdeen and Grampian Tourist Board,
27 Albyn Place, Aberdeen AB10 1DE
Tel: (01224) 288828
Fax: (01224) 581367
e-mail: info@castlesandwhisky.com
www.agtb.org

ABERDEENSHIRE CITY COUNCIL

Transport Department, Woodhill House,
Westburn Road,
Aberdeen AB16 5GB
Tel: (01224) 664580

BUSES

Freepark Community Service:
Tel: (01224) 680100.
4 minibuses with straps and ramps.
(Ronnie Devlin-Transport).
J.W.Coaches: Tel: (01330) 823300

TAXICARD OPERATORS LIST

Tel: (01224) 665566
Bluebird: Tel: (01224) 212266

Campbell Cars: Tel: (01224) 625444
Fyvie Taxis: Tel: (01224) 890937
Brian L Hay: Tel: (07802) 447202
Rainbow-City: Tel: (01224) 494949 or 878787

TRAINS

Scotrail: Telephone for disabled Assistance:
(0845) 6057021

GNER - Telephone for Special Needs:
(08457) 225444
Minicom: (0191) 2330173
Wheelchair space in first and standard class. Assistance at station when booked in advance. Aberdeen Station offers staff assistance and ramps available.

SHOPMOBILITY

Flourmill Lane Car Park, Flour Mill Lane,
Aberdeen AB10 1AG
Tel/Minicom: (01224) 630009
Fax: (01224) 640741

HOTELS

MARCLIFFE at PITFODELS
North Deeside Road, Aberdeen AB15 9YA
Tel: (01224) 861000   Fax: (01224) 868860
e-mail: reservations@marcliffe.com
No. of Accessible Rooms: 1
Accessible Facilities: Lounge, Restaurant.
Country hotel in the city, 20 minutes from airport. Dining room under glass.

SPEEDBIRD INNS
Aberdeen Airport, Argyll Road, Dyce,
Aberdeen AB21 0AF
Tel: (01224) 772884   Fax: (01224) 772560
No. of Accessible Rooms: 3
Accessible Facilities: Lounge, Restaurant.
Comfortable, modern airport hotel.

THISTLE ABERDEEN AIRPORT
Argyll Road, Dyce, Aberdeen AB21 0AF
Tel: (01224) 725252   Fax: (01224) 723745
No. of Accessible Rooms: 1
Accessible Facilities: Lounge, Restaurant.
Quality hotel located adjacent to the airport, just off the A96 with rail station.
Nine miles, 15 minutes' drive, to the city centre.

THISTLE ABERDEEN ALTENS
Souterhead Road, Aberdeen AB12 3LF

Tel: (01224) 877000   Fax: (01224) 896964
No. of Accessible Rooms: 1.
Accessible Facilities; Lounge, Restaurant
Located in the south of the city close to the
Altens Industrial Estate, popular with
visiting businessmen.

BRITANNIA HOTEL ABERDEEN
Malcolm Road, Bucksburn, Aberdeen AB21 9LN
Tel: (01224) 409988   Fax: (01224) 714020
No. of Accessible Rooms: 1.
Accessible Facilities: Restaurant, Bar.
Modern business hotel in north-west suburb.

ATTRACTIONS
ABERDEEN MARITIME MUSEUM
Shiprow, Aberdeen AB11 5BY
Tel: (01224) 337700   Fax: (01224) 213066
Housed in the city's oldest building (1593)
explore the history of the North Sea with
exciting exhibitions and multi-media displays
about the offshore oil industry, shipbuilding,
fishing and the story of Aberdeen harbour.
Centrepiece is the 8.5m high model of the
Murchison oil platform.

SD	CP n/a	E	L
C	S	WC	

CRUIKSHANK BOTANIC GARDENS
University of Aberdeen, Dept. of Plant and
Soil Sciences, St. Machar Drive,
Aberdeen AB24 3UU
Tel: (01224) 272704   Fax: (01224) 272703
The majority of the garden is level,
although some areas are grass and will
present some difficulty. 11 acres of rock
gardens, rose garden, herbaceous borders,
arboretum and patio garden.

CP (call in advance)	E	RF n/a
C n/a	S n/a	WC n/a

GORDON HIGHLANDERS MUSEUM
St. Lukes, Viewfield Road, Aberdeen AB15 7XH
Tel: (01224) 311200   Fax: (01224) 319323
e-mail: museum@gordonhighlanders.com
Story of this famous regiment which spans
200 years of world history, with interactive
displays, a unique collection of regimental
treasures, an AV theatre and detailed life-
size and scale reproductions of some of the
regiment's finest moments in battle.

SD n/a	CP	E	RF
C	S	WC	

BALLATER
Queen Victoria purchased Balmoral
Estate in 1852 and the it has been the
summer home of The Royal Family ever
since. Ballater is an old Deeside railway
town, almost 250m above sea level
with an impressive backdrop of forest
and mountain. Many of the shops have
royal warrants. It developed in the
C19th as a spa town, its waters
reputedly good for curing tuberculosis.

BALLATER ROYAL DEESIDE TOURISM
36 Golf Road, Ballater AB35 5RS
Tel: (013397) 55467   Fax: (013397) 55283
e-mail: ballaterroyaldeeside@compuserve.com
www.royal-deeside.org.uk

TOURIST INFORMATION CENTRE
The Old Royal Station, Station Square, Ballater
Tel: (013397) 55306

HOTEL
DARROCH LEARG HOTEL
Braemar Road, Ballater AB35 5UX
Tel: (013397) 55443   Fax: (013397) 55252
e-mail: nigel@darroch-learg.demon.co.uk
No. of Accessible Rooms: 1
Accessible Facilities: Lounge, Restaurant
Family run hotel built in 1888 as a
comfortable residence in Royal Deeside. It
became a hotel about 50 years ago. It is
set in four acres of wooded grounds on
the slopes of Craigendarroch. Located high
above Ballater with fine views of the
Grampians across the Dee Valley.

ATTRACTION
BALMORAL ESTATES
The Estate Office, Balmoral, Ballater AB35 5TB
Tel: (013397) 42334   Fax: (013397) 42034
e-mail: info@balmoralcastle.com
www.balmoralcastle.com
The castle is closed to the public, except
for the ballroom. Carriage hall exhibitions
are accessible with exhibitions of carriages,
commemorative china, plus wildlife display
in natural habitat. The three-acre gardens
contain a range of glasshouses and a
conservatory, plus a large kitchen garden
and a water garden created by the Duke of

339

Edinburgh. The garden cottage, where Queen Victoria used to write her diaries that was rebuilt in 1895, is not open to the public, but one can peek through the windows to view the unchanged interior.

SD n/a   CP 👨‍🦽   E ♿   RF ♿
C ♿   S 👨‍🦽   WC 🧍   RFE ♿

BALLINDALLOCH
Situated on a spur of the Speyside Way where the Glenlivet Estate is part of the Crown Estate.

SELF-CATERING
TORVUE COTTAGE   🧍
Achnascraw Farm, Braes of Glenlivet, Ballindalloch AB37 9JT
Tel: (01807) 590256
No. of Accessible Units: 1. Bath
No. of Beds per Unit: 5
Accessible Facilities: Lounge, Kitchen. Step from outside into porch and porch into kitchen. Modern bungalow with expansive views onto surrounding hills in peaceful, scenic countryside of secluded Braes of Glenlivet. 6 miles from Tomintoul.

ATTRACTION
GLENLIVET DISTILLERY VISITOR CENTRE
Glenlivet, Ballindalloch AB37 9DB
Tel: (01542) 783220   Fax: (01542) 783218
200 years ago, whisky was closely bound up in the lives of every family in the glen of the Livet. This whisky, favoured by aristocracy and royalty, can be made only in this single spot. An exhibition explores the turbulent history of whisky smugglers, teaches the intriguing mysteries of distilling and of course you must sample this true spirit of Scotland.

SD ♿   CP ♿   E ♿   RF ♿   L ♿
C ♿   S ♿   WC 🧍   RFE ♿

BANCHORY
Holiday town of elegant buildings with excellent salmon fishing on river Dee and trout on river Fengh.

TOURIST INFORMATION CENTRE
Bridge Street, Banchory
Tel: (01330) 822000

ATTRACTION
CRATHES CASTLE AND GARDENS
Banchory AB31 5QJ
Tel: (01330) 844525   Fax: (01330) 844797
Impressive C16th castle only accessible on the ground floor. Walled garden of three acres with unusual plants, and seven other gardens, extensive grounds and a disabled nature trail. Lower level of gardens only is accessible.

SD ♿   CP 🧍   RF ♿   C 🧍
S 🧍   WC 🧍   G 👨‍🦽

BUCKIE
One of the largest of the Moray towns, extending along three miles of coastline, its principal industry is fishing. The Fish Market operates daily with harbour particularly full of boats on Friday nights. Good bird watching along shore.

ATTRACTION
THE BUCKIE DRIFTER
MARITIME HERITAGE CENTRE
Freuchny Road, Buckie AB56 1TT
Tel: (01542) 834646   Fax: (01542) 835995
History of the herring-boom years in the Moray area during the 1890s and 1930s. Active participation includes finding out how to catch herring and packing fish in a barrel, plus hands-on displays and changing exhibits.

SD ♿   CP 👨‍🦽   E ♿   L ♿
C ♿   S ♿   WC 🧍   RFE ♿

CRAIGELLACHIE
ATTRACTION
SPEYSIDE COOPERAGE VISITOR CENTRE
Dufftown Road, Craigellachie, Aberlour AB38 9RS
Tel: (01340) 871108   Fax: (01340) 881437
e-mail: info@speyside-coopers.demon.co.uk
www.speysidecooperage.com
Unique "Acorn to Cask" exhibition with different skilled coopers practising ancient craft, repairing cask for the maturation of

different whiskies. Exhibition includes Victorian cooperage with life size models, speaking in local dialect.

SD   CP   E   L n/a
C   S   WC

N.B. Entrance is ramped at 1:10.

DUFFTOWN
On the malt whisky trail.

TOURIST INFORMATION CENTRE
The Clock Tower, The Square, Dufftown
Tel: (01340) 820501

ATTRACTION
THE GLENFIDDICH DISTILLERY
William Grant & Sons Ltd.,
Dufftown AB55 4DH
Tel: (01340) 820373   Fax: (01340) 822083
Founded in 1887 by William Grant this remains a family firm. View the stages of the whisky-making process and sample the finished product! Audio-visual display of the history and manufacture of whisky. Tasting takes place in the original malt barn which houses various interesting artifacts from the distillery's history.

SD   CP   E   RF
C   S   WC   RFE

ELGIN
Major town of Moray, famous as Scotland's malt whisky country. Retains its medieval layout with a cobbled market place and narrow lanes and the ruins of a C13th. cathedral. There are some C18th buildings with original arched facades.

TOURIST BOARD
17 High Street, Elgin IV30 1EG
Tel: (01343) 543388   Fax: (01343) 552982

SELF-CATERING
CARDEN SELF-CATERING
The Old Steading, Carden, Alves, Elgin,
Moray IV30 8UP
Tel: (01343) 850222   Fax: (01343) 850626
e-mail: smooth @carden.co.uk

www.carden.co.uk
No. of Accessible Units: 2, Bothy and Stables, both with Roll-in Showers.
No. of Beds per Unit: 2
Accessible Facilities: Open plan Lounge/Diner/Kitchen, Courtyard patio. Two of six courtyard cottages created from the original C18th farm steading. Open views of surrounding countryside with the hills of distant Sutherland visible over the Moray Firth to the north and farmland views to the south.

ATTRACTION
PLUSCARDEN ABBEY
Elgin IV30 8UA
Tel: (01343) 890257   Fax: (01343) 890258
Monastery founded in 1230, burnt down and restored in C14th and C19th. Once more it is a religious community. All services are open to the public, with Gregorian chant. Beeswax polish and natural apiary remedies can be purchased.

SD   CP   E   RF
S   WC   RFE

FORRES
Renouned for its many beautiful green parks, Forres has been an established settlement for at least 2000 years. See the topiary gardens in Grant Park, and Nelson's Tower that overlooks the town. It was built in 1806 to celebrate victory at Trafalgar. Easy access to the Moray Firth.

TOURIST INFORMATION CENTRE
116 High Street, Forres, IV30 0NP
Tel: (01309) 672938

ATTRACTION
BRODIE CASTLE (NT for S), Brodie, Forres
Tel: (01309) 641371
Owned and lived in by the Brodie family since 1160, this gabled castle offers fine furniture and a collection of C17th Dutch art, C19th English watercolours and French impressionists. Lovely grounds. Wheelchairs available for loan, and a wheelchair lift to the first floor but you have to book the support for this lift in advance.

SD   CP  E C S

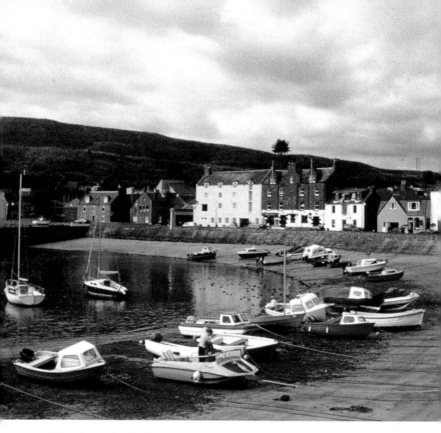

Stonehaven harbour

THE FALCONER MUSEUM
Tolbooth Street, Forres, IV36 1PH
Tel: (01309) 673701 Fax: (01309) 675863
e-mail: museums@moray.gov.uk
www.moray.org/museums
Delightful local museum containing a
treasure of Moray's heritage. N.B. Only
the ground floor is accessible.

SD   E   S

INVERURIE
Thriving market town and centre of
castle country with easy access to the
whisky trail. Progressive agricultural
centre with auctions daily.

TOURIST INFORMATION CENTRE
18 High Street, Inverurie AB51 3XQ
Tel: (01467) 625800

HOTEL
STRATHBURN HOTEL
Burghmuir Drive, Inverurie AB51 4GY

Tel: (01467) 624422   Fax: (01467) 625133
No. of Accessible Rooms: 2
Accessible Facilities: Lounge, Restaurant.
Built by the present owners in 1985, and
gradually extended to 25 rooms, this
pleasant property is located just off the
main A96 Aberdeen/Inverness road
overlooking Strathburn Park. 10 miles from
Aberdeen Airport.

KEITH
Fine 1830 catholic church and Auld
Brig. Built in 1609, it is among the
oldest bridges in Scotland.

SELF-CATERING
PARKHEAD COTTAGES
Drummuir, Keith, Banffshire AB55 5PQ
Tel/Fax: (01466) 794017
e-mail: LinCollins@tesco.net
No. of Accessible Units: 2. Roll-in Shower
No. of Beds per Unit: 6
Accessible Facilities: Open-plan living,

Dining, kitchen. Specially designed for both disabled and able-bodied holidaymakers, both cottages are double glazed and have electric central heating available if required. They also have other features which will suit most disabilities. Hospital beds are available for Garden Cottage but please book in advance. They are single storey detached stone houses set in well planted gardens in a secluded valley in the Grampian mountains midway between Dufftown and Keith.

MACDUFF

Former spa town and still a busy fishing and boat-building centre, looking out across the Moray Firth.

ATTRACTION
MACDUFF MARINE AQUARIUM
11 High Shore, Macduff AB44 1SL
Tel: (01261) 833369   Fax: (01261) 831052
e-mail: macduffaquarium@marine-aquarium.com
www.marine-aquarium.com
Offers a unique centrepiece display tank open to the sky in which a Moray firth kelp reef thrives, complete with kelp and other seaweeds and a whole community of fish – don't miss the divers feeding the fish.

SD ♿   CP ♿   E ♿   RF ♿
S ♿   WC ♿   RFE ♿

PETERHEAD

Famous for its harbour, fish-market and prison, it is the busiest whitefish port in Europe, its harbour is full of trawlers.

ATTRACTION
ABERDEENSHIRE FARMING MUSEUM
Aden Country Park, Mintlaw,
Peterhead AB42 5FQ
Tel: (01771) 622906   Fax: (01771) 622884
e-mail: heritage@aberdeenshire.gov.uk
Unique semi-circular steading surrounded by the beautiful woodlands of Aden Country Park, bringing alive the story of this region's farming history. There are three related interpretative themes: the Aden Estate Story: Well Worked Ground,

farming from 1780s to present day: and thirdly a video on the newly reconstructed Hareshowe Working Farm.

SD ♿   CP 🚶   E ♿   RF 🚶
C ♿   S 🚶   WC 🚶

PETERHEAD MARITIME HERITAGE
The Lido, South Road, Peterhead AB42 2UP
Tel/Fax: (01779) 473000
e-mail: itstrachan.er@aberdeenshire.gov.uk
The story of Peterhead's seafaring history told through an AV presentation, touch-screen computers and other displays, including period kitchen and tableaux of shipbuilding. Set by the shore of the Harbour of Refuge on south side of town, this is a fascinating visit.

SD ♿   CP ♿   E ♿   RF ♿
C ♿   S ♿   WC 🚶

STONEHAVEN

Holiday resort with lovely pebble and sand beach reached from the central Allardice Street. Oldest part of town is the charming little harbour, where Tolbooth Museum is to be found.

TOURIST INFORMATION CENTRE
66 Allardice Street, Stonehaven, AB39 2AA
Tel: (01569) 762806

ATTRACTION
TOLBOOTH MUSEUM
Old Pier, Stonehaven, Kincardineshire
Tel: (01771) 622906   Fax: (01771) 622884
e-mail: heritage@aberdeenshire.gov.uk
Stonehaven's oldest building – the Earl Marischal's C16th storehouse – served as the County Tolbooth from 1600-1767. Episcopal priests imprisoned here in 1748.

SD ♿   CP 🚶   E ♿   S ♿

TOMINTOUL

On the Glenlivet Estate, one of the highest villages in Britain and the highest north of the Highland line. Planned and laid out by the 4th Duke of Gordon in 1776.

TOURIST INFORMATION CENTRE
TOMINTOUL and GLENLIVET
HIGHLAND HOLIDAYS
The Square, Tomintoul AB37 9ET
Tel: (01807) 580285

ATTRACTION
TOMINTOUL MUSEUM
The Square, Tomintoul AB37 9ET
Tel: (01309) 673701   Fax: (01309) 675863
e-mail: museums@moray.gov.uk
Displays on local wildlife, history of the
town and local skiing industry with
reconstructed crofters kitchen and smithy.

SD   CP   E   S

TURRIFF
Historic town situated at confluence
of the Idoch Water and River
Deveron, and once a capital of the
Picts. The Old Church was built in
C11th and in 1179 the Knights
Templar were given land here. One of
the main centres of the Covenanter
Rebellion of mid C17th. Today Turriff
is a thriving community and a main
shopping centre for surrounding
farmlands.

SELF-CATERING
ELMWOOD
Delgatie Castle Estates Trust, Delgatie Castle,
Turriff AB53 8ED
Tel/Fax: (01888) 563479
No. of Accessible Units: 1
No. of Beds per Unit: 4 - 7
Accessible Facilities: Lounge, Dining Room,
Kitchen. North wing in C11th castle. One
of five houses in the grounds, Elmwood
has been adapted downstairs to
accommodate disabled people and has
accommodation for seven people with a
double bedroom downstairs along with
shower room and toilet. Very spacious
sitting room with large picture window.
The kitchen is very large and has lovely
views from the window. Delgatie was a
private home and has fine painted
ceilings, paintings, and furniture in a
parkland setting.

The coastline around Brora is magical.

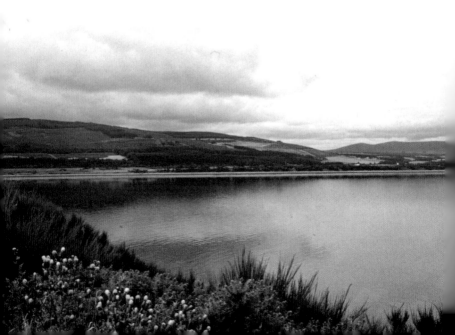

REGION 7
THE HIGHLANDS AND SKYE

ACHNASHEEN
Located just east of Loch a'Chroisg on the road to Torridon.

HOTELS
LOCH TORRIDON HOTEL   [&]
By Achnasheen IV22 2EY
Tel: (01445) 791242   Fax: (01445) 791296
e-mail: stay@lochtorridonhotel.com
www.lochtorridonhotel.com
No. of Accessible Rooms: 19
Accessible Facilities: Lounge, Restaurant
Former shooting lodge at the foot of the Torridon Mountains, on the shores of Loch Torridon.

LOCH MAREE HOTEL   [大]
Talladale, Loch Maree, by Achnasheen IV22 2HN
Tel: (01445) 760288   Fax: (01445) 760241
No. of Accessible Rooms: 2
Accessible Facilities: Lounge, Restaurant, Bar. Built in 1872 in superb scenery on Loch Maree, its restaurant is supplied daily by the fishing fleet of Gairloch.

AVIEMORE
Originally a small village, now the region's commercial centre. Its location in the foothills of the Cairngorm mountains means many concrete blocks accommodate tourists, particularly in the ski season, when buses transport visitors to ski area 13km away.

TOURIST INFORMATION CENTRE
Grampian Road, Aviemore PH22 1PT
Tel: (01479) 810363   Fax: (01479) 811063

SELF-CATERING
SILVERGLADES HOLIDAY HOMES   [大&]
Dalnaby, Aviemore PH22 1TD
Tel: (01479) 810165   Fax: (01479) 811246

No. of Accessible Units: 1
No. of Beds per Unit: 1 - 6
Accessible Facilities: Lounge/Diner, Room, Kitchen. The Macdui unit is one of six chalet-style units here, situated at the foot of the Cairngorms, surrounded by glorious scenery.

PINE BANK CHALETS   [大]
Shieling Apartment,
Dalfaber Road, Aviemore PH22 1PX
Tel: (01479) 810000   Fax: (01479) 811469
e-mail: pinebank@ntlworld.com
www.pinebankchalets.co.uk
No. of Accessible Units: 1
No. of Beds per Unit: 5
Accessible Facilities: Lounge, Kitchen
Chalets and apartments in lovely riverside location close to Aviemore village. Craigellachie Hill and nature reserve behind and Cairngorm Mountains in front.

BALLACHULISH
Located on Loch Linnhe, very close to Glencoe with fantastic scenery surrounding the Loch.

TOURIST INFORMATION CENTRE
Albert Road, Ballachulish PA39 4JR
Tel: (01855) 811866   Fax: (01855) 811720

HOTELS
THE ISLES OF GLENCOE HOTEL and
LEISURE CENTRE   [&]
Ballachulish PA39 4HL
Tel: (01855) 811602   Fax: (01855) 811770
No. of Accessible Rooms: 2
Accessible Facilities: Lounge, Restaurant. Located 250m from the village centre on Loch Leven, one is almost afloat! Set on an highland estate with two harbours and 3kms of water frontage and spectacular views.

BALLACHULISH HOTEL   [大&]
Ballachulish PA38 4YJ
Tel: (01855) 821582   Fax: (01855) 821463
e-mail: reservations@freedomglen.co.uk
www.freedomglen.co.uk
No. of Accessible Rooms: 1

345

Accessible Facilities: Lounge, Restaurant
One of Scotland's oldest and best known
hotels in fine lochside location.

BEAULY

Charming village with good range of
shops, restaurants, hotels, pubs, a craft
centre and ruins of C13th priory.
Established centre for salmon and
brown trout fishing and for Campbells
world famous wool shop.

SELF-CATERING

DUNSMORE LODGES   [♿]
Farley, by Beauly IV4 7EY
Tel: (01463) 782424   Fax: (01463) 782839
e-mail: inghammar@dunsmorelodges.co.uk
www.dunsmorelodges.co.uk
No. of Accessible Units: 1
No. of Beds per Unit: 3
Accessible Facilities: Open Plan
Lounge/Kitchen/Diner/BBQ/Wood burner
Scandinavian lodges, with Dornie being
accessible. Situated on two wooded
hillside sites, 0.25 mile apart, 100-300m.
above the Beauly river with great views of
hills and mountains. Four miles from
Beauly.

BRORA

Rather charming small town with
lovely beaches around Kintradwell Bay
and salmon and trout fishing on River
Brora. A good base for touring this
part of the north east.

BED AND BREAKFAST

GLENAVERON   [♿]
Golf Road, Brora, Sutherland KW9 6QS
Tel/Fax: (01408) 621601
e-mail: glenaveron@hotmail.com
www.glenaveron.co.uk
No. of Accessible Rooms: 1. Shower (slight
ramp).
Accessible Facilities: Lounge, Dining Room,
Gardens. Absolutely charming old stone
house built in 1904 in mature gardens.
Very spacious interior with warm
ambience, pine and oak furnishings and a

family atmosphere. One of our most
impressive visits.

CULLODEN

Desolate stretch of moorland, 6km east
of Inverness, looking as it did in April
1746.

ATTRACTION

CULLODEN BATTLEFIELD (NT for S)
Culloden Moor Visitor Centre, Culloden Moor,
Inverness IV2 5EU
Tel: (01463) 790607   Fax: (01463) 794294
www.nts.org.uk/culloden
Site of the last battle fought on mainland
Britain on 16 April 1746 when Bonny
Prince Charles Edward Stuart's army was
routed by the Duke Butcher of
Cumberland. The battlefield has been
restored to its state on that day. Visitor
Centre with Jacobite exhibition and audio-
visual show. Audio visual auditorium has
wide doors and ground level space for
wheelchairs. Electric scooter and manual
wheelchair available. Rough nature of the
site and its size means that those in
wheelchairs and the less-able may find it
tiring to go round the whole site.

SD [♿]	CP [♿]	E [♿]	RF [♿]
C [♿]	WC [♿]	RFE [♿]	S [♿]

DINGWALL

Established by Victorian penchant for
the Highlands, Dingwall is the main
centre for the region, and birthplace of
Macbeth.

HOTEL

KINKELL HOUSE HOTEL   [♿]
Easter Kinkell, Conon Bridge,
By Dingwall IV7 8HY
Tel: (01349) 861270   Fax: (01349) 865902
No. of accessible Rooms: 1
Accessible Facilities: Lounge, Restaurant
Small country house hotel in own grounds
surrounded by trees and pasture land.
Situated 10 miles north of Inverness on the
Black Isle with fine view of the Cromarty
Firth and West Ross hills.

DRUMNADROCHIT

Third of the way down Loch Ness with thriving monster mania through Monster Exhibition Centre, shops and crafts. 3km away is Urquart Castle offering good photographic access to the Loch.

HOTELS
CLUNEBEG LODGE   🦽
Clunebeg Estate, Drumnadrochit IV3 6US
Tel: (01456) 450387   Fax: (01456) 450854
No. of Accessible Rooms: 6
Accessible Facilities: Lounge, Restaurant. Comfortable modern lodge, set on quiet farm, overlooking the town by Loch Ness.

DRUMNADROCHIT HOTEL   🚶
Drumnadrochit IV63 6TU
Tel: (01456) 450202   Fax: (01456) 450793
e-mail: fraser@nessie.sol.co.uk
www.lochness.scotland.net
No. of Accessible Rooms: 1
Accessible Facilities: Dining Room/Shop with ramp. Award-winning hotel at Loch Ness with Travel Inn style rooms.

SELF-CATERING
LOCHLETTER LODGES   🦽
Balnain, Drumnadrochit,
Glenurquhart IV63 6TJ
Tel: (01456) 476313   Fax: (01456) 476301
No. of Accessible Units: 1
No. of Beds per Unit: 4 – 6
Accessible Facilities: Lounge, Kitchen, Full Disability equipment available free of charge. Glomach Lodge is one of four pine lodges situated in Glenurquhart which stretches from Loch Ness to Glen Affric. Well placed for highland touring. Located in mature birchwood with own access road.

DUNBEATH

Between Wick and Brora on the north-east coast.

ATTRACTION
LAIDHAY CROFT MUSEUM
Dunbeath KW6 6EH

Tel: (01593) 731244
Housed in a 200-year-old thatched Caithness longhouse, furnished as of 100 years ago. The visitor to Laidhay Croft can get a taste of what life was like for the C18th and C19th croft dwellers - their sparse furnishings, what they ate and drank and their spartan lifestyles. There is also a collection of early farm tools and machinery. Situated 2 miles north of Dunbeath, 18 miles south of Wick.

SD 🦽   CP 🚶   E 🚶   RF 🚶
WC 🚶   RFE 🚶

FORT GEORGE
Ardersier, by Inverness IV1 2TD
Tel: (01667) 462777

Although there has been a royal stronghold and military garrison at Inverness since C12th, Fort George dates back to 1725 when it was rebuilt and extended. It is one of the outstanding military fortifications in Europe and still an active army barracks. Within the Fort is the Regimental Museum of the Queen's own Highlanders (see below).
Many grassed areas that can be soft, but a wide path runs throughout. Battlements are accessible via a ramp.

CP 🦽 (although 200m from entrance, surface is good and slightly sloped)   E 🦽   RFE 🦽
S 🦽   WC 🚶

REGIMENTAL MUSEUM
Collection of the Queen's Own Highlanders (Cameron and Seaforth) located in the house of the former Lieutenant Governor. Fascinating displays of uniforms, medals, pictures and weaponry on three floors. Ground floor and first floor (stairlift) accessible. The second floor, dedicated to WWII, is not accessible.

FORT WILLIAM
Known for its location at the foot of Ben Nevis, this has always been a good base for touring this area of the Highlands. Stores for climbers, skiers and sightseers line the main street. Can get very busy in summer.

TOURIST INFORMATION CENTRE
Cameron Centre, Cameron Square,
Fort William PH33 6AJ
Tel: (01397) 703781   Fax: (01397) 705184

HOTELS
LODGE ON THE LOCH   ♿
Onich, by Fort William PH33 6RY
Tel: (01855) 821237
Fax: (01855) 821463
No. of Accessible Rooms: 1. Shower
Accessible Facilities: Lounge (Side
entrance), Restaurant.
Delightful country house hotel facing
south across a mile-wide bay off Loch
Linnhe, the sea loch at the south-western
end of the Great Glen. 10 miles south of
Fort William.

OLD PINES RESTAURANT WITH ROOMS ♿
Spean Bridge, by Fort William PH34 4EG
Tel: (01397) 712324   Fax: (01397) 712433
e-mail: smoothguides@oldpines.co.uk
No. of Accessible Rooms: 3
Accessible Facilities: Lounge, Restaurant
Warm family home built 20 years ago in
Scandinavian style with recent stone and
wood additions. Situated above the village
of Spean Bridge, it is set among mature
Scots Pines in 30 acres of ground with good
views across the Great Glen and Glen Spean
to Ben Nevis. Winner of 2000 Good Food
Guide, Restaurant of the Year. Legendary
Restaurant. Disabled British downhill ski
champion has been a guest here. Good
base for exploring West Highlands and
Islands. 10 miles from Fort William.

BED AND BREAKFAST
LOCHAN COTTAGE GUEST HOUSE   🚶
Lochyside, Fort William PH33 7NX
Tel: (01397) 702695
www.fortwilliam-guesthouse.co.uk
No. of Accessible Rooms: 1
Accessible Facilities: Lounge, Dining Room.
Situated in lovely gardens with panoramic
views over Ben Nevis.

SELF-CATERING
MOSSFIELD APARTMENTS   ♿
Lochyside, Fort William,
Invernesshire PH33 7NY
Tel/Fax: (01397) 703087

No. of Accessible Units: 1. Shower
No. of Beds per Unit: 2
Accessible Facilities: Lounge/Diner.
Kitchen
One of a group of seven holiday flats,
three miles from Fort William.

ATTRACTION
THE WEST HIGHLAND MUSEUM
Cameron Square, Fort William PH33 6AJ
Tel/Fax: (01397) 702169
Displays on traditional Highland life, with
Jacobite artefacts, including the famous
secret portrait of Bonnie Prince Charlie,
that looks like splash of paint but is
indeed a portrait when reflected in a
metal cylinder. N.B. Ground floor access
only for wheelchairs.
SD ♿   E ♿   RF 🚶
S 🚶 (Sales point at entrance)   WC ♿

GAIRLOCH
Traditional coastal crofting town and
holiday village, now rather tourist
conscious. The road through the
village leads to a campsite with good
views of the Torridon range and lovely
beaches.

TOURIST INFORMATION CENTRE
Achtercairn, Gairloch IV22 2DN
Tel: (01445) 712130   Fax: (01445) 712071

SELF-CATERING
WILLOW CROFT   ♿
Big Sand, Gairloch, Wester Ross
Tel: (01445) 712448
No. of Accessible Units: 1
No. of Beds per Unit: 6. Accessible
Facilities: Lounge, Dining room, Kitchen,
Sauna. Five miles from the village.

GLENCOE
Awesome scenery combines with a
savage history here with steep cliffs,
craggy peaks and the river Coe.
Famous for the Massacre of Glencoe
in 1692 in which the Glencoe
Macdonalds were betrayed and killed
by soldiers of William III.

ATTRACTION
GLENCOE & NORTH LORN FOLK MUSEUM
Glencoe PH49 4HS
Tel: (01855) 811664
Two thatched cottages in the main street
housing items relating to the Macdonalds
and Jacobite upisings, particularly the
Massacre at Glencoe.

SD   CP   E  RF
S   WC (0.25 miles from museum)

GRANTOWN-ON-SPEY
Victorian resort offering a peaceful
highland holiday with fishing and golf
popular.

TOURIST INFORMATION CENTRE
54 High Street, Grantown on Spey PH26 3EH
Tel/Fax: (01479) 872773

BED AND BREAKFAST
DUNALLAN HOUSE
Woodside Avenue,
Grantown-on-Spey PH26 3JN
Tel/Fax: (01479) 872140
e-mail: dunallan@mcmail.com
www.dunallan.mcmail.com
No. of Accessible Rooms: 1. Shower
Accessible Facilities: Lounge, Dining Room.
Lovely, traditional seven-bedroomed
Victorian villa.

KINROSS HOUSE
Woodside Avenue, Grantown-on-Spey,
Morayshire PH26 3JR
Tel: (01479) 872042   Fax: (01479) 873504
www.kinrosshouse.freeserve.co.uk
No. of Accessible Rooms: 1
Accessible Facilities: Lounge, Dining Room,
Sauna. Attractive Victorian villa, with warm
ambience, on the wooded southside of
Grantown, a good base for exploring this
part of the Highlands.

ATTRACTION
SPEYSIDE HEATHER GARDEN AND VISITOR
CENTRE
Skye of Curr, Dulnain Bridge,
by Grantown on Spey PH26 3PA
Tel: (01479) 851359   Fax: (01479) 851396
e-mail: enquiries@heathercentre.com

Heather Heritage Exhibition,
gallery/antique shop and show gardens.
Home of 'The Original Cloutie Dumpling
Restaurant'.

SD   CP   E RF
C S WC

HELMSDALE
Famous as holiday home destination of
authoress Barbara Cartland, the town
is set on craggy headland with small
harbour in north east Highlands.

ATTRACTION
TIMESPAN
Dunrobin Street, Helmsdale KW8 6JX
Tel: (01431) 821327
History of the Highlands from the Picts and
Vikings to the Highland clearances and the
oil industry. Re-creations with life-size sets,
sound effects and audio-visual material.

SD CP E L
C S WC RFE

INVERNESS
Highland capital, compact and easily
accessible centre, with unattractive
modern architecture softened by lovely
floral displays in summer. River Ness
flows through centre of the town,
which is dominated by Inverness
Castle, a Victorian red sandstone
building, now the court house.

TOURIST INFORMATION CENTRE
Castle Wynd, Inverness IV2 3BJ
Tel: (01463) 234353   Fax: (01463) 710609

BUSES
Scots City Link: Tel: (0870) 505050
2 journeys per day for local buses with
ramps and straps.

TRAINS
Scotrail: Disabled passengers no:
Tel: (0845) 6057021
Wheelchair unassisted access and ramps
available, with 24 hours' notice.

GNER – Special Needs: Tel: (0845) 7225444
Minicom: (0191) 2330173
Wheelchair space in first and standard class. Assistance available at stations if booked in advance.

SHOPMOBILITY
Eastgate Pedestrian Precinct, Inverness
Tel: (01463) 717624

HOTELS
INVERNESS MARRIOTT ♿
Culcabock Road, Inverness IV2 3LP
Tel: (01463) 237166   Fax: (01463) 225208
No. of Accessible Rooms: 2. Bath.
Accessible Facilities: Lounges, Restaurant.
(Conservatory has 4 steps). Delightful property set in 4 acres of gardens, a mile south of Inverness.

GLEN MHOR HOTEL and RESTAURANTS 🚶
9-12 Ness Bank, Inverness IV2 4SG
Tel: (01463) 234308   Fax: (01463) 713170
No. of Accessible Rooms: 2
Accessible Facilities: Lounge, 2 Restaurants.
Lovely quiet central riverside location near the historic sites.

ATTRACTIONS
STOREHOUSE OF FOULIS
Foulis Ferry Point, Easter Ross, Invernesshire IV16 9UX
Tel: (01349) 830000
Fax: (01349) 830033
e-mail: info@storehouseoffoulis.co.uk
www.storehouseoffoulis.co.uk
Opened in summer 1998, this excellent attraction, set on the shore of the Cromarty Firth, offers a fascinating history of the fully restored Girnal, which houses a series of entertaining and educational history and wildlife exhibitions. Unravel secrets of 7 centuries of land and people brought to life in Rogues Gallery theatre. Learn about the Munro Clanlands history and heritage. Fascinating Sealpoint exhibition. Outside are traditional fishing cobbles and picnic area. Located 20 minutes north of Inverness on main A9.

| CP ♿ | E ♿ | RF ♿ | C ♿ |
| S ♿ | WC ♿ | RFE ♿ | |

KINGUSSIE
Originally a weaving and spinning centre, the arrival of the railway in 1890 encouraged building of lovely Victorian homes for English families travelling to the Highlands by train. River Spey runs through the town.

TOURIST INFORMATION CENTRE
c/o Highland Folk Museum, Duke Street, Kingussie PH21 1JG
Tel: (01540) 661297

HOTEL
AVONDALE GUEST HOUSE 🚶
Newtonmore Road, Kingussie PH21 1HF
Tel: (01540) 661731
No. of Accessible Rooms: 1
Accessible Facilities: Lounge, Dining Room
Edwardian property, 5 minutes' walk from the town centre.

ATTRACTION
HIGHLAND WILDLIFE PARK
Kincraig, Kingussie PH21 1NL
Tel: (01540) 651270   Fax: (01540) 651236
e-mail: info@highlandwildlifepark.org
www.kincraig.com/wildlife
260-acre site with an amazing variety of native Scottish wildlife, visit the new Wolf Territory, herds of red deer, secretive roe deer, Highland cattle, bison, ancient breeds of sheep and Przewalski's horses, one of the world's rarest mammals. Clear driving route, although exploration on foot to themed habitats also available .

| SD ♿ | CP ♿ | E ♿ | RF ♿ |
| C ♿ | S ♿ | WC ♿ | |

HIGHLAND FOLK MUSEUM
Duke Street, Kingussie PH21 1JG
Tel: (01540) 661307   Fax: (01540) 661631
e-mail: highlandfolk@highland.gov.uk
www.highlandfolk.com
Touch, feel and smell the World of the Highlander as you walk through material remains of 400 years of Highland life from clansman to crofter. Unique collection of everyday domestic artefacts, plus countryside furniture, machinery and implements

KINLOCHLEVEN

One of the first industrial towns in the Highlands, where Scots and Irish workers constructed the Blackwater Dam. Situated at the head of Loch Leven at the foot of the Mamore Hills, with the West Highland way passing through the town.

GUEST HOUSE

TIGH-na-CHEO
Kinlochleven PA40 4SE
Tel: (01855) 831434   Fax: (01855) 831441
e-mail: reception@tighnacheo.co.uk
www.tighnacheo.co.uk
No. of Accessible Rooms: 1
Accessible Facilities: Lounge, Restaurant, Sauna. Family run delightful small hotel located between Fort William and Oban, close to Glencoe.

KINLOCHEWE

Village lying at foot of Glen Docherty, the road west from here leading into startling mountain scenery of Torridon Hills, Beinn Eighe National Nature Reserve bordered by Loch Maree and Loch Torridom, 50 miles W. of Inverness

BED AND BREAKFAST

CROMASAIG
Torridon Road, Kinlochewe IV22 2PE
Tel: (01445) 760234   Fax: (01445) 760333
e-mail: cromasaig@hotmail.com
www.cromasaig.com
No. of Accessible Rooms: 1
Accessible Facilities: Lounge, Dining Room Small family run accommodation surrounded by fine mountain scenery.

ISLE OF RAASAY

In his Hebridean Journals, Samuel Johnson recounts great tales of a stay on Raasay. Raasay is a small, close knit crofting community, who welcome visitors. With breathtaking views of Torridon peaks to the east and Cuillins of Skye to the west, Raasay is a treasure-trove for nature lovers. Wildlife, plants and archaeology are on the menu with wonderful walks for those who both wish and are able to do so.

ISLE OF RAASAY HOTEL

Raasay, by Kyle of Lochalsh,
Inverness-shire IV40 8PB
Tel/Fax: (01478) 660222
No. of Accessible Rooms: 6. Bath.
Accessible Facilities: Lounge, Restaurant. Small, family-run hotel with a blend of old and new. Modern wings have been added to the renovated old stone mansion house, with views across the glittering Narrows of Raasay to Skye. Lovely gardens. To get to Raasay, first you must get to Skye, and then by road to Sconser and from this village on Loch Sligachan you sail to Raasay. Several daily sailings (except Sundays) in each direction, duration of 15 minutes. NB No petrol on Raasay, so fill up in Broadford (Skye).

LAIDE

Situated above the shoreline of Gruinard Bay, between outflows of Little Gruinard and Inverianvie rivers.

SELF-CATERING

ROCKLEA
Little Gruinard, Laide, Wester Ross IV22 2NG
BOOK THROUGH: Mr/Mrs Gilchrist, Grassvalley Cottage, 12 Woodhall Road, Colinton, Edinburgh EH13 ODX
Tel: (0131) 441 6053   Fax: (0131) 441 4849
e-mail: aandagilchrist@onetel.net.uk
No. of Accessible Units: 1
No. of Beds per Unit: 5
Accessible Facilities: Lounge, Dining room, Kitchen. Log constructions standing in own grounds of about 5 acres. Uninterrupted outlook across bay towards Gruinard Island and beyond.

NAIRN

Refined Victorian holiday town on the shores of the Moray Firth with long sandy beaches.

TOURIST INFORMATION CENTRE
62 King Street, Nairn IV12 4DN
Tel/Fax: (01667) 452753

HOTEL
CLAYMORE HOUSE HOTEL 　&
Seabank Road, Nairn IV12 4EY
Tel: (01667) 453731　Fax: (01667) 455290
e-mail:
ClaymoreNairnScotland@compuserve.com
No. of Accessible Rooms: 1. Roll-in Shower
Accessible Facilities: Lounge, Restaurant
Quality hotel located in the centre of Nairn.

BED AND BREAKFAST
GREENLAWNS
13 Seafield Street, Nairn IV12 4HG
Tel/Fax: (01667) 452738
e-mail: greenlawns@cali.co.uk
No. of Accessible Rooms: 3
Accessible Facilities: Lounge, Dining Room, Bar. Will do packed lunch and dinner by arrangement. Large 100-year-old house restored to original Victorian past. Set in own grounds at the western end of town.

SELF-CATERING
BURNSIDE AND MILL LODGES
Raitloan, Geddes, Nairn IV12 5SA
Tel: (01667) 454635
No. of Accessible Units: 2
No. of Beds per Unit: 6
Accessible Facilities: Open plan Lounge/Diner/Kitchen, Patio (Burnside), Timber Deck (Mill).
Lovely situation in quiet wooded setting, 3 miles from Nairn.

LAIKENBUIE
Grantown Road, Nairn IV12 5QN
Tel: (01667) 454630
e-mail: muskus@bigfoot.com
No. of Accessible Units: 2
No. of Beds per Unit: 6
Accessible Facilities: Open plan Lounge, Dining Room, Kitchen.

NETHYBRIDGE

Lovely Highland village between Grantown-on-Spey and Boat of Garten.

SELF-CATERING
FHUARAIN FOREST COTTAGES
Badanfhuarain, Nethybridge,
Nr. Grantown-on-Spey PH25 3ED
Tel/Fax: (01479) 821642
e-mail: fhuarain.forestcottages@virgin.net
www.forestcottages.com
The owner writes disabled and access guides to Badenoch and Strathspey.
Flox and Badanfhuarain Cottages:
No. of Accessible Units: 2. Badanfhuarain -Roll-in shower,
Flox - Bath.
No. of Beds per Unit: 5
Accessible Facilities:
Flox: Kitchen/Dining/Living
Badanfhuarain: Kitchen, Dining/Living Room
Quite delightful C19th forest cottages with fenced gardens. Four miles from Grantown-on-Spey.

CREGGAN COTTAGE
Causer, Nethybridge.
Bookings: Speyside Holiday Cottages, 1 Chapelton Place, Forres, Moray IV36 2NL
Tel/Fax: (01309) 672505
e-mail: brian@speysidecottages.co.uk
www.speysidecottages.co.uk
No. of Accessible Units: 1. Bath
No. of Beds per Unit: 6
Accessible Facilities: Open plan Living room/Kitchen
Comfortable cottage in lovely Highland village close to river and forest, with private fenced gardens.

ATTRACTION
RSPB LOCH GARTEN OSPREY CENTRE
Forest Lodge, Abernethy Forest Reserve, Nethbridge PH25 3EF
Tel: (01479) 821409　Fax: (01479) 821069
Once widespread in the UK, egg-collectors and hunters almost wiped out the fish-eating osprey. Now, from a single pair in 1959, ospreys have returned

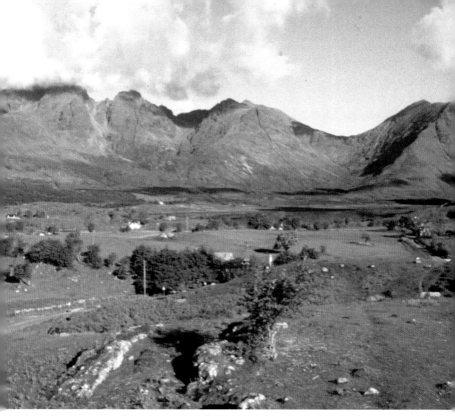

Over the sea to Skye. You can go by bridge now. It's well worth the effort.

to nest here, in trees, on the Loch and surroundings. The centre enables one to watch these superb birds of prey at close quarters. Centre located 400m from car park, use the set-down facility. Centre overlooks famous nesting ospreys with viewing slots at various heights, including low level ones for visitors in wheelchairs.

SD	CP n/a	E ♿	RF
S ♿	WC	RFE ♿	

NEWTOWNMORE

Situated in the heart of the Highlands, close to Kingussie and the facilities of Aviemore. A delightful village dominated by Creag Dubh and close to the River Spey, with secluded glens such as Glen Banchor less than a mile from the village centre.

HOTEL
BALAVIL SPORT HOTEL 🚶
Main Street, Newtonmore PH20 1DL

Tel: (01540) 673220   Fax: (01540) 673773
www.host.co.uk
No. of Accessible Rooms: 10 (ground floor) and 9 (via lift) Accessible Facilities: Lounge, restaurant. Family owned hotel in Newtonmore.

SELF-CATERING
CRUBENBEG FARM STEADING 🚶
Newtonmore PH20 1BE
Tel: (01540) 673566   Fax: (01540 673509
e-mail: enquiry@crubenbeg.com
www.crubenbeg.com
No. of Accessible rooms: 1. Roll-in Shower
No. of Beds per Unit: 2
Accessible Facilities: Lounge, Kitchen, Trout fishing from disabled platform. Original derelict farm buildings converted into seven holiday cottages of which one is accessible. Situated on a wooded hillside at the foot of Crubenbeg Hill above the River Trium as it tumbles toward the River Spey. Located 5 miles south of the village.

ATTRACTION
HIGHLAND FOLK MUSEUM
Autlarie Croft, Newtonmore
Tel: (01540) 661307 Fax: (01540) 661631
The world of the Highlander from early
C18th to mid C20th, from clansman to
crofter. Mile long site, transport via
wheelchair accessible bus (green) between
all three areas.
1) Central area with reception, accessible
with firm paths, old school particularly
interesting.
2) Steading area with stables, barns and
byres - exteriors accessible.
3) Highland township visible from bus
stop, but grassy, sloped and uneven area.
Well worth a bus tour alone.
N.B. Catering and WC on the first floor,
ramped at 1:19

SD   CP    E   RF
S [ ]   C [ ]   WC [ ]

WALTZING WATERS (SCOTLAND)
Balavil Brae, Newtownmore PH20 1DR
Tel/Fax: (01540) 673752
Elaborate water, light and music
production with thousands of dazzling
patterns of moving water synchronised
with music.

SD n/a   CP   E [ ]   RF [ ]
S [ ]   WC   RFE [ ]

POOLEWE
Located between Loch Ewe and Loch
Gairloch, 6 miles from Gairloch.
Famous for the popular Inverewe
Gardens (some parts difficult for
wheelchairs).

SELF-CATERING
AN BOTHAN
8 Naast, Poolewe IV22 2LL
Tel/Fax: (01445) 781360
e-mail: highlands.dreams@virgin.net
web: freespace.virgin.net/nicola.taylor/
highlands-dreams.htm
No. of Accessible Units: 1.Bath
No. of Beds per Unit: 5
Accessible Facilities: Lounge,
Kitchen/Diner, Garden (shared with

owner's bungalow)
Absolutely charming former croft house
in crofting community with just 8 houses
on the western shore of Loch Ewe, 3
miles north of Poolewe. Fine views across
Loch Ewe to mountains by Loch Maree
and those beyond Ullapool up to
Sutherland. Nearest shop is in
Inverasadale, 1 mile north of cottage.
Safe sandy beach at Firemore Beach, two
miles north of Naast.

INNES-MAREE BUNGALOWS
Poolewe IV22 2JU
Tel/Fax: (01445) 781454
e-mail: info@poolewebungalows.com
www.poolewebungalows.com
No. of Accessible Units: 1. Shower
No. of Beds per Unit: 6.
Accessible Facilities: Lounge, open plan
kitchen/dinette. One of 6 modern
purpose-built bungalows in lovely village.
Area around Poolewe offers mountain
and forest, loch and glen and safe sandy
beaches. The bungalows are a few
minuets from Inverewe Gardens.

SHIELBRIDGE
Tiny community just off the main A87
Kyle of Lochalsh road.

BED AND BREAKFAST
TIGH UR
MacInnes Park, Ratagan, Glenshiel,
Ross-shire IV40 8HR
Tel: (01599) 511292
e-mail: TIGHUR88@aol.com
No. of Accessible Rooms: 2. Roll-in
shower. Twin room - pneumatic height
adjusting bed and manual ARGO sling
lift. Accessible Facilities: Lounge, Dining
Room. Evening Meal available. Spacious,
unpretentious bungalow owned by
charming couple, she in a wheelchair,
who create a homely ambience. Superb
location in hamlet of Ratagan, metres
from, and with views of, the lovely Loch
Duich, in the foothills of Kintail. From
A87, Ratagan is 1.5 miles from
Shielbridge. Good location for touring
Skye and Western Highlands.

ISLAND OF SKYE

Largest of Inner Hebrides and reached by bridge linking Kyle of Lochalsh on mainland with Kyleakin. Varied dramatic scenery, divided by sea lochs, inland area never more than 8km from sea. Volcanic plateau in the north, grasslands in the south. Historically known for association with Bonnie Prince Charlie.

BUSES
Highland County Buses: Tel: (01463) 222244
Regular service with ramps and straps.
Citylink: Tel: (0870) 505050
National Express: Tel: (08705) 808080
www.gobycoach.com

TAXIS
Waterloo Taxis: (01471) 822630
Regular service with ramps and straps but please book in advance.

TRAINS
Scotrail: Tel: (0845) 6057021

SELF-CATERING
BROADFORD, SKYE
Second largest town on Skye in south-east.

TOURIST INFORMATION CENTRE
The Car Park, Broadford IV49 9AB
Tel: (01471) 822361   Fax: (01471) 822141

CORREIGORM BEAG
Bayview Crescent, Broadford,
Isle of Skye IV49 9AB
Tel: (01471) 822515   Fax: (01471) 822860
No. of Accessible Units: 1
No. of Beds per Unit: 1
Accessible Facilities: Lounge, Kitchen.

DUNVEGAN, SKYE
On Durinish Peninsula on western shores of island.

TOURIST INFORMATION CENTRE
2 Lochside, Dunvegan IV55 8WB
Tel: (01470) 521581   Fax: (01470) 521582

HOTEL/RESTAURANT
THE THREE CHIMNEYS
Colbost, Dunvegan IV55 8ZT
Tel: (01470) 511258   Fax: (01470) 511358
e-mail: eatandstay@threechimneys.co.uk
www.threechimneys.co.uk
No. of Accessible Rooms: 1.
Accessible Facilities: Restaurant.
A famous award-winning Restaurant with 6 luxurious rooms in the House Over-By, completed in 1999. Located in small village just SW of Dunvegan, 5 miles from Dunvegan Castle.

KILMUIR, SKYE
BED & BREAKFAST
WHITEWAVE ACTIVITIES
No. 19 Linicro, Kilmuir IV51 9YN
Tel: (01470) 542414   Fax: (01470) 542443
e-mail: info@whiteact.demon.co.uk
www.whiteact.demon.co.uk
No. of Accessible Rooms: 1
Accessible Facilities: Dining Room/Living Room. A cross between an outdoor centre, a ceilidh place and a family home with accessible activities of all kinds.

PORTREE, SKYE
TOURIST INFORMATION CENTRE
Bayfield House, Bayfield Road,
Portree IV51 9EL
Tel: (01478) 612137   Fax: (01478) 612141

BED & BREAKFAST
AUCHENDINNY GUEST HOUSE
Treaslane, by Portree IV51 9NX
Tel/Fax: (01470) 532470
www.stayskye.co.uk
No. of Accessible Rooms: 1. Bath
Accessible Facilities: Lounge, Dining Room
House in 2 acres of gardens with lawns and wooded areas, overlooking Loch Treaslane, a sea loch 70m. away. Located just off the Portree/Dunvegan road (A850).

SLEAT, SKYE
Adjacent to Armadale, with an active pier and ruins of Armadale Castle, built in 1815, adjoining the Clan Donald Centre.

ATTRACTION
ARMADALE CASTLE GARDENS & MUSEUM OFTHE ISLES (CLAN DONALD VISITOR CENTRE)
Armadale, Sleat IV45 8RS
Tel: (01471) 844305   Fax: (01471) 844275
e-mail: office@cland.demon.co.uk
www.cland.demon.co.uk

Clan Donald's history dates back 1300 years, a history of fighting, diplomacy, governing, clearances, triumph and defeat. Armadale Castle Gardens and Museum of the Isles is set in the heart of a 20,000 acre highland estate. This estate, once part of the traditional lands of Macdonald of Sleat was purchased by the Clan Donald Lands Trust in 1971. The Trust has restored the gardens and part of the castle, created the Museum of the Isles, founded a study centre, built holiday accommodation and established a Visitor Centre that appeals to all age groups. All facilities are on the ground floor and are accessible. Most of the gardens are also accessible. Reserved parking is available adjoining all of the buildings. Wheelchairs, including two electric scooters, one a three wheeler and the other a four wheeler, are available for visitors to borrow. Please ask when you purchase your ticket or in high season it is suggested that you phone and book in advance. There is a self-catering cottage that has a ramp and is suitable, with assistance, for people with wheelchairs.

SD ♿	CP ♿	E ♿	RF ♿
C ♿	S ♿	WC ♿	RFE ♿

WATERNISH, SKYE
SELF-CATERING
GREENBANK   ♿
Halistra, Waternish IV55 8GL
Tel/Fax: (01470) 592369
e-mail: greenbank@freewire.co.uk
www.greenbankonskye.co.uk
No. of Accessible Units: 1.Roll-in Shower
No. of Beds per Unit: 4
Accessible Facilities: Purpose built bungalow for wheelchair users which has been awarded four stars under the Quality Assurance Scheme of Scotland. Greenbank faces south-west and enjoys a spectacular and uninterrupted views over a large sea-loch with several islands and craggy Dunvegan Head. Also outstanding sea views across the Little Minch to the Outer Hebrides.

STRATHPEFFER
Located west of Dingwall, a popular spa town and health resort in C19th and now a quiet town with lots of huge hotels as residue. Sample the water at the Water Tasting Pavilion in the town centre.

HOTEL
ACHILTY HOTEL   ♿
Contin, by Strathpeffer IV14 9EG
Tel: (01997) 421355   Fax: (01997) 421923
No. of Accessible Rooms: 4
Accessible Facilities: Lounge, Restaurant. Renovated C18th coaching inn west of Contin. Owner-managed.

ATTRACTION
HIGHLAND MUSEUM OF CHILDHOOD
The Old Station, Strathpeffer IV14 9DH
Tel: (01997) 421031
e-mail: info@hmoc.freeserve.co.uk
Located in Victorian railway station of 1885, alongside various craft shops.

SD ♿	CP ♿	E ♿	RF ♿
C ♿	S ♿	WC ♿	RFE ♿

STROMFERRY
Close to Kyle of Lochalsh.

SELF-CATERING
GLENVIEW   ♿
Birchwood, Achmore, Stromeferry IV53 8UT
Tel: (01599) 577211
No. of Accessible Units: 1
No. of Beds per Unit: 4
Accessible Facilities: Lounge/Kitchen, Dining Room. Modern bungalow within grounds of owner's house in rural location. Nearest facilities at Balmacara and Plockton.

TALMINE

Three miles north of Tongue and off the main tourist route between John O'Groats and Cape Wrath. Seals, otter, deer and a variety of bird life can be observed here.

SELF-CATERING
CLOISTERS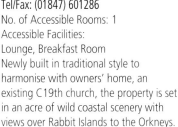
Church Holme, Talmine IV27 4YP
Tel/Fax: (01847) 601286
No. of Accessible Rooms: 1
Accessible Facilities:
Lounge, Breakfast Room
Newly built in traditional style to harmonise with owners' home, an existing C19th church, the property is set in an acre of wild coastal scenery with views over Rabbit Islands to the Orkneys.

THURSO

Located 32km west of John O'Groats, a well organised little town with shops and hotels leading off a main central square. Surfing and windsurfing are popular off local beaches. One can catch the ferry here from Scrabster to Stromness on Orkney. Close by is the gigantic white dome of Dounreay nuclear reprocessing plant, no longer open.

TOURIST INFORMATION CENTRE
Riverside, Thurso KW14 8BU
Tel: (01847) 892371   Fax: (01847) 893155

HOTEL
CASTLE ARMS HOTEL
Mey, by Thurso KW14 8XH
Tel/Fax: (01847) 851244
e-mail: info@castlearms.co.uk
www.castlearms.co.uk
No. of Accessible Rooms: 1
Accessible Facilities: Lounge, Restaurant, Wheelie fishing boat on nearby loch (trout). The Castle Arms Hotel is a former 19th century coaching inn situated in 6 acres of open parkland. It has a Royal Gallery with photographs of the late Queen Mother's life in Caithness. Situated on the John O'Groats peninsula in the north coast village of Mey.

FORSS COUNTRY HOUSE HOTEL
Forss, by Thurso KW14 7XY
Tel: (01847) 861201   Fax: (01847) 861301
www.host.co.uk
No. of Accessible Rooms: 6
Accessible Facilities: Lounge, Restaurant.
Lovely country house set in 25 acres of woodlands by River Forss with an abundance of wildlife.

SELF-CATERING
CURLEW COTTAGE
Hilliclay Mains, Weydale, Thurso KW14 8YN
Tel: (01847) 895638
No. of Accessible Units: 1
No. of Beds per Unit: 4
Accessible facilities: Lounge, Dining Room (includes a piano), Kitchen, Garden
Set amid high farmland, 4 miles from Thurso with grand views across Caithness to the distant mountains.
Good base for touring Caithness and Northern Sutherland with two-mile stretch of Dunnet Sands, other secluded beaches and fine coastal scenery within a short drive.

ULLAPOOL

Very pretty village with palm trees and white-washed houses on the west coast, planned and built as a fishing community in 1788, it juts into Loch Broom. Embarkation point for ferry to Stornoway on Isle of Lewis.

TOURIST INFORMATION CENTRE
Argyle Street, Ullapool IV26 2UB
Tel: (01854) 612135   Fax: (01854) 613031

BED AND BREAKFAST
DROMNAN GUEST HOUSE
Garve Road, Ullapool IV26 2SX
Tel: (01854) 612333   Fax: (01854) 613364
e-mail: dromnan@msn.com
www.dromnan.co.uk
No. of Accessible Rooms: 1. Shower
Accessible Facilities: Lounge, Dining Room

357

Family-run guest house in peaceful location overlooking Lochbroom.

WICK

The community grew on Wick as it became the busiest herring port in Europe, it is still a busy town.

TOURIST INFORMATION CENTRE
Whitechapel Road, Wick KW1 4EA
Tel: (01955) 602596   Fax: (01955) 604940

BED AND BREAKFAST
24 LINDSAY DRIVE
Wick KW1 4PG
Tel: (01955) 603001   www.host.co.uk
No. of Accessible Rooms: 1
Accessible Facilities: Lounge, Dining Room
Bungalow in quiet cul-de-sac en route to Sinclair and Girnigoe Castle. Good overnight stay for Orkneys.

REGION 8
OUTER ISLANDS

ORKNEY

Seventy flat, undulating islands, twenty inhabited. Two hours' sailing time from Scrabster. Spectacular coastline with famous landmark of 150m Old Man of Hoy. The islands are well known for the most dense concentration of archaeological sites in Britain, evidence of more than 5,000 years of settlements here. Notable are Skara Brae Prehistoric village, and many Iron Age brochs all along the coast. There also are traces of Vikings everywhere. Farming and fishing remain very important to the Orcadians.

ORKNEY DISABILITY FORUM
Mackays Buildings, Junction Road, Kirkwall, Orkney KW15 1LB
Tel/Fax: (01856) 870340
Publishes very useful book: *Holiday Accommodation for People with Disabilities.*

DIAL A BUS and SHOPMOBILITY KIRKWALL
Tel: (01856) 871515
You can join this on a temporary basis as a visitor.

BUSES
Highland Scott Omnibus/Tel: (01463) 233371
City Link: Tel: (0870) 505050

BIRSAY

Located on the north-west corner of the mainland, once an important Viking settlement. See the ruins of the C16th earl's palace.

BED AND BREAKFAST
PRIMROSE COTTAGE
Birsay KW17 2NB
Tel: (01856) 721384
No. of Accessible Rooms: 3
Accessible Facilities: Lounge, Dining Room
Bungalow overlooking Marwick Bay, close to RSPB reserves at The Loons and Marwick Head.

DOUNBY

Located north-east of Kirkwall on the mainland.

SELF-CATERING
LOCHLAND CHALETS
Dounby KW17 2HR
Tel: (01856) 771340
No. of Accessible Units: 1
No. of Beds per Unit: 4
Accessible Facilities: Open plan Lounge/Kitchen. Bird Hide on site.

EVIE

Located 10 minutes from Kirkwall and Stromness.

BED AND BREAKFAST
WOODWICK HOUSE
Evie, Orkney KW17 2PQ
Tel: (01856) 751330   Fax: (01856) 751383
www.woodwickhouse.co.uk

No. of Accessible Rooms: 2. Bath. Shower
Accessible Facilities: Lounge, Dining Room,
Gardens. Delightful house surrounded by
trees, secluded corners, lawns and
wonderful views overlooking the island of
Gairsay and beyond.

KIRKWALL

Main town, dominated by St. Magnus
Cathedral, c1140, yellow and red stone
church. Flag-stoned streets and a small,
busy harbour.

ATTRACTION
THE ORKNEY MUSEUM
Broad Street, Kirkwall KW15 2DH
Tel: (01856) 873191   Fax: (01856) 871560
C16th building, 'A' listed, with exhibits on
Orkney's history and archaeology.

SD ♿   CP ♿   E ♿   RF ♿
L ♿ (Stairlift from ground to first floor and another to
extension area).   S ♿   WC ♿

NORTH RONALDSAY

Remote island lying at the north eastern
extremity of Orkney with open sea beyond
towards Shetland and Norway. Farming
and kelp sustain the island's economy.

BED AND BREAKFAST
NORTH RONALDSAY BIRD OBSERVATORY ♿
North Ronaldsay KW17 2BE
Tel: (01857) 633200   Fax: (01857) 633207
e-mail: alison@nrbo.prestel.co.uk
No. of Accessible Rooms: 1
Accessible Facilities: Lounge, Dining Room.
Established in 1987, the bird observatory
provides comfortable, inexpensive
accommodation with special opportunities
for visitors interested in birds and natural
history. Set on the crofts of Twingness and
Lurand, its 30 acres follow traditional
farming practice. Rich grassland and
remnant coastal heath are combined with
bere barley and a flock of sheep.

STROMNESS
ATTRACTION
STROMNESS MUSEUM

52 Alfred Street, Stromness KW16 3DF
Tel: (01856) 850025
e-mail: museum@orkney.gov.uk
www.billrobertson.orknt.co.uk/smuseum
Museum focuses on Orkney's maritime
connections, the accessible lower gallery
display reflects the fishing industry,
German fleet in Scapa Flow, Arctic
exloration and Hudson Bay Company.

SD ♿   CP ♿   E ♿   RF n/a
S ♿   WC ♿

SHETLAND

Over 100 cliff-edged islands, (15
inhabited), closer to Norway than mainland
Scotland and nowhere more than 5km
from the sea. Fishing and salmon fishing
are still important while North Sea oil has
had a great impact on the economy. Fine
beaches and a striking coastline.

DISABILITY SHETLAND
Toll Clock Centre, Lerwick,
Shetland ZE1 0DE
Tel/fax: (01595) 692196
Free and independent advice on holidays,
aid, equipment.

SOCIAL WORK DEPARTMENT
92 St. Olaf's Street, Lerwick, Shetland ZE1 0ES
Tel: (01595) 744400
Provide temporary badges for car parks but
please write in advance.

BUSES
John Leask and Son, Lerwick:
Tel: (01595) 693162
Wheelchair accessibility en route between
Lerwick – North and South Sandwick –
Sumburgh Airport.
Shalder Coaches, Scalloway:
Tel: (01595) 880217
Wheelchair accessibility en route Lerwick -
Scalloway; Lerwick - Mossbank Brae and
Hillswick

LERWICK

Mainland Shetland's major town with
flag-stones narrow lanes, grey stone
buildings.

HOTEL
SHETLAND HOTEL

Holmsgarth Road, Lerwick ZE1 0PW
Tel: (01595) 695515   Fax: (01595) 695828
No. of Accessible Rooms: 1. Roll-in Shower
Accessible Facilities: Lounge, Restaurant
Modern purpose-built hotel located
opposite main ferry terminal at northern
end of the town.

BED AND BREAKFAST
WHINRIG

12 Burgh Road, Lerwick ZE1 0LB
Tel: (01595) 693554
No. of Accessible Rooms: 1
Accessible Facilities: Dining Room
Attractive house, centrally located, but in a
quiet area.

SUMBURGH HEAD
Located at southern tip of the
mainland, famous for seabird colonies.
RSPB has a site here. Within three
miles of Jarlshof archaeological site.

SELF-CATERING
PRINCIPAL LIGHTHOUSE-KEEPER'S
HOUSE

Sumburgh Head Lighthouse, Sumburgh Head.
Bookings: c/o T. Johnson-Ferguson,
Solwaybank, Canonbie,
Dumfries-shire DG14 0XS.
Tel: (013873) 72240
No. of Accessible Units: 1. Bath
No. of Accessible Beds: 6
Accessible Facilities: Lounge/Diner, Kitchen.
Fascinating property, 1 of 4 lighthouse
keepers' cottages in spectacular clifftop
location, along with fields and land
enclosed within drystone walls. In summer
puffins and fulmars come within a few
metres of the dining/sitting room. Within
three miles are wonderful white sandy
beaches, the RSPB site and the Pool of
Virkie (for birds).

ATTRACTION
RSPB SUMBURGH HEAD SEABIRD
VIEWPOINT
About 13,000 guillemots breed here,
laying their single egg directly onto the
cliff ledges. Razorbills, shags and gannets
can also be seen. In the seas around there
are harbour porpoises and white-beaked
dolphins, orcas (killer whales), minke and
humpback whales can sometimes be seen.
Lighthouse compound separated from cliffs
by high dry-stone dykes: at one point the
dykes are low enough for wheelchair users
to see over the top and view the birds on
the cliffs. This low section of dyke is
adjacent to where a car may be parked.
The reserve is not ideal for wheelchair
users, but with some assistance, certain
areas of the reserve can be enjoyed.
SD n/a
CP [♿] Use small car park near the lighthouse.   E [♿]

UPPER SCALLOWAY
Second town to Lerwick. Standing
over an attractive bay looking out to
the Atlantic. Large catches of cod and
haddock brought in daily. The town is
dominated by ruins of C7th
Scalloway Castle.

WALLS
Main village in the western area of the
mainland. With attractive shoreline
both here and nearby at Sandness that
has views of the island of Papa Stour.

GUEST HOUSE
BURRASTOW HOUSE

Walls, Shetland ZE2 9PD
Tel: (01595) 809307   Fax: (01595) 809213
www.users.zetnet.co.uk/burrastow-house
No. of Accessible Rooms: 1
Accessible Facilities: Lounge, Restaurant.
C18th house on a promontory facing the
island of Vaila. Otters and seals can be seen
from the windows and wild orchids flourish
in the grounds.

ISLAND OF FETLAR
SELF-CATERING
2 CHALETS

Tigh Sith, Fetlar
Tel/Fax: (01957) 733303
Bookings: Society of our Lady of the Isles,

Aithness, Fetlar ZE2 9DJ
No. of Accessible Units: 1
No. of Beds per Unit: 2
Set on the headland of Aithness, ideal for a peaceful break and for an opportunity of living alongside and worshipping with the community.

ISLAND OF UNST

Britain's most northerly inhabited island is one of the most spectacular, varied and interesting in Europe. Just 12 miles long by five miles wide there are stupendous cliffs, jagged sea stacks, sheltered inlets, golden beaches, heathery hills, freshwater lochs, peat bogs and fertile farmland. Rich variety of wildlife include Shetland ponies and seabirds. Lying north of the 60 degree parallel, Unst experiences perpetual daylight at midsummer. Modern roads and frequent roll-on/roll-off vehicle ferries link Shetland mainland to Unst via neighbouring island of Yell. From Lerwick it is a 45-minute drive north on main A970 to Toft ferry terminal: crossing to Yell takes 20 minutes, then follow main road to Gutcher ferry terminal (30-minute drive) for 10-minute crossing to Unst. It is always advisable to book well in advance for ferries, particularly in summer. Ferry Booking Office – Ulsta, Yell Tel: (01957) 722259/722268. www.unst.shetland.co.uk

HOTEL
BALTASOUND HOTEL
Baltasound, Central Unst, Shetlands ZE2 9DS
Tel: (01957) 711334   Fax: (01957) 711358
e-mail: balta.hotel@zetnet.co.uk
No. of Accessible Rooms: 3
Accessible Facilities: Lounge, Restaurant. Britain's most northerly hotel, an old stone house and pine log chalets in the garden, with great views over Baltasound. Village has shops, post office, marina and leisure centre. The Keen of Hamar nature reserve with its abundance of rare plants, is very close.

ATTRACTION
UNST HERITAGE CENTRE-BOAT HAVEN

Haroldswick, Shetland ZE2 9ED
Tel: (01957) 711528
Unst Heritage Centre is Unst's permanent link to its rich history. It preserves fine examples of traditional Shetland working boats, together with artefacts and photographs, capturing a glimpse of Shetlands' fishing history. The Boat Haven is dedcicated to the maritime history of the Shetland boats. There are currently 17 boats, mainly traditional Shetland, but including one each from Faroe and Norway, a Welsh coracle and a Berhon folding dingy. A privately owned replica of a C19th sixareen is based in the Baltasound during the summer.

SD CP E RF WC

WESTERN ISLES

Comprising Lewis, Harris, North Uist, South Uist, Benbecula and Barra. Stornaway, on Lewis, is the only town in the islands and is the main administrative and shopping centre. Ullapool ferry sails into Stornaway and the airport has regular flights to and from Glasgow and Inverness.

WESTERN ISLES TOURIST BOARD
26 Cromwell Street, Stornoway,
Isle of Lewis HS1 2DD
Tel: (01851) 703088
Fax: (01851) 705244

LOCAL AUTHORITY TRANSPORT DEPARTMENT
Tel: (01851) 703773

MINIBUSES.
Graham Minibus Hire: Tel: (01851) 705716
8-seater minibus with wheelchair facilities and ramp.

ISLE OF HARRIS
Separated from Lewis by two sea lochs, Harris has a craggy east coast dominated by An Clisham, the highest mountain in the outer islands. Rocky landscape can be rather desolate, but there are superb sandy beaches.

361

TOURIST INFORMATION CENTRE
Pier Road, Tarbert
Tel: (01859) 502011 (Seasonal)

SELF-CATERING
CABHALAN COTTAGE
Quidinish, Harris HS3 3JQ
Tel/Fax: (01359) 530255
BOOK THROUGH: Mr/Mrs Luty, 35 Telford
Road, Inverness IV3 8JA on the same
number or by email:jsluty@hotmail.com
No. of Accessible Units: 1 with roll-in
shower. No. of Beds per Unit: 4
Accessible Facilities: Lounge, Dining Room,
Kitchen. Very secluded stone cottage
overlooking the sea.

LEWIS
Largest in 130-mile long chain of
islands, this is low lying with moors
and meadows. The capital, Stornaway,
hosts many Gaelic events. Don't miss
the broch at Carloway and the bronze
age Standing Stones at Callanish.

ATTRACTION
COLL POTTERY
Back, Isle of Lewis, Western Isles HS2 0JP
Tel: (01851) 820219   Fax: (01851) 820565
e-mail: admin@scotia-ceramics.com
www.scotia-ceramics.com
Manufacture of widest range of ceramics
in Scotland made in crofting town of Coll.
Famous for earthenware figurines
reflecting Hebridean life and marbled ware
representing lands, sea and sky of locale.
Stunning domestic and artistic pieces.

SD   CP   E   RF
C ⍟   S ⍟   WC ⍟

NORTH UIST
Linked to South Uist by a causeway
through Benbecula, the main centre
here is Lochmaddy, a good touring
base. The island is dominated by sea
lochs birds, there are also standing
stones, chambered caves and stone
circles, all worth viewing.

TOURIST INFORMATION CENTRE
Pier Road, Lochmaddy
Tel: (01876) 500321 (Seasonal)

ATTRACTION
UIST ANIMAL VISITORS CENTRE
Kyle Road, Bayhead, North Uist,
Outer Hebrides
Tel: (01876) 510706   Fax: (01876) 510223
Meet some exotic animals, pot-bellied
pigs, llama which children can pet and
feed, rare poultry and game breeds with
much of the centre undercover.

CP   E    C ⍟
S ⍟   WC ⍟

SOUTH UIST
Hill island with a mountainous spine
running down the eastern side. Many
historical and archaeological sites,
wonderful beaches, abundance of wild
life, including many rare breeding birds
and rich variety of plant life. Worth
visiting village of Howmore.

TOURIST INFORMATION CENTRE
Pier Road, Lochboisdale
Tel: (01878) 700286 (Seasonal)

HOTEL
ORASAY INN
Lochcarnan, South Uist HS8 5PD
Tel: (01870) 610298   Fax: (01870) 610267
e-mail: orasayinn@btinternet.com
No. of Accessible Rooms: 2
Accessible Facilities: Lounge, Dining Room
Small, privately owned hotel, with views
across the Minch in an area of outstanding
natural beauty.

BED & BREAKFAST
CROSS ROADS
Stoneybridge, South Uist HS8 5SD
Tel: (01870) 620321
No. of Accessible Rooms: 2
Accessible Facilities: Dining Room.
This Category 1 house was the first on
the island to have facilities for disabled
visitors.

362

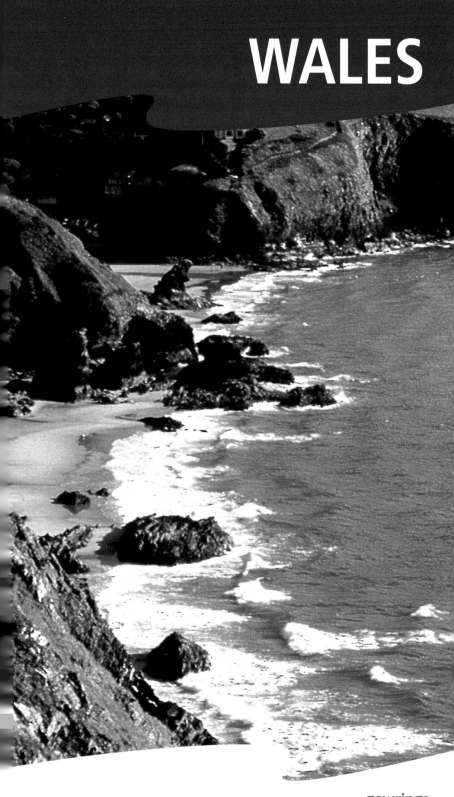

WALES

Rugged splendour of Cardigan Bay.

gowrings
mobility

WALES TOURIST BOARD
Brunel House, 2 Fitzaland Road,
Cardiff CF2 1UY
Tel: 012922 499909   Fax: 012922 485031
e-mail: info@tourism.wales.gov.uk
www.visitwales.com

REGIONAL WALES TOURIST BOARDS
THE ISLE OF ANGLESEY
Llangefni LL77 7TW
Tel: (01248) 752411   Fax: (01248) 752192
e-mail: brxpl@anglesey.gov.uk

LLANDUDNO, COLWYN BAY
Tourism & Leisure Dept. Civic Offices
Colwyn Bay LL29 8AR
Tel: (01492) 575387   Fax: (01492) 513664
e-mail: tourism@conwy.gov.uk

RHYL & PRESTATYN
Coastal Tourism Unit, West Promenade
Rhyl LL18 1HZ
Tel: (01745) 344515   Fax: (01745) 342255

NORTH WALES BORDERLANDS
Economic Development and Tourism,
Flintshire County Council, County Hall,
Mould CH7 6NB
Tel/Fax: (01352) 759331

SNOWDONIA MOUNTAINS & COAST
Gwynedd Council, Cae Penarlag
Dolgellau LL40 2YB
Tel: (01341) 423558   Fax: (01342) 424440
e-mail: tourism@gwyness.gov.uk
www.gwynedd.gov.uk

MID WALES LAKES & MOUNTAINS
Powys Tourism, Neuadd Maldwyn,
Severn Road, Welshpool SY21 7AS
Tel: (01938) 551255
e-mail: tourism@powys.gov.uk

MID WALES TOURISM
The Station, Machynlleth SY20 8TG
Tel: Freephone: (0800) 273747
Fax: (01654) 703855
e-mail: info@brilliantbreaks.demon.co.uk

CEREDIGION-CARDIGAN BAY
Ceredigion Tourism,
Lisburn House, Terrace Road,
Aberystwyth SY23 2AG

Tel: (01970) 612125   Fax: (01970) 626566
e-mail: econ@ceredigion.gov.uk

PEMBROKESHIRE
PO Box 103, Pembroke Dock SA72 6TQ
Tel: (01646) 682278   Fax: (01646) 682281
e-mail: tourism@pembrokeshire.gov.uk

CARMARTHENSHIRE-COAST &
COUNTRYSIDE IN WEST WALES
Carmarthenshire County Council Tourism,
Economic Development Division,
Parc Amanwy, New Road,
Ammanford,
Carmarthenshire SA18 3EP
Tel: (01269) 590200   Fax: (01269) 590290
e-mail: tourism@carmarthenshire.gov.uk

SWANSEA BAY
Swansea Tourist Information Centre,
Plymouth Street, Swansea SA1 3Q
Tel: (01729) 468321   Fax: (01729) 464602
e-mail: swantrsm@cableol.co.uk

NORTH WALES TOURISM
77 Conway Road, Colwyn Bay LL29 7LN
Tel: (01492) 531731   Fax: (01492) 530059
e-mail: croeso@nwt.co.uk.
www.nwt.co.uk

VALLEY OF SOUTH WALES
Valley Breaks, Tourism S & W Wales
Charter Court, Enterprise Park,
Swansea SA7 9DBA
Tel: (01792) 781212   Fax: (01792) 781300
e-mail: valleys@tsww.com

GLAMORGAN HERITAGE COAST
& COUNTRYSIDE
Tourism Unit, Vale of Glamorgan Council,
Dock Office, Barry CF63 4RT
Tel: (01446) 709328   Fax: (01446) 704892
e-mail: tourism@valeofglamorgan.gov.uk
www.valeofglamorgan.gov.uk

WYE VALLEY & VALE OF USK
Tourism Section, Monmouthshire County
Council
County Hall, Cwmbran NP44 2XH
Tel: (01633) 644842   Fax: (01633) 644800
e-mail: tourism@monmouthshire.gov.uk

DISABILITY ORGANISATIONS

ARTS DISABILITY WALES
Sbectrwm, Bwlch Road,
Fairwater, Cardiff, CF5 3EF
Tel: (029) 20 377885
arts.disability@btconnect.com
www.artsdisabilitywales.com

DISABILITY WALES
Wernddu Court, Caerphilly Business Park,
Van Road, Caerphilly CS83 3ED
Tel: (029) 20 887325
Freephone: (0800) 731 6282
All Wales disability information and
campaigning organisation.

DISABILITY HELPLINE WALES
3 Links Court, Business Park, St. Mellons,
Cardiff CF3 0SP
Tel: (029) 20 798633
Information and advice for disabled people.

DISCOVERING ACCESSIBLE WALES
Welsh Tourist Board
Dept VOW 2, PO Box 1
Cardiff CF1 2XN
Free booklet packed with information for
visitors who have impaired movement or
are in a wheelchair.

TRAVEL FREEDOM WALES
Unit 2b. St. David's Industrial Estate,
Pengam NP2 1SW
Tel: (01443) 831000
Fax: (01443) 839800
Provides detailed information on aspects of
travel, transport, accommodation and
services for disabled visitors.

TRANSPORT

RAIL
WALES AND WEST PASSENGER TRAINS
Brunel House, 2 Fitzalan Road,
Cardiff CF2 1SU
Special Needs: Tel: (0845) 300 3005
Minicom: (0845) 758 5469

CARDIFF

Welsh capital with fusion of ancient
heritage and successful modernity.
Dominated by a splendid Norman
castle, converted in mid C19th to
present medieval appearance. Cardiff
Bay is a striking combination of old
dock buildings and spectacular new
developments. Barrage across the
rivers Taff and Ely has created a huge
500-acre lake. Other major
developments include the demise of
the much-loved Cardiff Arms Park
Stadium and its re-birth as the
Millennium Stadium, built for the
Rugby World Cup in 1999. Shopping
here is fun in eight delightful Victorian
and Edwardian arcades and a
Victorian market. A thriving city. Not
to be missed.

TOURIST INFORMATION CENTRE
16 Wood Street, Cardiff CF10 1ES
Tel: (029) 20 227281   Fax: (029) 20 239162

CARDIFF BAY VISITOR CENTRE
Harbour Drive, Cardiff Bay,
Cardiff, CF10 4AA
Tel: (029) 20 463833

PUBLIC TRANSPORT INFORMATION
Tel: (029) 20 873252

TRAVELINE
Tel: (0870) 6082608

TRAINS
First Great Western: Special Needs:
Tel: (0845) 7413775
Valley Line: Special Needs:
Tel: (029) 20 449944
Virgin Trains: Special Needs:
Tel: (0845) 7443366
Minicom: (0845) 7443367
Wales and West: Special Needs:
Tel: (0845) 3003005

CAR PARKS
Free unlimited disabled badge parking.
Tel: (029) 20 872000

SHOPMOBILITY
Oxford Arcade Car Park, Bridge Street,
Cardiff CF2 2EB
Tel: (029) 20 399355

HOTELS
COPTHORNE CARDIFF ♿
Copthorne Way, Culverhouse Cross,
Cardiff CF5 6DH
Tel: (029) 20 599100   Fax: (029) 20 599080
No. of Accessible Rooms: 2
Accessible Facilities: Lounge, Restaurant.
Quality hotel in picturesque lakeside
setting four miles from the city centre.

CARDIFF MARRIOTT HOTEL ♿
Mill Lane, Cardiff CF10 1EZ
Tel: (029) 20 399944   Fax: (029) 20 395578
Web: www.marriott.com/marriott/cwldt
No. of Accessible Rooms: 2
Accessible Facilities: Lounge, Restaurant,
bar, disabled changing rooms in leisure
club. Quality hotel located in the heart of
the city opposite colourful café quarter.

CARDIFF WEST TRAVELODGE ♿
Moto Hospitality, M4 Junction 33,
Pontyclun, Cardiff CF72 8SA
Tel: (029) 20 891141   Fax: (029) 20 892497
No. of Accessible Rooms: 2
Accessible Facilities: Restaurant.
Located 11 miles from Cardiff city centre.

CARDIFF MOAT HOUSE ♿
Circle Way East, Llanederyn, Cardiff CF3 7XF
Tel: (029) 20 589988   Fax: (029) 20 549092
No. of Accessible Rooms: 2
Accessible Facilities: Lounge, Restaurant,
Bar. Conveniently located for M4 also
with easy access to the city centre.

SELF-CATERING
PARC-COED-MACHEN
COUNTRY COTTAGES ♿
St. Brides Super-Ely, Nr. Cardiff CF5 6EZ
Tel: (01446) 760684
Fax: (01446) 760289
No. of Accessible Units: 2
No. of Beds per Unit: 3
Accessible Facilities: Lounge, Dining
Room, Kitchen, Patio with garden
furniture. Situated in the north-east of
the Vale of Glamorgan, this is a working

organic stock farm with cottages around
a central courtyard of original farm
buildings, six miles from Cardiff. Easily
accessible conductive education
summer school.

ATTRACTIONS
CARDIFF BAY VISITOR CENTRE
Harbour Drive, Cardiff Bay
Tel: (029) 20 463833 Fax: (029) 20 486650
e-mail: viscen@cardiff-bay.co.uk
web: www.cardiff-bay.co.uk
Known locally as The Tube, the visitor
centre was designed by avant-garde
architect William Alsop, creating a
futuristic giant telescope offering
panoramic views of the bay. Also a large-
scale model of Cardiff Bay, the largest
architectural model in the UK.

| SD ♿ | CP ♿ | E ♿ | RF ♿ |
| S ♿ | WC ♿ | RFE ♿ | |

DYFFRYN GARDENS
St. Nicholas, Nr. Cardiff CF5 6SU
Tel: (029) 20 593328   Fax: (029) 20 591966
A superb landscaped garden of 55 acres,
with small themed gardens, kitchen
garden, arboretum and glass house.

| SD ♿ | CP ♿ | E ♿ | RF ♿ |
| C ♿ | S ♿ | WC ♿ | RFE |

NATIONAL MUSEUM AND GALLERY
Cathays Park, Cardiff CF1 3NP
Tel: (029) 20 397951   Fax: (029) 20 573321
Neo-classic building, a treasure house,
with extensive range of art and science
displays. Art Galleries – works by famous
artists, including the Impressionists in the
fine Davies collection. Evolution of Wales
exhibition traces the country's development from 4,600 million years ago. Also
the Natural History of Wales exhibition as
well as displays of bronze age gold,
Christian monuments and Celtic treasures.

| SD ♿ | CP ♿ | E ♿ | RF ♿ |
| L ♿ | C ♿ | S ♿ | WC ♿ |

TECHNIQUEST
Stuart Street, Cardiff CF1 6BW
Tel: (029) 20 475475 Fax: (029) 20 482517
e-mail: gen@tquest.org
UK's leading Science Discovery Centre,
located in waterfront site in the heart of

Cardiff Bay. Over 160 hands-on exhibits: freeze your own shadow, launch a hot-air balloon or even film your own animation. 1996 award for most accessible building for disabled visitors in Cardiff.

SD ♿ CP ♿ E ♿ RF ♿ L ♿
C 🚹 S ♿ WC 🚹 RFE ♿

THEATRE
THE SHERMAN THEATRE
Sendhennydd Road, Cathays, Cardiff CF2 4YE
Admin: (029) 20 646901
Fax: (029) 20 646902
Booking-Box Office: (029) 20 646900
Minicom: (029) 20 646909

SD ♿ L ♿
CP 🚹 Public CP-Dumfries Place, 5-10 minutes walk
Taxi Rank -Outside main entrance. RE ♿ ED ♿
INT 🚹 WC ♿ (main foyer)
AUD – Main Theatre ♿ studio – n/a
B/R ♿ forms part of Foyer

SPORTS VENUE
THE MILLENNIUM STADIUM
CARDIFF ARMS PARK
A Millennium Project
1st Floor St. David's House, Wood Street, Cardiff CF1 1ES
Tel: (029) 20 232661
Fax: (029) 20 232678
e-mail: info@cardiff-stadium.co.uk
web: www.cardiff-stadium.co.uk
Produces comprehensive leaflet on access for disabled visitors. 20 designated spaces in basement car park, access across level plazas with no ramp steeper than 1:20. Entrances from north along riverwalk to Gate 1. From east across Westgate Plaza to Gate 3: from south across Millennium Plaza to Gates 6 and 7: Wheelchair-accessible terraces at level 3 (324 spaces + 206 companion spaces): Level 4 (28 spaces + 24 companion spaces): Level 6 (28 spaces + 24 companion spaces). Lifts access spaces on upper levels (lift size unknown). Adapted WCs available on Levels 3, 4, 6, plus private boxes level 5 (boxes and WCs adapted). NB. Quality of adaptation not known. Catering close to accessible viewing areas at all levels. 10 wheelchairs available for loan.

CARMARTHENSHIRE
www.carmarthenshire.gov.uk

CARMARTHEN
Centre of West Wales' agricultural community with flourishing cattle market and excellent covered market; pork butchers a speciality. Built cAD74 around the Roman fortress of Maridunum, the town was an important administration centre in Roman Britain. Reputed to be the birthplace of Merlin, the wizard of Arthurian folklore.

TOURIST INFORMATION CENTRE
Lammas Street SA31 3AQ
Tel: (01267) 231557   Fax: (01267) 221901

PUBLIC TRANSPORT INFORMATION
Tel: (01267) 231817

TRAVELINE
Tel: (0870) 6082608

TAXIS
Chris Cars: Tel: (01267) 234438
2 adapted vehicles.

TRAINS
Wales and West: Special Needs:
Tel: (0845) 3003005
Minicom: (0845) 7585469

CAR PARKS
Free unlimited disabled badge parking:
Tel: (01267) 231557

WHEELCHAIR HIRE
British Red Cross. Tel: (01686) 626663

HOTEL
CWMTWRCH HOTEL ♿
Nantgaredig, Nr. Carmarthen SA32 7NY
Tel: (01267) 290238 Fax: (01267) 290808
No. of Accessible Rooms: 3
Accessible Facilities: Restaurant, Garden, Indoor Pool. Set in 30 acres off the beaten track in lovely countryside. Nantgaredig is between Carmarthen and Llandeilo.

BED AND BREAKFAST
ALLT-Y-GOLAU UCHAF ♿
Felingwm Uchaf, Nantgaredig,
Nr. Carmarthen SA32 7BB
Tel: (01267) 290455
No. of Accessible Rooms:1
Accessible Facilities: Dining Room Georgian
stone-walled farmhouse built in 1812 with
many original features. Panoramic views
over Tywi Valley and beyond to Black
Mountains.

GOLDEN GROVE
Located in the lovely Towy valley,
overlooked by Dinefwr Castle, close to
Llandeilo.

SELF-CATERING
HAMDDEN LLETY MEIRI ♿
Golden Grove, Carmarthen, SA32 8NL
Tel/Fax: (01558) 823059
e-mail: patmcl@btinternet.com
No. of Accessible Units: 3
No. of Beds per Unit: 4
Accessible Facilities: Lounge/ Kitchen/Diner,
Games room, Fitness room, Laundry,
Gardens, fishing from specially constructed
platforms. Located in lovely countryside in
the Towy Valley, 3 cottages, all accessible,
built of traditional Welsh stone, set around
a central courtyard next to a large orchard.

KIDWELLY
Historic town with a magnificent
C11th. Norman castle, one of the best
preserved in Wales. Nine miles south of
Carmarthen. Also lovely river walks.

ATTRACTION
KIDWELLY CASTLE
5 Castle Road, Kidwelly SA17 5BQ
Tel: (01554) 890104
Fine example of late C13th design with
defensive system of walls within walls. Later
additions, including chapel from about
1400. Approach to castle entrance gently
sloping, with slightly steeper stretch on
approach to drawbridge.

SD ♿   CP ♿   E ♿
RF ♿ from car park   S ♿   WC ♿

KIDWELLY INDUSTRIAL MUSEUM
Broadford, Kidwelly SA17 4LW
Tel: (01554) 891078
Established in 1980 on the site of the
second oldest tinplate works in Britain to
preserve and interpret the nation's sole
surviving pack mill. Tinplate production
started here in 1737, the works closing in
1941. Fascinating displays include Engine
House and Coal Museum, Brynlliw Locomotive and Bessie, a steam-powered crane.

SD ♿   CP ♿   E ♿   RF ♿
C 🚶   S 🚶

LLANDEILO
The former capital of West Wales
retains its old world atmosphere with
narrow streets and historic buildings.
Many reflect the agricultural prosperity
of the C18th and early C19th.
Charming market on the last Saturday
of every month. Best enjoyed from the
south across the many-arched bridge
of 1848.

TOURIST INFORMATION CENTRE
Municipal Car Park, Crescent Road,
Llandeilo SA19 6HN
Tel/Fax: (01558) 824226

HOTEL
THE PLOUGH INN AT RHOSMAEN ♿
Rhosmaen, Llandeilo SA19 6NP
Tel: (01558) 823431   Fax: (01558) 823969
e-mail: ploughinn@rhosmaen.demon.co.uk
No. of Accessible Rooms: 1
Accessible Facilities: Restaurant, End of
Towy Lounge (1 step).
Situated on the A40, a mile north of
Llandeilo and within the heart of the
Towy Valley. Wonderful views of the
Black Mountains.

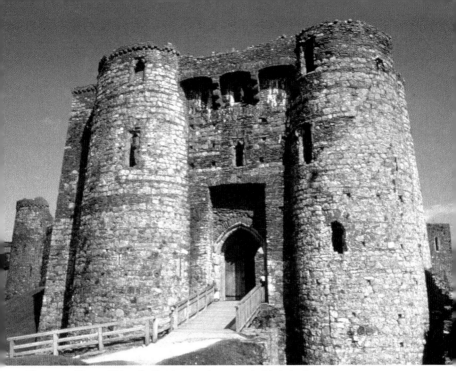

The magnificent Kidwelly Castle remains remarkably intact.

LLANDOVERY

Small grey-stone town that had a Roman fort, fragments of bricks are still visible in the walls of the site now covered by St. Mary's Church. Cattle drovers stopped here en route from the grazing area in the west to Smithfield Market in London. Located in north-west corner of Brecon Beacons National Park.

TOURIST INFORMATION CENTRE
Kings Road, Llandovery SA20 0AW
Tel/Fax: (01550) 720693

HOTEL
LLANERCHINDDA FARM 🚶
Cynghordy, Llandovery SA20 0NB
Tel: (01550) 750274   Fax: (01550) 750300
e-mail: nick@cambrianway.com
www.cambrianway.com
No. of Accessible Rooms: Several. Roll-in Showers. Accessible Facilities: Lounge, Library Dining Room. West wing of old farmhouse in tranquil location on working sheep farm at 200m on southern slopes of Cambrian Mountains foothills. Fine views.

Awarded Best B & B in Wales in 1997.

ATTRACTION
LLANDOVERY HERITAGE CENTRE/TOURIST INFORMATION CENTRE/BRECON BEACONS NATIONAL PARK
Tyllwyd, Kings Road, Llandovery SA20 0AW
Tel/Fax: 01550 720693
SD ♿   CP ♿   E ♿   WC 🚶
Heritage Centre – 1 Wheelchair/stair lift to upper floor.

LLANELLI

Originally the tinplate capital of the world although coal from the Amman Valley and copper are equally important industries now. Its rapid industrial growth in the C19th meant much of the town was based on the Victorian terraced house. The town centre and market are pedestrianised.

TOURIST INFORMATION CENTRE
The Central Library, Vaughan Street, Llanelli SA15 3AS
Tel: (01554) 772020   Fax: (01554) 750125
Seasonal, in winter contact Carmarthen.

ATTRACTION
THE WILDFOWL AND WETLANDS TRUST
Llanelli Centre, Penclacwydd, Lewynhandy,
Llanelli SA14 9SH
Tel/Fax: (01554) 741087
e-mail: wwtllanelli@aol.com
www.wwt.org.uk

Excellent visitor centre with fine views to
Gower Peninsula. This is the only WWT
centre in Wales and has a resident
population of over 1,000 wildfowl from
across the world. The centre recently
developed two new projects as part of the
Millennium Coastal Park development; the
Millennium Discovery Centre, an indoor
discovery centres that informs people
about the importance and misuse of water
and wetlands through imaginative and
interactive interpretation, and the
Millenium Wetland, the largest wetland
habitat creation in the UK.

| SD ♿ | CP ♿ | E ♿ | RF ♿ |
| C ♿ | S 🚶 | WC 🚶 | RFE ♿ |

WHITLAND
Market town with remains of
C12th Abbey.

SELF-CATERING
HOMELEIGH COUNTRY COTTAGES ♿
Red Roses, Whitland SA34 0PN
Tel: (01834) 831765
No. of Accessible Units: 3.
No. of Beds per Unit: 4, 5, 7
Accessible Facilities: Lounge,
Dining Room, Kitchen.
Small friendly complex designed around
ease and accessibility of wheelchair users
and their families. Set in picturesque village
amid many farm animals. Located on the
edge of the Pembrokeshire National Park.

CEREDIGION
TOURIST INFORMATION
e-mail: econ@ceredigion.gov.uk
www.ceredigion.gov.uk
Tel: (01239) 613230   Fax: (01239) 614853

ABERAERON
Striking harbour and neat Georgian
layout, purpose-built in early 1800s.
Poor beach.

TOURIST INFORMATION CENTRE
The Quay, Aberaeron SA46 0BT
Tel: (01545) 570602   Fax: (01545) 626566
e-mail: aberaeron.tic@ceredigion.gov.uk

ATTRACTION
SEA AQUARIUM/COASTAL VOYAGES
2 Quay Parade, Aberaeron SA46 0BT
Tel: (01545) 570142   Fax: (01545) 570160
Insight into marine life in coastal waters of
Cardigan Bay with various tanks stocked
with local fish and shellfish, plus own
small lobster and fish hatcheries. Large
screen AV presentation describes a
fisherman's working life, past and present.
Wheelchair users are welcome on Atlantic
Leopard, a rigid inflatable boat, on 1 and
2-hour trips around the bay to see many
sea birds and mammals such as puffin and
dolphin.

| SD ♿ | CP n/a | E ♿ | RF ♿ |
| C n/a | S n/a | WC 🚶 | |

ABERPORTH
Small seaside village, traditionally
depending on farming and fishing, but
now a delightful holiday base for some
of the finest scenery on Ceredigion's
Heritage Coast with its award-winning
beaches.

BED AND BREAKFAST
FFYNONWEN COUNTRY GUEST HOUSE ♿
Aberporth SA43 2HT
Tel: (01239) 810312
No. of Accessible Rooms: 1
Accessible Facilities: Lounge/Bar, Dining
Room, Tarmac area with close access to
farm animals and views over small lakes.
Farmhouse, about 300 years old, set in 20
acres with unspoiled coastline.

ABERYSTWYTH

A favourite traditional seaside resort with many visitor attractions and easy access to the open hills, coastline and beaches.

TOURIST INFORMATION CENTRE
Terrace Road, Aberystwyth SY23 2AG
Tel: (01970) 612125   Fax: (01970) 612125
e-mail: aberystwythtic@ceredigion.gov.uk
Will hire out Red Cross wheelchairs.

PUBLIC TRANSPORT INFORMATION
Tel: (01545) 572504

TRAVELINE
Tel: (0870) 6082608

BUSES
Arriva Cymru: Tel: (01970) 617951

TRAINS
Central Trains: Assistance:
Tel: (0845) 7056027
www.centraltrains.co.uk

CAR PARKS
Some free unlimited disabled badge parking on-street and in car parks.
Tel: (01545) 572413/572440

HOTEL
GWEST MARINE HOTEL
Marine Terrace, The Promenade,
Aberystwyth SY23 2BX
Tel: (01970) 612444   Fax: (01970) 617435
No. of Accessible Rooms: 1.
Accessible Facilities: Restaurant, Bar.
Large seafront hotel with disabled entrance.

ATTRACTIONS
BWLCH NANT YR ARIAN
Ponterwyd, Aberystwyth SY23 3AD
Tel: (01970) 890500   Fax: (01970) 890340
Forest enterprise.

SD   CP   E 🔽   RF 🔽
C 🔽   S   WC

NATIONAL LIBRARY OF WALES
Penglais, Aberwystyth SY23 3BU
Tel: (01970) 632800   Fax: (01970) 615709
e-mail: mgm@llgc.org.uk
Huge library, one of Britain's six copyright libraries, specialising in Welsh and Celtic literature. There are maps, manuscripts and drawings plus books and a permanent exhibition on A Nation's Heritage.

SD n/a   CP 🔽   E 🧍   RF 🔽   L 🔽
C 🔽   S 🔽   WC 🧍   RFE 🔽

RHEIDOL POWER STATION
Cwm Rheidol, Aberystwyth SY23 3NF
Tel: (01970) 880667   Fax: (01970) 880670
Power station lying in a secluded valley with a visitor centre. Also fish farm, forest trails and lakeside picnic area. Free guided tour of station and fish farm.

SD 🔽   CP   E   RF
C 🔽   WC 🧍   RFE 🔽

BORTH

Popular holiday village with lovely firm sandy beach. Fine views from Ynyslas dunes to the north across the Dovey Estuary. Lies to the north of Aberystwyth on a scenic coastline.

TOURIST INFORMATION CENTRE
Cambrian Terrace, Borth SY24 5HU
Tel: (01970) 871174   Fax: (01970) 871365
e-mail: borth.tic@ ceredigion.gov.uk
Seasonal, winter contact Aberystwyth.

SELF-CATERING
ABERLERI FARM COTTAGES
Dept.C. Cambrian Coast Park, Borth SY24 5JU
Tel: (01970) 871233   Fax: (01970) 871124
No. of Accessible Units: 2
No. of Beds per Unit:6
Accessible Facilities: Lounge, Kitchen
Complex of farmhouse and 4 cottages adjoining quality holiday park facilities. Close to sandy beach.

CARDIGAN

Second largest town in the county where in 1176, the very first National Eisteddfod was held. Handsome C18th bridge, ruined castle on its mound and long, curving Victorian High Street.

TOURIST INFORMATION CENTRE
Theatr Mwldan, Bath House Road, Cardigan SA43 2YJ
Tel: (01239) 613230   Fax: (01970) 626566
e-mail: cardigantic@ceredigion.gov.uk

HOTEL
PENBONTBREN FARM HOTEL
Glynarthen, Nr. Cardigan SA44 6PE
Tel: (01239) 810248   Fax: (01239) 811129
No. of Accessible Rooms: 2
Accessible Facilities: Lounge, Restaurant
Old farm buildings now a hotel in the secluded valley of the river Dulais. Award winning restaurant accredited by Welsh Rarebits. Three Star rating by Welsh Tourist Board; AA Rosette Award; RAC Dining Award; Victorian farmhouse overlooks the complex. Surrounded by 90 acres of livestock-raising farm.

SELF-CATERING
GORSLWYD FARM
Tanygroes, Cardigan SA43 2HZ
Tel: (01239) 810593
e-mail: steve.roni@talk21.com
www.gorslwyd.com
No. of Accessible Units: 7/1
No. of Beds per Unit: 6/4
Accessible Facilities: Lounge, Games Room, Laundry Facilities, Adventure play area, Gardens, Barbecue. Comfortable cottages in attractive gardens, 7 miles from Cardigan and sandy beaches.

CANLLEFAES GANOL COTTAGES
Penparc, Cardigan SA43 1SG
Tel/Fax: (01239) 613712
e-Mail: Canllefaes@clara.co.uk
No. of Accessible Units: 2
No. of Beds per Unit: 2 – 8, + cot
Accessible Facilities: Lounge, Dining Room, Kitchen, Outdoor Pool (2 steps).

CROFT FARM AND CELTIC COTTAGES
Croft Farm, Nr. Cardigan SA43 3NT
Tel: (01239) 615179   Fax: (01239) 615179
No. of Accessible Units: 1
No. of Beds. Per Unit: 4.
Accessible Facilities: Lounge, Kitchen
Comfortable accommodation in unspoilt countryside.

ATTRACTION
FELINWYNT RAINFOREST & BUTTERFLY CENTRE
Felinwynt, Cardigan SA43 1RT
Tel/Fax: (01239) 810882
Wander among free-flying exotic butterflies, observe their life history and how they use both tropical and native plants for breeding and feeding. Waterfall, ponds and streams provide humidity. Accompanied by recorded sounds of the Peruvian Amazon.

SD 🦽	CP 🦽	E 🦽	RF 🦽
C 🚹	S 🦽	WC 🚹	RFE 🦽

LAMPETER

Situated on River Teifi amid rolling farmland, Lampeter is both a university and a market town. The centre of St. David's College is a single Tudor-style quadrangle in attractive grounds. Mostly Georgian and Victorian in character with a large livestock market held on Tuesdays generally.

BED AND BREAKFAST
BRYNCASTELL FARMHOUSE
Llanfair Road, Lampeter SA48 8JY
Tel: (01570) 422447
No. of Accessible Rooms: 2
Accessible Facilities: Lounge, Dining Room. Join this traditional bilingual Welsh farming family on their 140-acre riverside farm overlooking the Teifi valley. Located a mile from Lampeter.

SELF-CATERING
TY GLYN DAVIS TRUST
1 Dolfor, Cilia Aeron, Lampeter SA48 8DE
Tel: (01545) 571604
No. of Accessible Units: 1

No. of Beds per Unit: 18
Accessible Facilities: Lounge, Dining Room, Kitchen, Wild Life Garden. Purpose- built centre for young people with disabilities just outside the seaside town of Aberaeron. Situated in woodlands on the banks of the River Aeron.

LLANDYSUL

Teifi-side village in historic textile-producing area where woollen mills still exist. Salmon fishing is popular here.

ATTRACTION
MUSEUM OF THE WELSH WOOLLEN INDUSTRY
Drefach Felindre, Llandysul SA44 5UP
Tel: (01559) 370929   Fax: (01559) 371592
Exhibits tracing history of the woollen industry include C19th textile machinery with demonstrations of fleece to fabric.

CONWY

BETWS-Y-COED
Nestling among the forested slopes of Snowdonia, the town's glorious mountain backdrop draws many ramblers and rock-climbers. Full of rather severe slate-roofed houses in local stone, rather like a Victorian mountain resort. It lies just within the eastern boundary of Snowdonia National Park and is an excellent centre from which to explore.

TOURIST INFORMATION CENTRE
Snowdonia National Park,
Royal Oak Stables LL24 0AH
Tel: (01690) 710426   Fax: (01690) 710665

ATTRACTION
CONWY VALLEY RAILWAY MUSEUM
The old Goods Yard, Betws-y-Coed LL24 0AL
Tel: (01690) 710568   Fax: (01690) 710132
Two large museum buildings with displays on North Wales railways, including stock and other memorabilia. Working model

railway layouts, steam-powered 4-acre miniature railway in the grounds and tramway to the woods.

SD ♿	CP ♿	E ♿	RF ♿
C ♿	S ♿	WC 🧍	RFE ♿

COLWYN BAY/RHOS-ON-SEA
Late-Victorian and Edwardian seaside resort with beautiful sands and curving promenade running three miles from Rhos-on-Sea in the north to the village of Old Colwyn in the east. Rhos has a mixture of red brick villas and hotels with some older cottages, producing the ambience of an old fishing village.

TOURIST INFORMATION CENTRE
(Colwyn Bay)
Imperial Buildings, Station Square, Princes Drive, Colwyn Bay LL29 8LA
Tel: (01492) 530478   Fax: (01492) 534789
RHOS. TOURIST INFORMATION CENTRE
The Promenade, Rhos on Sea LL28 4EP
Tel: (01492) 548778
Seasonal, in winter contact Colwyn Bay.

SHOPMOBILITY
44 Sea View Road, Colwyn Bay LL29 8DG
Tel: (01492) 533822   Fax: (01492) 535372
Small collection/delivery charge and small daily charge.

HOTELS
NORTHWOOD HOTEL 🧍
47 Rhose Road, Rhos-on-Sea,
Colwyn Bay LL28 4RS
Tel: (01492) 549931
No. of Accessible Rooms: 1
Accessible Facilities: Lounge, Dining Room, Bar. Small family-run hotel in the centre of Rhos-on-Sea, 175m from shops and Promenade. Rhos is a charming resort at the western end of Colwyn, but retains a quiet atmosphere with a backcloth of the Pwllcrochan Woods and Clwydian Hills.

SELF-CATERING
BEACHMOUNT
67 Colwyn Avenue, Rhos-on-Sea,
Colwyn Bay LL28 4NN
Tel: (01492) 549314

No. of Accessible Units: 1
No. of Beds per Unit: 2
Accessible Facilities: Lounge/Diner,
Kitchen. Delightful Victorian residence
50m from sea front in pleasant quiet
avenue with award-winning garden. Five
minutes' level walk to the village centre.

CONWY

A World Heritage Site, Conwy has a
C13th castle, complete town walls and
many historic buildings including a
C14th merchant's house, a fine
Elizabethan town house, the smallest
house in Britain. There is also a
charming harbour full of yachts and
fishing boats.

TOURIST INFORMATION CENTRE
Cadw Visitor Centre, Castle Entrance,
Conwy LL32 8LD
Tel: (01492) 592248
Can supply Conwy Public Transport
Information booklet which gives all
information on buses and trains.

CAR PARKS
Tel: (01492) 592248 (same number as above)
Free unlimited disabled badge spaces

BUSES
Tel: (01492) 57541
Some low-floor buses on some routes.

TAXIS
Castle Cabs: Tel: (01492) 593398
3 adapted vehicles.

TRAINS
First North Western: Special Needs:
Tel: (0845) 6040231

SHOPMOBILITY
44 Sea View Road, Colwyn Bay,
Conwy LL29 8DG
Tel: (01492) 533822   Fax: (01492) 535372
Small collection/delivery charge and small
daily charge.

HOTEL
THE LODGE HOTEL

Tal-y-Bont, Conwy LL32 8YX
Tel: (01492) 660766
Fax: (01492) 660534
e-mail: b.baldon@lodgehotel.co.uk
www.lodgehotel.co.uk
Number of Accessible Rooms: 6. Bath
Accessible Facilities: Lounge, Restaurant,
Bar. Built in 1974 on the site of a
smallholding and well converted into a
charming small hotel, with 3.5 acres of
gardens. Located on the B5106 six miles
south of Conwy. Tal-y-Bont is a peaceful
rural village in the heart of the lovely
Conwy Valley, on the edge of Snowdonia
National Park. The hotel is framed by the
Cardeddau mountains.

ATTRACTION
THE SMALLEST HOUSE IN GREAT BRITAIN
The Quay, Conway LL32 8BB
Tel/Fax: (01492) 593484
Occupied until 1900, this house is only
72 inches (180cm) wide and 122 inches
(305cm) high. There is a tiny fireplace
where cooking was done: a settle with a
lift-up seat that doubled as a coal
bunker, a small round table, a water tap
hidden behind the stairs and a minute
bedroom with a long single bed. WC
used to be at the back. The last occupant
was a mussel fisherman standing 6ft 3in.
(187.5cm). Access to downstairs room
only.

SD 🔓   CP ♿   E 🔓

LLANDUDNO

Wales' largest resort, located
between the Great and Little Ormes,
with the award-winning North Shore
beach and the quiet sand-duned
West Shore beach. Although full of
modern attractions, Llandudno
retains much Victorian and
Edwardian elegance.

TOURIST INFORMATION CENTRE
1/2 Chapel Street, Llandudno LL30 2NY
Tel: (01492) 876413   Fax: (01492) 872722

HOTEL
THE WEST SHORE HOTEL

Grooms Holidays.
West Parade, Llandudno LL30 2BB
Tel: (01492) 876833   Fax: (01492) 875461
No. of Accessible Rooms: All
Accessible Facilities: Lounge, Dining Room,
Bar. Situated at the foot of the magnificent
Great Orme and a short walk from the
ornate Victorian Pier and Promenade.

BEDFORD HOTEL & RESTAURANT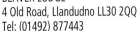
The Promenade, Craig-y-Don,
Llandudno LL30 1BN
Tel: (01492) 876647   Fax: (01492) 860185
No. of Accessible Rooms: 2. Bath
Accessible Facilities: Lounge, Italian
Restaurant.
On the promenade, many rooms enjoy fine
views of the sweeping bay.

BELMONT HOTEL
21 North Parade, Llandudno LL30 2LP
Tel: (01492) 877770
No. of Accessible Rooms: 6
Accessible Facilities: Lounge, Restaurant.
Hotel owned by Henshaw's Society for the
Blind close to the beach (100m) and 300m
from the town centre.

THE ROYAL HOTEL
Church Walks, Llandudno LL30 2HN
Tel: (01492) 876476   Fax: (01492) 870210
No. of Accessible Rooms: 6. Bath
Accessible Facilities: Lounge, Restaurant.

Established in 1857, this is the oldest hotel
in Llandudno, retaining an air of Victorian
elegance. Situated at the foot of the Great
Orme within easy distance of both North
and West shores and the town centre.
Large, secluded gardens.

SELF-CATERING
BEAVER LODGE
4 Old Road, Llandudno LL30 2QQ
Tel: (01492) 877443
No. of Accessible Units: 2
No. of Beds per Unit: 2
Accessible Facilities: Lounge, Open Plan
Kitchen. Steep driveway but flat parking
outside bungalow.

DENBIGHSHIRE

DENBIGH
Pretty walled and old market town
dominated by the scanty remains of a
huge castle begun in 1282. There are
narrow streets, piazza and historic
buildings, plus C16th hall now
housing a good museum. Denbigh
was once the centre of glove-making
in Wales. Famous as the birthplace of
Henry Morton Stanley who uttered the
immortal words "Dr. Livingstone, I
presume."

375

Llandudno bay from Great Orme.

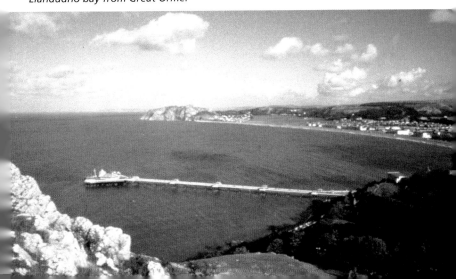

HOTEL
BRYN GLAS HOTEL
St. Asaph Road, Trefnant,
Nr. Denbigh LL16 5UD
Tel: (01745) 730868   Fax: (01745) 730590
e.mail:enqbrynglas@aol.com
www.brynglashotel.co.uk
No. of Accessible Rooms: 8
Accessible Facilities: Lounge, Restaurant,
Bar, Lawn, Grounds. Privately owned hotel
purpose built in 1988, previously the site
of an old farm. The proprietor's son is a
spinal injured person and the hotel is
staffed by the family who are very familiar
with special requirements.

CORWEN
Market town in Vale of Edeyrnion with
regular livestock market. Located 12
miles from Llangollen, it is a good
centre for Snowdonia.

ATTRACTION
LLYN BRENIG VISITOR CENTRE
Cerrigydrudion, Corwen LL21 9TT
Tel: (01490) 420463   Fax: (01490) 420694
A 1,800 acre estate with archaeological
and nature trails. Specially adapted fishing
boat for disabled anglers, the centre has
an exhibition on geology, archaeology,
history and natural history of the region.

SD	CP-	E	RF
C	S	WC	RFE

EWLOE
Located 10 miles west of Chester with
a castle that is proudly Welsh, built by
native princes in a wooded hollow to
attack the English.

HOTEL
ST. DAVID'S PARK HOTEL
St. David's Park, Ewloe,
Nr. Chester CH5 3YB
Tel: (01244) 520800   Fax: (01244) 520930
e-mail: reservations@st.davids-park-hotel.co.uk
web: www.st.davids-park-hotel.co.uk
No. of Accessible Rooms: 6
Accessible Facilities: Bar, Restaurant,
Leisure Club
Quality hotel in delightful grounds, with
nearby Northrop Country Park Golf Club.

HOLYWELL
Associated with a virtuous virgin of
C7th St. Winefride was restored to life
after her head had been chopped off
by the holy water of the Holywell
stream. The buildings associated with
the spring are set into a steep hillside
and there is a well and chapel in her
name.

ATTRACTION
GREENFIELD VALLEY COUNTRY PARK MUSEUM AND FARM
Administration Centre, Basingwerk House,
Greenfield, Holywell CH8 7QB
Tel: (01352) 714172   Fax: (01352) 714791
www.greenfieldvalley.co.uk
Set in 50 acres of woodland, within the
Abbey Farm complex is a museum
complete with machinery, equipment and
animals, restored cottages depicting a way
of life long gone and a Victorian school.
Explore further for ruined mills, good picnic
spots and silent pools.

SD	CP	E	RF	C
S	WC	RFE	MOLD	

LLANGOLLEN
Situated on the banks of the River Dee,
this lovely town is famous for its steam
railway and horse-drawn canal boats.
In the town, a C14th bridge spans the
river, and there are many historical
buildings.

TOURIST INFORMATION CENTRE
Town Hall, Castle Street, Llangollen LL20 5PD
Tel: (01978) 860828   Fax: (01978) 861563

LOCAL TRANSPORT INFORMATION
Tel: (01824) 706968

TRAVELINE
Tel: (0870) 6082608

TRAINS
Nearest station is Ruabon, Central Trains.

CAR PARKS
Disabled badge spaces available in off-street car park, but chargeable at normal rate.
3-hour free parking on-street.

WHEELCHAIR HIRE
Red Cross North Wales
Tel: (01492) 877886

HOTEL
BRYN HOWEL HOTEL AND RESTAURANT
Llangollen LL20 7UW
Tel: (01978) 860331
Fax: (01978) 860119
e-mail: hotel@brynhowel.co.uk
No. of Accessible Rooms: 1
Accessible Facilities: Lounge Bar, Restaurant. Built in 1896 as a private home, a lovely red brick property family owned and managed. Good location for exploring Vale of Llangollen.

ATTRACTION
LLANGOLLEN WHARF CANAL MUSEUM AND HORSEDRAWN BOATS
Wharf Hill, Llangollen LL20 8TA
Tel (01978) 860702
The museum offers imaginative displays on canal life in its heyday. New horse-drawn boats accessible via ramp in order to take full advantage of a 45-minute boat trip along the lovely Llangollen valley.

SD	CP	E	RF
C	S	WC	RFE

PRESTATYN
Seaside resort on which vast amounts of money have been spent to make the town an oasis of family fun, so there is much to do. Don't miss Offa's Dyke trail, stretching from the town to Chepstow. The poet Philip Larkin wrote a poem Sunny Prestatyn that captures the flavour of the resort.

TOURIST INFORMATION CENTRE
Offa's Dyke Centre, Central Beach, Prestatyn LL19 7EY
Tel: (01745) 889092

HOTEL
TRAETH GANOL HOTEL
41 Beach Road West, Prestatyn LL19 7LL
Tel: (01745) 853594   Fax: (01745) 886687
No. of Accessible rooms: 3
Accessible Facilities: Lounge, Restaurant, Bar. Located opposite the sea at Central Beach with Promenade access by the Nova Leisure Centre 100m. away. Small and personal family-owned hotel.

Pontcysyllte aquaduct, Llangollen canal .

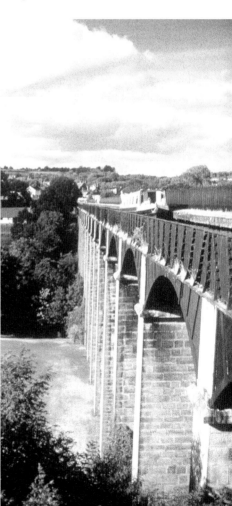

GWYNEDD

ABERSOCH
Popular small resort, calling itself the Welsh Riviera. There are two sandy bays full of dinghies and windsurfers, and offshore are St. Tudwal's Islands with seals and seabirds.

TOURIST INFORMATION CENTRE
Abersoch LL53 7AP
Tel/Fax: (01758) 712929

SELF-CATERING
RHYDOLION
Llangian, Abersoch, LL53 7LR
Tel/Fax: (01758) 712342
No. of Accessible Units: 1. Roll-in shower.
No. of Beds per Unit: 6
Accessible Facilities: Lounge/Diner, Kitchen.
Cottage on working farm.

BALA
Market town on the edge of Snowdonia with a single street lined with trees. In the deep valley to the SW of the town is Bala Lake, the largest natural body of water in Wales. Originally founded as an English borough in 1310, the back lanes running parallel to the High Street show the limits of the original burbage plots.

TOURIST INFORMATION CENTRE
Pensarn Road, Bala LL23 7NH
Tel/Fax: (01678) 521 021
e-mail: bala.tic@gwynedd.gov.uk

ATTRACTION
BALA LAKE RAILWAY
The Station, Llanuwchllyn, Bala LL23 7DD
Tel: (01678) 540666   Fax:(01678) 540535
www.bala-lake-railway.co.uk
Narrow gauge train running along the shores of Wales' largest natural lake. Lovely nine-mile return journey through Snowdonia national park with fine views of the lake and surrounding pastoral and woodland scenery and nearby mountains.

SD ⬚   CP   E   RF
C ⬚   S ⬚   WC ⬚
RFE ⬚   Platform – Direct Access at Llanuwchllyn, but NOT AT BALA. Train- Ramped Access

BANGOR
Cathedral and university city overlooking the scenic Menai Strait. A wide variety of architectural styles, a Victorian pier and its cathedral, founded in AD525, said to be the oldest in Britain. The city began to grow at the end of the C18th when Penrhyn slate was exported. The university arrived in 1884 and Bangor is now a small metropolis.

TOURIST INFORMATION CENTRE
Town Hall, Deiniol Road, Bangor LL57 7RE
Tel: (01248) 352786   Fax: (01248) 362701
e-mail: bangor.tic@gwynedd.gov.uk

PUBLIC TRANSPORT INFORMATION
Tel: (01286) 679535

TRAVELINE
Tel: (0870) 6082608

TRAINS
First North Western: Special Needs:
Tel: (0845) 6040231
Virgin Trains: Special Needs:
Tel: (0845) 7443366

HOTEL
THE BRITISH HOTEL
High Street, Bangor LL57 1NP
Tel: (01248) 364911   Fax: (01248) 370569
e-mail: BritishHotelBangor@compuserve.com
web: www.S-H-Systems.co.uk/Hotels/Brit,Html
No. of Accessible Rooms: 40 (via lift)
Accessible Facilities: Lounge, Restaurant, Buttery and Cocktail Bar. Purpose-built property close to university halls, main shopping and entertainment areas.

ATTRACTION
PENRHYN CASTLE (NT)
Bangor LL57 4HN
Tel: (01248) 353084   Fax: (01248) 371281
Neo-Norman castle with towers and

battlements commissioned in 1827 as a sumptuous family home. Notable rooms include the Great Hall, Library and Dining Room with a fine collection of paintings. Also an industrial railway museum in the Stableyard, and Victorian terraced walled garden in the 40-acre grounds. Ground floor rooms only are accessible. Wheelchairs available and volunteer-driven 3-passenger vehicles to assist in viewing the grounds.

SD ♿ CP ♿ E ♿ RF ♿
C ♿ S ♿ WC ♿ RFE ♿

GREENWOOD FOREST PARK CENTRE
Y Felinheli, Nr. Bangor LL56 4QN
Tel: (01248) 671493 Fax: (01248) 670069
e-mail: info@greenwood-centre.co.uk
Set up to provide an insight into the extraordinary world of trees, with conservation a priority. Forest and Adventure Park with herb garden, sculpture trail, tree world in the great hall, adventureland, Welsh crafts and animals. Film show on the Forgotten Forests of Snowdonia and inter-active exhibition. Located a few miles SW of Bangor.

SD ♿ CP ♿ E ♿ RF ♿
C 🚶 S 🚶 WC 🚶 RFE ♿

BLAENAU FFESTINIOG

TOURIST INFORMATION CENTRE
Unit 3, High Street,
Blaenau Ffestiniog LL41 3ES
Tel: (01690) 710426 Fax: (01690) 710665
Seasonal, in winter contact Betws-y-Coed.

ATTRACTION
LLECHWEDD SLATE CAVERNS
Blaenau Ffestiniog LL41 3NB
Tel: (01766) 830306 Fax: (01766) 831260
e-mail: llechwedd@aol.com
Discover the working conditions of Victorian slate mines where primitive tools were used to move millions of ton of rock. Surface exhibitions on mine tramways and slate mining, old smithy, slate mill and Victorian shops. All surface attractions, except Miners Arms, are accessible. For the mine take the Miner's Tramway guided tour through an 1846 network of amazing man-made caverns of cathedral

proportions, supplemented with tableaux and demonstrations of ancient mining skills. Folding wheelchairs can be carried on the train, but transfer from wheelchair to train seat for journey and at several points underground is required.
NB: Entrance ramped at 1:9: Route to features is ramped at 1:10. The Deep Mine tour is not accessible.

SD ♿ CP ♿ E n/a RF ♿
C ♿ S ♿ WC 🚶 RFE n/a

DOLGELLAU
Quiet, historic market town with narrow streets once famed for the mining of Welsh gold. An excellent touring centre.

PUBLIC TRANSPORT INFORMATION
Tel: (01286) 679535
41) 422888 Fax: (01341) 422576

TRAVELINE
Tel: (0870) 6082608

CAR PARKS
Free unlimited disabled badge parking.
Tel: (01341) 422341

WHEELCHAIR HIRE
British Red Cross: Tel: (01341) 422620

BED AND BREAKFAST
GRAIG-WEN HOUSE ♿
Arthog, Nr. Dolgellau LL39 1BQ
Tel: (01341) 250482 Fax: (01341) 250482
www.craig-wen@supanet.com
No. of Accessible Rooms: 1
Accessible Facilities: Lounge, Dining Room, Snooker Room. Set in 45 acres of woodland and pasture reaching down the spectacular Mawddach Estuary with views of surrounding mountains. Located five miles from Dolgellau and between there and Fairbourne on the A493.

SELF-CATERING
PEN Y LON ♿
Pentre Bach, Llwyngwril,
Nr Dolgellau LL37 2JU
Tel: (01341) 250294 Fax: (01341) 250885

e-mail: ride@pentrebach.com
www.pentrebach.com
No. of Accessible Units: 1, shower with seat
No. of Beds per Unit: 7 + cot
House in seaside village in the southern part of Snowdonia National Park. At the end of a 250m private, tree-lined drive, 12 miles from Dolgellau, with glorious views across Cardigan Bay to Lleyn Peninsula. Village at top of drive with Post Office, shops and pub.

HARLECH
Small town on SW border of Snowdonia and a good base from which to explore the mountains inland. Against an amazing sea and mountain background, Harlech Castle is the epitomy of a medieval stronghold. It was erected as one of the Iron Ring of defences by Edward I in the late C13th.

TOURIST INFORMATION CENTRE
Bro Gynton, Porkington Place,
High Street, Harlech LL46 2YE
Tel/Fax: (01766) 780658

MOTEL
ESTUARY MOTEL
Talsarnau, Harlech LL47 6TA
Tel: (01766) 771155 Fax: (01766) 771697
No. of Accessible Rooms: 10 Accessible Facilities: Lounge, Restaurant.Located midway between Harlech and Portmeirion.

SELF-CATERING
YSTUMGWERN FARM
Dyffryn Ardudwy, Nr. Harlech LL44 2DD
Tel: (01341) 247249 Fax: (01341) 247171
No. of Accessible Units: 1
Accessible Beds per Unit: 8
Accessible Facilities: Lounge, Dining Room, Kitchen. Farmhouse 5 miles from Harlech.

LLANBERIS
Lively mountain town and a popular touring centre at the foot of Snowdon, with two lakes and the craggy Llanberis Pass.

TOURIST INFORMATION CENTRE
41b High Street, Llanberis LL55 4EU
Tel: (01286) 870765 Fax: (01286) 871924

ATTRACTIONS
LLANBERIS LAKE RAILWAY
Gilfach Ddu, Llanberis LL55 4TY
Tel/Fax: (01286) 870549
www.lake-railway.co.uk
e.mail:info@lake-railway.co.uk
Enjoy spectacular views of Snowdon and surrounding mountains. Starting at Gilfach Ddu station, the train takes about 40 minutes to run to Penllyn through Padarn Country Park and back with a short stop at Cei Llydan for sightseeing. Stop here for a picnic and catch a later train back to Llanberis. Extention to line in progress.

SD | CP | E | RF
C | S | WC
RFE TRAIN Specially adapted carriage to take 6 wheelchairs. Graded by WTB as accessible for unaccompanied wheelchair users.

SNOWDON MOUNTAIN RAILWAY
Llanberis LL55 4TY
Tel: (0870) 4580033 Fax: (01286) 872518
www.snowdonrailway.co.uk
email: info@snowdonrailway.co.uk
For passengers with some limited mobility who can leave their wheelchairs, staff recommend these be left in Llanberis and use be made of the ones kept at the summit. Disembarkation at the summit is not possible for powered chairs.

SD | CP | E (Platform) | RF
C | S | WC
TRAIN – 2 trains able to accommodate either 2 manual or 1 powered wheelchair. Wheelchairs have to be carried from platform to carriage, but staff advise they will always help.

WELSH SLATE MUSEUM
Padarn Country Park, Llanberis LL55 4TY
Tel: (01286) 870630 Fax: (01286) 871906
Set among towering slate quarries, this is a living working site, a pocket of the past. There is a quarry workshop with demonstrations and the largest working waterwheel on mainland Britain. Plus spectacular 3-D presentation of life in the quarries, restored Chief Engineer's house and unique working slate incline.

Quarrymens' houses and pattern loft not accessible.

SD ⚿ CP ⚿ E ⚿ RF ⚿
C ⚿ S ⚿ WC ⚿ RFE ⚿

PANT GLAS
Located on the SW edge of Snowdonia

HOTEL
HEN YSGOL OLD SCHOOL ⚿
Bwlch-Derwin, Pant Glas,Gwynedd, LL51 9EQ
Tel: (01286) 660701
e-mail: OldSchoolPantGlas@Talk21.com
No. of Accessible Rooms: 3
Accessible Facilities: Lounge, Dining Room, Gardens, Grounds. Historic country school built in 1858 now converted and retaining much of the traditional features. Situated on the NW boundary of the Snowdonia National Park, an ideal base for touring Snowdon and neighbouring area. Beaches of Criccieth and Pwllheli within 6-10 miles.

PORTHMADOG
Pretty town lying on the Glaslyn estuary on the Llyn Peninsula, designated an "Area of Outstanding Natural Beauty", with a number of beaches managed by the National Trust. The town has a fascinating maritime heritage and a lovely harbour.

TOURIST INFORMATION CENTRE
High Street, Porthmadog LL49 9LP
Tel: (01766) 512981   Fax: (01766) 515312
e-mail: porthmadog.tic@gwynedd.gov.uk

ATTRACTION
FFESTINIOG RAILWAY
Harbour Station, Porthmadog LL49 9NF
Tel: (01766) 516073   Fax: (01766) 516006
e-mail: info@festrail.co.uk
www.festrail.co.uk
Famous railway with little steam-hauled narrow-gauge trains running along 13.5 miles main line in miniature from coastline at Porthmadog into the mountains at Blaenau Ffestiniog with wonderful views. Also on the sister railway between

Caernarfon and Waunfawr, there are gentle pastoral views of the Menai Strait. Porthmadog and Blaenau Ffestiniog stations have ramped access routes and partially adapted WCs. Caernarfon and Waunfawr have ramped access. Coaches on some trains have extra wide doors (not electric chairs).

SD ⚿ CP ⚿ E ⚿ RF ⚿
C ⚿ S ⚿ WC ⚿

PWLLHELI
Historic market town, also on the Llyn Peninsula, has many buildings dating back to early C17th. It has a 420-berth marina and 5 miles of sand and shingle beaches.

TOURIST INFORMATION CENTRE
Min y Don, Sgwar yr Orsaf,
Pwllheli. LL53 5HG
Tel/Fax: (01758) 613000
e-mail: pwllheli.tic@gwynedd.gov.uk

BED AND BREAKFAST
RHOSYDD ⚿
26 Glan Cymerau, Pwllheli LL53 5PU
Tel: (01758) 612956
No. of Accessible Rooms: 1
Accessible Facilities: Dining room.
Detached bungalow situated 1/4 mile from beach, on outskirts of town. Leisure Centre and golf nearby.

Full steam ahead for the top of Snowdon.

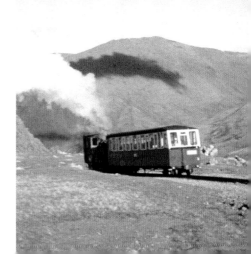

SELF-CATERING
AFONWEN FARM
Pwllheli LL53 6TX
Tel/Fax: (01766) 810939
No. of Accessible Units: 4
No. of Beds per Unit: 4 – 8
Accessible Facilities: Lounge, Kitchen, Games Room, Nature Trail around farm. Converted in 1995, 4 cottages and farm-house on owner's working farm between Snowdonia National park and Lyn Peninsula. Surrounded by farmland, lovely mountain views and within five minutes' of the beach.

CEFN COED
Chwilog, Pwllheli LL53 6NX
Tel: (01766) 810259
No. of Accessible Units: 1
No. of Beds per Unit: 6
Accessible Facilities: Lounge, Dining Room, Kitchen. C18th cottages on farm in quiet countryside with panoramic views of Cardigan Bay coast.

TRAWSFYNYDD
Located in heart of Snowdonia National Park midway between Dollgellau and Porthmadog.

BED AND BREAKFAST
OLD MILL FARMHOUSE
Trawsfynydd LL41 4UN
Tel/Fax: (01766) 540397
No. of Accessible Rooms: 1 Roll-in shower.
Accessible Facilities: Lounge, Dining Room, Garden. Holiday Care Award winning property, once the home of the village corn miller, dating back to early C18th. The farm land allows families plenty of open space and contact with safe friendly animals. Accommodation in converted old farm building adjacent to farmhouse, where breakfast is served.

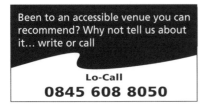
Been to an accessible venue you can recommend? Why not tell us about it... write or call
Lo-Call
0845 608 8050

TYWYN
Seaside resort on Cardigan Bay with important Christian monuments of St. Cadfan's Stone and Llanegryn Church. Located west of Dolgellau and Machynlleth at the SW tip of Snowdonia National Park.

TOURIST INFORMATION CENTRE
High Street, Tywyn LL36 9AD
Tel/Fax: (01654) 710070
e-mail: tywyn.tic@gwynedd.gov.uk
Seasonal, in winter contact Dolgellau.

ATTRACTION
TALYLLYN RAILWAY
Wharf Station, Tywyn LL36 9EY
Tel: (01654) 710472   Fax: (01654) 711755
Narrow gauge line using steam locomotives that opened in 1865 and runs inland from Tywyn on the mid Wales coast to Nant Gwernol. A journey of just under an hour, much of it within Snowdonia National Park with waterfalls at Dolgoch.
NB No road access at Nant Gwernol terminus and so the main starting point is Abergynolwyn.

| SD | | E | | RFE | | C | |
| S | | WC | | RFE | | | |

TRAIN – entrance to compartment by ramp assisted by staff.

ISLE OF ANGLESEY
www.anglesey.gov.uk

HOLYHEAD TOURIST INFORMATION CENTRE
The Kiosk, Stena Line, Terminal 1, Holyhead LL65 1DR
Tel: (01407) 762622

CENTRE FOR INTEGRATED LIVING:
Tel: (01248) 750249
Information on accommodation and transport in the area.

TRAVELINE
Tel: (0870) 6082608

COMMUNITY TRANSPORT
(01248) 751312
If you get in touch before you travel they can help with travel arrangements.

ISLE OF ANGLESEY COUNTY COUNCIL
Transport Department
Tel: (01248) 752459
Tel: (01248) 750444

AMLWCH
Parys Mountain is the most spectacular hill in Anglesey, site of greatest copper mines in the world in the late C18th, with Amlwch as their port. Widened in the 1790s to make a harbour, the little port retains its late C18th appearance and is still used by various types of boat. The catholic church, Our Lady Star of the Sea, is built in the shape of an overturned boat, emphasising the area's seafaring tradition.

BEAUMARIS
Small town in glorious setting, overlooking the Menai Strait which is very broad at this point, the south shore rises to the mountains of Snowdonia. Popular with holidaymakers from late Georgian times it is an elegant resort with a pier, seafront green and brightly painted terraces facing the water.

HOTEL
BEST WESTERN BULKELEY
Castle Street, Beaumaris LL58 8AW
Tel: (01248) 810415   Fax: (01248) 810146
www.consorthotels.com
Accessible Facilities: Lounge, Restaurant. Built for the young Princess Victoria in 1832, retains the style and elegance. Very close to the beach and pier with views of Menai Straits to Snowdonia mountains.

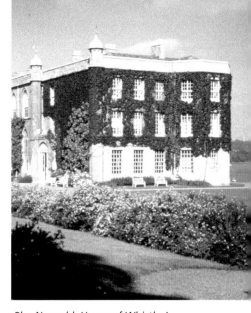

Plas Newydd. Home of Whistler's largest mural.

BENLLECH
Popular holiday village above a sweeping bay on the east coast. Long and sandy beach for families with beach shops and cafes. Nearby cliffs rich in fossils.

BED AND BREAKFAST
BRYN MEIRION GUEST HOUSE
Amlwch Road, Benllech LL74 8SR
Tel: (01248) 853118
No. of Accessible Rooms: 6
Accessible Facilities: Lounge, Dining Room, Gardens. Panoramic views across the sea to Llandudno and Snowdonia mountains beyond. Family run guest house, set in lovely lawned gardens on fine coastal site on east coast of Anglesey. The owners, having worked in a residential school for children with disabilities, established this property to cater for all.

BRYNSIENCYN
Hamlet near shores of Menai Strait, looking across to Snowdonia.

ATTRACTION
ANGLESEY SEA ZOO
Brynsiencyn LL61 6TQ
Tel: (01248) 430411   Fax: (01248) 430213
e-mail: FISHANDFUN@SEAZOO.demon.co.uk
www.angleseyseazoo.co.uk
Gaze at local creatures as they live and
grow undisturbed in one of Britain's
largest single underwater viewing stations.
Wander through a shipwreck and a new
exhibition on how pearls are bred and
used. See, touch, smell and breathe the
sea.

SD   CP   E   RF
C   S   WC

LLANFAIRPWLL
It's compulsory to visit this village –
Llanfairpwllgwyngyllgogerychwyrndrob
wllllantysiliogogogoch – the longest
name in Britain. It was a C19th hoax
by a tailor from the Menai Bridge to
attract tourists to the station. Get a
souvenir platform ticket from James
Pringle Weavers centre. Llanfair means
St. Mary's.

TOURIST INFORMATION CENTRE
Station Site, Llanfairpwll LL61 5UJ
Tel: (01248) 713177   Fax: (01248) 715711

ATTRACTION
PLAS NEWYDD (NT)
Llanfairpwll LL61 6DQ
Tel: (01248) 714795   Fax: (01248) 713673
e-mail: ppnmsn@smtp.ntrust.org.uk
C18th house with a mixture of classical and
Gothic architecture. Re-styled interior of
1930s, famous for Rex Whistler whose
largest wall painting is housed here plus an
exhibition about his work. Military museum
with relics of Battle of Waterloo and a fine
garden.

SD   CP   E   RF
C   S   WC

LLANGEFNI
County town of Anglesey standing
on the island's longest river, the Cefni.
Many leisure facilities and weekly
open air markets on Thursday and
Saturdays. The nearby Llyn Cefni
reservoir offers trout fishing and bird
watching.

HOTEL
TRE-YSGAWEN HALL
Capel Coch, Llangefni LL77 7UR
Tel: (01248) 750750   Fax: (01248) 750035
No. of Accessible Rooms: 3
Accessible Facilities: Lounge, Restaurant.
Country house mansion, built in 1882,
and renovated in 1990. Set in the heart of
a 3,000-acre estate

RED WHARF BAY
Superb sands make this one of
Anglesey's most popular beaches.

HOTEL
BRYN TIRION HOTEL
Red Wharf Bay, LL75 8RZ
Tel: (01248) 852366   Fax: (01248) 852013
bthotel@btinternet.com
No. of Accessible Rooms: 1
Accessible Facilities: Lounge, Restaurant
Family run hotel enjoying superb views
over the bay.

SELF-CATERING
YR HEN YSGOL
Rhoscolyn, Nr. Trearddur Bay LL65 2RQ
Tel: (01407) 741593
No. of Accessible Units: 2
No. of Beds per Unit: 6
Accessible Facilities:
2 bungalows in unspoilt countryside,
close to beaches.

MERTHYR TYDFIL

High up the Taff Vale, for many years the Iron Capital of the World, much of the early industrial heritage remains. The last foundry was shut down by British Steel in 1987, but this is still a proud, if rather bleak town.

MERTHYR TYDFIL
TOURIST INFORMATION CENTRE
14A Glebeland Street,
Merthyr Tydfil CF47 8AU
Tel: (01685) 379884   Fax: (01685) 350043

PUBLIC TRANSPORT INFORMATION
Merthyr Tydfil County Borough Council,
Technical Services
Tel: (01685) 726256

BUSES
Stagecoach Red & White: Tel: (01685) 385539
Some low-floor buses.

TAXIS
A & P Cars: Tel: (01685) 374326
1 adapted vehicle.
First Class Cars: Tel: (01685) 373737
1 adapted vehicle

TRAINS
Valley Line: Special Needs:
Tel: (029) 20 449944
All trains have ramps – ring a few days before travel – also provides park & ride.

SHOPMOBILITY
St. Tydfil's Square, Shopping Centre,
Merthyr Tydfil
Tel/Fax: (01685) 373237
Minicom: (01685) 373400

HOTEL
TREGENNA HOTEL
Park Terrace, Merthyr Tydfil CF47 8RF
Tel: (01685) 723627   Fax: (01685) 721951
e-mail: treghotel@aol.com
No. of Accessible Rooms: 2 Accessible

Facilities: Lounge, Restaurant. Family run in the heart of the National Park on the edge of the Brecon Beacons.

ATTRACTIONS
BRECON MOUNTAIN RAILWAY CO.
Plant Station, Merthyr Tydfil, CF48 2UP
Tel: (01685) 722988   Fax: (01685) 384854
Located 3 miles north of town. All-weather observation coaches behind vintage steam locomotive through beautiful scenery into the Brecon Beacons National Park along the full length of Taf Fechan Reservoir to Dol-y-Gaer.
Access positively described in literature.
Carriages: 1, specially designed to carry wheelchairs.

P & A	E	C tables not accessible
S	WC	Features: Platform

CYFARTHFA CASTLE MUSEUM and ART GALLERY
Brecon Road, Merthyr Tydfil   CF47 8RE
Tel/Fax: (01685) 723112
Gothic mansion built in 1825 with wonderful surviving gardens. Houses fine collection of decorative arts, archaeological and natural history items and social and industrial history of the region. Basement gallery has chairlift and wheelchair available at foot.

SD	CP	E	RF
S	WC	RFE	

TREHARRIS
Located 8 miles from Merthyr Tydfil.

ATTRACTION
LLANCAIACH FAWR MANOR
LIVING HISTORY MUSEUM
Plas Llancaiach Fawr, Nelson,
Treharris CF46 6ER
Tel: (01443) 412248   Fax: (01443) 412688
Civil War period museum: 1645 invitation to meet the servants of the then Lord of the Manor, Colonel Edward Pritchard. Access to ground floor only.

SD	CP	E	RF
C	S	WC	RFE

MONMOUTHSHIRE

ABERGAVENNY
One of the prettiest gateways to the Brecon Beacons with The Sugar Loaf, Blorenge and Skirrid Fawr mountains providing a dramatic backdrop to the town. This is a market town: Livestock on Tuesdays and crowded Market Hall on Tuesdays and Fridays. Fine parish church, St. Mary's, referred to as the Westminster Abbey of Wales for its amazing collection of beautifully carved tombs. A C19th hunting lodge in the Norman ruins of the castle is now home to the town's museum. Wales' oldest pub, The Skirrid Inn is here.

TOURIST INFORMATION CENTRE
Bus Station, Swan Meadow, Monmouth Road, Abergavenny NP7 5HH
Tel: (01873) 857588   Fax: (01873) 850217

TRAVELINE
Tel: (0870) 6082608

TRAINS
Wales and West: Special Needs:
Tel: (0845) 3003005

CAR PARKS
Free three-hour parking in all council car parks and some on-street parking.

SELF-CATERING
LOWER GREEN FARM
Llanfair Green, Crosh Ash,
Abergavenny NP7 8PA
Tel/Fax: (01873) 821219
No. of Accessible Units: 1. Shower
No. of Beds per Unit: 6
Accessible Facilities: Open plan Lounge/kitchen/diner.
Swallow Cottage is 1 of 2 converted barns on 170-acre farm, set in tranquil countryside. Guests are welcome to explore the farm and meet the farm animals.

ATTRACTION
ABERGAVENNY CASTLE AND MUSEUM
Castle Street, Abergavenny,

Monmouthshire   NP7 5EE
Tel: (01873) 854282   Fax: (01873) 736004
Displays on the town's development and its surroundings. Almost every room in the Museum has steps to or from it and is not suitable for visitors who must remain in their wheelchairs.

SD [♿]   CP [♿]   E [♿]   RF [♿]
S [♿]   WC [♿]   RFE [♿]

CHEPSTOW
Standing on the Monmouthshire/Gloucestershire border, overlooking the lower reaches of the River Wye before it flows into the Severn. Mid C11th castle, built after the Norman conquest, stands above a bend in the Wye. The castle is at the centre of many attractions in this walled town. There is a restored gatehouse and charming narrow streets lead to the castle.

TOURIST INFORMATION CENTRE
Castle Car Park, Bridge Street,
Chepstow NP16 5EY
Tel: (01291) 623772   Fax: (01291) 628004

SELF-CATERING
BYRE COTTAGE   [♿]
Cwrt-y-Gaer, Wolvesnewton,
Chepstow NP16 6PR
Tel: (01291) 650700
No. of Accessible Units: 1
No. of Beds per Unit: 2 – 4
Accessible Facilities: Kitchen, Lounge, patio with furniture.
One of 3 stone cottages converted from farm buildings, in lovely location on the site of an ancient Welsh hill-top fort with 20 acres of woods and meadows.

ATTRACTION
CALDICOT CASTLE MUSEUM
Church Road, Caldicot,
Nr Chepstow NP26 4HU
Tel: (01291) 420241   Fax: (01291) 435094
Well preserved Norman fortification, fully developed by late C14th and restored as Victorian family home. Set down is directly in front of Museum – route from CP to the entrance is very steep. Located

just south of Chepstow at western end of Second Severn Crossing (M4).

SD   CP n/a   E   RF [⌖]
C [⌖]   S [⌖]   WC [⌖]

MONMOUTH

Famous for its C13th gateway, on the Monnow Bridge, the only complete monument of its kind in Britain. There are well preserved Tudor and Georgian buildings around Agincourt Square. High street connects here with narrow shopping lanes and courtyard eating areas. King Henry V was born at the town's castle in 1387, as was Sir Charles Rolls of Rolls-Royce fame.

TOURIST INFORMATION CENTRE
Shire Hall, Agincourt Square,
Monmouth NP25 3DY
Tel: (01600) 713899   Fax: (01600) 772794

SELF-CATERING
HARVEST HOME   [⌖]
The Hill, Bryngwyn, Raglan,
Nr. Monmouth NP5 2JH
Tel/Fax: (01291) 690007/691207
e.mail: harvesthome@freeuk.com
www.harvest-home.co.uk
No. of Accessible Units: 1
No. of Beds per Unit: 2-4
Accessible Facilities: Lounge, Kitchen.
Set in lovely countryside with fine mountain and lovely garden views. Located 7 miles from Monmouth.

TINTERN

"The most romantic valley in Wales"
William Wordsworth. Riverside village in lovely stretch of Wye Valley.

HOTEL
THE ROYAL GEORGE HOTEL   [⌖]
Tintern NP6 6SF
Tel: (01292) 689205   Fax: (01291) 689448
No. of Accessible Rooms: 1
Accessible Facilities: Lounge, Restaurant, Bar. Built in 1598, converted in C17th to a coaching inn and extended and improved

over the years into a 16 - bedroom hotel. The ruins of Tintern Abbey (inaccessible) are a minute away as are the Forest of Dean and the River Wye. The hotel has an award-winning restaurant overlooking lovely gardens.

USK

At the heart of rural Monmouthshire this pretty town is famous for wonderful floral displays. A past winner of Britain in Bloom and constant winner of Wales in Bloom. It also offers antique furniture shops, painted cottages and lovely pubs and restaurants. A great place to browse.

SELF-CATERING
THE PHEASANT PENS
Brace Farm, Llandenny, Nr. Usk NP5 1DN
Tel: (01291) 690216
No. of Accessible Units: 1
No. of Beds per Unit: 2-4
Accessible Facilities: Open plan Living room/Kitchen.
1 of 2 cottages converted from farm buildings on working farm. Situated in Usk Valley within easy reach of the Wye Valley.

ATTRACTION
USK RURAL LIFE MUSEUM
The Malt Barn, New Market Street,
Usk NP5 1AU
Tel: (01291) 673777
The museum portrays life in the Welsh Border country from Victorian times until the end of WWII. All aspects of country life shown and explained with thousands of exhibits donated by local people over the past 30 years. Fascinating experience.

SD- [⌖]   CP   E [⌖]   RF
S [⌖]   WC n/a

NEATH AND PORT TALBOT

NEATH
Located where the Vale of Neath opens out into an industrial spread. Given a new look, the town is at its best in September at its annual fair, the oldest in Wales. There are ruins of its 1280-1330 abbey and boat trips on the spruced up canal.

BED AND BREAKFAST
CWMBACH COTTAGES
Cwmbach Road, Cadoxton, Neath SA10 8AH
Tel: (01639) 639825
No. of Accessible Rooms: 1
Accessible Facilities: Lounge, Dining Room. The Primrose Room (accessible) has its own car park and is next to Dining Room. Located on a hillside overlooking Neath and in a woodland area, six old miners' cottages converted. On the doorstep is Craig Gwladys Country Park, Penscynor Wildlife Park and Aberdulais Falls.

ATTRACTION
ABERDULAIS FALLS (NT)
Aberdulais, Neath, Port Talbot, SA10 8EU
Tel: (01639) 636674 Fax: (01639) 645069
For over 300 years the Falls have powered the wheels of industry, grinding corn, refining copper and manufacturing tinplate. This has the largest waterwheel generating electricity in Europe. The Falls roar down the rock in a rustic landscape, surrounded by thick vegetation. Much loved by C18th and C19th landscape painters, including Turner. Since 1981 it has been cleared by the National Trust.

SD  CP   E   RF   L
C ⬡ S ⬡ WC ⬡ RFE ⬡

PORT TALBOT
One of the largest of Welsh towns, where the growing iron and copper industries flourished in the mid C19th. The port was extended in 1972 to allow for a deep-water harbour. The town is squeezed between the shore and rising hills, stretching for miles. This, with the chemical works to the west, complete a mainly industrial landscape.

TRAVELINE
(0870) 6082608

TRAINS
First Great Western: Special Needs:
Tel: (0845) 7413775
Wales & West: Special Needs:
Tel: (0845) 3003005

SHOPMOBILITY
Unit 43, Aberavon Shopping Centre, Port Talbot
Tel: (01639) 894949

HOTEL
ABERAVON BEACH HOTEL
Port Talbot SA12 6QP
Tel: (01639) 884949   Fax: (01639) 897885
www.sales@aberavonbeach.com
No. of Accessible Rooms: 1
Accessible Facilities: Lounge, Restaurant, Pool, Sauna, Spa. Modern hotel opposite wide sandy beach with fine views across Swansea Bay. All weather leisure centre

NEWPORT
Medieval cathedral and castle compete with Victorian architecture here: Roman walls and amphitheatre with modern developments. The most famous landmark, the Transporter Bridge, has been restored to working order.

TOURIST INFORMATION CENTRE
Museum and Art Gallery,
John Frost Square, Newport NP20 1PA
Tel: (01633) 842962   Fax: (01633) 222615

HOTELS
HILTON NEWPORT
Chepstow Road, Langstone, Newport NP6 2LX
Tel: (01633) 413737   Fax: (01633) 413713
e-mail: reservations@newport.co.uk
web: www.hilton.com
No. of Accessible Rooms: 4
Accessible Facilities: Bar, Restaurant, Courtyard Garden.
Quality hotel located close to M4 (J24).

BEST WESTERN PARKWAY HOTEL AND
CONFERENCE CENTRE
Cwmbran Drive, Cwmbran, Newport NP18 2LX
Tel: (01633) 871199   Fax: (01633) 869160
No. of Accessible Rooms: 3
Accessible Facilities: Lounge, Restaurant.
Privately owned quality hotel, developed on a Mediterranean theme all 70 bedrooms enjoying Welsh countryside views. Located at M4 West (J25A), M4E (J26), between Newport and Cwmbran.

ATTRACTION
CAERLEON FORTRESS BATHS
High Street, Caerleon, Nr. Newport
Tel: (01633) 422518
An important Roman military base, Caerleon's Fortress Baths were excavated in the 1970s and show the most complete example of Roman Legionary bath building in Britain.

SD [⌖]   CP [⌖]   E [⌖]   RF [⌖]
C n/a   S [⌖]   WC n/a

PEMBROKESHIRE

PHYSICALLY IMPAIRED PEOPLE OF PEMBROKESHIRE ASSOCIATION
The Coach House, Bridgend Square
Haverfordwest SA61 2NO
Tel/Fax: (01437) 760999
Information and Advice plus Wheelchair Hire Scheme and RADAR toilet keys.

HAVERFORDWEST
Dominated by the ruins of its Norman Castle which was rebuilt during Georgian times, with little still standing. The coming of the railway destroyed much of its sea trade and in 1920 the last steamer sailed down the western Cleddar River. The town's maritime past is still evident in some old warehouses. Close by is the spacious sandy beach of Broad Haven.

PEMBROKESHIRE COAST NATIONAL PARK VISIT CENTRE
40 High Street, Haverfordwest
Tel: (01437) 760136

TOURIST INFORMATION CENTRE
19 Old Bridge, Haverfordwest
Tel: (01437) 763110   Fax: (01437) 767738
www.visitpenprokeshire.com

SELF-CATERING
KEESTON HILL COTTAGE
Keeston Kitchen, Keeston,
Haverfordwest SA62 6EJ
Tel: (01437) 710440
www.keestonhill.cottage@virgin.net
No. of Accessible Units: 1. Bath.
No. of Beds per Unit: 1 double, 2 singles
Accessible Facilities: Living Room with galley-style Kitchen. Ground floor apartment in lovely converted cottage set in own large garden, set back from main Haverfordwest/St. David's road in quiet layby. 4 miles from Haverfordwest. Next door to family-run restaurant.

MILLMOOR FARM COTTAGES AND
ROCKSDRIFT APARTMENTS
Broad Haven, Haverfordwest SA62 3JH
Tel: (01437) 781507   Fax: (01437) 781002
No. of Accessible Units: Rocksdrift
No. of Beds per Unit: 6
Accessible Facilities: Lounge/Diner, Kitchen, Gardens. Located in heart of Pembrokeshire Coast National Park. Award winning property. The beach-side apartments at Rocksdrift are converted from C18th coach house into two apartments. Rocksdrift is on the ground floor.

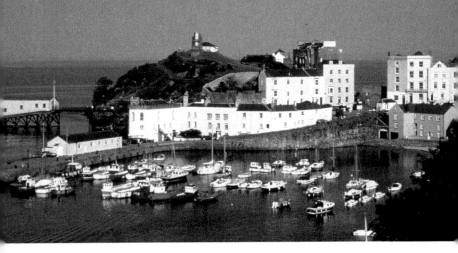

Picturesque Tenby harbour.

ROSEMOOR

Walwyn's Castle, Haverfordwest SA62 3ED
Tel: (01437) 781326   Fax: (01437) 781080
No. of Accessible Units: 1
No. of Beds per Unit: 2 - 9
Accessible Facilities: Lounge,
Kitchen/Diner, Lawns facing west.
Within the grounds are other cottages
and all are surrounded by open country,
trees and fields.

DREENHILL FARM

Dale Road, Haverfordwest SA62 3XG
Tel/Fax: (01437) 764494
No. of Accessible Units: 1
No. of Beds per Unit: 2. Shower.
Accessible Facilities: Living/Dining Room,
Kitchen, Patio.
"Fledracks" is 1 of 2 self-contained
properties attached to, and separated by,
the main farmhouse. Situated in large
gardens with fields and private nature
trail. 120m from road. 2.5m from
Haverfordwest.

ATTRACTION
SCOLTON MANOR MUSEUM VISITOR CENTRE

Spittal, Haverfordwest SA62 5QL
Tel: (01437) 731328   Fax: (01437) 731743
Exhibits in Victorian mansion and stables
on history and natural history of the
region and environmentally friendly visitor
centre and 60 acres of grounds.

SD   CP   E   RF
C   S   WC

NARBETH

Small market town, convenient for
beaches of Carmarthen Bay and resorts
of Tenby and Saundersfoot. Many
attractions nearby.

ATTRACTION
OAKWOOD PARK LEISURE

Canaston Bridge, Narbeth SA67 8DE
Tel: (01834) 891373   Fax: (01834) 891380
e-mail: park@oakwood-leisure.com
www.oakwood-leisure.com
Theme park with numerous activities and
rides, both undercover and outdoor.
Includes Europe's largest wooden roller-
coaster, pirate ship, boating lake, waterfall
and bobsleigh rides amongst others.

SD   CP   E   RF
C- Restaurant   Acorn Tearoom
S   WC   RFE

PEMBROKE

A Norman town, still retaining an
ancient street pattern and long
burbage plots which run down to the
last vestiges of the medieval walls.
There is an imposing Norman castle,
founded in 1090, one of the best-
preserved in Britain. Pembroke was a
Naval Dockyard until 1924.

TOURIST VISITOR CENTRE
Commons Road, Pembroke SA71 4EA
Tel: (01646) 622388   Fax: (01646) 621396
Seasonal, in winter contact Tenby.

BED AND BREAKFAST
ROSEDENE GUEST HOUSE   [♿]
Hodgeston, Pembroke SA71 5JU
Tel: (01646) 672586 Fax: (01646) 672855
Mobile: 07799 282025
www.rosedeneguesthouse.co.uk
e.mail:eileen@rosedeneguesthouse.co.uk
No. of Accessible Rooms: 1
Accessible Facilities: Lounge, Dining Room,
Garden, accessible by ramp. Charming
property in peaceful village with private
patio. Located midway between Tenby and
Pembroke.

ST. DAVID'S
Tiny city, dominated by a fine cathedral
on whose site as early as C6th a
religious order was founded, the oldest
cathedral settlement in Britain. The
present building was completed in
1176. The city has many attractions
relating to its coastal position, for,
although a wild and remote spot, it is
busy with more facilities than one
would expect; the hub of activity is
centred around the C14th market
cross.

ATTRACTION
BISHOPS PALACE
St. Davids SA62 6PE
Tel: (01437) 720517
Sheltering in a grassy hollow this
outstanding religious site, even in ruins
conveys the affluence and power of the
medieval church. This great palace is
unequalled elsewhere in Wales. The Great
Hall built, in early C14th, shows worldly life
reflected in extravagance of architecture
and lavish stone carvings. Ground floor at
grass courtyard level, including 2 exhibition
rooms, is accessible, the first floor is not.

SD [♿]   CP [♿]   E [♿]   RF [♿]
S [🚶]   WC [♿]

ST. DAVID'S CATHEDRAL
The Close, St. Davids SA62 6PE
Tel: (01437) 720202   Fax: (01437) 721885
Varied architecture, built in the C12th
and altered several times, including C20th
extension. Fine ceilings and stone vaulting.

SD [♿]   CP [♿]   E [♿]   RF [♿]
S [🚶]   WC [🚶]

391

STACKPOLE (NT)
The old Home Farm, Stackpole SA71 5DQ
Tel: (01646) 661359   Fax: (01646) 661639
Stackpole Estate is set in an area of
outstanding natural beauty and much of it is
designated as a Site of Special Scientific
Interest. There are beaches, cliffs, limestone

St. David's Cathedral.

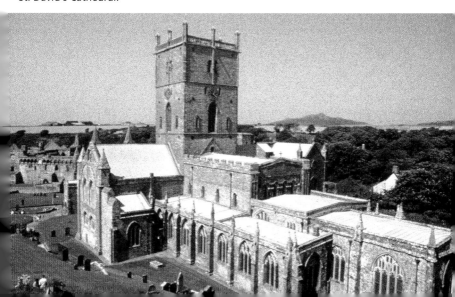

grassland and dunes, lakes and woods. Wheelchair-accessible lakeside and woodland footpath and bird watching hide at the boat house, are shown clearly on the comprehensive map for visitors with disabilities. Strong companion pusher needed.

SD ♿ CP ♿ RF ♿
C ♿ S N/A WC ♿

TENBY

Very popular holiday resort with pastel Georgian houses running down to lovely harbour and 3 great beaches. Medieval town walls are almost intact enfolding a maze of tiny streets and alleyways. Originally a fishing port, now offering much to see and many interesting excursions in the area.

TOURIST INFORMATION CENTRE
The Croft, Tenby SA70 8AP
Tel: (01834) 842402   Fax: (01834) 845439

HOTEL
GREENHILLS COUNTRY HOTEL ♿
St. Florence, Tenby SA70 8NB
Tel: (01834) 871291   Fax: (01834) 871948
No. of Accessible Rooms: 4
Accessible Facilities: Lounge, Restaurant, Pool, Sauna.
Lovely hotel in own grounds within floral award winning village. 3 miles from Tenby.

ATLANTIC HOTEL ♿
The Esplanade, Tenby SA70 7DU
Tel/Fax: (01834) 842881
e.mail:enquiries@atlantic-hotel.uk.com
www.atlantic-hotel.uk.com
No. of Accessible Rooms: 1
Accessible Facilities: Lounge, Restaurant.
Charming family-owned property fronted by lovely natural gardens with cliff top terraces and fine sea views.

SELF CATERING
HOMELEIGH COUNTRY COTTAGES ♿
Red Roses, Whitland, Nr Tenby SA34 0PN
Tel: (01834) 831765
e-mail: enquiries@holmleigh.org
www.homeleigh.org
No. of Accessible units 3. Bath.

No of Beds per unit 6-8.
Accessible facilities – open plan.
Attractive cottages in peaceful Pembroke countryside in small village on A477, midway between St. Clears and Tenby.

ATTRACTION
MANOR HOUSE WILDLIFE PARK
St. Florence, Tenby SA70 8RJ
Tel/Fax: (01646) 651201
Central feature here is the Manor House itself, built in 1750s and now housing the Natural History Museum and the refreshment area. Wide collection of animals, birds, fish and reptiles, with bird of prey displays and snake handling. Go-karts, astroglide and remote boats and cars for children. Fine floral gardens.

SD ♿ CP 🚶 E ♿ RF ♿
C ♿ S ♿ WC 🚶 RFE ♿

POWYS

ABECRAF

Located in the Upper Swansea Valley, on southern edge of Brecon Beacons National Park.

HOTEL
MAES-Y-GWERNEN HOTEL ♿
School Road, Abercraf,
Swansea Valley SA9 1XD
Tel: (01639) 730218   Fax: (01639) 730765
e-mail: maesyg@globalnet.co.uk
No. of accessible Rooms: 1
Accessible Facilities: Lounge, Restaurant, Sauna, Whirlpool, Bar, Conservatory, Gardens. Country hotel in private grounds, on the southern edge of the National Park, convenient for mountains and Gower coast.

ATTRACTION
CRAIG-Y-NOS COUNTRY PARK
Pen-y-cae, Nr. Abercraf,
Swansea Valley SA9 1GL
Tel/Fax: (01639) 730395
40 acres of countryside to enjoy in this lovely part of the upper Tawe valley. Access to Visitor Centre with displays and activity areas explaining what can be found, and accessible

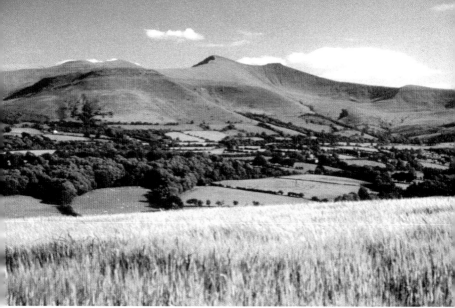

Pen-y-fan. One of the stars of the Brecon Beacons.

Welcome Point and map near parking area. Wheelchair available free of charge. Located north of Abercraf on A 4067.

SD ♿ CP ♿ E ♿ RF ♿
S ♿ WC ♿

BRECON

Fascinating medieval street plan still remains here, although many of the older houses are rebuilt or were given fashionable Georgian facades in the C18th and C19ths. Remains an important agricultural centre and good base for exploring the Brecon Beacons National Park.

TOURIST INFORMATION CENTRE
Cattle Market Car Park, Brecon LD3 9DA
Tel: (01874) 622485   Fax: (01874) 625256

TRAVELINE
(0870) 6082608

TAXIS
Wye Valley Taxis: Tel: (01982) 553142
1 adapted vehicle.

TRAINS
Valley Lines: Special Needs:
Tel: (029) 20 449944

CAR PARKS
Parking in council car parks.
Tel: (01597) 826529

HOTEL
THE CASTLE OF BRECON   ♿
The Castle Square, Brecon LD3 9DB
Tel: (01874) 624611   Fax: (01874) 623777
e-mail: hotel@breconcastle.co.uk
www.breconcastle.co.uk
No. of Accessible Rooms: 2
Accessible Facilities: Lounge, Restaurant
A listed building, originally a coaching inn in late C18th and one of the first hotels in Wales in early C19th. Occupying site and remains of Brecon Castle, it stands on a bluff of lands between two rivers, commanding fine views along valley of the River Usk, but 200m only from centre of town. Privately owned and managed.

ATTRACTION
BRECKNOCK MUSEUM
Captain's Walk, Brecon LD3 7DW
Tel: (01874) 624121   Fax: (01874) 611281
Exploration of area history with archaeological and historical artefacts, folklore and decorative arts.

SD ♿ CP ♿ E ♿ AT REAR
L ♿ S ♿ WC ♿ RFE ♿

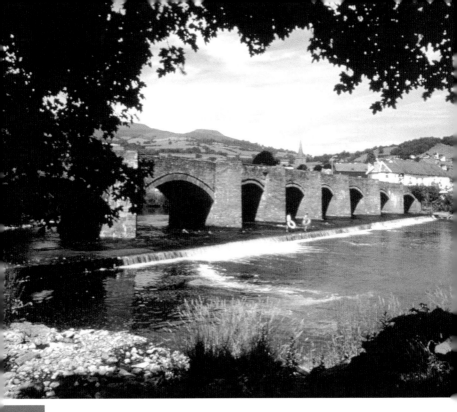

The magnificent 13 arched bridge at Crickhowell which spans the River Usk.

BRECON BEACONS NATIONAL PARK AUTHORITY

7 Glamorgan Street, Brecon LD3 7DP
Tel: (01874) 624437   Fax: (01874) 622574
e-mail: enquiries@breconbeacons.org

The highest mountains in southern Britain, together with 500 square miles of the surrounding countryside, became a National Park in 1957. This is a landscape dominated by wildness, natural variety and farming tradition. It is a landscape of contrasts with open moorland and hidden waterfalls, windswept mountains and sheltered valleys, bustling market towns and isolated farmsteads. Welsh cultural traditions are very strong and the agricultural landscape is rich in wildlife habitats with a great variety of plants and animals. A strong sense of history pervades in the legacy of ancient monuments and buildings telling the story of the people who have lived and worked here during the past five thousand years.

NATIONAL PARK VISITOR CENTRE (MOUNTAIN CENTRE)

Libanus, Nr. Brecon LD3 8ER
Tel: (01874) 623366   Fax: (01874) 624515

The Mountain Centre, 5.5 miles southwest of Brecon is run so that visitors can enjoy the spectacular scenery, discover what to see and do in the area, learn about local features of interest and find out about the role of a National Park.

SD ♿   CP 🚶   E ♿   RF ♿
C ♿   S ♿   WC ♿

BUILTH WELLS

Small castle town on the banks of the Wye. Best known as home of the Royal Welsh Show, the country's largest agricultural event. There is no evidence of the spa which flourished in the C19th.

TOURIST INFORMATION CENTRE

The Groe Car Park. Builth Wells LD2 3BT
Tel: (01982) 553307

Seasonal, in winter contact
Llandrindod Wells.

HOTELS
CAER BERIS MANOR HOTEL
Builth Wells LD2 3NP
Tel: (01982) 552601   Fax: (01982) 552586
No. of Accessible Rooms: 2. Roll-in Shower
(1)
Accessible Facilities: Lounge, Restaurant,
Bar. Country house hotel situated in 27
acres of beautiful woodland on River Irfon.

PENCERRIG GARDENS HOTEL
Llandrindod Road, Builth Wells LD2 3TF
Tel: (01982)553266   Fax: (01982) 552347
e-mail: info@pencerrig.co.uk
www.pencerrig.co.uk
No. of Accessible Rooms: 5
Accessible Facilities: Lounge, Restaurant.
Reputedly of C15th origin, the property
has grown from farmhouse to country
house with many original, unique features
retained. Set in beautiful gardens and
rolling hills of mid Wales, it is a perfect
place to relax and enjoy Welsh hospitality.

CRICKHOWELL
"The most cheerful-looking town I ever
saw" Richard Fenton, 1804. Small and
urban, little has changed since then
with fine Crickhowell Bridge along the
Usk and a square with The Bear, a
Georgian inn.

TOURIST INFORMATION CENTRE
Beaufort Chambers, Beaufort Street,
Crickhowell NP8 1AA
Tel: (01873) 812105
Seasonal, in winter contact Brecon.

HOTEL
THE OLD RECTORY HOTEL
Llangattock, Crickhowell NP8 1PH
Tel/Fax: (01873 810373
No. of Accessible Rooms: 2
Accessible Facilities: Lounge, Restaurant,
Family owned and run C17th building
situated in a small hamlet. Set in 12 acres of
grounds with 9-hole private golf course.

KNIGHTON
The town began as a Saxon settlement
and is as old as Offa's Dyke, standing
mid-way along its 172 miles of National
Trail from Prestatyn to Chepstow. Now
a market centre for the Tene Valley.

TOURIST INFORMATION CENTRE
Offas Dyke Centre, West Street,
Knighton LD7 1EN
Tel: (01547) 529424   Fax: (01547) 529242
e-mail: oda@offasdyke.demon.co.uk

HOTEL
KNIGHTON HOTEL
Broad Street, Knighton LD7 1BL
Tel: (01547) 520530   Fax: (01547) 520529
No. of Accessible Rooms: 15
Accessible Facilities: Lounge, Restaurant.
Hotel has narrow lift and ramps.

LLANDRIDNOD WELLS
Elegant Victorian spa town where you
can still take the waters at the Pump
Room in Rock Park. It plays on its
Victorian heyday with an annual
Victorian Festival in August. A good
touring centre for central Wales.

TOURIST INFORMATION CENTRE
Old Town Hall, Memorial Gardens,
Llandrindod Wells LD1 5DL
Tel: (01597) 822600

BUSES
Cross Gates: Tel: (01597) 851226
Some low-floor buses.

TAXIS
Adey's Taxis: Tel: (01597) 822118
1 adapted vehicle.

Wye Valley Taxis: Tel: (01982) 553142
1 adapted vehicle.

TRAINS
Wales and West: Special Needs:
Tel: (0845) 3003005
Minicom: (0845) 7585469

Llandrindod Wells Station is accessible to wheelchairs by ramp access.

CAR PARKS
Car park information.
Tel: (01597) 826529

HOTEL
THE BELL COUNTRY INN 〔♿〕
Llanyre, Llandrindod Wells LD1 6DY
Tel: (01597) 823959 Fax: (012597) 825899
No. of Accessible Rooms: 1
Accessible Facilities: Lounge, Restaurant, During C17th and C18th, the hostelry provided stabling and nourishment for drovers, the original building being replaced by current stone building of 1890s. Now a charming country inn.

CORVEN HALL 〔♿〕
Howey, Llandrindod Wells LD1 5RE
Tel: (01597) 823368
No. of Accessible Rooms: 1
Accessible Facilities: Lounge, Restaurant, Bar, Garden. Victorian country house in large grounds and peaceful setting.

ATTRACTION
GILFACH FARM NATURE RESERVE
St. Harmon, Rhayader,
Nr. Llandrindod Wells LD6 5LF
Tel: (01597) 870301 Fax: (01597) 823274
e-mail: radnorshirewt@cix.co.uk
Restored Welsh longhouse at the centre of a 418-acre nature reserve. Upland River, oak woodland meadows and upland moorland. Live film of wildlife from the reserve and history of Gilfach.

| SD ♿ | CP ♿ | E ♿ | RF ♿ |
| C ♿ | S ♿ | WC 🚶 | |

LLANFAIR CAEREINION
Tiny country town in which development has meant that the urban section of the railway, creeping past backyards and across roads, can never be linked to the main line.

ATTRACTION
WELSHPOOL and LLANFAIR LIGHT RAILWAY
The Station, Llanfair Caereinion SY21 0SF

Tel: (01938) 810441 Fax: (01938) 810861
8-mile trip through lovely scenery on narrow-gauge steam train. Many carriages and coaches from around the world on view. Two locations for boarding.

SD ♿	CP ♿	E ♿	RF ♿
C ♿	S ♿	WC 🚶	
RFE ♿ Platform access via ramp			

LLANGAMMARCH WELLS
Sleepy little town 185m. above sea level, renowned for fine trout fishing on River Irfon. Once a spa with water believed to cure gout and heart disease. Close to Epynt mountain.

HOTEL
THE LAKE COUNTRY HOUSE 〔♿〕
Llangammarch Wells LD4 4BS
Tel: (01591) 620202 Fax: (01591) 620457
No. of Accessible Rooms: 2
Accessible Facilities: Lounge, Restaurant. Welsh country house furnished with antiques and set in 50 acres with sweeping lawns, a par-3 golf course, croquet lawn, putting green, clay pigeon shooting, archery and tennis. Fishing close by.

MACHYNLLETH
Capital of the lower Dowey valley and surrounded by parkland rising into the hills of mid Wales. Busy and popular in summer. In 1404 Owain Glyn Dwr was crowned Prince of Wales here and held a parliament, though not in what is now called Parliament House, a good example of a late medieval town house.

TOURIST INFORMATION CENTRE
Canolfan Owain Glyndwr,
Machynlleth SY20 8EE
Tel: (01654) 702401 Fax: (01654) 703675

BED AND BREAKFAST
CWMDYLLUAN 〔🚶〕
Forge, Machynlleth SY20 8RZ
Tel: (01654) 702684 Fax: (01654) 700133

e-mail: dylluan@clara.co.uk
No. of Accessible Rooms: 3, Bath
Accessible Facilities: Lounge, Dining room
House built on elevated site in 1983,
standing in an acre of land in quiet country
location bordered by River Dulas. Forge is
a small village a mile from Machynlleth
along a quiet mountain road.

ATTRACTION
CELTICA
Y Plas, Aberystwyth Road,
 Machynlleth SY20 8ER
Tel: (01654) 702702   Fax: (01654) 703604
e-mail: celtica@celtica.wales.com
www.celtica.wales.com
Unique attraction relaying history of the
Celts, housed in restored mansion which
was once the country home of the
Marquis of Londonderry. The sights and
sounds of Wales' Celtic past are brought
alive through audio-visual technology as
you discover the Celtic settlement and
the Roundhouse where the characters tell
their own stories. An interpretative centre
with artefacts, photographs and books
gives insight into the Celtic way of life.

SD 🚹 CP 👨‍🦽 E 🚹 RF 🚹 L 👨‍🦽
C 🚹 S 🚹 WC 🚹 RFE 🚹

CENTRE FOR ALTERNATIVE TECHNOLOGY
Machynlleth SY20 9AZ
Tel: (01654) 702400   Fax: (01654) 702782
e-mail: info@cat.org.uk
www.cat.org.uk
Wales Tourism Award Winner. Seven
acres of environmental solutions to
inspire, inform and entertain. Tranquil
organic garden: transport maze: wind,
water and solar power displays: animals
on small-holding: discover how to save
energy – and money! Vegetarian
restaurant.

SD 🚹 CP 🚶 E 👨‍🦽 RF 👨‍🦽
C 🚶 S 🚶 WC 🚶

YNYS-HIR RSPB RESERVE
Cae'r Berllan, Eglwysfach, Machynlleth
Tel: (01654) 781265   Fax: (01654) 781328
Although much of the reserve is
unsuitable for wheelchair access due to
the terrain, there is a ramp overlooking
the estuary where visitors may drive down

and park, with good views of many of the
estuary birds, especially at high tide.
Please contact in advance for this facility.
Ynys-Hir Nature Reserve lies just off the
main road between Aberystwyth and
Machynlleth.

SD 🚹 CP 🚶 E 🚹

NEWTOWN
Once the centre of Welsh flannel and
textiles industry and now the most
populous town in Powys with the
best shopping. The flourishing
Tuesday market has been active since
1279.

TOURIST INFORMATION CENTRE
The Park, Back Lane, Newtown SY16 2PW
Tel: (01686) 625580   Fax: (01686) 610066

TRAVELINE
(0870) 6082608

TRAINS
Virgin Trains: Special Needs:
Tel: (0845) 7443366

CAR PARKS
Free unlimited disabled badge parking in
all council car parks.
Tel: (01597) 826529

PRESTEIGNE
Located right on Herefordshire border
and seems rather English in character,
although it was the county town of
Radnorshire from the C16th-C19th.
A prosperous market town, it
declined after 1899, but evidence of
its importance is shown in the large
parish church, some fine inns and the
Venetian Gothic Market Hall built in
1865. The streets are Georgian in
character with older structures,
possibly C17th.

TOURIST INFORMATION CENTRE
Shire Hall, Broad Street, Presteigne LD8 2AD
Tel: (01544) 260650   Fax: (01544) 260652

ATTRACTION
THE JUDGE'S LODGING
(as TIC above.)
The Old Shire Hall, now known as the Judge's Lodging, is an elegant Victorian building. Contrasting with the upstairs grandeur of the judge's well furnished lodging rooms and vast courtroom, were the downstairs services or servants' hall, kitchen and cells for prisoners awaiting trial upstairs. After much research, repair and restoration, the Shire Hall now captures the Victorian heyday of a most unusual household, by gaslight, lamp and candle, for visitors to savour. Visitors are accompanied by an audio-tour of voices from the past as room by room, you hear the inside story. A delightful and unique museum. Entrance via a lift at the rear of the building. Wheelchair lift takes 1 chair and occupant and 1 other standing person.

SD 🚹 E 🚹 RF 🚹 L 🚹
S 🚹 WC 🚹

WELSHPOOL
Attractive town with numerous half-timbered buildings typical of upper Severn Valley. The most unusual is the hexagonal cockpit used until cockfighting was outlawed in 1849. Nearby is Powis Castle, built in C12th, and added to ever since, plus lovely Glansevern Hall.

TOURIST INFORMATION CENTRE
Vicarage Garden, Church Street, Welshpool SY21 7DD
Tel: (01938) 552043 Fax: (01938) 554038

SELF-CATERING
MADOG'S WELLS 🚹
Llanfair Caereinion, Welshpool SY21 0DE
Tel/Fax: (01938) 810446
No. of Accessible Units: 2
No. of Beds per Unit: 5/6
Accessible Facilities: Lounge/Dining Room, Kitchen, Games Room.
Small hill farm in quiet secluded valley. Accessible bungalow adjacent to beamed farmhouse in secluded valley. Watch the birds from your breakfast table.

ATTRACTION
GLANSEVERN HALL GARDENS
Glansevern, Berriew, Welshpool SY21 8AH
Tel: (01686) 640200 Fax: (01686) 640829
18 acres of garden surrounding C18th Greek Revival house, set in wider parkland on the banks of the River Severn. Mostly level ground, and retaining warm and intimate ambience of family garden. Large number of unusual species of trees, 4 acre lake, profusely water, rock and rose gardens and herbaceous borders and beds. Plants for sale.

SD 🚹 CP 🚹 E 🚹 RF 🚹
C 🚹 S 🚹 WC 🚹

RFE Garden – powered wheelchairs move more easily over grass.

RHONDDA CYNON TAFF

PONTYPRIDD
Market town of substance on south outlet of the Rhondda into the Taff Vale. The river here is crossed by an elegant C18th bridge, and two fine chapels stand at the Bridgehead.

TOURIST INFORMATION CENTRE
Historical Centre, The Old Bridge, Pontypridd CF37 3PE
Tel: (01443) 409512

HOTEL
HERITAGE PARK HOTEL 🚹
Coed Cae Road, Trehafod, Nr. Pontypridd CF37 2NP
Tel: (01443) 687057 Fax: (01443) 687060
e-mail:info@rhonddaheritagepark.co.uk
www.rhonddaheritagepark.co.uk
No. of Accessible Rooms: 1. Bath
Accessible Facilities: Restaurant, Lounge Bar.
Intimate and smallish hotel with large rooms and attractive dining room situated in Rhondda Valley just west of Pontypridd and adjacent to the Heritage Park centre and museum, 20 miles from Cardiff.

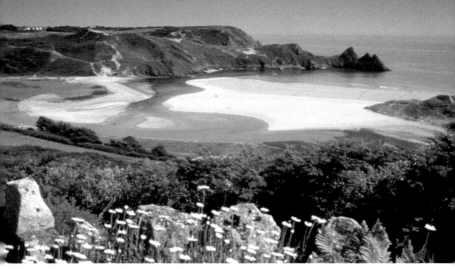

The stunning Three Cliffs Bay on the Gower Peninsular.

ATTRACTION
RHONDDA HERITAGE PARK
Lewis Merthyr Colliery, Coed Cae Road,
Trehafod, Nr. Pontypridd CF37 7NP
Tel: (01443) 682036   Fax: (01443) 687420)
e-mail: rhonpark@netwales.co.uk

It is hard now to imagine the impact coal had on Wales. This living history museum tells the story of coal mining in the valleys through visual and aural narrative in two winding houses and a ride down a shaft to the pit bottom guided by an ex-miner. There is a visitor centre with shop, indoor street reconstruction and art gallery and coffee shop on the first floor accessible by lift. Only area inaccessible is the final part of the mine tour, a simulated ride back to the surface. An excellent visit.

SD   CP   E   RF   L
C   S   WC   RFE

ATTRACTION
GOWER HERITAGE CENTRE
Parkmill, Gower, Swansea SA3 2EH
Tel: (01792) 371206 Fax: (01792) 371471
e-mail:
info@gowerheritagecentre.sagehost.co.uk
www.gowerheritage.sagehost.co.uk

Located 8 miles from Swansea, the centre is based around a water-powered corn and saw mill complex with craft workshops. Farming museum, fishpond and animal farm, puppet theatre and picnic and adventure play areas. The mill was built around 1160AD by the Norman rulers of Gower, grinding corn to provide flour and foods for nearby Pennard Castle estate. It is a Grade II ancient monument and one of very few complete and working mills in Wales.

SD   CP   E   RF
C   S   WC

SWANSEA

GOWER
The Gower Peninsular is 19 miles long, dipping into the Bristol Channel, with wonderful beaches and Britain's first designated "Area of Outstanding Natural Beauty" in 1957. The dramatic cliffs, sweeping marshlands and ancient farmland and commons, combine with glorious bays, Rhossili Bay, being notably spectacular.

SWANSEA
Dramatically set in the crescent moon of Swansea Bay, Wales' second largest city is modern and cosmopolitan, but with a splendid coastline, rural landscape and mountains. Fine shopping in The Quadrant and covered market. The bay is a fine natural harbour with busy docks and shipping lanes. An award-winning yachting

marina has been created in the former south dock and there is a constant buzz of cafes, restaurants and pubs in the Maritime Quarters. Much to see and do here.

TOURIST INFORMATION CENTRE
Plymouth Street, Swansea SA1 3QG
Tel: (01792) 468321   Fax: (01792) 464602
www.visitswanseabay.com

TRAVELINE
(0870) 6082608

TAXIS
Data Cabs: Tel: (01792) 474747/545454
50 Adapted vehicles.
Yellow Cabs: Tel: (01792) 700400
1 adapted minibus.

TRAINS
First Great Western: Special Needs:
Tel: (0845) 7413775
Virgin Trains: Special Needs:
Tel: (0845) 7443366
Minicom: (0845) 7443367
Wales and West: Special Needs:
Tel: (0845) 3003005

CAR PARKS
Badge holder information.
Tel: (01792) 636795

SHOPMOBILITY
12 St. David's Square, Swansea SA1 3LG
Tel: (01792) 461785

ATTRACTIONS
SWANSEA MARITIME and
INDUSTRIAL MUSEUM
Museum Square, Maritime Quarter,
Swansea SA1 1SN
Tel: (01792) 650351   Fax: (01782) 654200
e-mail:
swansea.maritime.museum@business.ntl.com
www.
swansea.gov.uk/culture/museums/maritime.htm
Swansea Maritime and Industrial Museum is situated in the heart of Swansea's waterfront development, the marina area

of the Maritime Quarter. 25 years ago the dock and its surroundings were completely derelict - the Museum was just one of two buildings left standing. Now there is a thriving modern residential and recreational development, established as a visitor centre for both locals and tourists. Selection of floating boats and displays relating to the history of the Port of Swansea, plus complete working woollen mill. Also programme of temporary exhibitions.

| SD 🚻 | CP 🚻 | E 🚻 | RF 🚻 |
| C 🚹 | S 🚹 | WC 🚹 | |

TORFAEN

BLAENAFON
A rather bleak village. 300m up on the eastern rim of South Wales coalfield are 2 important sites which summarise much of the regions' industrial history – Blaenafon ironworks and the Big Pit.

TOURIST INFORMATION CENTRE
Blaenafon Ironworks, North Street,
Blaenafon NP4 9RQ
Tel: (01495) 792615
Seasonal, in winter contact Abergavenny.

ATTRACTION
BIG PIT MINING MUSEUM
Blaenafon NP4 9XP
Tel: (01495) 790311   Fax: (01495) 792618
e-mail: bigpit@nmgw.ac.uk
Closed as a working mine in 1980, but visitors can don safety helmets and lamps and go down the 300ft shaft to discover what life was like. Pithead exhibition and reconstructed miner's cottage also displayed.

SD 🚻	CP 🚹	E 🚻	RF 🚹
C 🚻	S 🚹	WC 🚻	
RFE- 🚻 Underground Tour			

CWMBRAN
Sixth largest town in Wales and the only example of the comprehensively planned new towns initiated after

WWII. Designated a new town in 1949, it is unexciting architecturally with sweeping roads, housing neighbourhoods, industrial estates and pedestrianised shopping areas.

WYE VALLEY AND VALE OF USK TOURISM
Floor 6, County Hall, Cwmbran NP44 2XH
Tel: (01633) 644847   Fax: (01633) 644800
e-mail: mcc_tourism_@compuserve.com

ATTRACTION
GREENMEADOW COMMUNITY FARM
Greenforge Way, Cwmbran NP44 5AJ
Tel: (01633) 862202   Fax: (01633) 489332
Major farm attraction with milking demonstrations, tractor rides, farm and nature trails and adventure play area.

SD   CP   E   C
S   WC   RFE

PONTYPOOL
Easternmost of the Valleys towns, rather hilly. Considerable Italian influence from emigrants coming to South Wales in C19th.

ATTRACTION
PONTYPOOL MUSEUM
Park Buildings, Pontypool NP4 6JH
Tel: (01495) 752036   Fax: (01495) 752043
Housed in the Georgian stable block of the Hanbury mansion. Explore effects of man's relationship with the land and look at land formation from the primeaval landscape to the hey-day of the coal industry.

SD   CP   E   C
S   WC

VALE OF GLAMORGAN

COWBRIDGE
Notable for good shopping, particularly fashion boutiques and a Tuesday cattle market which reinforces its agricultural traditions. Excellent centre for exploring the Vale, which has hamlets, thatched cottages and pubs.

HOTEL
JANE HODGE RESORT HOTEL
Grooms Holidays
Trerhyngyll, Nr. Cowbridge CF71 7TN
Tel: (01446) 772608   Fax: (01446) 775831
No. of Accessible Rooms: 39
Accessible Facilities: Lounge, Restaurant, Hydrotherapy Pool, Sauna, Whirlpool, Multi Gym, Sports Hall.
Located in quiet village, just outside Cowbridge, equidistant between Cardiff and Bridgend, and within the Gower Peninsula. Excellent facilities.

PENARTH
Genteel Victorian seaside resort with period charm and fine town houses built for ship owners and master mariners in the C19th. Describes itself as a "garden by the sea", with lovely sea views and lush green parks. No funfairs or "tat" usually associated with such resorts.

ATTRACTION
COSMESTON COUNTRY PARK LAKES AND MEDIEVAL VILLAGE
Lavernock Road, Penarth CF64 5UY
Tel: (02920) 701678   Fax: (01222) 708686
Original village of Comeston decimated by first Great Plague of C14th. Strolls along wooden boardwalks through acres of parkland and 2 lovely lakes. Take a tour around the medieval village with costumed guides in the cottages, byres and barns, reconstructed on the site of an original C14th settlement. The boardwalks are inevitably slightly uneven and the surrounds of the cottages in the village are mainly uneven paving. Path to each individual building, but doorways are narrow.

SD   CP   E   (visitor centre)
RF   C   S
WC   visitor centre. 2 others on RADAR key
RFE

WREXHAM

Large, busy town which grew up around local coal and iron industries. Mineral-rich uplands enhanced its prosperity in C18th and C19th, but only Erdig remains. There is a fine parish church, St. Giles, with splendid 3-storey tower completed in 1506. Founder of Yale University, Elihu Yales, was born in Wrexham and is commemorated in St. Giles.

TOURIST INFORMATION CENTRE
Lambpit Street, Wrexham LL11 1WN
Tel: (01978) 292015   Fax: (01978) 292467

TRAVELINE
(0870) 6082608

TAXIS
Apollo Taxis: Tel: (01978) 262600
1 adapted vehicle.
Atax: Tel: (01978) 262380
3 adapted minibuses.
Prestige Taxis: Tel: (01978) 291999
1 black cab.
Wrexham Taxis: Tel: (01978) 357777
1 black cab.

TRAINS
Central Trains: Assistance:
Tel: (0845) 7056027
www.centraltrains.co.uk
First North Western: Special Needs:
Tel: (0845) 6040231

CAR PARKS
Some unlimited disabled badge parking
Tel: (01978) 292000

SHOPMOBILITY
21 Egerton Street, Wrexham LL11 1ND
Tel: (01978) 312390

ATTRACTIONS
ALYN WATERS COUNTRY PARK
Mold Road, Gwersyllt, Wrexham LL11 4AG
Tel: (01978) 761222

Situated in the lovely Alyn Valley, the park is in 2 halves. Within the Gwersyllt half is the visitor centre with exhibitions on history and wildlife of the area and on the Llay side is a new cycle way with good access for wheelchair users. Located 3 miles north of Wrexham between Gwersyllt, Bradley and Llay.
SD 👤 CP 👤 E 👤 S 👤
WC 👤 RFE 👤 (Circular walk with disabled access – 500m. long)

BERSHAM HERITAGE CENTRE
Bersham, Wrexham LL14 4HT
Tel: (01978) 261529   Fax: (01978) 361703
The furnaces and foundries which produced cannons for the American War of Independence and cylinders for James Watt's steam engines are brought alive here in the story of this C18th ironworks. Limited access to actual ironworks.
SD 👤 CP 👤 E 👤 RF 👤
S 👤 WC 👤

TY MAWR COUNTRY PARK
Cae Gwilym Lane, Cefn Mawr,
Wrexham LL14 3PE
Tel: (01978) 822780
On the banks of the River Dee overlooking the Vale of Llangollen and the Pontcysyllte Aqueduct, this 35-acre grassland park offers a variety of wildlife plus rare breeds of sheep, donkeys, ponies and goats. Farmed organically Ty Mawr still manages hay meadows along the river in the traditional way. Informative visitor centre and surfaced paths for easier access. Great for picnics or barbecues.
SD 👤 CP 👤 E 👤 RFE 👤
S 👤 WC 👤 RFE 👤

SPORTING VENUE
BANGOR-ON-DEE RACECOURSE
Bangor-on-Dee, Wrexham LL13 0DA
Tel: (01978) 780323   Fax: (01978) 780985
CP 👤
RE 👤 ED 👤 INT 👤
WC 👤 (1 adapted WC in each toilet block – 6 in total)
SS – Viewing platform for wheelchairs   B/R 👤

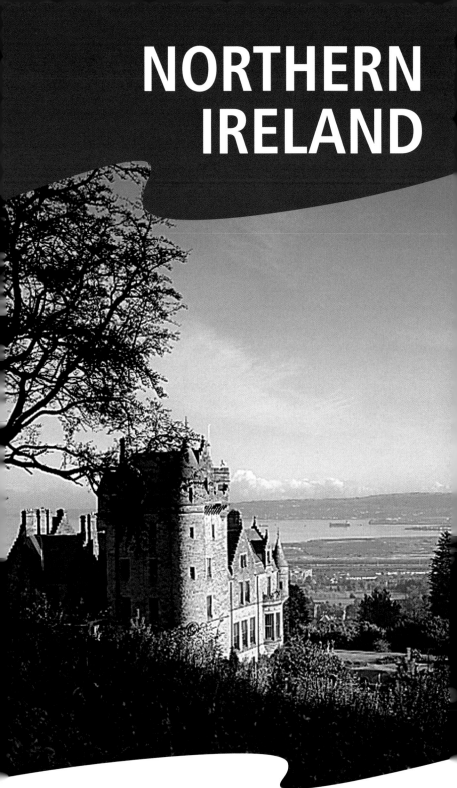

NORTHERN IRELAND

Belfast Castle with Belfast Lough in the background.

gowrings
mobility

TOURIST BOARDS

BELFAST WELCOME CENTRE
47 Donegal Place, Belfast
(028) 9024 6609

DISABILITY ORGANISATIONS
ASSOCIATION FOR SPINA BIFIDA &
HYDROCEPHALUS (ASBAH)
Graham House, Knockbracken Healthcare
Park, Saintfield Road, Belfast BT8 8BH
Tel: (028) 90 798878
Similar to ASBAH in introduction

DISABILITY ACTION (HEAD OFFICE)
Portside Business Park, 189 Airport Road
West,Belfast BT3 9ED
Tel: (028) 90 297880   Fax: (028) 90 297881
This organisation works to ensure that
people with disabilities attain their full
rights as citizens. Currently very involved
in accessible transport. Will supply
information as required.
Publishes Getting Out and About.

IRISH DISABLED FLY FISHING ASSOCIATION
6 Grouse Hill Park,
Altnagelvil
Londonderry BT74 2LZ
Tel: (028) 7134 7199

NORTHERN IRELAND PARAPLEGIC
ASSOCIATION
c/o Disability Action (see above)

NORTHERN IRELAND REGIONAL ACCESS
COMMITTEE
c/o Disability Action (see above)

PHAB NORTHERN IRELAND
Unit 25, Townsend Enterprise Park,
Townsend BT13 2ES
Tel: (028) 90 796565   Fax: (028) 90 796070
e-mail: info@phabni.org
www.phabni.org
Provides range of services to encourage
those with disabilities to achieve equal
opportunities, including fully accessible
residential activity centre in Ballinran,
Co. Down.

ACCESSIBLE TRANSPORT
DRD Transport (Policy and Support) Division

12th Floor, River House, 48 High Street,
Belfast BT1 2AR
Tel: (028) 90 251300   Fax: (028) 90 257333
e-mail: chris.malone@drdni.gov.uk

TRANSLINK
Tel: (028) 90 666630
Integrated public transport operations of
Citybus, NI Railways and Ulsterbus.
    www.translink.co.uk
    www.citybus.co.uk
    www.ulsterbus.co.uk
    www.nirailways.co.uk

COUNTY ANTRIM

BALLYCASTLE
Lying at the heart of the Causeway
Coast and renowned as the site of
the Ould Lammas Fair, Ballycastle has
been designated an architectural
conservation area. A medium sized
resort town with an attractive
harbour and central sandy beach.

TOURIST INFORMATION CENTRE
Sheskburn House, 7 Mary Street,
Ballycastle BT54 6QH
Tel: (028) 207 62024 Fax: (028) 207 62515
e-mail: ballycastle@hotmail.com

HOTEL
MARINE HOTEL
North Street, Ballycastle BT54 6BN
Tel: (028) 207 62222   Fax: (028) 207 69507
No. of Accessible Rooms: 2
Accessible Facilities: Restaurant, Bar.
Attractive hotel on the sea front,
overlooking a fine bay across to Rathlin
Island and the Scottish Isles.

BALLYCLARE

BED AND BREAKFAST
RUA-WAI FARM
149 Templepatrick Road,
Ballyclare BT39 9RW
Tel: (028) 93 352417

No. of Accessible Rooms: 3
Accessible Facilities: Dining Room.
Bungalow with large garden on 20 acre
horse farm, 2 miles from Ballyclare.

BALLYGALLEY
On the Antrim coast, a few miles north
of Larne.

BED AND BREAKFAST
CAIRNVIEW
13 Croft Heights, Ballygalley BT40 2QS
Tel: (028) 28 583269
No. of Accessible Rooms: 1
Accessible Facilities: Dining Room, Lounge.
Modern house in quiet residential area of
Ballygalley with fine views.

BALLYMENA
Prosperous town surrounded by some
of the richest farmland in Northern
Ireland. Good Saturday livestock
market. Close by is Gracehill, a small
Moravian settlement with some C18th
buildings still standing.

TOURIST INFORMATION CENTRE
76 Church Street, Ballymena, BT43 6DF
Tel: (028) 2563 8494   Fax: (028) 2563 8495

HOTELS
TULLYGLASS HOUSE HOTEL
178 Galgorm Road, Ballymena BT42 1HJ
Tel: (028) 256 52639   Fax: (028) 256 46938
No. of Accessible Rooms: 1. Shower
Accessible Facilities: Lounge, Restaurant,
Bar. Converted period house set in private
own grounds on outskirts of town.

CAIREAL MANOR GUEST HOUSE
90 Glenravel Road, Martinstown,
Ballymena BT43 6QQ
Tel/Fax: (028) 217 58465/58344/58221
No. of Accessible Rooms: 2. Shower
Accessible Facilities: Lounge, Dining Room
Detached villa located on A43 gateway to
the Glen of Glenariffe, within 15 minutes
drive of Ballymena and surrounded by
lovely countryside.

GALGORM MANOR
136 Fenaghy Road, Ballymena BT42 1EA
Tel: (028) 25 881001   Fax: (028) 25 880080
No. of Accessible Rooms: 1.
Accessible Facilities: Restaurant. C19th
gentleman's residence in 85 acres with
various activities on site including fishing.

BALLYMONEY
Busy town in the Bann Valley.

TOURIST INFORMATION CENTRE
Riada House, 14 Charles Street,
Ballymoney BT53 6DZ
Tel: (028) 276 62280   Fax: (028) 276 67659

BED AND BREAKFAST
GLEN LODGE
93a Frocess Road, Ballymoney BT53 7EJ
Tel: (028) 276 63800
No. of Accessible Rooms: 1 with roll-in
shower
Accessible Facilities: Dining room/Lounge.
Television and tea and coffee making
facilities in all rooms. Tea and scones on
arrival. Modern detached chalet bungalow
with spacious gardens. Situated on the
A26 Belfast to Portrush Road near
Ballymoney.

ATTRACTION
BANVARDEN GARDENS
Benvarden, Dervock, Ballymoney, BT53 6NN
Tel: (028) 207 41331   Fax: (028) 276 41955
www.ballymoney.gov.uk/benvarden
2-acre walled garden ranging from rose
beds to kitchen garden, the grounds
stretching down to a river bank and
Woodland Pond. Cobbled Stable Yard
contains stables, coach and cart houses
and tea room.

LESLIE HILL OPEN FARM
Ballymoney BT53 6QL
Tel/Fax: (028) 276 66803
An C18th estate with lovely grounds.
Extensive collection of rare breeds, poultry,
horsedrawn machinery, museum, working
forge and walled garden.

SD ♿ CP ♿ E ♿ RF ♿
C ♿ S ♿ WC 🚹 RFE ♿

BELFAST
Only city in Ireland to experience the full force of the Industrial Revolution and its ship-building, rope-making and tobacco industries caused massive rise in population by the end of WW1. The legacy of imposing buildings is still evident, although the Troubles and industrial decline have damaged economic lift. Still a handsome city.

BELFAST VISITOR & CONVENTION BUREAU
Tel: (028) 90 239026   Fax: (028) 90 249026
www.belfastvisitor.com

DRD Transport (Policy and Support) Division
12th Floor, River House, 48 High Street
Belfast BT1 2AR
Tel: (028) 90 251300   Fax: (028) 90 257333
e-mail: chris.malone@drdni.gov.uk

BUSES
Translink (Citybus, NI Rail, Ulsterbus -latter does not operate in Belfast City)
New buses have been fitted with ramps and low-floor level wheelchair accessibility/
Citybus: Tel: (028) 90 666630
NI Rail: Tel: (028) 90 899411
Ulsterbus: Tel: (028) 90 666630
Centrelink: Every 15 minutes. Low-floor buses.

TAXIS
For all queries call: (028) 90590300
Community Black Taxis, London style, operate in certain areas of Belfast and Londonderry - not all are accessible. This is a bus type of service. Public hire taxis in Belfast are identified by a yellow plate at the rear and front of the vehicle. Private hire taxis are identified by a roof sign with white front panel and a green licence disc on the windscreen.

TRAINS
NI Railways
Central Station, Belfast BT1 3PB
Enquiries: Tel: (028) 90 899411

The glittering lights of nightime Belfast Waterfront complex.

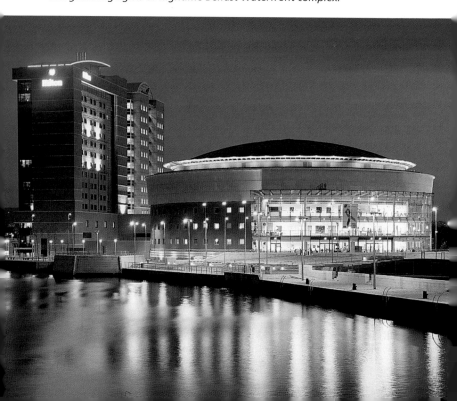

Wheelchair users well catered for with dedicated space in carriage plus call button facilities. Ramps available. One carriage in each train has space set aside for wheelchairs users.

SHOPMOBILITY
Unit 26, Victoria Centre, Victoria Square, Belfast BT1 4TL
Tel: (028) 90 808090   Fax: (028) 90 808099

HOTEL
ALDERGROVE AIRPORT HOTEL
Belfast International Airport, Crumlin, Belfast BT29 4ZY
Tel: (028) 94 422033   Fax: (028) 94 423500
No. of Accessible Rooms: 3
Accessible Facilities: Lounge, Restaurant. Modern airport hotel.

BALMORAL HOTEL
Blacks Road, Dunmurry, Belfast BT10 0ND
Tel: (028) 90 301234   Fax: (028) 90 601455
No. of Accessible Rooms: 8
Accessible Facilities: Lounge, Restaurant. Modern purpose-built hotel in its own grounds three miles from the centre of Belfast, adjacent to the M1 motorway

HASTINGS EUROPA HOTEL
Great Victoria Street, Belfast BT2 7AP
Tel: (028) 90 327000   Fax: (028) 90 327800
e-mail: res@eur.hastingshotels.com
www.hastingshotels.com
No. of Accessible Rooms: 2
Accessible Facilities: Lounge, Restaurants 2.
Quality hotel situated in the heart of the city on the Golden Mile.

HOLIDAY INN EXPRESS
106 University Street, Belfast BT7 1HP
Tel: (028) 90 311909   Fax: (028) 90 311910
e-mail: express@holidayinn-ireland.com
www.holidayinn-ireland.com
No. of Accessible Rooms: 6
Accessible Facilities: Lounge, Restaurant. Business hotel situated 1km from the city centre. All bedrooms fitted with workstations and computer points.

STORMONT HOTEL
Upper Newtownards Road, Belfast BT4 3LP

Tel: (028) 90 658621   Fax: (028) 90 480240
e-mail: res.stor@hastingshotels.com
www.hastingshotels.com
No. of Accessible Rooms: 1
Accessible Facilities: Lounge, Restaurants 2, Bar. Quality modern hotel located opposite the Parliament Buildings, 4 miles east of the city centre.

JURYS BELFAST INN
Fisherwick Place, Gt. Victoria Street, Belfast BT2 7AP
Tel: (028) 90 533500 Fax: (028) 90 533511
No. of Accessible Rooms: 1. Roll-in Shower
Accessible Facilities: Lounge, Restaurant, Bar. Modern hotel in city centre adjacent to the Opera House. All public areas are level, carpeted and wide with much natural light. Bedrooms are notably spacious. Room 104 (accessible) on the first floor is accessed by an accessible lift. There are 4 other semi-accessible rooms.

THE McCAUSLAND HOTEL
34-38 Victoria Street, Belfast BT1 3GH
Tel: (028) 90 220200   Fax: (028) 90 220220
e-mail: info@mccauslandhotel.com
www.mccauslandhotel.com
No. of Accessible Rooms: 3
Accessible Facilities: Restaurant
Formerly 2 warehouses designed in Italianate classical style in the 1850s, and opened late 1999 as a prestigious 60-bedroom hotel. Original cast-iron pillars, high arched ceilings and oak beams have all been retained.

BED AND BREAKFAST
GREENWOOD HOUSE
25 Park Road, Belfast BT7 2FW
Tel: (028) 90 202525   Fax: (028) 90 202530
e-mail: greenwood.house@virgin.net
No. of Accessible Rooms: 1
Accessible Facilities: Lounge, Dining Room. The house faces a quiet park with paved paths.

ATTRACTIONS
BELFAST ZOO
Antrim Road, Belfast BT36 7PN
Tel: (028) 90 776277   Fax: (028) 90 370578
50-acre zoo with award-winning primate house, penguin enclosure and free-flight

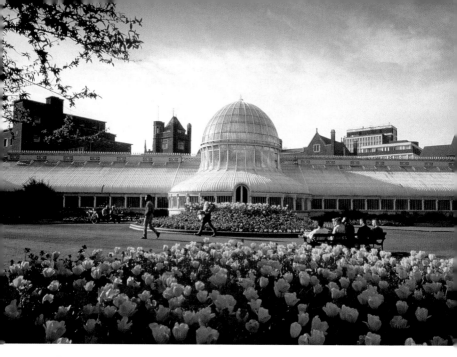

The tropical house at the Botanic Gardens, Belfast

aviary. Red pandas and rare spectacled bears, free-ranging lemurs and an African enclosure also. As an outdoor facility, levels do vary and some are hilly

SD ♿ CP ♿ E ♿ RF ♿
C ♿ S ♿ WC 🚶 RFE ♿

BOTANIC GARDENS
Stranmillis Road BT7 1JB
Tel: (028) 90 324902 Fax: (028) 90 237070
A rose garden, colourful herbaceous and shrub borders and children's playground are complimented by the Tropical Ravine House and the Palm House.

SD ♿ CP ♿ E ♿ RF (Ravine) ♿
L 🚶 C ♿ S ♿
WC: (Museum/Bowling Green) 🚶
RFE: (Palm House/Ravine) ♿

LAGAN LOOKOUT VISITOR CENTRE
1 Donegal Quay, Belfast BT1 3EA
Tel: (028) 90 315444 Fax: (028) 90 311955
Tells story of the important role of the River Lagan in Belfast's development via models, interactive displays and videos.

SD ♿ CP ♿
E ♿ (warning -very long ramp at 1:11)
L ♿ WC 🚶

ULSTER MUSEUM
Within, but separate from, the Botanic Gardens
Tel: (028) 90 383000 Fax: (028) 90 383003
www.ulstermuseum.org.uk
Collection of fine and decorative arts, archaeology, local history and natural sciences.

SD ♿ CP 🚶 E ♿ RF ♿ L ♿
C ♿ S ♿ WC ♿ RFE ♿

BUSHMILLS
Small town with an attractive square and fine River, but its main claim to fame is whiskey.

TOURIST INFORMATION CENTRE
See Giant's Causeway Visitor Centre (page 405).

BED AND BREAKFAST
VALLEY VIEW
6a Ballyclough Road, Bushmills BT57 8TU
Tel/fax: (028) 207 41608/41319
e-mail: valerie.mcfall@btinternet.com
No. of Accessible Rooms: 1
Accessible Facilities: Lounge, Dining Room
Comfortable family-run country house overlooking the Bush River Valley and Antrim Mountains.

BROWN'S COUNTRY HOUSE 🚶
174 Ballybogey Road, Bushmills BT52 2LP
Tel: (028) 207 32777 Fax: (028) 207 31627
No. of Accessible Rooms: 3
Accessible Facilities: Lounge, Restaurant
Attractive property with long established
reputation for fine food. Close to Giant's
Causeway.

THE POACHERS REST 🚶
11 Cozies Road, Castlecatt,
Bushmills BT57 8YG
Tel: (028) 207 42125
No. of Accessible Rooms: 1
Accessible Facilities: Lounge, Dining
Room.
Very quiet location 2.5 miles from
Bushmills and close to Bushmills Distillery
and Giants Causeway.

SELF-CATERING
BALLYLINNEY COTTAGES 🚶♿
7 Giants Causeway, Bushmills BT57 8SU
Tel/Fax: (028) 207 31683
info@giantscauseway.co.uk
www.giantscauseway.co.uk
No. of Accessible Units: 1. Roll-in Shower
No. of Beds per Unit: 6
Accessible Facilities: Lounge, Dining
Room, Kitchen. Weirs Snout is one of six
quality self-contained cottages set
alongside the Laverty farm. Cottages are
grouped together around landscaped
garden. Fine views over the Causeway,
sleepy seaside village of Portballintrae and
the Donegal Coastline beyond. Located a
mile from Bushmills.

ATTRACTIONS
THE OLD BUSHMILLS DISTILLERY CO.
Bushmills BT57 8XH
Tel: (028) 207 31521 Fax: (028) 207 33256
www.bushmills.com
World's oldest licensed whiskey distillery
to which James I granted the original
license in 1608. For over four centuries
the art of distillation has been passed
down through the generations. The tour
is not accessible, but an excellent video is
shown in the accessible viewing room,
where chairs are moveable, will allow
those in wheelchairs to gain some sense
of the distillery tour, joining up with able-
bodied friends at the shop afterwards.
From the visitor centre to the shop there's
a downward gradient of 1:15, staff will
assist.

SD n/a	CP ♿	E ♿	Visitor Centre
RF ♿	C ♿	S ♿	WC ♿ Shop
VC 🚶			

GIANT'S CAUSEWAY VISITOR CENTRE
44 Causeway Road, Bushmills BT57 8SU
Tel: (028) 207 31855 Fax: (028) 207 32537
Unique rock formations stand as natural
rampart against ferocity of Atlantic
storms. The rugged hexagonal symmetry
of the columns is amazing. Now generally
accepted that the Causeway was a result
of intense volcanic activity which took
place when continents were separating
and oceans forming some 60 million years
ago. VC has shops, WC, café, video
cinema and exhibition. The Ulster Bus or
Translink Bus taking visitors down to the
Causeway from the VC, 0.75 mile, has
space for one wheelchair at the rear, but
no actual tailgate lift. During our visit,
some visitors in wheelchairs were pushed
down by companions and bused back.

SD ♿	CP ♿	E ♿	RF ♿
C ♿	S ♿	WC ♿	
RFE 🚶	Causeway Bus		

CARNLOUGH
Long farmed area with dry-stone
walls, located at the foot of the
Glencoy. Good base for touring the
Glens, particularly Garron Moor, and
Giant's Causeway, with a fine sandy
beach and delightful harbour.

HOTEL
THE LONDONDERRY ARMS HOTEL ♿
20 Harbour Road, Carnlough BT44 0EU
Tel: (028) 28 885255 Fax: (028) 28 885263
e-mail: lda@glensofantrim.com
No. of Accessible Rooms: 1
Accessible Facilities: Lounge, Restaurant
Family run hotel, built in 1848, once
owned by Sir Winston Churchill.

BED AND BREAKFAST
BETHANY HOUSE
5 Bay Road, Carnlough, BT44 0HQ
Tel: (028) 28 885667
No. of Accessible Rooms: 1
Accessible Facilities: Lounge, Dining Room.
Detached house in the centre of the village with good sea views.

CARRICKFERGUS
The town grew up around the massive castle begun in 1180, which, sadly, due to an entrance ramped at a gradient of 1:7, is not accessible. Worth viewing from the harbour.

TOURIST INFORMATION CENTRE
Heritage Plaza, Carrickfergus BT38 7DQ
Tel: (028) 93 366455
Fax: (028) 93 350350

BED AND BREAKFAST
HILLCREST
66 Bellahill Road, Carrickfergus BT38 9DB
Tel/Fax: (028) 93 367342
No. of Accessible Rooms: 2
Accessible Facilities: Lounge, Dining Room.
Large, modern bungalow set in its own grounds of five acres with extensive landscaped gardens. Rural location overlooking Belfast Lough, three miles from Carrickfergus, 15 from Belfast. Good base for touring Antrim Glens and coast.

ATTRACTION
THE HERITAGE PLAZA, Antrim Street, Carrickfergus BT38 7DG
Tel: (028) 93 366455
Fax: (028) 93 350350
Accessible trip through time, experiencing over 1,000 years of the town's stormy history, see, feel and smell the past of one of Ulster's liveliest towns.

SD 🦽   E 🦽   S 🦽
WC 🚹   L 🦽

Features: Knight Ride: In a wheelchair enter the shop and go up to the Ride via the lift. Technician will put you, in your chair, into a specially designed helmet/car to enjoy the ride. NB: This attraction is going to be updated in 2003

CUSHENDALL
Attractive village in the Heart of the Glens of Antrim between the hills and the sea of Moyle. Located at the bottom of Ballyeamon, one of the nine glens. One of the first villages in Northern Ireland to be declared a Conservation Area it has retained its character and charm.

BED AND BREAKFAST
THE MEADOWS
79-81 Coast Road, Cushendall BT44 0QW
Tel: (028) 217 72020
No. of Accessible Rooms: 1. Shower
Accessible Facilities: Lounge, Dining Room
Detached house on Larne side of town.

THE BURN
63 Ballyeamon Road, Cushendall BT44 0SN
Tel: (028) 217 71733   Fax: (028) 25646111
e-mail: the burns63@hotmail.com
N. of Accessible Rooms: 2
Accessible Facilities: Lounge, Dining Room.
Detached bungalow a mile from Cushendall.

CULLENTRA HOUSE
16 Cloughs Road (off Gault's Road), Cushendall BT44 0SP
Tel/Fax: (028) 217 71762
e-mail: cullentra@ireland-holidays.net
No. of Accessible Rooms: 2 . Showers
Accessible Facilities: Lounge, Dining Room
Award-winning country guesthouse with fine scenery of Antrim coast, overlooking the sea of Moyle with views of Scottish hills in the background. Situated to at the end of Gault's Road - the last one on the left!

GARRON VIEW
14 Cloghs Road, Cushendall BT44 0SP
Tel: (02821) 771018
No. of Accessible Rooms: 3
Accessible Facilities: Lounge, Dining Room
Working farm situated just off main road

outside village. Fine views of Red Bay and Garron Point.

CUSHENDUN

At the foot of the River Dun and at the mouth of Glendun, the village has unique Cornish architecture and is an area of outstanding beauty. The heart of the village is rather a surprise with its main street of whitewashed dwellings, a shop, teahouse and pub (reputedly the smallest in Ireland). The street continues across the bridge over the River Dun. Long attracted many of Ireland's best known artists.

BED AND BREAKFAST
CLONEYMORE BED & BREAKFAST
103 Knocknacarry Road,
Cushendun BT44 0NT
Tel: (028) 2176 61443
e-mail: ann.cloneymore@btinternet.com
www.ireland/holidays.net
No. of Accessible Rooms: 1. Roll-in Shower
Accessible Facilities: Lounge,
Dining Room.
Attractive old house, family owned, in lovely surroundings.

LARNE

Not the prettiest of towns, but it does lie on the threshold of the fine Antrim coastline. The sheltered waters of Larne Lough have been a landing point for 9,000 years, most recently in 1914 when the UVF landed a huge cache of German arms here during its campaign against Home Rule.

TOURIST INFORMATION AND INTERPRETIVE CENTRE
Narrow Gauge Road, Larne BT40 1XB
Tel/Fax: (028) 28 260088
admin@larne.gov.uk

BED AND BREAKFAST
CAIRNVIEW
13 Croft Heights, Ballygalley, Larne BT40 2QS
Tel: (028) 28 583269   Fax: (028) 28 583269

No. of Accessible Rooms: 1. Bath
Accessible Facilities: Lounge, Dining Room.
Lovely modern house 4 miles north of Larne in village of Ballygalley.

ATTRACTIONS
CARRFUNNOCK COUNTRY PARK
Coast Road, Larne
Tel: (028) 28 270541
Beautiful woodland and fine gardens with unique collection of sundials and maze in the shape of N.I. Superb children's activity centre.

SD ⟨⟩   CP ⟨⟩   E ⟨⟩   C ⟨⟩
S ⟨⟩   WC ⟨⟩   RFE ⟨⟩

LARNE INTERPRETIVE CENTRE (see TIC)
Story of the building of the Antrim Coast Road.

LISBURN

Located in the Lagan Valley, this was an important centre for linen-making during C18th, established in Lisburn by Louis Cromell, a French Hugenot and refugee. He is buried in the planters gothic cathedral here.

TOURIST INFORMATION CENTRE
Irish Linen Centre and Lisburn Museum,
Market Square, Lisburn BT28 1AG
Tel: (028) 92 660038

BED AND BREAKFAST
HILLTOP
60 Tullyard Road, Drumbo, Lisburn BT27 5JN
Tel: (028) 92 826021   Fax: (028) 92 826061)
No. of Accessible Rooms: 1
Accessible Facilities: Lounge, Dining Room.
Modern bungalow off Hillhall Road.

ATTRACTION
IRISH LINEN CENTRE & LISBURN MUSEUM
Market Square, Lisburn BT28 1AG
Tel: (028) 92 663377   Fax: (028) 92 672624
Follow the history of linen from C17th: visit a spinner's cottage: see and hear Victorian mill girls: watch damask linen being prepared in the traditional way: learn how linen was made from flax and watch spinning – and more. Truly fascinating.

SD ♿ CP ♿ E ♿ RF ♿
L ♿ C ♿ S ♿ WC ♿

NEWTOWNABBEY

Located seven miles north of Belfast, major site for out of town shopping with huge mall, on main road between Glengormley and Templepatrick. Known for Ballyclare May Fair, traditionally a hiring fare for the farming community, and still renowned as a horse fair.

NEWTOWNABBEY LEISURE AND TECHNICAL SERVICES DEPT.
Glenmount, 49 Church Road, NewtownAbbey BT36 7LG
Tel: (028) 90 868751   Fax: (028) 90 365407

HOTEL
CORR'S CORNER HOTEL ♿
315 Ballyclare Road, Newtown Abbey BT36 4TQ
Tel: (028) 90 849221   Fax: (028) 90 832118
No. of Accessible Rooms: 1
Accessible Facilities: Restaurant
Originally opened in 1919 as a bar for travellers between Belfast and the coast and more recently a roadhouse. In mid 1997 30 bedrooms were added, making this a small, comfortable property. Family-owned and operated.

CHIMNEY CORNER HOTEL 🚶
630 Antrim Road, NewtownAbbey BT36 4RH
Tel: (028) 90 844925   Fax: (028) 90 844352
No. of Accessible Rooms: 1
Accessible Facilities: Lounge, Restaurant, Garden. Located on main road from Glengormley to Templepatrick.

PORTRUSH

A rather brash resort with an abundance of souvenir shops and amusement arcades.

TOURIST INFORMATION CENTRE
Dunluce Centre, Sandhill Drive, Portrush
Tel: (028) 70 823333   Fax: (028) 70 822256

HOTEL
MAGHERABUOY HOUSE HOTEL 🚶
41 Magheraboy Road, Portrush BT56 8NX
Tel: (028) 70 823507   Fax: (028) 70 824687
e-mail:
administration@magherabuoy.freeserve.co.uk
No. of Accessible Rooms: 20
There are 16 rooms on the ground floor and four chalets accessed by small step and ramp. Accessible Facilities: Breakfast room, Dining Room. The hotel overlooks the Atlantic Ocean and is a short distance from the Giant's Causeway.

BED AND BREAKFAST
DUKES LODGE
6 - 7 Kerr Street, Portrush BT56 8DG
Tel/Fax: (028) 70 824159
No. of Accessible Rooms: 1
Accessible Facilities: Dining Room, 2 Lounges, Lift. House along the seafront beside Barrys and the train/bus station.

HAYESBANK KANTARA 🚶
5/6 Ramore Avenue, Portrush BT56 8BB
Tel: (028) 70 823823   Fax: (028) 70 822741
No. of Accessible Rooms: 1. Bath, first floor, accessible by chair lift.
Accessible Facilities: Dining Room
Family run guest house in pleasant area overlooking bowling greens and convenient to amenities.

ATTRACTION
THE DUNLUCE CENTRE
10 Sandhill Drive, Portrush BT56 8BF
Tel: (028) 70 824444   Fax: (028) 70 822256
Fine inter-active hi-tec family entertainment.
SD ♿ CP ♿ E ♿ C 🚶
S ♿ WC 🚶 RFE ♿

TEMPLEPATRICK
ATTRACTION
PATTERSON'S SPADE MILL (NT)
751 Antrim Road, Templepatrick BT38 9AP
Tel/Fax: (028) 94 433619
Only surviving water-driven spade mill in Ireland. Restored by National Trust and back in production.
SD   CP   E   RF
WC 🚶 RFE ♿

COUNTY ARMAGH

ARMAGH

One of Ireland's oldest cities, dating back to the age of St. Patrick in the C5th. Narrow streets in the centre follow the ditches which once ringed the church, founded by the saint in 455AD. There are 2 cathedrals, both called St. Patrick's, one catholic, one protestant, sitting on opposing hills. The elegant mall surrounding a peaceful park, is full of dignified Georgian houses.

TOURIST INFORMATION CENTRE
Old Bank Buildings,
40 English Street, Armagh
Tel: (028) 37 521800   Fax: (028) 37 528329

BUSES
Ulsterbus: Tel: (028) 37 522266

BED AND BREAKFAST
HILLVIEW LODGE
33 Newtownhamilton Road,
Armagh BT60 2PL
Tel: (028) 37 522000   Fax: (028) 37 528276
e-mail: alice@hillviewlodge.com
www.hillviewlodge.com
No. of Accessible Rooms: 1
Accessible Facilities: Lounge, Dining Room
Set in rolling hills, enjoying lovely rural location, 1 mile from Armagh. Guesthouse of the Year Finalist 1998.

NI EOGHAIN LODGE
32 Ennislare Road, Armagh BT60 2AX
Tel/Fax: (028) 37 525633
E-mail: nieoghainlodge@amserve.com
No. of Accessible Rooms: 3
Accessible Facilities: TV Lounge, Dining Room. Farmhouse set amid award-winning gardens, located two miles off A29 Keady/Armagh road.

ATTRACTIONS
ARMAGH COUNTY MUSEUM
The Mall East, Armagh BT61 9BE
Tel: (028) 37 523070   Fax: (028) 37 522631

Located on the Mall, an area of urban parkland in the city centre, this is the oldest County museum in Ireland with a distinctive Greek classical design although built in 1834. Extensive collection of artefacts include military costumes, ceramics, natural history specimens, railway material and historic household items. Ever changing temporary exhibitions.
SD ♿ | CP n/a – Street parking only, very close.
E ♿ | RF ♿ | L ♿ | S ♿ | WC ♿

ARMAGH PLANETARIUM
College Hill, Armagh BT61 9DB
Tel: (028) 37 524725   Fax: (028) 37 526187
Multimedia Star-Show with 3-D effects and tour of the Hall of Astronomy and Eartharium, Weather Room and School's Internet Centre. N.B. Exhibitions change so it is recommended to telephone first to see what is available.
SD ♿ | CP ⚠ | E ♿ (Main E. has disabled lift)
RF ♿ | C ⚠ | S ♿ | WC ⚠ | RFE ⚠

THE NAVAN CENTRE
81 Killylea Road, Armagh BT60 4LD
Tel: (028) 37 525550   Fax: (028) 37 522323
e-mail: navan@anterprise.net
Navan Fort is a famous Celtic site: seat of ancient Kings of Ulster. The Centre tells the history and archaeology of the fort in superb visual interactive display. NB: Access to Navan Fort Ancient Monument is difficult for wheelchairs.
SD ♿ | CP ♿ | E ♿ | RF ♿
C ♿ | S ♿ | WC ⚠

PALACE STABLES HERITAGE CENTRE
The Palace, Demesne, Armagh BT60 4EL
Tel: (028) 37 529629   Fax: (028) 37 529630
Housed in Georgian stables and courtyard where visitors can experience stable life in the C18th via life-like models, audio-commentary and colour murals.
SD ♿ | CP ♿ | E ♿ | RF ♿ | L ♿
C ⚠ | S ♿ | WC ♿ | RFE ♿

SAINT PATRICK'S TRIAN VISITOR COMPLEX
40 English Street, Armagh BT61 7BA
Tel: (028) 37 521801   Fax: (028) 37 510180
Name derives from three distinct districts or Trians - here there are three major

exhibitions. The Armagh Story with AV presentation: exhibition on Saint Patrick and the Land of Lilliput where adventures of Gulliver are narrated, Jonathan Swift having spent time in Armagh. Much to see.

SD ♿ CP ♿ E ♿ RF ♿
L ♿ C ♿ S ♿ WC ♿

CRAIGAVON

Located in the NE area of the County, this is a new town, not beautiful, but with two large artificial lakes and close to Lough Neagh.

LOUGH NEAGH DISCOVERY CENTRE
Oxford Island National Nature Reserve, Nr. Craigavon BT66 6NJ
Tel: (028) 38 322205   Fax: (028) 38 347438
History and wildlife of the Lough through audio-visual shows, interactive games and exhibitions and then experience it all for yourself.

SD ♿ CP ♿ E ♿ RF ♿
C ♿ S ♿ WC ♿

NEWRY

Old prosperous town on the River Clanrye with imposing houses and public buildings. Newry Canal, the oldest in Britain, now well stocked with fish.

TOURIST INFORMATION CENTRE
Town Hall, Newry BT35 6HR
Tel: (028) 302 68877   Fax: (028) 302 68833

BED AND BREAKFAST
GREEN VALE 🚶
141 Longfield Road, Forkhill, Newry BT35 9SD
Tel: (028) 30 888314
No. of Accessible Rooms: 2
Accessible Facilities: Lounge, Dining Room.
Bungalow on farm, 1.5 miles from Forkhill.

PORTADOWN

Old linen town in the industrial NE area of the county. Close to Lough Neagh and the river Bann.

HOTEL
SEAGOE HOTEL 🚶
22 Upper Church Lane, Portadown BT63 5JE
Tel: (028) 38 333076
Fax: (028) 38 350210
No. of Accessible Rooms: 2. Bath
Accessible Facilities: Restaurant, Bar.
Situated close to Lough Neagh.
Contemporary 34 bedroom hotel in attractive grounds.

COUNTY DOWN

BALLYNAHINCH
BED AND BREAKFAST
NUMBER THIRTY 🚶
30 Mountview Road,
Ballynahinch BT24 8JR
Tel: (028) 97 562956
No. of Accessible Rooms: 1. Bath
Accessible Facilities: Dining Room
Modern chalet bungalow situated in quiet country area overlooking the Mournes.

BANBRIDGE

Main gateway to the famous Mourne Mountains, with a great hill on the south of the river Bann. In 1834 the main street of Banbridge was divided into 3 sections with an underpass cut out in the middle to lower the hill and a bridge built over the gap.

GATEWAY TOURIST INFORMATION CENTRE
200 Newry Road, Banbridge, BT32 3NB
Tel: (028) 406 23322

BED AND BREAKFAST
MOURNEVIEW 🚶
32 Drumnascamph Road, Laurencetown, Banbridge BT63 6DU
Tel/Fax: (028) 406 26270
e-mail: N.W.79@dial.pipex.com
No. of Accessible Rooms: 4
Accessible Facilities: Lounge, Dining Room.
Detached bungalow 2 miles from Banbridge.

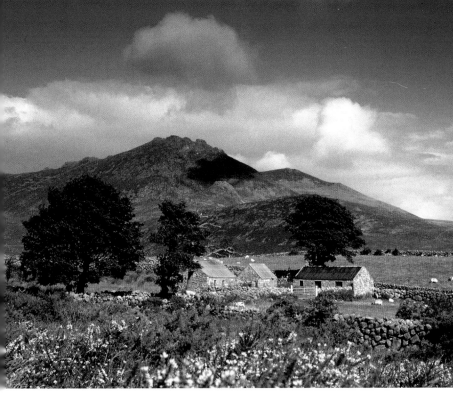

The Mountains of Mourne. You can almost taste the Guinness!

BANGOR
Resort town with modern marina and well known yacht clubs. A little south of the town is Donaghadee from where boats sail to the uninhabited Copeland Islands.

TOURIST INFORMATION CENTRE
Tower House, 34 Quay Street,
Bangor BT20 5ED
Tel: (028) 91 270069   Fax: (028) 91 274466

BUSES
Translink Bangor
Abbey Street, Bangor, BT20 4JA
Ulsterbus: Tel: (028) 91 271143
Majority of buses in Co. Down are NOT wheelchair accessible, the fleet is being renewed. Call Ulsterbus before travelling.

RAIL
NI Railways, Bangor Rail Station,
Abbey Street, Bangor
Tel: (028) 91 271143

One carriage on each train is wheelchair accessible and has ramps.

SHOPMOBILITY
55-59 The Arcade, High Street,
Bangor BT20 5BE
Tel: (028) 91 456586

HOTELS
CLANDEBOYE LODGE HOTEL
10 Estate Road, Clandeboye, Bangor BT19 1UR
Tel: (028) 91 852500   Fax: (028) 91 852772
e-mail: info@clandeboye.co.uk
www.clandeboyelodge.com
No. of Accessible Rooms: 2
Accessible Facilities: Lounge, Restaurant, Lift. Set in woodland overlooking Clandeboye Estate. Furnished and decorated to reflect relaxed rural setting. 3 miles from Bangor,11 from Belfast.

MARINE COURT HOTEL
The Marina, 18-20 Quay Street,
Bangor BT20 5ED
Tel: (028) 91 451100   Fax: (028) 91 451200
No. of Accessible Rooms: 1. Shower

Accessible Facilities: Lift, Lounge, Restaurant, Pool, Sauna, Spa.
Purpose-built hotel in centre of Bangor with seafront location overlooking Marina.

CASTLEWELLAN

Hill top market town in foothills of the Mournes with 2 large market places. The town is surrounded by private woods.

BED AND BREAKFAST
TREETOPS ⛹
39 Circular Road, Castlewellan BT31 9ED
Tel: (028) 437 78132
No. of Accessible Rooms: 1
Accessible Facilities: Dining Room.
Two-storey modern house set in spacious gardens.

SELF-CATERING
COAST VIEW COTTAGE ⛹
41 Ballywillwill Road, Castlewellan BT31 9LF
Tel: (028) 437 78006
e-mail: murray@unite.co.uk
No. of Accessible Units: 1. Bath
No. of Beds per Unit: 5
Accessible Facilities: Dining room, lounge, kitchen.
Charming cottage with stunning views from Mountains of Mourne to Belfast Lough.

COMBER

A pleasant town with a prominent statue of Robert Gillespie, Ulster military hero in Indian campaigns.

BED AND BREAKFAST
THE OLD SCHOOLHOUSE INN ⛹
100 Ballydrain Road, Castle Espie, Comber BT23 6EA
Tel: (028) 97 541182 Fax: (028) 97 542583
E-mail: info@theoldschoolhouseinn.com
www.theoldschoolhouseinn.com
No. of Accessible Rooms: 12
Accessible Facilities: Lounge, Dining Room.
The last bell rang in the playground 14 years ago. Now a guest house and

restaurant in a rural location, three miles from Comber.

ATTRACTION
THE WILDFOWL AND WETLANDS TRUST
Castle Espie, Ballydrain Road, Comber BT23 6EA
Tel: (028) 91 874146 Fax: (028) 91 873857
www.wwt.org.uk
Home to Ireland's largest collection of ducks, geese and swans. Three hides, landscaped gardens and 30 acres of woodland to explore.

| SD ♿ | CP ♿ | E ♿ | RF ⛹ |
| C ♿ | S ♿ | WC ⛹ | RFE ♿ |

HOLYWOOD

History dates back to 700AD, when townland of Balleyderry (town of the wood), was renamed by the Normans to Sanctus Boscus – the Holy Wood. Situated on shores of Lough Belfast with good restaurants, pubs and excellent shopping. High street has one of few remaining Maypoles in Ireland - a ship's mast presented to the town by grateful Dutch sailors after a shipwreck.

BED AND BREAKFAST
ARDSHANE COUNTRY HOUSE ⛹
5 Bangor Road, Holywood BT18 0NU
Tel: (028) 90 422044 Fax: (028) 90 427506

No. of Accessible Rooms: 2
Accessible Facilities: Lounge, Dining Room.
Built at turn of C19th on 800-year-old camp site of King John's army as it marched through Ireland. Ardshane means Hill of John. Guest house on the outskirts of the town amidst mature gardens and glens. Main reception area restored to reflect living styles of 1902 .

ATTRACTION
ULSTER FOLK AND TRANSPORT MUSEUM
Cultra, Holywood BT18 0EU
Tel: (028) 90 428428 Fax: (028) 90428728
e-mail: uftm@talk21.com
www.magni.org.uk

Irish Railway Collection, Transport and Folk Galleries, Town and Rural Areas. All exhibition galleries are ramped throughout: buildings in the open-air museum are all original, brought from original locations and re-erected in the Museum – their interiors therefore are inaccessible. Given the nature of the museum, distances involved and some gradients on the site, DISABLED VISITORS MAY GO ROUND THE OPEN-AIR MUSEUM BY CAR, AFTER 3PM. The Transport Museum covers many aspects including the Titanic exhibition and the Irish Railway collection.

SD ⬥ CP ⬥ E ⬥ RF ⬥ S ⬥
WC ⬥ Irish Railway Collection & Road Transport Galleries:
RF ⬥ C ⬥ WC ⬥ Folk Galleries:
RF ⬥ S ⬥ WC ⬥

KILKEEL

Busy, prosperous town and fishing port, home to the coast's main fishing fleet. Built on the site of a prehistoric fort, the ruins of a C14th castle stand in the square located in the heart of the Mourne Mountains, there are great views of coastal and mountain scenery on the Spelga Pass towards Hilltown.

TOURIST INFORMATION CENTRE
28 Bridge Street, Kilkeel BT34 4AD
Tel/Fax: (028) 417 62525

HOTEL
KILMOREY ARMS
41-43 Greencastle Street, Kilkeel BT34 4BH
Tel: (028) 417 62220   Fax: (028) 417 65399
No. of Accessible Rooms: 2
Accessible Facilities: Lounge, Restaurant.
Original building 250 years old. Located in the town centre .

BED AND BREAKFAST
SHARON FARM
6 Ballykeel Road, Ballymartin,
Nr. Kilkeel BT34 4PL
Tel: (028) 417 62521
No. of Accessible Rooms: 1. Bath
Accessible Facilities: Lounge, Dining Room.
Modern bungalow situated on outskirts of Ballymartin, with lovely sea & mountain views.

HILL VIEW BED AND BREAKFAST
18 Bog Road, Attical, Kilkeel BT34 4HT
Tel: (028) 417 64269
No. of Accessible Rooms: 2
Accessible Facilities: Lounge, Dining Room.
Farmhouse located in the Mourne countryside.

417

Strangford Lough.

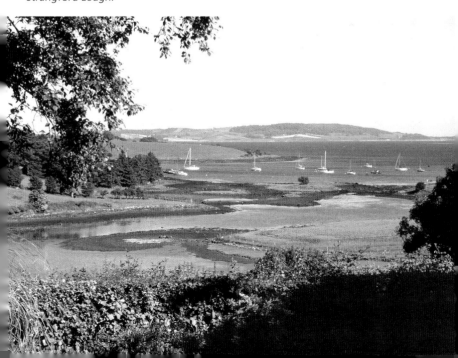

LISBURN

BED & BREAKFAST
BROOK LODGE
79 Old Ballynahinch Road, Lisburn BT27 6TH
Tel: (028) 92 638454
No. of Accessible Rooms: 1.
Accessible Facilities: Dining Room
Modern guest house on 65-acre mixed
farm with views of Dromara Hills and
Mourne Mountains. 3 miles from Lisburn.

NEWCASTLE
Attractive, lively town and a popular
resort since the early C19th,
Newcastle's promenade overlooks
golden beaches and rolling hills. Close
by is forest park of Tullmore.

TOURIST INFORMATION CENTRE
Annesley Mansions, Central Promenade,
Newcastle BT33 0AA
Tel: (028) 437 22222   Fax: (028) 437 22400

HOTELS
BURRENDALE HOTEL & COUNTRY CLUB
51 Castlewellan Road, Newcastle BT33 0JY
Tel: (028) 437 22599   Fax: (028) 437 22328
No. of Accessible Rooms: 12
Accessible Facilities: Lounge, Bar,
Restaurant (2), Country Club with poolside
lift for pool and jacuzzi. The hotel provides
an excellent guide to its facilities for
disabled guests. Delightful, modern hotel
located between Mourne Mountains and
Irish Sea, one hour from Belfast and close
to Newcastle.

HASTINGS SLIEVE DONARD HOTEL
Downs Road, Newcastle BT33 0AH
Tel: (028) 437 21066   Fax: (028) 437 24830
e-mail: res.sdh@hastingshotels.com
www.hastingshotels.com
No. of Accessible rooms: 4. Bath.
Accessible Facilities: Lounge, Restaurant
Quality hotel in 6 acres of grounds leading
to beach. Close to Tullymore Forest Park.

BED AND BREAKFAST
MOURNE VIEW HOUSE
16 off Main Street, Dundrum,
Nr. Newcastle BT33 0LU
Tel: (028) 437 51457
No. of Accessible Rooms: 1
Accessible Facilities: Dining Room
Cottage-style property situated in its own
grounds. Located just off the main
Dundrum street at the entrance to the
Quay. 4 miles from Newcastle.

NEWTOWNARDS
Popular for medievalists, there is an
impressive town square. Best known
as home of Mt. Stewart.

TOURIST INFORMATION CENTRE
31 Regent Street, Newtownards BT23 4AD
Tel: (028) 91 826846   Fax: (028) 91 826681

BED & BREAKFAST
ERNSDALE
120 Mountstewart Road, Carrowdore,
Newtownards BT22 2ES
Tel: (028) 91 861208
No. of Accessible Rooms: 3. Bath
Accessible Facilities: Dining Room.
Working farm located close to
Mountstewart House. 6.5 miles from
town.

SELF-CATERING
BEECH COTTAGE
20 Mountstewart Road, Newtownards
BT22 2AL
Tel/Fax: (028) 42788357
e-mail: ballycastlehouse@breathemail.net
www.ballycastlehouse.com
No. of Accessible Units: 1
No. of Beds per Unit: 1 - double
Accessible Facilities: Lounge, Dining
Room, Kitchen. Quiet rural setting 2.5
miles from Restaurant, pub and groceries.

ATTRACTION
MOUNT STEWART HOUSE AND GARDENS
(NT)
Portaferry Road, Newtownards BT22 2AD
Tel: (028) 4278 8387   Fax: (028) 42788569
E-mail: mountstewart@ntrust.org.uk
Charming C18th house with C19th
additions, the childhood home of Lord
Castlereagh and famous for its fine

garden. Wheelchairs and 2 self-drive
buggies available.

SD ♿   CP 🚹   E ♿   RF ♿
C ♿   S ♿   WC ♿

SOMME HERITAGE CENTRE
233 Bangor Road, Newtownards BT23 7PH
Tel: (028) 91 823202
Examines Ireland's contribution to WW1
through 10th & 16th (Irish) Divisions and
36th (Ulster) Division. Reconstructed trench
system, museum and audio-visual
recreation of the Battle of the Somme.

SD ♿   CP ♿   E ♿   RF ♿
C ♿   S ♿   WC 🚹

PORTAFERRY
Conservation village with brightly
painted houses on the shores of
Strangford Lough, one of the most
important marine sites in Europe. On
the waterfront look across to
Strangford village.

TOURIST INFORMATION CENTRE
The Stables, Castle Street, Portaferry BT22 1NZ
Tel: (028) 427 29882   Fax: (028) 427 29822
(Seasonal)

BED AND BREAKFAST
THE NARROWS   ♿
8 Shore Road, Portaferry BT22 1JY
Tel: (028) 427 28148   Fax: (028) 427 28105
e-mail: info@narrows.co.uk
www.narrows.co.uk
No. of Accessible Rooms: 8
Accessible Facilities: Lounge, Dining Room,
Sauna. National Holiday Care Award
Winner 1996. Highest proportion of
accessible bedrooms of any small
mainstream hotel in UK. Seafront location,
all rooms having wonderful views of
Strangford Lough, Ireland's first Marine
Nature Reserve. Exceptional variety of
marine life and colonies of common seals.

ATTRACTION
EXPLORIS
The Ropewalk, Castle Street, Portaferry, BT22 1NZ
Tel: (028) 427 28062   Fax: (028) 427 28396
www.exploris.org.uk

Aquarium with Open Sea Tank, Shoal Ring.
Journey from Strangford Lough through
the neck of the Lough – the Narrows.

SD ♿   CP ♿   E ♿   RF ♿   L ♿
C ♿   S 🚹   WC ♿   RFE 🚹

SAINTFIELD
ATTRACTION
ROWALLANE GARDEN (NT)
Saintfield BT24 7LH
Tel: (028) 97 510131   Fax: (028) 97 511242
e-mail: liroest@smtp.ntrust.org.uk
21 hectare shrub and tree garden
containing many exotic species from
around the world. Fine displays of azaleas
and rhododendrons. Accessed by
compacted gravel or mown grass paths.
Some areas undulating.

SD ♿   CP ♿   E ♿   RF ♿
C- ♿   WC ♿   RFE 🚹

COUNTY FERMANAGH

FERMANAGH
TOURIST INFORMATION CENTRE
Wellington Road, Enniskillen BT74 7EF
Tel: (028) 66 323110   Fax: (028) 66 325511
www.fermanaghlakelands.com

BELLEEK
Northern Ireland's most westerly
village, close to Lower Lough Erne.
Famous for its pottery.

ATTRACTION
BELLEEK POTTERY VISITOR CENTRE
Belleek Pottery, Belleek, County Fermanagh
Tel: (028) 686 59300   Fax: (028) 686 58625
e-mail: customerservices@belleek.ie
Lining walls of reception in Centre are
photographs telling the Belleek story since
its establishment in 1857. Museum
contains some pieces dating back over 100
years: AV theatre presentation takes you
through production process, followed by
20 minute tour, all on one level. Visit the
Casting and Fettling Shops, and Flowering
rooms and see craftsmen design, mould
and shape the intricate basketware. Quite
fascinating.

| SD ♿ | CP ♿ | E ♿ | RF ♿ |
| C ♿ | S ♿ | WC 🚹 | RFE-TOUR ♿ |

DERRYGONNELLY
BED AND BREAKFAST
NAVAR GUEST HOUSE   🚹
Derryvarey, Derrygonnelly BT93 6HW
Tel: (028) 686 41384
No. of Accessible Rooms: 5. Bath
Accessible Facilities: Lounge, Dining Room.
(1 step at front entrance). Modern
bungalow on working farm, in rural
setting close to Lough Melvin and Erne.
Located 1.5 miles from Derrygonnelly
toward Enniskillen.

ENNISKILLEN
Dominated by its C15th castle, the
town appears initially medieval, but
modern buildings rather spoil the
illusion. Before the plantation, the
Maguires ruled this lakeland area. The
centre of Enniskillen is rather a jumble,
with a winding main street and an old
buttermarket, known for hand-crafted
goods. The centre occupies an island
between Upper and Lower Lough
Erne. The C17th Church of Ireland
cathedral was re-constructed in C19th.

TOURIST INFORMATION CENTRE
Wellington Road, Enniskillen, BT74 7EF
Tel: (028) 66 323110

BUSES
Ulsterbus: Tel: (028) 66 322633

HOTEL
KILLYHEVLIN HOTEL   ♿
Dublin Road, Enniskillen BT74 6RW
Tel: (028) 66 323481   Fax: (028) 66 324726
E-mail: info@killyhevlin.com
www.killyhevlin.com
No. of Accessible Rooms: 1
Accessible Facilities: Lounge, Restaurant
Family run hotel situated on the shores of
beautiful Lough Erne, in extensive
grounds. 05.miles from town centre.

BED AND BREAKFAST
BRINDLEY GUEST HOUSE   🚹
Tully, Killadeas, Enniskillen BT94 1RE
Tel: (028) 66 28065
No. of Accessible Rooms: 3
Accessible Facilities: Lounge, Dining
Room.
Modern property with fine views over
Lower Lough Erne.

LACKABOY FARM HOUSE   🚹
Tempo Road, Enniskillen BT74 6EBA
Tel: (028) 66 322488
No. of Accessible Rooms: 1
Accessible Facilities: Lounge, Dining
Room.
60-acre dairy farm, 2 miles from
Enniskillen centre and close to Castle
Coole.

THE POINT   🚹
Tempo Road, Enniskillen BT74
Tel: (028) 66 323595
No. of Accessible Rooms: 1
Accessible Facilities: Lounge, Dining Room
Spacious modern house located 1 mile
outside town boundary.

SELF-CATERING
BELMORE COURT HOTEL   ♿
Tempo Road, Enniskillen BT74 6HX
Tel: (028) 66 326633
Fax: (028) 66 326362
e-mail: book@motel.co.uk
www.motel.co.uk
No. of Accessible Units: 1. Shower
No. of Beds per Unit: 2
Accessible Facilities: Kitchenette. Quality
apartments situated on the edge of town,
at junction of Dublin and Temp roads,
close to main amenities.

ATTRACTIONS
CASTLE COOLE (NT)
Dublin Road, Enniskillen BT74 6JY
Tel: (028) 66 322690   Fax: (028) 66 325665
e-mail: castlecoole@ntrust.org.uk
One of finest neo-classical buildings in
British Isles, built between 1789/95 by
architect James Wyatt, with wonderful
plasterwork ceilings and superb Regency
furniture. Outside lawns slope gently
toward Lough Coole.

WARNING: Entrance is ramped at 1:5, but staff are very caring and an electric buggy is OK - otherwise, make sure you have a very strong pusher!

SD ♿   CP 🚶   E n/a (see above)
RF ♿   C ♿   S ♿   WC 🚶

ENNISKILLEN CASTLE
Castle Barracks, Enniskillen BT74 7HL
Tel: (028) 66325000   Fax: (028) 66 327342
www.enniskillencastle.co.uk
Three-storey keep surrounded by huge barracks with C17th water gate, which houses two museums and a heritage centre. Exhibits on Royal Enniskillen Fusiliers regiment and area antiquities.

SD ♿   CP 🚶   E ♿   RF ♿
L 🚶   S ♿   WC 🚶   RFE ♿

ADAPTIVE CRUISERS
ERINCURRACH CRUISERS
Blaney, Enniskillen BT93 7EQ
Tel: (028) 66 68641737   Fax: (028) 66 864173
www.boatingireland.com
Accessible Cruiser Class: Blaney
No. of Accessible Cruisers: 1
No. of Berths: 6
Sedan style cruiser specially adapted for access to wheelchairs to all compartments via interior lifts. Explore the waterways and lakes of the Lough Erne and River Shannon systems.

FLORENCECOURT
ATTRACTION
MARBLE ARCH CAVES/
CUILCAGH MOUNTAIN PARK
Marlbank Scenic Loop, Florencecourt BT92 1EW
Tel: (028) 66 348855   Fax: (028) 66 348928
The Caves are unsuitable for wheelchair users, but Reception/Exhibition building is accessible with audio-visual facility.

SD ♿   CP ♿   E ♿   RF ♿
L 🚶   C ♿   S ♿   WC 🚶

GARRISON
Charming village on shores of Lough Melvin.

BED AND BREAKFAST
LOUGH MELVIN HOLIDAY CENTRE   ♿
Garrison BT93 4ET
Tel: (028) 686 58142   Fax: (028) 686 58719
No. of Accessible Rooms: 3
Accessible Facilities: Dining Room, TV Lounge. Modern holiday centre on the shores of Lough Melvin, central to the county's top attractions with quality restaurant and coffee shop on site. Caters for range of activities that include accessible boating on the Lough.

KESH
Busy little fishing village where one can learn the old skills of spinning and weaving nearby at Ardress.

BED AND BREAKFAST
DRUMRUSH LODGE   ♿
Drumrush, Kesh
Tel: (028) 686 31578
No. of Accessible Rooms: 1
Accessible Facilities: Lounge, Dining Room. Purpose built complex overlooking Muckross Bay in Lower Lough Erne beside marina.

CLAREVIEW   🚶
Scenic Route, 85A Crevenish Road, Kesh BT93 1RQ
Tel: (028) 686 31455
e-mail: kesh@clareview.swinternet.co.uk
No. of Accessible Rooms: 2. Bath
Accessible Facilities: Lounge, Dining Room. Modern bungalow on elevated site on scenic route between Kesh and Castle Archdale with fishing and boating close by.

LISNASKEA
Interesting market town with restored market cross and ruined C17th castle in the town centre.

SELF-CATERING
SHARE HOLIDAY VILLAGE   ♿
Smith's Strand, Lisnaskea BT92 0EQ
Tel: (028) 677 22122   Fax: (028) 677 21893

e-mail: info@sharevillage.org
www.sharevillage.org
No. of Accessible Chalets: 17
No. of Accessible Guesthouse Rooms: 13
Charity promoting integration between able-bodied people and those with special needs. The village is a lakeside activity centre with purpose-built accommodation for use by physically challenged guests. Wide range of outdoor sports and wheelchair accessible coaches for trips to local places of interest.

NEWTOWNBUTLER
Located on Upper Lough Erne

ATTRACTION
CROM ESTATE (NT)
Newtownbutler BT92 8AP
Tel/Fax: (028) 677 38118
e-mail: cromw@smtp.ntrust.org.uk
An important conservation area with woodland, parkland and wetland on the shores of Upper Lough Erne. Wheelchair and self-drive buggy available.

COUNTY LONDONDERRY

AGHADOWEY
Located a few miles south of Coleraine and 10 miles from the coast.

HOTEL
BROWN TROUT GOLF & COUNTRY INN ♿
209 Agivey Road, Aghadowey BT51 4AD
Tel: (028) 70 868209
Fax: (028) 70 868878
e-mail: bill@browntroutinn.com
www.browntroutinn.com
No. of Accessible Rooms: several
Accessible Facilities: Lounge, Bar, Restaurant (accessed by stair lift). Situated on banks of River Agivey, one of the country's oldest hostelries. A family affair, the first record dating from 1817, this is a charming property, the first golf hotel in Northern Ireland. Owner's sister, returning to help with staff training and catering, used to be with London Tara Hotel, well-known for its facilities for disabled guests.

COLERAINE
Home to the Coleraine campus of the University of Ulster, with the ambience of a university town. Founded by St. Patrick, most of the town was developed by the Irish Society of London. The river Bann runs through the centre, and a rare collection of daffodils and narcissi bloom here in late April.

TOURIST INFORMATION CENTRE
Railway Road, Coleraine
Tel: (028) 703 44723
Fax: (028) 703 51756

CAUSEWAY COAST AND GLENS
11 Lodge Road, Coleraine,
Co. Londonderry BT52 1LU
Tel: (028) 70 327720
Fax: (028) 70 327719
e-mail: mail@causewaycoastandglens.com
www.causewaycoastandglens.com

HOTEL
BOHILL HOTEL & COUNTRY CLUB ♿
69 Cloyfin Road, Coleraine BT52 2NY
Tel: (028) 703 52424   Fax: (028) 703 55873
No. of Accessible Rooms: 37
Accessible Facilities: Lounge, Restaurant, Gardens, Grounds.
Modern hotel with chalet type rooms.

BED AND BREAKFAST
COOLBEG ♿
2e Grange Road, Coleraine BT52 1NG
Tel: (028) 703 44961   Fax: (028) 703 43278
No. of Accessible Rooms: 2
Accessible Facilities: Lounge, Dining Room, Garden access. Modern bungalow situated in quiet residential area. Surrounding area is flat and town centre under a mile. Plenty of Restaurants and eating places in the area.

THE LODGE HOTEL AND TRAVELSTOP
Lodge Road, Coleraine BT52 1NF
Tel: (028) 703 44848   Fax: (028) 70354555
e-mail: info@thelodgehotel.com
www.thelodgehotel.com
No. of Accessible Rooms: 2
Accessible Facilities: Restaurants (2)
Accessible rooms in Travelstop adjacent
main hotel with facilities available. Located
0.5 mile from town centre and close to
Giant's Causeway and Mussendum Temple
- 1770s, maintained by National Trust with
cliff top views.

SELF-CATERING
KINGS COUNTRY COTTAGES
"Ballyvennox" 66 Ringrash Road, Macosquin,
Coleraine BT51 4LJ
Tel/Fax: (028) 703 51367
No. of Accessible Units: 1. Roll-in Shower
No, of Beds per Unit: 6
Accessible Facilities: Lounge, Kitchen
1 of 6 cottages in quiet farmyard setting,
in village just south-west of Coleraine.

KILREA
In the Bann Valley on B64 between
Coleraine and Maghera, before the
Bann broadens out into Loch Beg and
then Loch Neagh. Attractive farming
landscape, highly cultivated.

BED AND BREAKFAST
PORTNEAL LODGE
75 Bann Road, Kilrea BT51 5RX
Tel: (028) 295 41444   Fax: (028) 295 41424
E-mail: info@portneal.com
www.portneal.com
No. of Accessible Rooms: 2. Roll in shower.
Accessible Facilities: Dining room.
Homely B & B situated in seven acres of
woodland overlooking a stretch of the
Lower Bann River, very close to town.
Evening meals available. Known for coarse
and game angling.
Disabled rooms fully customised for
visitors.

LIMAVADY
Largely of modern character but some
Georgian evidence in early streets.
Beautifully located in the Roe Valley
with glorious mountain landscapes to
the north and south-east.

TOURIST INFORMATION CENTRE
Council Offices, 7 Connell Street, Limavady
Tel: (028) 777 22226   Fax: (028) 777 22010

HOTEL
GORTEEN HOUSE HOTEL
187 Roe Mill Road, Limavady BT49 9EX
Tel: (028) 777 22333
No. of Accessible Rooms: 6. Shower
Accessible Facilities: Lounge, Restaurant,
Bar. Former C18th residence located on
outskirts of the town, close to Derry
Airport.

RADISSON ROE PARK
HOTEL & GOLF RESORT
Roe Park, Limavady BT49 9LB
Tel: (028) 777 22222
Fax: (028) 777 22313
e-mail: reservation@radissonroepark.com
No. of Accessible Rooms: 1
Accessible Facilities: Lounge, Restaurants
(2). Quality hotel set within private 18-hole
golf course and surrounded by lovely
tranquil countryside of Roe Valley
Country Park.

BED AND BREAKFAST
THE POPLARS GUEST HOUSE
352 Seacoast Road, Limavady BT49 0LA
Tel: (028) 777 50360
No. of Accessible Rooms: 1. Bath
Accessible Facilities: Dining Room.
Evening Meal available. Detached modern
farm bungalow in mature gardens with
good views of Donegal Hills. Close to
Benone Strand, 6 miles from Limavady.

(LONDONDERRY) DERRY
Derry is the only completely walled city
in Ireland. Developed by the City of
London in the early C17th, it took on
the London prefix and the city's walls

and inner city were the showpiece development of the Plantation era in Ulster. There are many Georgian streets, some fine buildings, including St. Columb's Cathedral of 1633 (sadly not very accessible) and the lavish neo-Gothic Guildhall.

VISITOR AND CONVENTION BUREAU
44 Foyle Street, Derry BT48 6AT
Tel: (028) 71 377577   Fax: (028) 71 377992
e-mail: info@derryvisitor.com
www.derryvisitor.com

BUSES
Ulsterbus: Tel: (028) 90 333000
10 low-floor buses for city service wheelchair assisted access.
Translink (Citybus, NI Rail, Ulsterbus)
New buses have been fitted with ramps and low-floor level wheelchair accessibility.
Citybus: Tel: (028) 9666650
NI Rail: Tel: (028) 90 899411
Ulsterbus: Tel: (028) 90 33300

TAXIS
For all queries call: (028) 71260247 Community Black Taxis -London style- operate in certain areas of Londonderry – not all are accessible. This is a bus type of service. Public hire taxis are identified by yellow plate at rear and front of vehicle. Private hire taxis identified by car roof sign with white front panel and green licence disc on windscreen.

RAIL
NI Railways: Tel: (028) 71 342228
Ramps available and one carriage in each train is wheelchair accessible. 24 hours notice to book assistance.

HOTEL
WATERFOOT HOTEL & COUNTRY CLUB
14 Clooney Road, Londonderry BT47 1TB
Tel: (028) 71 345500   Fax: (028) 71 311006
No. of Accessible Rooms: 2
Accessible Facilities: Dining Room, Bar (2 steps). Lovely hotel situated at eastern end of the Foyle Bridge with fine views of both the River and Co. Donegal

ATTRACTION
FOYLE VALLEY RAILWAY MUSEUM
Foyle Road Station, Londonderry BT48 6SQ
Tel: (028) 71 265234
Londonderry was once the meeting point of 4 railway systems and this museum hosts a fine collection of relics from the past. Majestic steam locomotives, railcars and wagons with hands-on activities. Ramp onto train.

PORTSTEWART
Originally popular with the Victorian middle-classes, this seaside resort remains rather sedate. It has a long crescent-shaped seafront promenade and west of the town is the Strand, a fine long sandy beach protected by the National Trust.

BED AND BREAKFAST
NORTHGATE
13 Old Coach Road, Portstewart BT55 7BX
Tel: (028) 70 832497
No. of Accessible Rooms: 1. Shower
Accessible Facilities: Lounge, Dining Room. Quiet family run home overlooking lovely sea views and golf course with small garden.

COUNTY TYRONE

CLOGHER
Clogher Valley Agricultural Show in Augher and in Clogher the William Carleton Summer School, a five-day arts event. Several places of interest nearby.

BED AND BREAKFAST
CORICK HOUSE
20 Corick Road, Clogher BT76 0BZ
Tel: (028) 855 48216   Fax: (028) 855 49531
No. of Accessible Rooms: 1. Roll in shower.
Accessible Facilities: Lounge, Dining Room Charmingly restored 10-bedroomed C17th

William and Mary house set in 20 acres of gardens overlooking River Blackwater. Tower and Garden Front added in 1863. Located 0.5 mile off main A4 Belfast to Enniskillen road between village of Augher and Clogher.

COOKSTOWN

Well known for its stately central thoroughfare 2km long and totally straight. A C17th Plantation town, the countryside around is rich in Neolithic and early Christian monuments.

TOURIST INFORMATION CENTRE
48 Moleworth Street, Cookstown BT80 4DL
Tel: (028) 867 66727 (Seasonal)
(028) 867 62205 (all year-Council offices)

HOTEL
GLENAVON HOUSE HOTEL   [♿]
52 Drum Road, Cookstown BT80 8JQ
Tel: (028) 867 64949 Fax: (028) 867 64396
No. of Accessible Rooms: 1
Accessible Facilities: Lounge, 2
Restaurants. Situated on the outskirts of town in nine acres of mature gardens. Located at the foot of the Sperrins.

TULLYLAGAN COUNTRY HOUSE   [♿]
40b Tullylagen Road, Cookstown BT80 8UP
Tel: (028) 867 65100 Fax: (028) 867 61715
No. of Accessible Rooms: 2
Accessible Facilities: Restaurant, Lounge. Early C19th property in style of late Georgian classic villa. Rural setting in 30 acres of mature grounds with Tullylagan River flowing through the estate. Located midway between Dungannon and Cookstown.

ATTRACTIONS
DRUM MANOR FOREST PARK
Oaklands, Cookstown
Tel: (028) 87 759311 Fax: (028) 87 759181
Small, yet varied and attractive, forest estate with Butterfly Garden with wide variety of wildflower and shrubs specially grown to attract native butterflies. High fertility of soil means wide tree variety can be grown. 4 wayside trails, No.2 being an

Adapted trail of 0.8 mile – gentle trail following promenade path to Butterfly Gardens, continuing to half-way picnic table and view point with easy return to car park. Car parking, with excellent spacing, is 400m from entrance.

| SD [♿] | CP n/a | E [♿] | RF [♿] |
| C [♿] | S n/a | WC [♿] | RFE [♿] |

KINTURK CULTURAL CENTRE
7 Kinturk Road, Cookstown, BT80 0JD
Tel: (028) 867 36512

| SD [♿] | CP [♿] | E [♿] | RF [♿] |
| L- [♿] | C [♿] | S [♿] | |

DUNGANNON

Hilly location and site of government of the O'Neill dynasty from C14th until Plantation. The town's Royal School, opened in 1614, claims to be the oldest in Northern Ireland. Originally known for its linen manufacture, the best known factory now is Tyrone Crystal.

HOTEL
COHANNON INN & AUTO LODGE   [♿]
212 Ballynakilly Road, Dungannon BT71 6HJ
Tel: (028) 87 722215 Fax: (028) 87 752217
No. of Accessible Rooms: 1
Accessible Facilities: Restaurant
Located at the A45 Filling Station, convenient to M1 Motorway (J.14), close to Lough Neagh and Sperrins foothills.

ATTRACTION
US GRANT ANCESTRAL HOMESTEAD
Dergenagh Road, Dungannon BT70 1TW
Tel: (028) 855 57133 Fax: (028) 855 767911
Ancestral homestead of Ulysses S. Grant, 18th President of the USA, restored to appearance of C19th Irish smallholding. Visitor Centre offers exhibitions on American Civil War and Ulster Scots Plantation.

| SD [♿] | CP [♿] | E [♿] | RF [♿] |
| C [♿] | S [♿] | WC [♿] | RFE [♿] |

FIVEMILETOWN
Deep in the heart of the Clogher Valley, surrounded by fine lakelands.

HOTEL
VALLEY HOTEL   [♿]
60 Main Street, Fivemiletown BT75 0PW
Tel: (028) 895 21505 Fax: (028) 895 21688
No. of Accessible Rooms: Several, accessible by Lift. Accessible Facilities: Lounge (2 steps), Restaurant, Bar. Well established family run hotel in town centre.

OMAGH
Capital of Tyrone, separated from Cookstown by the Black Bog, a nature reserve, which explains the turfcraft (compressed and heated peat). Lovely twin-spired church. Good for fishing on the Camowen and Owenreach Rivers.

TOURIST INFORMATION CENTRE
1 Market Street, Omagh BT78 1EE
Tel: (028) 82 247831

BUSES
Ulsterbus: Tel: (028) 82 242711

BED AND BREAKFAST
GREENMOUNT LODGE
COUNTRY HOUSE   [♿]
58 Greenmount Road, Gorlaclare, Omagh BT79 0YE
Tel: (028) 82 841325 Fax: (028) 82 840019
No. of Accessible Rooms: 1
Accessible Facilities: Lounge, Dining Room. Former C18th estate building which was rebuilt in 1970.

ATTRACTIONS
ULSTER-AMERICAN FOLK PARK
Mellon Road, Castletown, Omagh BT78 5QY
Tel: (028) 82 243292 Fax: (028) 82 242241
e-mail: mail@folkpark.com
Outdoor museum tracing Ulster's links with USA and emigration during C18th and C19th. 70-acre site divided into old and New Worlds, the former centred around restored farmhouse of Thomas Mellon, who emigrated to Pennyslvania in 1818, and the latter around log houses and outbuildings. Visitor Centre with exhibitions, AV presentations and Emigration Gallery complete with dockside buildings and emigrant ship. A must.

SD [♿] CP [♿] E [♿] RF [♿]
C [♿] S [♿] WC [♿] RFE [♿]

THE ULSTER HISTORY PARK
Cullion, Omagh BT79 7SU
Tel: (028) 8164 8188 Fax: (028) 8164 8011
e-mail: tourism@omagh.gov.uk
Access Award-winning museum with excellent visitor centre including accessible exhibition area, telling of first 10,000 years of Irish history with displays and video. EXTERIOR – Neolithic section with uneven, steep gravel paths – is not accessible. Plantation is accessible with reconstructed houses and exhibition telling of first settlers. Fascinating.

SD [♿] CP [♿] E [♿] RF [♿] Visitor Centre
C [♿] S [♿] WC [♿]

STRABANE
Bustling border town where the River Finn joins the River Foyle. Birthplace of John Dunlap, printer of the American Declaration of Independence. East of the town one passes into the lovely Tyrone Hills.

TOURIST INFORMATION CENTRE
Abercorn Square, Strabane BT82 8AW
Tel: (028) 71 883735 (Seasonal)
(028) 71 382204 (all year-Council offices).

BED AND BREAKFAST
HOLLYBUSH   [♿]
421a Victoria Road, Ballymagorry, Strabane BT82 0AT
Tel: (028) 71 382370
No. of Accessible Rooms: 2. Bath
Accessible Facilities: Lounge, Dining Room. Adjacent accessible restaurant. Chalet-style bungalow with large garden behind Ballymagorry Arms in village centre

Against each town are letters relating to the following facilities:
A: Accommodation   B: Attraction   C: Tourist Information Centre   D: Transport Information   E: Theatre   F: Sports
The bold figure at the end of each line denotes the page on which the town will be found.

427

Against each town are letters relating to the following facilities:
A: Accommodation   B: Attraction   C: Tourist Information Centre   D: Transport Information   E: Theatre   F: Sports
The bold figure at the end of each line denotes the page on which the town will be found.

Against each town are letters relating to the following facilities:
A: Accommodation   B: Attraction   C: Tourist Information Centre   D: Transport Information   E: Theatre   F: Sports
The bold figure at the end of each line denotes the page on which the town will be found.

429

Against each town are letters relating to the following facilities:
A: Accommodation   B: Attraction   C: Tourist Information Centre   D: Transport Information   E: Theatre   F: Sports
The bold figure at the end of each line denotes the page on which the town will be found.

Against each town are letters relating to the following facilities:
A: Accommodation   B: Attraction   C: Tourist Information Centre   D: Transport Information   E: Theatre   F: Sports
The bold figure at the end of each line denotes the page on which the town will be found.

Against each town are letters relating to the following facilities:
A: Accommodation   B: Attraction   C: Tourist Information Centre   D: Transport Information   E: Theatre   F: Sports
The bold figure at the end of each line denotes the page on which the town will be found.

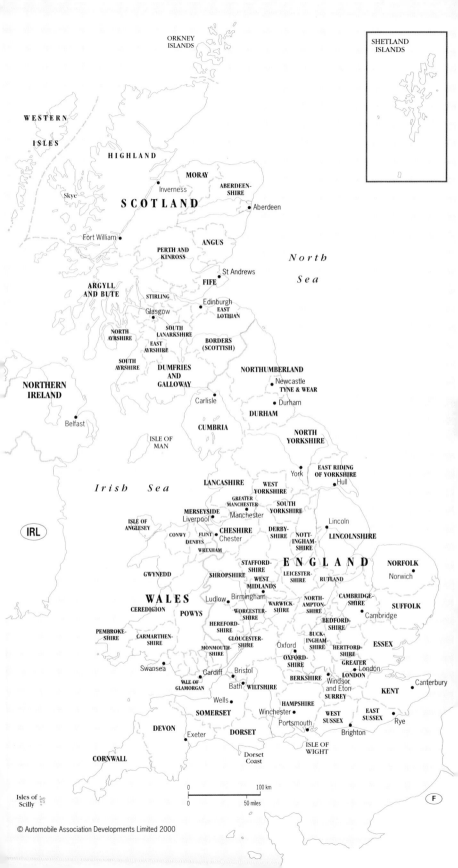

ORKNEY ISLANDS

SHETLAND ISLANDS

WESTERN ISLES

HIGHLAND

MORAY

Inverness

ABERDEEN-SHIRE

Aberdeen

Skye

SCOTLAND

Fort William

ANGUS

PERTH AND KINROSS

North Sea

St Andrews

ARGYLL AND BUTE

FIFE

STIRLING

Edinburgh

Glasgow

EAST LOTHIAN

NORTH AYRSHIRE

SOUTH LANARKSHIRE

EAST AYRSHIRE

BORDERS (SCOTTISH)

SOUTH AYRSHIRE

DUMFRIES AND GALLOWAY

NORTHUMBERLAND

Newcastle

TYNE & WEAR

NORTHERN IRELAND

Carlisle

Durham

DURHAM

Belfast

CUMBRIA

NORTH YORKSHIRE

ISLE OF MAN

Irish Sea

York

LANCASHIRE

WEST YORKSHIRE

EAST RIDING OF YORKSHIRE

Hull

GREATER MANCHESTER

SOUTH YORKSHIRE

MERSEYSIDE

Liverpool

Manchester

IRL

ISLE OF ANGLESEY

CONWY FLINT DENBYS

CHESHIRE

Chester

DERBY-SHIRE

NOTT-INGHAM-SHIRE

Lincoln

LINCOLNSHIRE

WREXHAM

GWYNEDD

SHROPSHIRE

STAFFORD-SHIRE

WEST MIDLANDS

LEICESTER-SHIRE

ENGLAND

RUTLAND

NORFOLK

Norwich

WALES

Ludlow

Birmingham

WARWICK-SHIRE

NORTH-AMPTON-SHIRE

CAMBRIDGE-SHIRE

SUFFOLK

CEREDIGION

POWYS

WORCESTER-SHIRE

BEDFORD-SHIRE

Cambridge

PEMBROKE-SHIRE

CARMARTHEN-SHIRE

HEREFORD-SHIRE

GLOUCESTER-SHIRE

MONMOUTH-SHIRE

Oxford

BUCK-INGHAM-SHIRE

HERTFORD-SHIRE

ESSEX

Swansea

Cardiff

Bristol

OXFORD-SHIRE

GREATER LONDON

London

VALE OF GLAMORGAN

Bath

WILTSHIRE

BERKSHIRE

Windsor and Eton

SURREY

KENT

Canterbury

Wells

HAMPSHIRE

WEST SUSSEX

EAST SUSSEX

Rye

SOMERSET

Winchester

Portsmouth

Brighton

DEVON

Exeter

DORSET

ISLE OF WIGHT

CORNWALL

Dorset Coast

0   100 km
0   50 miles

Isles of Scilly

F

© Automobile Association Developments Limited 2000

YOUR OWN NOTES:

YOUR COMMENTS AND SUGGESTIONS

Did we get it right? We need to know, so we can help you. Write to us with your comments, suggestions, corrections and news. Please fill in the coupon and send to our address below.

**Gowrings Mobility
Bone Lane, Newbury,
Berkshire, RG14 5EU,
England.**

Name

Company (if applicable)

Address

Postcode

Tel

Fax

Email

YOUR COMMENTS AND SUGGESTIONS

Request further Information

Please use this reply paid post
card to Request information on
Gowrings Mobility products:

(Please ✓ appropriate box)

☐ Wheelchair passenger
cars and minibuses

☐ Scooters and swivel
seats for cars

☐ More copies of the Smooth
Ride Guide

Name

Company (if applicable)

Address

Postcode

Tel

Fax

Email

Lo-Call **0845 608 8050**
www.gowringsmobility.co.uk

**gowrings
mobility**

Request further Information

Please use this reply paid post
card to Request information on
Gowrings Mobility products:

(Please ✓ appropriate box)

☐ Wheelchair passenger
cars and minibuses

☐ Scooters and swivel
seats for cars

☐ More copies of the Smooth
Ride Guide

Name

Company (if applicable)

Address

Postcode

Tel

Fax

Email

Lo-Call **0845 608 8050**
www.gowringsmobility.co.uk

**gowrings
mobility**

Request further Information

Please use this reply paid post
card to Request information on
Gowrings Mobility products:

(Please ✓ appropriate box)

☐ Wheelchair passenger
cars and minibuses

☐ Scooters and swivel
seats for cars

☐ More copies of the Smooth
Ride Guide

Name

Company (if applicable)

Address

Postcode

Tel

Fax

Email

Lo-Call **0845 608 8050**
www.gowringsmobility.co.uk

**gowrings
mobility**

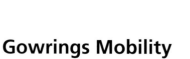

**Gowrings Mobility
FREEPOST**
Bone Lane,
Newbury,
Berkshire
RG14 5ZW

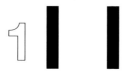

**Gowrings Mobility
FREEPOST**
Bone Lane,
Newbury,
Berkshire
RG14 5ZW

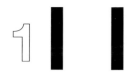

**Gowrings Mobility
FREEPOST**
Bone Lane,
Newbury,
Berkshire
RG14 5ZW

Request further Information

Please use this reply paid post
card to Request information on
Gowrings Mobility products:

(Please ✓ appropriate box)

☐ Wheelchair passenger
   cars and minibuses

☐ Scooters and swivel
   seats for cars

☐ More copies of the Smooth
   Ride Guide

Name

Company (if applicable)

Address

Postcode

Tel

Fax

Email

Lo-Call **0845 608 8050**
www.gowringsmobility.co.uk

**gowrings
mobility**

Request further Information

Please use this reply paid post
card to Request information on
Gowrings Mobility products:

(Please ✓ appropriate box)

☐ Wheelchair passenger
   cars and minibuses

☐ Scooters and swivel
   seats for cars

☐ More copies of the Smooth
   Ride Guide

Name

Company (if applicable)

Address

Postcode

Tel

Fax

Email

Lo-Call **0845 608 8050**
www.gowringsmobility.co.uk

**gowrings
mobility**

Request further Information

Please use this reply paid post
card to Request information on
Gowrings Mobility products:

(Please ✓ appropriate box)

☐ Wheelchair passenger
   cars and minibuses

☐ Scooters and swivel
   seats for cars

☐ More copies of the Smooth
   Ride Guide

Name

Company (if applicable)

Address

Postcode

Tel

Fax

Email

Lo-Call **0845 608 8050**
www.gowringsmobility.co.uk

**gowrings
mobility**

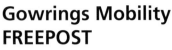

Gowrings Mobility
FREEPOST
Bone Lane,
Newbury,
Berkshire
RG14 5ZW

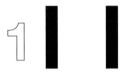

Gowrings Mobility
FREEPOST
Bone Lane,
Newbury,
Berkshire
RG14 5ZW

Gowrings Mobility
FREEPOST
Bone Lane,
Newbury,
Berkshire
RG14 5ZW